Behavioral Pediatric Healthcare for Nurse Practitioners

Donna Hallas, PhD, PPCNP-BC, CPNP, PMHS, FAANP, is a clinical professor and director of the Pediatric Nurse Practitioner (PNP) Program at New York University Rory Meyers College of Nursing. She is a pediatric primary care mental health specialist (PMHS) and has provided comprehensive healthcare to medically complex children and adolescents, many of whom had behavioral health problems. Her research focuses on improving healthcare outcomes for young children. She implemented a funded study on oral healthcare for newborns and young children for mothers on the postpartum unit. At research conferences, Dr. Hallas has presented the results of a randomized controlled trial (RCT) to improve the social–emotional development of toddlers and improve maternal confidence in caring for toddlers. She is currently the principal investigator (PI) of a Health Resources and Services Administration (HRSA) grant for preceptor development and the PI for an RCT on vaccine hesitancy in prenatal and postpartum women.

Dr. Hallas is the digital editor for *Contemporary Pediatrics*, writing a monthly column titled "The PNP Corner." She is a faculty scholar of the International Qualitative Institute at Alberta, Canada. Dr. Hallas is an active member of several nurse practitioner organizations and is a Fellow of the American Academy of Nurse Practitioners and the National Association of Pediatric Nurse Practitioners.

Behavioral Pediatric Healthcare for Nurse Practitioners

A Growth and Developmental Approach to Intercepting Abnormal Behaviors

DONNA HALLAS, PhD, PPCNP-BC, CPNP, PMHS, FAANP

Editor

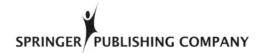

SPRINGER PUBLISHING COMPANY

Springer Publishing Company, LLC
11 West 42nd Street
New York, NY 10036
www.springerpub.com

Acquisitions Editor: Elizabeth Nieginski
Compositor: Exeter Premedia Services Pvt Ltd.

ISBN: 978-0-8261-1867-7
ebook ISBN: 978-0-8261-1681-9
Case Study Discussion Questions ISBN: 978-0-8261-3836-1
PowerPoint ISBN: 978-0-8261-3848-4

Instructor's Materials: Qualified instructors may request supplements by emailing textbook@springerpub.com

18 19 20 21 22 / 5 4 3 2 1

The author and the publisher of this Work have made every effort to use sources believed to be reliable to provide information that is accurate and compatible with the standards generally accepted at the time of publication. Because medical science is continually advancing, our knowledge base continues to expand. Therefore, as new information becomes available, changes in procedures become necessary. We recommend that the reader always consult current research and specific institutional policies before performing any clinical procedure. The author and publisher shall not be liable for any special, consequential, or exemplary damages resulting, in whole or in part, from the readers' use of, or reliance on, the information contained in this book. The publisher has no responsibility for the persistence or accuracy of URLs for external or third-party Internet websites referred to in this publication and does not guarantee that any content on such websites is, or will remain, accurate or appropriate.

Library of Congress Cataloging-in-Publication Data

Names: Hallas, Donna, editor.
Title: Behavioral pediatric healthcare for nurse practitioners : a growth and
    developmental approach to intercepting abnormal behaviors / Donna Hallas,
    editor.
Description: New York, NY : Springer Publishing Company, LLC, [2018] |
    Includes bibliographical references.
Identifiers: LCCN 2018012702| ISBN 9780826118677 | ISBN 9780826138361 (case
    study discussion questions) | ISBN 9780826116819 (e-book)
Subjects: | MESH: Child Behavior Disorders | Pediatric Nursing | Child |
    Infant | Adolescent | United States
Classification: LCC RJ245 | NLM WS 350.6 | DDC 618.92/00231—dc23
LC record available at https://lccn.loc.gov/2018012702

Contact us to receive discount rates on bulk purchases.
We can also customize our books to meet your needs.
For more information please contact: sales@springerpub.com

Printed in the United States of America.

I dedicate this book to my three outstanding children who were so much fun to raise and now are such fabulous young adults. I am so proud of each of you, all of your accomplishments, and all that you do and will do to improve the lives of others.

I also dedicate this book to all of my pediatric and adolescent patients and their parents, grandparents, aunts, and foster parents who were and are so dedicated to the well-being of their children. It was and is my privilege to be your pediatric nurse practitioner.

Contents

SECTION V: SCHOOL-AGE POPULATION

SECTION VI: ADOLESCENT POPULATION

SECTION VII: CHILD POPULATION

Contributors

Samar Mohsen Ashmawi, MS, PNP, Pediatric Nurse Practitioner, NYU Rory Meyers College of Nursing, New York, New York

Julie Baldyga, MS, NYU Rory Meyers College of Nursing, New York, New York

Paula Barbel, **PhD, PNP,** Assistant Professor, The College at Brockport, SUNY, Brockport, New York

Alexandra Barber, MS, BSN, RN, CLC, PNP, Pediatric Nurse Practitioner, NYU Rory Meyers College of Nursing; Nurse Clinician, NYU Langone Health, New York, New York

Caroline Bourassa, MS, BSN, RN, CPN, PNP, Pediatric Nurse Practitioner, NYU Rory Meyers College of Nursing, New York, New York

Traci R. Bramlett, DNP, RN, FNP-C, Assistant Professor of Nursing and Family Nurse Practitioner, University North Carolina Wilmington, College of Health and Human Services, Wilmington, North Carolina

Stephanie Brown, DNP, MSN, CPNP, PHMS, BSN, RN-BC, Pediatric Nurse Practitioner, Pediatric Primary Care Mental Health Specialist, Clinical Director, Starlight Pediatrics, Rochester, New York

Amelia Burke, MS, BSN, RN, PNP, Pediatric Nurse Practitioner, NYU Rory Meyers College of Nursing, New York, New York

Kimberly Cifelli, MS, BSN, RN, CPN, CPEN, CLC, PNP, Pediatric Nurse Practitioner, NYU Rory Meyers College of Nursing; Nurse Clinician, NYU Langone Health, New York, New York

Maura Coburn, MS, BSN, RN, CLC, PNP, Pediatric Nurse Practitioner, NYU Rory Meyers College of Nursing; Nurse Clinician, NYU Langone Health, New York, New York

Sally S. Cohen, PhD, RN, FAAN, Clinical Professor, NYU Rory Meyers College of Nursing, New York, New York

Nina B. Colabelli, DNP, RN, APN, CPNP-PC, Director of Child Health Program, Francois Xavier Bagnoud Center, Rutgers University, School of Nursing, Newark, New Jersey

Ingrid G. Cook, MSN, APRN, CPNP-PC, PMHS, Pediatric Nurse Practitioner, Pediatric Primary Care Mental Health Specialist, Clinical Adjunct Nursing Faculty, Northwestern State University College of Nursing, Graduate Studies Program, Shreveport, Louisiana; Captain, United States Navy Nurse Corps Reservist, Bossier City, Louisiana

Eileen Corcoran, DNP, APN, PPCNP-BC, Assistant Director of Child Health Program, Francois Xavier Bagnoud Center, Rutgers University, School of Nursing, Newark, New Jersey

Katelyn Dalina, MS, BSN, RN, CPN, PNP, Pediatric Nurse Practitioner, NYU Rory Meyers College of Nursing, New York, New York

Shayleigh K. Dickson, MSN, CPNP-AC, Pediatric Nurse Practitioner–Acute Care, Children's Specialized Hospital, Newark, New Jersey

Caroline Dorsen, PhD, FNP-BC, Assistant Professor, Family Nurse Practitioner, NYU Rory Meyers College of Nursing, New York, New York

Hillary Fairbanks, MS, RN, CPNP, Pediatric Nurse Practitioner, NYU Rory Meyers College of Nursing, New York, New York

Jane A. Fox, EdD, PPCNP-BC, FAANP, Professor and Pediatric Nurse Practitioner, University of North Carolina, Wilmington College of Health and Human Services, Wilmington, North Carolina

Isabel Gonzalez, MS, BS, RN, PNP, Pediatric Nurse Practitioner, NYU Rory Meyers College of Nursing, New York, New York

Jeanette F. Green, PhD, ARNP, CPNP-PC, PMHS, Pediatric Nurse Practitioner and Pediatric Primary Care Mental Health Specialist, Administrative Director of Nursing Research, University of Florida and University of Florida Health, Gainesville, Florida

Deborah Gutter, DNP, APN, CPNP-PC, RN, Assistant Director of Child Health Program, Francois Xavier Bagnoud Center; Pediatric Nurse Practitioner, Rutgers University, School of Nursing, Newark, New Jersey

Donna Hallas, **PhD, PPCNP-BC, CPNP, PMHS, FAANP,** Pediatric Nurse Practitioner and Pediatric Primary Care Mental Health Specialist, Clinical Professor, and Director Pediatric Nurse Practitioner Program, NYU Rory Meyers College of Nursing, New York, New York

Miles Harris, FNP-BC, MS, AAHIVS, Family Nurse Practitioner, Center for Transgender Medicine and Surgery, Mount Sinai Hospital System, New York, New York

Therese W. Harrison, MSN, APRN, CPNP, CPHMS, Pediatric Nurse Practitioner, Pediatric Primary Care Mental Health Specialist, St. Christopher's, Inc, Valhalla, New York

Kristen Hay, MS, BSN, RN, CPN, CLC, PNP, Pediatric Nurse Practitioner, NYU Rory Meyers College of Nursing; Nurse Clinician, NYU Langone Health, New York, New York

Kelsey Heiner, RN, BSN, PNP, Pediatric Nurse Practitioner, Pediatric Intensive Care Unit, NYU Langone Health, New York, New York

Jennifer Hensley, DNP, CPNP-PC, PMHS, Developmental Behavioral Pediatric Nurse Practitioner, Pediatric Primary Care Mental Health Specialist, Clinical Assistant Professor, Uniformed Services University, Fort Belvoir, Virginia

Beth Heuer, DNP, CRNP, CPNP-PC, PMHS, Pediatric Nurse Practitioner, Pediatric Primary Care Mental Health Specialist, Child Development Unit, Children's Hospital of Pittsburgh of UPMC, Pittsburgh, Pennsylvania

Mary Elizabeth Katinas, MS, BSN, RN, PNP, Pediatric Nurse Practitioner, NYU Rory Meyers College of Nursing, New York, New York

Jennifer Kiehl, MS, BSN, RN, PNP, Pediatric Nurse Practitioner, NYU Rory Meyers College of Nursing, New York, New York

Erica D. Kierce, DNP, PMHNP, PMHS, Assistant Clinical Professor, Psychiatric Nurse Practitioner, Pediatric Primary Care Mental Health Specialist, Auburn University School of Nursing, Auburn, Alabama

Yini Kong, MS, BSN, RN, PNP, Pediatric Nurse Practitioner, NYU Rory Meyers College of Nursing, New York, New York

Mary Koslap-Petraco, DNP, PPCNP-BC, CPNP, FAANP, Pediatric Nurse Practitioner, Adjunct Clinical Assistant Professor, Stony Brook University School of Nursing, Stony Brook, New York; Nurse Consultant Immunization Action Coalition; CEO, Pediatric Nurse Practitioner House Calls, Massapequa Park, New York

Nancy Kramer, EdD, CPNP, PMHS, CNE, ARNP, ANEF, Pediatric Nurse Practitioner, Vice Chancellor of Academic Affairs & Professor, Allen College, Waterloo, Iowa

Alexandra Laurenzano, MS, RN, PNP, Pediatric Nurse Practitioner, NYU Rory Meyers College of Nursing, New York, New York

Elizabeth Mandel, MS, BS, RN, PNP, Pediatric Nurse Practitioner, NYU Rory Meyers College of Nursing, New York, New York

James T. Mulholland, DNP, CPNP, Pediatric Nurse Practitioner, Starlight Pediatrics, Rochester, New York

Amanda Neilan, MS, RN, PNP, Pediatric Nurse Practitioner, NYU Rory Meyers College of Nursing, New York, New York

James Nguyen, BS, Instructional Design, NYU Rory Meyers College of Nursing, New York, New York

Susan R. Opas, PhD, CPNP, CPMHS, CNS, CHES, Pediatric Nurse Practitioner, Pediatric Primary Care Mental Health Specialist, Southern California Kaiser Permanente Medical Group, Woodland Hills, California

Shyvon Paul, MS, FNP-BC, Family Nurse Practitioner, Maimonides Health Center, Brooklyn, New York

Audra N. Rankin, DNP, APRN, CPNP, PMHS CNE, Pediatric Nurse Practitioner, Pediatric Primary Care Mental Health Specialist, Johns Hopkins University School of Nursing, Baltimore, Maryland

Mary M. Rock, DNP, CRNP, FNP, CNS-PMH-C, Family Nurse Practitioner and Clinical Nurse Specialist, Psychiatric Mental Health-Certified, Geisinger Holy Spirit Hospital, Camp Hill, Pennsylvania

LeAnne Elizabeth Rohlf, MSN, APRN, CPNP, PMHS, Pediatric Nurse Practitioner, Pediatric Primary Care Mental Health Specialist, St. Catherine University, Minneapolis, Minnesota

Bobbie Salveson, PhD, CPNP, PMHS, Advanced Registered Nurse Practitioner, Pediatric Nurse Practitioner, Pediatric Primary Care Mental Health Specialist, Mary Bridge Children's Hospital Genetics Clinic, Tacoma, Washington; Clinical Assistant Professor, University of Washington School of Nursing, Seattle, Washington

Emily Schadt, DNP, RN, CPNP-BC, PMHS, Pediatric Nurse Practitioner, Pediatric Primary Care Mental Health Specialist, University of South Alabama, Franklin Pediatrics, Blue Grass, Iowa

Julie Schreiner, DNP, PMHNP, FNP, PMHS, RN, Psychiatric Mental Health Nurse Practitioner, Family Nurse Practitioner, Pediatric Primary Care Mental Health Specialist, Surfside Pediatrics, Ventura County Behavioral Health Youth and Family Division, Ventura, California

Katie Pink Tolley, RN, MSN, CPNP, PMHS, Pediatric Nurse Practitioner, Pediatric Primary Care Mental Health Specialist, Holistic Health and Wellness Consultant, Cambridge, Maryland

Mary Weglarz, DNP, RN, APN, CPNP, CPMHS, Family Nurse Practitioner, Psychiatric Mental Health Nurse Practitioner, Assistant Director of Child Health Program, Francois Xavier Bagnoud Center, Rutgers University, School of Nursing, Newark, New Jersey

James J. Weidel, PhD, FNP-BC, PMHNP-BC, Clinical Assistant Professor, NYU Rory Meyers College of Nursing, New York, New York

Foreword

The first edition of *Behavioral Pediatric Healthcare for Nurse Practitioners: A Growth and Developmental Approach to Intercepting Abnormal Behaviors*, edited by Donna Hallas, PhD, PPCNP-BC, CPNP, PMHS, FAANP, is destined to have a high impact on the pediatric primary care community. This groundbreaking publication, using the innovative Intercepting Behavioral Health (IBH) model developed by Dr. Hallas, establishes a new generation of pediatric nursing scholarship. Most important is its reaffirmation of the importance of whole-child care that integrates behavioral health as a cornerstone of pediatric primary care.

Behavioral health issues and problems in infants, children, and adolescents has been a long-standing population health issue. The Surgeon General's Report in 2000, focused on the integration of mental health services and primary care, was one of the first documents to highlight the integral nature of mental health and overall health. Mental health is an important population health and public health issue. Current data reveal that, at any time, 13% to 20% of children in the United States are diagnosed with a mental health problem. The IBH model makes a compelling case that early recognition, intervention, and active monitoring by competent primary care providers are the answers, rather than watch, wait, and wait some more because there is a paucity of available developmental, behavioral, and mental health referral resources. Immediate recognition and evidence-based action by primary care providers is a positive paradigm shift for addressing covert or emerging problems before they escalate.

Because the majority of children, from infancy through adolescence, receive healthcare in primary care settings provided by pediatric and family nurse practitioners, RNs, physicians, and physician assistants, it makes sense to build interprofessional workforce capacity prepared to integrate behavioral health into their primary care practice. The IBH model provides a platform for pediatric and family nurse practitioners, and their colleagues, to provide whole-person care in primary care settings where they include physical, emotional, and social components of care to intercept potential common behavioral health problems using evidence-based approaches to assessment, diagnosis, treatment, and evaluation of care. As Dr. Hallas points out, the prevalence of behavioral health problems is quite alarming! The number of behavioral health specialists, psychiatrists, psychiatric nurse practitioners, psychologists, and social workers is insufficient to meet the demand for behavioral health services. Pediatric and family nurse practitioners can fill this gap.

The IBH model proposes use of evidence-based approaches that include, but are not limited to, screening, assessment, diagnosis, interventions (i.e., parent–child education through anticipatory guidance), psychoeducation, parenting effectiveness, motivational interviewing, coping skills, brief psychotherapeutic interventions such as cognitive behavioral therapy (CBT), psychopharmacologic medication management, as well as collaboration and referral. Integrating the social determinants of health surrounds the IBH model as clinicians collaborate with schools, day-care centers, after-school programs, and providers of more complex care. Optimizing primary care for the whole child, family, and community is the objective of integrating behavioral health in primary care.

Today, primary care providers are challenged to regard behavioral health as an essential competency fundamental to advanced nursing practice. Validation about the importance of behavioral health is evident in major professional documents that guide 21st-century implementation of advanced practice clinical practice roles. Recognition goes to the 2017 *Core Competencies for Nurse Practitioners* developed by the National Organization for Nurse Practitioner Faculties (NONPF) that affirm the integration of mental health into primary care for children and families. The Pediatric Nursing Certification Board (PNCB) should be saluted for developing the Pediatric Primary Care Mental Health Specialist (PMHS) certification exam. A joint statement by the American Psychiatric Nurses Association (APNA) and PNCB states that the PMHS certification exam validates the added knowledge, skill, and expertise of pediatric advanced practice nurses in the early identification, intervention, and collaboration of care for children, adolescents, and their families with developmental, behavioral, or mental health issues.

Dr. Hallas and the pediatric, family, and mental health nursing leaders she has chosen as contributors reflect a strong complement of clinical and academic talent; outstanding nursing professionals whose wealth of clinical and teaching experience informs the behavioral health discussion presented in each chapter. The in-depth discussion of screening, assessment, intervention, and evaluation models used to achieve quality clinical outcomes is enhanced by the presentation of the "best available evidence" to support the efficacy of the IBH model.

The unique consideration of the social determinants of health, that is, awareness of the racial/ethnic, gender, education, and socioeconomic differences, addresses how those forces interface with the behavioral and overall health of infants, children, adolescents, their families, and communities. From a teaching–learning perspective, the rich examples in each chapter and case studies provide learning anchors that facilitate contextual learning for students that supports integration of theory and clinical practice.

I am confident that the premier edition of *Behavioral Pediatric Healthcare for Nurse Practitioners: A Growth and Developmental Approach to Intercepting Abnormal Behaviors* will make an important contribution to the academic and clinical practice literature. As an advanced practice psychiatric nurse for more than four decades, I salute Dr. Hallas, a close colleague for more than 10 years, for launching this innovative project.

Judith Haber, PhD, APRN, FAAN
The Ursula Springer Leadership Professor in Nursing
Rory Meyers College of Nursing
New York University
New York, New York

Preface

It would be wonderful if babies were born with instructions for parents to raise them to be healthy and happy little wonders and truly bundles of joy throughout infancy, toddlerhood, preschool age, school age, and adolescence. It would also be ideal if the instructions just continued to flow as babies and children are raised by their parents, relatives, or even in out-of-home care through "the kindness of strangers" (Kittle, 2006) because something has gone terribly wrong in their young life. Oh wait! That is part of our role as pediatric nurses, pediatric and family nurse practitioners, pediatricians and family physicians, social workers, and school teachers—to help individuals and families understand the role of parenting a child and to raise children within a happy home to become socially and emotionally healthy adults.

Anticipatory guidance is a routine component of each well-child healthcare visit, but how much time do we, the pediatric primary care providers (P-PCPs), actually spend providing high-quality anticipatory guidance to each individual parenting a child and/or with the individual child or adolescent? We may delegate providing the routine anticipatory guidance to the office nursing staff and refer parents and family members to web-based parenting information, and recommend parenting books and literature. Are these anticipatory guidance strategies successful? What happens when the infant's/child's/adolescent's behavior disrupts the family dynamics? What can parents and providers do to identify and correct disruptive behaviors?

Statistics obtained from the National Survey of Child's Health in 2011–2012 revealed that one out of seven children between the ages of 2 and 8 had a diagnosis of mental, behavioral, or developmental health problems (Centers for Disease Control and Prevention, 2017). These statistics are more than concerning. P-PCPs in primary care are in a position to take definitive actions to reduce the prevalence of behavioral health problems in the United States. Thus, the question becomes, how can P-PCPs effectively reverse these statistics? Is the answer for P-PCPs to focus a portion of each primary care visit on infant, child/adolescent, and family behavioral health?

For the parents and families whose children fit the "norm," that is, meet their milestones as expected, receive and give love daily, are easy to raise, and enhance the family dynamics, family life is relatively easy, and it is expected that the primary care focus will also be easy. *But* for those parents and families whose children do not meet their milestones as anticipated, who place untoward demands on the family dynamics, cause parents to question their own parenting skills, are disruptive in social environments and at school, life is not easy. As P-PCPs, we must use our knowledge, judgment, communication skills, diagnostic skills, and the best available evidence-based treatment management strategies to *identify and intercept* presenting behavioral health problems to restore as much order and behavioral health for the infant, child/adolescent, and family dynamics as possible (see Chapter 1 for the conceptual model of Intercepting Behavioral Health [IBH]).

How often do you as a P-PCP consider the theoretical frameworks for mental health versus the concepts for behavioral health during routine office visits? To enable P-PCPs to consider behavioral health in every primary care visit and child/adolescent setting, the focus of each chapter is on assessment, diagnosis, and management of behavioral health norms and problems in pediatric primary care settings. Chapter authors provide strategic evidence-based measures for evaluating the behavioral health status during each well-child visit. Likewise, chapter authors provide strategies and resources for the evaluation of the parents' mental health status as part of our routine office practice. If P-PCPs are to provide care that is patient- and family-centric to ensure unmitigated mental and behavioral health, they must assess and evaluate the mental and behavioral health status for each child/adolescent in primary care settings. A major premise of this book is that a significant role of P-PCPs is to *intercept behaviors* that are "outside the norm" by implementing evidence-based strategies to restore order for the infant's, child's, and adolescent's well-being, after analysis of the developmental stage, behavioral development, and family dynamics.

In 2000, the Surgeon General's report discussed the integration of mental health services and primary care (U.S. Department of Health and Human Services, 2001). The Centers for Disease Control and Prevention recognized the need for pediatric and family primary care providers to be educated in care for children with behavioral health problems in primary care settings (Chowdhury, Kulcsar, Gilhrist, & Hawkins, 2012). Thus, programs that prepared pediatric nurse practitioners (PNPs) began to implement behavioral mental health concepts, case studies, treatment, and management strategies for these children and families. National organizations increased the numbers of continuing educational programs related to behavioral mental health in primary care settings. The Pediatric Nursing Certification Board (PNCB) analyzed the problem and created a new certification for pediatric, family, and psychiatric nurse practitioners, to acquire the recognition as a pediatric mental health specialist (PMHS). These providers have acquired the knowledge, skills, and abilities to care for children with specific behavioral health problems in primary care settings. Psychiatric-mental health nurse practitioner education and practice changed from child/adolescent to a family focus. The majority of the chapters in this book are written by PNPs, many of whom are also certified as PMHS by the PNCB, and who have extensive experience in treating children with behavioral health problems in primary care settings.

Chapters are also written by family nurse practitioners and psychiatric-mental health nurse practitioners who have also completed the PMHS examination.

This book uses a developmental approach to behavioral health for the entire pediatric population. Each section of this book is dedicated to the traditional developmental ages (i.e., infants, toddlers, preschoolers, school-age, and adolescents). Each opening chapter within the specific developmental age provides information for P-PCPs to assess, identify, and *intercept* potential behavioral health problems through the use of a developmental approach to behavioral health assessments (infants, Chapter 6; toddlers, Chapter 12; preschool-age children, Chapter 17; school-age children, Chapter 20; and adolescents, Chapter 23).

Within each developmental topic section, pediatric experts discuss common behavioral problems and strategies for implementing evidence-based care for children within the commonly accepted developmental age ranges (infancy, toddler, preschool-age, school-age, and adolescence). Assessment, screening, intervention, and treatment strategies are provided through analysis of the best available evidence by experts in the field of pediatric practice. Cutting-edge topics written by experts in the fields of pediatric primary care and pediatric behavioral health are highlighted in this book and include: infant brain development and outcomes from ineffective parenting (Chapter 2); social determinants of health and effect on behavioral health (Chapter 4); building resiliency in children (Chapter 5); infant depression (Chapter 7); behavioral problems in children with inborn errors of metabolism (Chapter 10); autism, global developmental delays, and genetic syndromes (Chapter 14); attention deficit hyperactivity disorder (ADHD) and comorbidities (Chapter 18); bullying (Chapter 21); social media and behavioral health (Chapter 22); eating disorders (Chapter 24); the autistic adolescent in residential treatment facilities (Chapter 27); child behaviors within military families (Chapter 29); foster care (Chapter 31); toxic stress (Chapter 32); trauma-informed care (Chapter 33); lesbian, gay, bisexual, and transgender adolescent (Chapter, 34); and holistic and integrative care, holistic and integrative medicine, and behavioral health (Chapter 35).

Within each developmental section, there are case studies that provide exemplary practices for assessing, diagnosing, and evaluating children presented with the particular behavioral health problem. Case studies include the following topics: failure to thrive in infancy (Chapter 9); infant colic (Chapter 11); toilet training (Chapter 13); sleep disorders in children with autistic spectrum disorder and ADHD (Chapter 15); toddler impulsive behaviors (Chapter 16); nail biting (Chapter 19); and adolescent substance abuse (Chapter 28).

Additionally, there are chapters on neurological disorders discussing mental health problems that are often referred by P-PCPs to psychiatric mental health specialists, such as psychiatric mental health disorders (Chapter 25); neurofibromatosis type 1 and Tourette syndrome (Chapter 26).

Psychotropic medications are discussed as appropriate in many of the chapters. Additionally, Chapter 3 describes best practices for prescribing and safe use of psychotropic medications in primary care settings and the primary care management of children and adolescents prescribed psychotropic medications by a P-PCP or a psychiatric specialist.

Faculty using this textbook to enable students to have an in-depth understanding of ways for early identification of behavioral health problems, with implementation of evidence-based treatment plans and evaluation of these plans, have digital access to multiple-choice questions for many chapters, discussion questions for chapters that are written as case studies, and a PowerPoint presentation. Qualified faculty can obtain this material by emailing textbook@springerpub.com.

The foundation for P-PCPs to *identify* behavioral health problems through evidence-based assessment strategies is described throughout the book, but especially in Chapter 1. Once the behavioral problems are identified, the authors provide P-PCPs evidence-based practice strategies for the diagnosis, treatment, and evaluation of infants, children, and adolescents to *intercept* the identified problems and to work with parents to better understand and raise behaviorally healthy children. Strategies for P-PCPs to work with parents to develop and/or improve their coping skills, parenting skills, and interactions within and outside of the family unit are presented. The conceptual model of IBH for this book is described in Chapter 1. It is believed that P-PCPs who implement the concepts of *intercepting* behavioral health problems in pediatric primary care settings will enable infants, children, and adolescents to achieve improved behavioral health outcomes throughout childhood and adolescent years, entering adulthood with the necessary coping skills to achieve behavioral health and happiness throughout the adult life span.

Donna Hallas

▨ REFERENCES

Centers for Disease Control and Prevention. (2017). *Mental, behavioral, and developmental health of children aged 2 to 8 years*. Retrieved from https://www.cdc.gov/childrensmentalhealth/data.html

Chowdhury, F. M., Kulscar, M., Gilchrist, S., & Hawkins, N. A. (2012). News from the CDC: Integrating behavioral health into the patient-centered medical home. *TBM*, 2, 257–259. doi:10.1007/s13142-012-0147-2

Kittle, K. (2006). *The kindness of strangers*. New York, NY: William Morrow.

U.S. Department of Health and Human Services. (2001). *Report of a Surgeon General's working meeting on the integration of mental health services and primary cares*. Atlanta, Georgia, Rockville, MD: U.S. Department of Health and Human Services, Public Health Service, Office of the Surgeon General.

Acknowledgments

I would like to acknowledge the dedication of all the pediatric, family, and psychiatric nurse practitioners who not only authored and coauthored chapters in this book but also provide primary care behavioral health services to children and adolescents with the hopes of improving their lives and long-term healthcare outcomes. It was my pleasure to work with each of you as each chapter was written, revised, and prepared to offer new insights in the care of children and adolescents with behavioral health problems.

Intercepting Behavioral Health Problems

CHAPTER 1

Intercepting Behavioral Health Problems: A Conceptual Model

DONNA HALLAS

■ INTERCEPTING BEHAVIORAL PROBLEMS IN PEDIATRIC PRIMARY CARE

In 2000, an initial trailblazing meeting to advance and support the integration of mental health services in primary care settings was held in Atlanta, Georgia (U.S. Department of Health & Human Services [DHHS], 2001) in response to the Surgeon General's report (DHHS, 1999) on the status of mental health in the United States. The meeting addressed the complexities of the mental health crisis and recommended an innovative initiative to provide mental health services to all populations in primary care settings. One major goal for this meeting was to develop a "national action strategy for the integration of mental health services in primary health care" (DHHS, 2001, p. 1). If accomplished, this goal had the potential to reduce access to care problems encountered by individuals and families in need of mental health services by providing immediate mental health services embedded within the primary healthcare settings. Since that meeting, there have been many calls to integrate mental health services within primary care settings as well as recommendations for practice models that may be able to successfully integrate mental health services within primary care settings (Boat et al., 2016; Chowdhury, Kulcsar, Gilchrist, & Hawkins, 2012; Jellineck, 2017). However, much work needs to be done to successfully integrate mental health and, in particular, behavioral health services, within pediatric primary care settings.

The overarching goal for providing behavioral and mental health services in pediatric primary care settings is to provide immediate and effective services to children, adolescents, and their families to change the course from potential adverse behavioral health outcomes to supportive positive directions in growth and developmental behavioral health. This textbook provides an analysis of evidence-based behavioral health practices to foster growth and developmental behavioral health through early behavioral health screenings and assessments with the goal of *intercepting* behavioral development and characteristics that are not within the "norm" of pediatric and adolescent development.

This conceptual model called Intercepting Behavioral Health (IBH; Hallas, 2017) has the potential to change the current practice of pediatric healthcare from one of "observing, watching, and waiting" to one which provides immediate recognition of potential problems based on detailed family and child behavioral health history and direct observation of behaviors followed by immediate implementation of specific evidence-based interventions to address the presenting and potential for presentation of behavioral health problems. In this model, the desired long-term outcome for early recognition and treatment of pediatric behavioral health disorders focuses on raising children to enter adulthood as healthy adults, with coping skills that support continued behavioral health when confronted with challenging life events. A basic premise of the IBH model is that adult behavioral health is contingent upon experiences throughout the pediatric and adolescent years that foster the attainment of normal behavioral growth and developmental behavioral health patterns.

A major question for all pediatric primary care providers (P-PCPs) and one that is considered and analyzed throughout this book is: How can we, as P-PCPs, successfully impact the direction of behavioral health in pediatric and adolescent populations to achieve positive behavioral health outcomes throughout childhood and adulthood?

▪ STATISTICAL DATA ON MENTAL HEALTH DISORDERS

In 2013, the Centers for Disease Control and Prevention (CDC) released the first report on the status of mental health disorders in children based on a review of data from 2005 to 2011 (CDC, 2013; Perou et al., 2013). The authors identified mental health as a central component of overall health and, in addition, as an important public health issue. No one age, ethnic, or racial background, or region in the United States, was found to be free of children presenting with mental health disorders. In fact, the authors estimate that each year, 13% to 20% of children living in the United States experience a mental health problem (CDC; National Research Council and Institute of Medicine, 2009; World Health Organization [WHO], 2011). Table 1.1 lists the disorders identified in the 2013 CDC's report on the mental health status of children in the United States.

▪ CONCEPTUAL MODEL: INTERCEPTING BEHAVIORAL HEALTH

The framework for the IBH conceptual model (Hallas, 1991–2017) is integrated as the foundation for primary care behavioral health practices throughout this textbook. IBH includes screening for early identification of the potential for and/or presenting behavioral health problems, a detailed and focused behavioral health assessment, and evidence-based interventions targeted toward the potential or identified problem, with planned follow-up care to achieve the primary behavioral healthcare goal of intercepting covert and/or emerging potentially problematic and/or abnormal behaviors *before* the behaviors escalate and undermine the normal patterns for behavioral development in the child or adolescent which disrupts the dynamics of the family unit. The principles of primary prevention are

TABLE 1.1

DIAGNOSIS OF MENTAL HEALTH DISORDERS IN CHILDREN

Disorder	Occurrence in U.S. population
Children Aged 3–17 years	
ADHD	6.8%
Behavioral or conduct problems	3.5%
Anxiety	3.0%
Depression	2.1%
Autism spectrum disorder	1.1%
Tourette syndrome (children 6–17 years)	0.2%
Adolescents Aged 12–17 years	
Illicit drug use disorder in the past year	4.7%
Alcohol use disorder in the past year	4.2%
Cigarette dependence in the past month	2.8%

ADHD, attention deficit hyperactivity disorder.

Source: Data obtained from Perou, R., Bitsko, R. H., Blumberg, S. J., Pastor, P., Ghandour, R. M., Gfroerer, J. C., . . . Huang, L. N. (2013). Mental health surveillance among children—United States, 2005–2011. *Morbidity and Mortality Weekly Report, 6*(2), 1–35. Retrieved from https://www.cdc.gov/mmwr/preview/mmwrhtml/su6202a1.htm?s_cid=su6201a1_w

embedded within the IBH conceptual model. It is hypothesized that implementation of interventions prior to presentation of behavioral health problems is a *key factor* in the success of preventing behavioral symptoms from escalating into problematic behavioral problems and/or mental health disorders.

Definitions Within the IBH Conceptual Model

The terms behavioral health and mental health are often used interchangeably by individuals in the health professions. The CDC uses the terms mental health, behavioral health, and child development as congruent phrases and thoughts; however, over time, the majority of their website information has focused on mental health disorders without a clear focus on *behavior, behavioral health*, and *behavioral health problems* within the construct of a "whole child" approach to behavioral developmental health. In 2017, the CDC defined mental health in childhood as "reaching developmental and emotional milestones, and learning health social skills and how to cope when there are problems" (CDC, Division of Human Development and Disabilities, National Center on Birth Defects and Developmental Disabilities, 2017, para. 1), which represents a shift in focus from mental health disorders to behavioral health for children and adolescents. In this textbook, chapter authors present behavioral health problems commonly encountered in pediatric primary care settings and identify evidence-based practices to move current perceptions of "mental health and mental health disorders" to "behavioral health via behavioral change" strategies to improve behavioral health outcomes for children, adolescents, and their families. Will this shift forfend mental health disorders? *The answer is most likely no*. However, the IBH model postulates that the sooner untoward behaviors are recognized and interventions implemented, the more likely adverse behaviors can be altered to improve behavioral healthcare outcomes. The tenets of the IBH model are based on the need to intercept behaviors *prior to* (through analysis of a comprehensive family and child health history) *and as soon as they emerge* (first sign of a potential behavioral health problem) to either prevent or control behaviors that are not within the expected norm for child/adolescent and family behavioral health.

Characteristics for children and adolescents who grow and develop displaying behavioral health are individuals who are dynamic, socially and emotionally responsive to persons and environmental stimuli, interpersonal, reflective, and normative. Thus, behavioral health is enmeshed with social, emotional, and cognitive health. The term social health has evolved over time from an overall societal definition to one that has discrete characteristics for infants and young children, and now, in the age of advanced global technology, the term for social health is evolving and constantly changing for school-age children, adolescents, young adults, and the entire adult populations. Raver and Ziegler (1997) defined social competence for young children as groups of behaviors that allow each child to develop and engage in interactions with other people. The identified behaviors for social competence included responding and initiating interactions, participating in cooperative and social activities, managing behaviors and resolving conflicts, displaying empathy, and developing a positive self-image (Raver & Ziegler, 1997). The definition of social health is embedded in the IBH conceptual model (Hallas, 2017).

Emotional health is broadly defined by the CDC (2013) within the context of mental health as to one who experiences life satisfaction, happiness, cheerfulness, and peacefulness. Emotional health in the IBH conceptual model (Hallas, 2017) is simultaneously a narrow and broad concept: narrow in that emotional health as an individual emotion is dependent upon developmental age and specific interactions within that age range, and broad in that without emotional health, the infant/child/adolescent may struggle throughout life to find a true sense of health and well-being, as emotional turmoil adversely affects behavior and physical health.

Cognitive health is defined by the CDC (n.d.) as a healthy brain in which an individual has the ability to learn new things, intuition, judgment, language, and remembering. Cognitive health for children is critical to meeting the developmental milestones and achieving normal growth and development within all parameters of physical, social, emotional, behavioral, and mental health. The definition and descriptors for emotional health are embedded in the IBH conceptual model (Hallas, 2017).

In summary, behavioral health is a complex, all-encompassing phenomenon—one that begins at the time of conception and needs to be nurtured throughout the infant, child, and adolescent years to ensure that adolescents enter adulthood as behaviorally healthy individuals. The role of the parents and P-PCPs in supporting behavioral health for each and every child cannot be overemphasized.

In particular, P-PCPs must make every effort to intercept adverse behaviors to enable each infant/child/adolescent to achieve behavioral health.

Understanding the Concept of Intercept as Applied to Behavioral Health

The mathematical term "intercept" is defined as the point where a curve intersects an axis with positive and negative points above and below the x-axis ("Intercept," n.d.). In the IBH conceptual model, the mathematical intercept equation and related solutions are directly applied to child and adolescent behaviors as they emerge with a contemporaneous healthcare focus on changing the direction from negative to positive behaviors by intercepting the negative behavior with immediate implementation of evidence-based interventions followed by an evaluation of the effectiveness of the interventions (Figure 1.1).

ANALOGY FOR INTERCEPTING BEHAVIORAL HEALTH PROBLEMS

In football, an interception occurs when a player on the opposite team catches the ball intended for the same-team player resulting in an unintended and undesirable change in possession of the football. This unintended and undesirable football interception is analogous to the IBH conceptual model (Hallas, 2017). The infant/child/adolescent (the quarterback), with the help of parents, teachers, and all significant adults, desires to maintain control of his or her personal behavioral health by acclimating to family and societal norms. The infant/child/adolescent (the quarterback) who is experiencing behavioral health problems and emits the problem in various environments with out-of-control behaviors benefits when the behavioral health problem is intercepted (by the parent, teachers, caretaker, or P-PCP) with the implementation of evidence-based interventions recommended by the P-PCPs who are working with the parents, teachers, and all significant

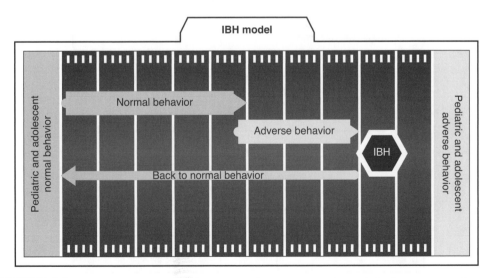

FIGURE 1.1 Intercepting behavioral health conceptual model: Core concepts.

IBH, intercepting behavioral health.

Figure design by James Nguyen.

adults to care for the infant/child/adolescent. The intent of the "quarterback displaying adverse behaviors" (analogy: infant/child/adolescent) is to control the ball regardless of the presenting behavior; the intent of the opposing receiver (analogy: parents, teachers, caretakers, and/or P-PCPs) is to swiftly identify adverse behaviors, react quickly, and effectively intercept adverse behaviors, thus transforming the presenting negative behaviors to positive behavioral health outcomes (Figure 1.2).

UNDERPINNINGS FOR THE IBH CONCEPTUAL MODEL

The initial underpinnings for the IBH conceptual model emerged from personal clinical practice observations over a period of 20 years while caring for infants/children/adolescents presenting not only with behavioral health problems but also with significant mental health disorders (personal clinical practice experience 1991–present). The infant/children/adolescents and their parents often presented

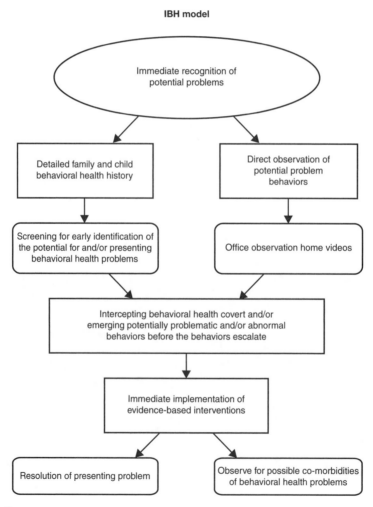

FIGURE 1.2 Intercepting behavioral health conceptual model: Analogy.

Figure design by James Nguyen.

with out-of-control behaviors. Despite comprehensive medical and mental health-care services, beneficial behavioral changes were infrequent. The basic assumption was that behaviors were permitted to "full expression" without efforts to encourage control of the behavior, thus missing early opportunities to change the course of the observed adverse behaviors.

Work by Shonkoff (2009) and later by Shonkoff et al. (2012) further supports the IBH conceptual model as the researchers reported that interventions for young people, in particular, 3- to 5-year-olds, present the greatest opportunity to reduce the risk of lifetime behavioral and related physical health problems seen in the adult population.

An initial study with adolescents parenting toddlers provided further insight into the emergence of behavioral problems in young children (Hallas & Koslap-Petraco, 2004). Observations and discussions with teenage mothers revealed that teenage mothers often viewed their toddler behaviors as problematic without truly understanding the normalcy of toddler behaviors or true behavioral problems and corrective actions. A concept that emerged from this study (Hallas & Koslap-Petraco, 2004) that is directly applicable to the IBH conceptual model (Hallas, 2017) included the identification of the "mirror image" of toddler behaviors that were reflective of his or her mother's behaviors, without the recognition by the teenage mother that her personal behaviors were mirrored by the toddler (Hallas & Koslap-Petraco, 2004). For example, the teenage mothers frequently responded "No" to requests for healthcare and behavioral changes for themselves or for their toddlers. The mirror image was observed by the researchers as their toddlers responded "No" more frequently than the normally anticipated response of "No" from toddlers. Additionally, the researchers observed that if the mother's affect was flat, then the toddler's affect mirrored the mother's and was also flat. In contrast, if the mother's affect was light and agreeable, the toddler's behavior was more agreeable and social—thus supporting the identification of the mirror image behavioral reflection between teen parents and their toddlers who participated in the study (Hallas & Koslap-Petraco, 2004).

The IBH conceptual model can also be applied to physical health that is directly related to physical–behavioral healthcare practices. Results from evidence-based literature search and a randomized controlled study (RCT; Hallas, Koslap-Petraco, & Fletcher, 2017) further confirmed the basic tenets of the IBH conceptual model (Hallas, 2017) that early interception of problematic behaviors leads to more positive outcomes for young children.

Overweight and obesity are complex medical problems and have a behavioral health component. A growing body of evidence demonstrated that implementing nutritional intake strategies in primary care practices, based on analysis of maternal history and weight, positively affects infant growth when interventions are implemented to intercept overweight and obesity in the first 1000 days of life by providing examples of behavioral changes needed by mothers when feeding their infants and toddlers (Cataldo et al., 2015; Hallas, 2017).

Another study that provided support for the IBH conceptual model was an RCT conducted to assess the effectiveness of brief office-based interventions by mothers to improve the social–emotional development of toddlers primarily from lower socioeconomic backgrounds. Study results revealed that P-PCPs who provided brief office-based educational interventions to mothers who struggle to care for impulsive toddlers not only improved maternal confidence in raising toddlers but also improved the mothers' understanding of normal toddler growth and developmental patterns (Hallas, Koslap-Petraco, & Fletcher, 2017).

■ COMPARISON OF PEDIATRIC PRACTICE MODELS TO IBH PRACTICE

Current pediatric and adolescent primary care practices provide anticipatory guidance, most often with each health maintenance healthcare visit (American Academy of Pediatrics [AAP], 2017). Anticipatory guidance provides educational information to parents and to adolescents on what to expect in the areas of growth and development between healthcare visits. The goal is for parents to know the norms and, if any issues outside of the anticipated norms are recognized, to inform the P-PCP so that further assessments and interventions can be initiated. Much of the anticipatory guidance is based on the norms for growth and development with little attention on the potential for behavioral health issues and problems.

Pediatric practice within the current mental health model allows for extended lapses in time before making a referral to a psychiatric mental health provider. For example, the current practice guideline for attention deficit hyperactive disorder (ADHD; AAP, 2011) calls for symptoms to be present for 6 months in more than one setting before the diagnosis is confirmed. The outcome for a "watch and wait" practice permits 6 months of hyperactive and impulsive symptoms in which the child's behavior is not effectively managed. Most often this 6-month time frame frustrates and angers the child, the parent, and all those who encounter the child, including peers, teachers, and community members. In the IBH model, the focus is on early recognition of symptoms, immediate screening and assessment of presenting symptoms, and immediate interventions for symptom management at home and in all environments in which the child learns and plays. Intercepting potential adverse behaviors at the earliest time point provides opportunities to implement immediate behavioral health strategies that focus on behavioral modification strategies for the entire family unit, enabling the child to learn appropriate skills to control his personal behaviors and perhaps offset the previously anticipated ADHD diagnosis. It must be noted that this approach immediately addresses presenting symptoms and interventions for presenting behavioral health symptoms and *not* the diagnostic criteria or length of time for observation to make the diagnosis as recommended in the ADHD clinical practice guideline (AAP, 2011). The IBH model supports continued behavioral health interventions for children/adolescents who do not meet diagnostic criteria.

■ INTEGRATING BEHAVIORAL HEALTH IN PRIMARY CARE

A key to the success of integrating pediatric primary healthcare and behavioral health within one setting is either to offer primary care and behavioral health services in one setting by one healthcare provider who is educated in pediatric primary healthcare and pediatric behavioral health, or offer these services in one setting by two or more providers who closely collaborate with one other to achieve the goal for each child/adolescent to achieve physical, behavioral, and social–emotional health and well-being.

In 2016, Boat et al. published a discussion paper on workforce development to address the issues of caring for the rising population of children and adolescents within the pediatric primary care settings who were experiencing a mental health disorder or behavioral health disorder. The authors recommended integrating primary care and behavioral health practices and providers with a focus on interprofessional, family-centered care for children and families. They further recommended educational preparation changes to create an integrated workforce in various disciplines that work with children and families.

Pediatric, family, psychiatric nurse practitioners, and pediatric clinical nurse specialists have the opportunity to include behavioral health management within their pediatric primary care practices by obtaining the Pediatric Primary Care Mental Health Specialist (PMHS) certification offered by the Pediatric Nursing Certification Board (PNCB). The PNCB website (www.pncb.org) provides detailed information on the application process and the role of the PMHS in primary care. Hawkins and Van Cleve (2013) describe the research base for the creation of the role. In addition, specific recommendations were made for a nursing education collaborative to strengthen PNP curriculum to prepare PNPs to care for the increased population of children who present with behavioral health problems in primary care practices (Hawkins et al., 2011).

To attain the overarching goal of raising infants, children, and adolescents to enter adulthood as behaviorally competent individuals, P-PCPs must be knowledgeable about behavioral health throughout the pediatric population and intercept adverse behavioral health problems quickly through the implementation of behavioral health evidence-based interventions.

■ METHODS FOR INTEGRATING BEHAVIORAL HEALTH IN PRIMARY CARE

Motivational interviewing (MI; Rollnick, Miller, & Butler, 2008), cognitive behavioral therapy (CBT), and parent and child education through anticipatory guidance are three methods that can be implemented in primary care settings to immediately intercept a problem and intervene with evidence-based interventions (Erickson, Gerstle, & Feldstein, 2005). The intent of this brief discussion on MI and CBT (anticipatory guidance is discussed above) is to inform the reader of strategies for using MI and CBT in pediatric primary care practices and recommend further training, if the training was not a part of the reader's educational curriculum. Additional information on MI can be found at www.motivation alinterviewing.org and for CBT at www.nacbt.org/whatiscbt-htm. Parent education has been a part of educational curriculum as anticipatory guidance for many years and is commonly used in pediatric practices. Parent education concerning behavioral modification is discussed throughout each subsequent chapter in this book.

Motivational Interviewing

MI (Rollnick et al., 2008) is a popular tool for facilitating positive behavioral change in many settings, and has been shown to be an effective tool in 5-minute brief office-based encounters (Erickson, Gerstle, & Feldstein, 2005; Midboe, Cuccuare, Trafton, Ketroser, & Chardos, 2011). MI is a method for conducting a *collaborative* interview with the child, adolescent, and/or parent(s) (identified in this discussion on MI as the individual), with a focus by the interviewer (provider) on motivating and inspiring the individual to change a behavior to improve healthcare outcomes, including but not limited to smoking cessation (Myhre & Adelman, 2013), sexual health behaviors (Day, 2015), diet, overweight and obesity, exercise, substance abuse, medication compliance, and reduction of risky behaviors for adolescents (Booth, 2015; Rollnick et al., 2008).

There are several key components to establish an effective MI encounter, especially with adolescents and parents who are struggling with their infant/child/adolescent's behaviors. *Collaboration* in MI is the process for eliciting and conveying respect for the child's, adolescent's, or parent's ideas, opinions, and autonomy. Collaboration is "nonauthoritarian, ever-present, supportive, and exploratory" (Sciacca, 2009, p. 2). Collaboration is especially important when using MI to enable an adolescent or parent to consider how the individual feels about beginning a behavioral change in which the individual makes the choices and maintains the control. Open-ended questions begin the conversation, permitting the individual to think about the problem and plan behavioral changes that will lead toward and enable problem resolution based on how the individual can make personal changes in his or her lifestyle. Asking the adolescent or parent to "think out loud" during the interprofessional communication interaction is an important way to communicate with an adolescent, as this may be the first time the individual actually "hears his or her own voice" and can consider what that voice is saying, while the provider remains empathic and nonjudgmental, and the adolescent feels safe in a nonpressured environment, with assurance of confidentiality and nonpunitive consequences.

Four specific strategies used during MI are open-ended questions, affirmation, reflective listening, and summarization (Rollnick, Miller, & Butler, 2008). Rollnick et al. (2008) also use the acronym RULE: R–Resist the righting reflex, in which the clinician leads the thinking and makes recommendations for change, rather than providing the opportunity for the individual to think about the problem and suggest changes that are reasonable for the individual to achieve; U–Understand the individual's motivations to even consider a behavioral change; L–Listen intently to the individual throughout the interaction; E–Empower the individual to consider the problem, the potential options that fit the individual's lifestyle, and make the decision to change a behavior. Rollnick et al. (2008) provide numerous examples for communicating strategies with individuals to support positive healthcare outcomes. These authors also provide many references in their book from authors who describe their use of MI in clinical practice settings.

MI provides a unique way to communicate with children, adolescents, and parents about many problems and risky behaviors that they are confronted with each day in our complex world. The motivation for establishing a successful behavioral change must come from the individual, but the provider who uses MI techniques has the opportunity to motivate the individual to begin a behavioral change. Behavioral health problems are amenable to change through MI; thus P-PCPs need to acquire the MI skill set, use the skill set in clinical practice, reflect on the successes and failures while personally using the MI of skill set, and make improvements, with the goal of guiding each individual to achieve their personal goals for physical, social, emotional, and behavioral health.

Cognitive Behavioral Therapy

CBT is a form of psychotherapy that can be used by P-PCPs in brief office-based interventions and is used by psychiatric mental health specialists or therapists to treat emotional, behavioral, and thought problems with talk therapy ("Cognitive Behavioral Therapy," 2017). The approach of CBT differs from MI in that CBT is led by the P-PCP or psychiatric mental health specialist, not by the patient. The patient is an active participant, but the P-PCP or therapist is more active in the role of the problem-solver. The underlying principles of CBT make the assumption that the individual's problems are based on the way the individual takes in and processes the information (Beck Institute for Cognitive Behavior Therapy, n.d.). Individuals are helped to uncover the backstory for their presenting problem, and then practice alternative ways to think about the problem. The P-PCP or therapist may ask the individual to record their thoughts and feelings when a particular problem is presented and then to review with the P-PCP or therapist the connections between the thoughts and the emotions. CBT is often used for a variety of behavioral presentations, including but not limited to, anxiety, depression, drug and alcohol use, anger management, and in the care of children and adolescents who have been exposed to various traumatic events.

CBT programs have been studied and reported in the literature. P-PCPs who plan to use the principles of CBT in brief office-based interventions must be knowledgeable about the processes and use effective strategies to promote a positive behavioral change in the child or adolescent. Research of evidence-based studies on CBT is readily available in the literature. Examples of CBT research with children include such topics as depression in children (Wannachaiykul, Thapinta, Sethabouppha, Thungiaroenkul, & Likhitsathian, 2017), anxiety in children (Rapee et al., 2017), and children who are victims of sexual abuse (Soringer, Misurell, & Hiller, 2012).

P-PCPs who use CBT in the office must receive training in CBT, practice using CBT, and determine the effectiveness of their interventions in reducing the individual's presenting problem. P-PCPs must make a timely referral to a psychiatric mental health provider if the individual who receives office-based CBT does not show evidence of the anticipated improvement.

■ SUMMARY

The conceptual model for IBH problems focuses on identifying the very earliest presentation of even one symptom that may lead to a behavioral health problem and immediately beginning the process for intercepting the potential problem with evidence-based treatments. This interception may enable the child or adolescent to develop coping skills and other strategies to identify and solve the problem before escalation of the problem into out-of-control behaviors. MI is one strategy that can be used with children, adolescents, and/or parents to not only identify the problem but also to place the responsibility for change on the individual via his or her own motivation and desire to change to improve healthcare outcomes. CBT is another strategy used to change behaviors. Education via anticipatory guidance is also a recognized way for helping children, adolescents, and parents understand a problem and possible solutions. P-PCPs in primary care settings play a unique role in caring for children with behavioral health problems with the goal of enabling each individual and family to achieve healthy social, emotional, and behavioral health.

■ REFERENCES

American Academy of Pediatrics. (2011). ADHD: Clinical practice guideline for the diagnosis, valuation, and treatment of attention-deficit/hyperactivity disorder in children and adolescents. *Pediatrics, 128*. Retrieved from http://pediatrics.aappublications.org/content/pediatrics/early/2011/10/14/peds.2011-2654.full.pdf

Beck Institute for Cognitive Behavior Therapy. (n.d.). *Beck institute for cognitive behavioral therapy.* Retrieved from https://beckinstitute.org/about-beck

Boat, T. F., Land, M. L., Leslie, L. K., Hoagwood, K. E., Hawkins-Walsh, E., McCabe, M. A., . . . Sweeney, M. (2016). *Workforce development to enhance the cognitive, affective, and behavioral health of children and youth: Opportunities and barriers in child health care training.* [Discussion paper]. Washington, DC: National Academy of Medicine. Retrieved from https://nam.edu/wp-content/uploads/2016/11/Workforce-Development-to-Enhance-the-Cognitive-Affective-and-Behavioral-Health-of-Children-and-Youth.pdf

Booth, J. (2015). Motivational interviewing: Helping patients make life style changes. *NURSE.com OnCourse Learning.* Retrieved from https://www.nurse.com/ce/motivational-interviewing

Cataldo, R., Huang, J., Calixte, R., Wong, A. T., Bianchi-Hayes, J., & Pati, S. (2015). Effects of overweight and obesity on motor and mental development in infants and toddlers. *Pediatric Obesity, 11*, 389–396. doi:10.1111/ijpo.12077

Centers for Disease Control and Prevention. (n.d.). Healthy aging. Retrieved from https://www.cdc.gov/aging/pdf/perceptions_of_cog_hlth_factsheet.pdf

Centers for Disease Control and Prevention. (2013). *Mental health basics.* Retrieved from https://www.cdc.gov/mentalhealth/basics.htm

Centers for Disease Control and Prevention, Division of Human Development and Disabilities, National Center on Birth Defects and Developmental Disabilities. (2017). *Children's mental health.* Retrieved from https://www.cdc.gov/childrensmentalhealth/index.html

Chowdhury, F. M., Kulcsar, M., Gilchrist, S., & Hawkins, N. A. (2012). News from the CDC: Integrating behavioral health into the patient-centered medical home. *Translational Behavioral Medicine, 2*, 257–259. doi:10.1007/s13142-012-0147-2

Cognitive behavioral therapy. (n.d.). *Psychology Today.* Retrieved from https://www.psychologytoday.com/basics/cognitive-behavioral-therapy

Day, P. (2015). Using motivational interviewing to support sexual health. *British Journal of School Nursing, 9*, 506–509. doi:10.12968/bjsn.2014.9.10.506

Erickson, S. J., Gerstle, M., & Feldstein, S. W. (2005). Brief interventions and motivational interviewing with children, adolescents, and their parents in pediatric health care settings. *Archives of Pediatric and Adolescent Medicine, 159*, 1173–1180. doi:10.1001/archpedi.159.12.1173

Hagan, J. F., Shaw, J. S., & Duncan, P. M. (Eds.). (2017). *Bright futures: Guidelines for health supervision of infants, children, and adolescents* (4th ed.). Elk Grove, IL: American Academy of Pediatrics.

Hallas, D. (1991–2017). Personal clinical practice: Pediatric primary care and pediatric mental health specialty practice within primary care settings.

Hallas, D. (2017, Mar 17). *Preventing overweight and obesity in the first 1000 days of life: The evidence-base for NP practice in primary care.* Presented at the 2017 Annual Conference of the National Association of Pediatric Nurse Practitioners. Denver, CO.

Hallas, D., & Koslap-Petraco, M. (2004, July 21). *Implementing evidence-based practice in pediatric primary care*. Presented as a peer reviewed invited poster presentation at the Sigma Theta Tau International Honor Society of Nursing 15th International Nursing Research Congress & International Evidence-Based Practice Preconference. Dublin, Ireland.

Hallas, D., Koslap-Petraco, M., & Fletcher, J. (2017). Social emotional development of toddlers: A randomized controlled trial of an office based intervention. *Journal of Pediatric Nursing, 33*, 33–40. doi:10.1016/j.pedn.2016.11.004

Hawkins-Walsh, E., Crowley, A., Mazurek Melnyk, B., Beauschense, M., Brandt, P., & O'Haver, J. (2011). Improving health-care quality through AFPNP national nursing education collaborative to strengthen PNP curriculum in mental/behavioral health and EBP: Lessons learned from academic faculty and clinical preceptors. *Journal of Professional Nursing, 27*(1), 10–18. doi:10.1016/j.profnurs.2010.09.004

Hawkins, E., & Van Cleve, S. (2013). The pediatric mental health specialist: Role delineation. *The Journal for Nurse Practitioners, 9*, 142–148. doi:10.1016/j.nurpra.2012.11.017

Intercept. (n.d.). *iCoachMath*. Retrieved from http://www.icoachmath.com/math_dictionary/intercept.html

Jellineck, M. (2017). A path beyond advocacy to improve mental health services for children and families: Population health management. *JAMA Pediatrics, 171*, 615–616. doi:10.1001/jamapediatrics.2017.0216

Midboe, A. M., Cuccuare, M. A., Trafton, J. A., Ketroser, N., & Chardos, J. F. (2011). Implementing motivational interviewing in primary care: The role of provider characteristics. *Translational Behavioral Medicine, 1*, 588–594. Retrieved from https://www.ncbi.nlm.nih.gov/pmc/articles/PMC3717678

Myhre, K. E., & Adelman, W. (2013). Motivational interviewing: Helping teenaged smokers to quit. *Contemporary Pediatrics, 30*(10), 18–23. Retrieved from http://www.happyhealthyteeth.com/wpt/blog-docs/contpeds-2013-10.pdf

National Research Council and Institute of Medicine. (2009). *Preventing mental, emotional, and behavioral disorders among young people: Progress and possibilities*. Washington, DC: National Academies Press.

Perou, R., Bitsko, R. H., Blumberg, S. J., Pastor, P., Ghandour, R. M., Gfroerer, J. C., . . . Huang, L. N. (2013). Mental health surveillance among children United States, 2005–2011. *Morbidity and Mortality Weekly Report, 6*(2), 1–35. Retreived from https://www.cdc.gov/mmwr/preview/mmwrhtml/su6202a1.htm?s_cid=su6201a1_w

Rapee, R. M., Lyneham, H. J., Wuthrich, V., Chatterton, M. L., Hudson, J. L., Kangas, M., & Mihalopoulos, C. (2017). Comparison of stepped care delivery against a single, empirically validated cognitive behavioral therapy program for youth with anxiety: A randomized clinical trial. *Journal of the American Academy of Child & Adolescent Psychiatry, 56*, 841–848. doi:10.1016/j.jaac.2017.08.001

Raver, C. C., & Ziegler, E., F. (1997). Social competence: An untapped dimension in evaluating Head Start's success. *Early Childhood Research Quarterly, 12*, 363–385. doi:0.1016/S0885-2006(97)90017-X

Rollnick, S., Miller, W. R., & Butler, C. C. (2008). *Motivational interviewing in health care: Helping patients change behavior*. New York, NY: Guilford Press.

Sciacca, K. (2009). Motivational interviewing – MI, glossary & fact sheet. Retrieved from https://www.researchgate.net/profile/Kathleen_Sciacca/publication/280236508_Motivational_Interviewing_Glossary_and_Fact_Sheet_Kathleen_Sciacca/links/55ae8a8a08ae98e661a6eb7d/Motivational-Interviewing-Glossary-and-Fact-Sheet-Kathleen-Sciacca.pdf

Shonkoff, J. P. (2009). Investment in early childhood development lays the foundation for a prosperous and sustainable society. In R. E. Tremblay, M. Boivin, & R. DeV. Peters (Eds.), *Encyclopedia on early childhood development* [online]. Montreal, Quebec: Centre of Excellence for Early Childhood Development and Strategic Knowledge Cluster on Early Child Development. Retrieved from http://www.childencyclopedia.com/documents/ShonkoffANGxp.pdf

Shonkoff, J. P., Garner, A. S., Siegel, B. S., Dobbins, M. I., Earls, M. F., Garner, A. S., . . . Wood, D. L. The committee on psychological aspects of child and family health, committee on early childhood, adoption, and dependent care, and second on developmental and behavioral pediatrics. (2012). The lifelong effects of early childhood adversity and toxic stress. *Pediatrics, 129*, e232–e246. doi: 10.1542/peds.2011-2663.

Soringer, C., Misurell, J. R., & Hiller, A. (2012). Game-based cognitive-behavioral therapy (GB-CBT) group program for children who have experienced sexual abuse: A three-month follow-up investigation. *Journal of Sexual Abuse, 21*, 646–664. doi:10.1080/10538712.2012.722592

U.S. Department of Health & Human Services. (1999). *Mental health: A report of the surgeon general*. Bethesda, MD: National Institute of Mental Health.

U.S. Department of Health & Human Services. (2001). *Report of a Surgeon General's working meeting on the integration of mental health services and primary health care* (November 30–Dec 1). Atlanta, GA and Rockville, MD: U.S. Department of Health & Human Services, Public Health Service, Office of the Surgeon General.

Wannachaiykul, S., Thapinta, D., Sethabouppha, H., Thungjaroenkul, P., & Likhitsathian, S. (2017). Randomized controlled trial of computerized cognitive behavioral therapy program for adolescent offenders with depression. *Pacific Rim International Journal of Nursing Research, 21*, 32–43. Retrieved from Retrieved from https://www.tci-thaijo.org/index.php/PRIJNR/article/view/62508

World Health Organization. (2011). *Mental health: A state of well-being.* Geneva, Switzerland: Author Retrieved from http://www.who.int/features/factfiles/mental_health/en/index.html

CHAPTER 2

Brain Development and Compelling Outcomes of Ineffective Parent-Child Bonding

EMILY SCHADT

Ineffective child-rearing practices and parental bonding have negative, lifelong impacts on children. Poor parental bonding and lack of effective parenting is related to adverse physical, psychological, and social–emotional hardships for the entire pediatric population who experiences them. Although inadequate parenting has been linked to psychological issues with older children, few studies have investigated the negative effects ineffective bonding in the infant and toddler periods have on brain development (Jefferis & Oliver, 2006). This chapter discusses the compelling outcomes of ineffective parenting and provides insights for assessing the parent–child relationship and interventions that may *intercept* behavioral disorders in children and adolescents as a direct result of ineffective parenting.

■ SECURE ATTACHMENT

The foundation for secure attachment in infancy is directly related to parental bonding (see Chapter 7). Appropriate social–emotional development is dependent upon behaviors and attitudes toward infants expressed by their caregivers, which begins during the natal period. Mothers who are unable to adequately bond with newborns and infants in the natal period have been found to have higher associations of fewer prenatal visits with an obstetric provider or no prenatal care, poorer nutrition, and increased alcohol and nicotine consumption when compared to mothers who bond appropriately after birth (Rossen et al., 2017). Beginning with the immediate post-delivery experience, newborns whose caregivers are *unable* to bond appropriately and parent effectively throughout infancy have been found to have higher levels of toxic stress and increased probabilities of adverse childhood experiences (ACEs; Felitti et al., 1998). Inappropriate initial bonding then sets the stage for a cyclical and sizable descending spiral into both psychological and physical disease states throughout life.

Healthy physical and psychological development of the newborn begins at the point of conception, and either strengthens or worsens over time. Children need appropriate environmental exposures and parental support to establish positive reactions to life experiences. Early experiences set the stage for proper brain development, which can be adversely affected by inappropriate parental interactions. Basic foundations, which include a stable environment with appropriate and nurturing caregiver interactions, as well as nonviolent and supportive physical and psychological surroundings must be established early in the newborn period to assure healthy brain development without architectural demise (Center on the Developing Child at Harvard University, 2017a).

■ BRAIN ARCHITECTURE

Absence of parental–newborn secure attachment and appropriate child-rearing practices poses a serious threat to child health, growth, and development. Salubrious physical and psychological development is directly associated with healthy adult relationships. Brain architecture is reliant on appropriate attachment and healthy responses from caregivers during stressful situations. Caregivers who do not bond with their newborns, infants, and young children appropriately, and fail to provide variable responses to critical needs in sensitive time periods of brain development are more likely to disrupt neurodevelopment, and activate potentially harmful stress hormone cascades, in their infants and children. Thus, children whose brain architecture is negatively impacted during these sensitive time periods can have disparities in physical, psychological, social, and emotional health throughout their life (Center on the Developing Child at Harvard University, 2017b).

■ BRAIN DEVELOPMENT

The recent paradigm shift between the roles that *nature* and *nurture* play in the developing brain has changed the way medical professionals should view brain formation. The constant interaction between genes and environmental experiences has been shown to have significant effects on brain development as early as conception. The brain should be viewed as a collective structure whose development is reliant on social interactions, daily experiences, and outward opportunities that permit the brain to make connections and formations throughout childhood. Early synapses, which can occur up to thousands of times per second in the infancy period, provide for the foundational aptitude of a child to learn, adapt, and be resilient throughout life. Due to the extreme overdevelopment of brain formation in the early childhood years, when inadequate parenting and child-rearing practices occur, especially during critical periods of time, development is easily sidetracked and difficult to reroute (Britto, 2014).

Brain development begins and solidifies in a hierarchical pattern, beginning with the brainstem, and concluding with the cortex. Innate tasks like respiration, heart contraction, temperature regulation, sleep/wake cycles, motor movements, speech, coordination, and appetite and satiety are brain stem and cerebellar functions that develop quickly and are ingrained into life from the time of conception.

The hippocampus, amygdala, and hypothalamus, which make up the limbic system, develop more slowly and are responsible for emotions, learning, memory, and motivation. Finally, the most advanced part of the brain develops latest. The cerebral cortex (frontal, parietal, occipital, and temporal lobes) allows humans to think, understand, and perceive information. Skills developed through the cortex, like critical thinking, affiliation, and secure attachment, can be easily swayed by child-rearing and take a tremendous amount of time and effort to obtain (Center on the Developing Child at Harvard University, 2017a).

The most rapid phase of brain development occurs in utero. By age 4, a child's brain is almost the size of an adult's. During the first years of life, experiences positively or negatively shape brain architecture; the brain is extremely plastic and is actively dependent on experiences and environment. Normal brain development is dependent upon the establishment of critical connections throughout infancy and early childhood. Unfortunately, the process of brain building can be structurally altered by negative experiences such as stress, abuse, and neglect. Although important neurodevelopment processes continue throughout adulthood, brain rewiring is significantly more difficult to achieve with age (Burgess-Chamberlin, 2008). Thus, infant and young children need positive infant/child attachment and bonding without undue negative stressors for brain development to achieve maximum human potential.

■ SERVE AND RETURN EXPERIENCES

One of the most indispensable ways to foster a developing child's brain is through serve and return mechanisms, which are essentially appropriate interactions between a child and his or her caregiver. Children distinctively desire physical touch and emotional interaction, and when their fundamental desires are unmet, neuronal connections are not made, leading to altered brain architecture. As young children attempt to interact by babbling, crying, or gesturing, if caregivers respond correctly, the brain sends signals that offer supportive development of communication and social skills. As early as 18 months of age, environmental exposure and early experiences have already shaped brain formation. Children with adverse early childhood experiences display difficulties in educational achievement by 18 months of age.

By 3 years of age, vocabulary development in children with proper *serve and return experiences* has been reported to be two to three times greater than same-age children with poor serve and return experiences. At school-age, children with positive serve and return experiences have been shown to be fundamentally ahead of their cohorts who were not able to make appropriate neuronal connections as a direct result of inadequate parenting. Unfortunately, for children with poorer child-rearing practices and increased adversities, by age 3, there are significant alterations in their brain development that may negatively affect their physical, psychological, social, and emotional development throughout their lifetime. Developmental delays in language, behavior, and cognition may be solidified before the child even reaches school-age. Therefore, it is imperative to intercept these negative factors and provide the adequate loving care in the early developmental years to decrease the potential for developmental delay (Center on the Developing Child at Harvard University, 2017b).

■ ACEs AND TOXIC STRESS

Currently, nearly half of the nation's children will incur at least one or more ACEs before their 18th birthday. This means that one out of two children will live in a world where toxic stress is normal for them; 50% of children will be abused, neglected, or live in a dysfunctional environment (Stevens, 2013). Although adversities affect all ages, children are more at risk of developing negative associations. Constant stress and adversities physically modify children's brains by disrupting neurodevelopment, which causes physical impairments, increases risky behaviors, instills inappropriate coping, and eventually leads to premature death. As little as one adversity increases rates of substance abuse, sexually transmitted diseases, promiscuity, cigarette smoking, depression, suicide, heart disease, diabetes, and numerous other mental and physical diseases (Centers for Disease Control and Prevention [CDC], 2014).

The introduction of ACEs and toxic stress began in the late 1990s following a groundbreaking analysis conducted by Robert Anda and Vincent Felliti, in association with the Kaiser Permanente Foundation (Felitti et al., 1998). Chapter 32 provides details about this study as well as screening tools and interventions for children exposed to ACEs throughout childhood and adolescence.

A paradigm shift of the critical understanding between adversities and poor health has occurred in relation to the ACE study. Recent advances in the field of epigenetics (see Chapter 35) have helped solidify the link between ACEs, toxic stress, and trauma, with the latter two being identified as key components of origin (Shonkoff, Garner, Siegel, Dobbins, & Earls, 2011). Toxic stress and trauma are unique terms that are closely intertwined with adversities, yet are completely distinctive to every individual. Although the general impression of trauma is violent mayhem, in all actuality, trauma is any experience where an individual is physically and/or emotionally left in a vulnerable state. If traumatic experiences occur repetitively and without intervention, they become toxic. Over time, the accumulation of toxic stress then leads to physical and psychological abnormalities due to a maladaptation of the stress cascade system known as allostatic load (Harris & Renschler, 2015).

Though stress is generally thought to be a negative occurrence, there are essentially three different types of stress that affect the body in different ways: positive, tolerable, and toxic (Alberta Family Wellness Initiative, 2017). Positive stressors are necessary and important for development; they nurture secure relationships by triggering activation of the hypothalamic-pituitary-adrenal (HPA) axis and neuro-endocrine-immune (NEI) network, which initiates the autonomic nervous system (Shonkoff et al., 2011). Positive stress stimulates the "fight-or-flight" response in children, training their bodies to self-adjust through negative feedback systems. Positive stressors are short-lived; examples might include meeting new people, or preparing for exams at school. Tolerable stressors are unavoidable circumstances where allostatic load is increased and altered over a slightly longer period of time. Negative effects can occur from tolerable stress, but with positive, supportive relationships from caregivers, children are able to recover; tolerable stress does not have to alter brain development if nurturing environments are present. Instances of tolerable stress include the loss of a loved one or a natural disaster. Unfortunately, however, without the protection and support of a caring provider, tolerable stress can lead to toxic stress—stress that occurs when there is prolongation of allostatic load, leading to an imbalance of the NEI system and causing a chronic surge of the sympathetic nervous system (Purewal et al., 2016). The persistence of homeostasis imbalance affects body and brain stability, leading to alterations in brain architecture and increased susceptibility to physical and psychological adversities in adult life (Payne, Levine, & Crane-Godreau, 2015).

■ CAUSE AND EFFECT RELATIONSHIP OF ACEs

Chronic proliferation of the sympathetic nervous system can occur for a variety of different reasons, but for the purpose of the ACE study, adversities were caused from 10 distinct instances: physical, emotional, and sexual abuse, physical and emotional neglect, caregiver mental illness, caregiver separation, maternal abuse, incarceration of a caregiver, and/or substance abuse by a caregiver. Overwhelming data gleaned from the initial study, as well as research outside of the ACE questionnaire, identified that adversities continue to be extremely common and affect every age, sex, and ethnicity group. Data also revealed that if a person has one ACE they are over eight times more likely to experience two or more ACEs (Starecheski, 2015).

Although it may sound insignificant to have more than one ACE score, the consequences of adversities have been found to be astronomical. Research has identified an exposure–reaction response between adversities and poor health outcomes. The belief of an over accumulation of circulating cortisol secondary to toxic stress is the foundation of structural brain formation variations (Purewal et al., 2016). Although the exact cause–effect relationship of ACEs varies between individuals due to patient experience, chronic restructuring of the brain due to toxic stress has been well studied and linked to an underdevelopment of temporal lobe activity. Therefore, due to brain matter underdevelopment secondary to increased allostatic load, ACEs have a direct link to an overwhelming proliferation of risky behaviors, as well as increased diagnoses of physical and psychological diseases for the majority of patients who incur them (Stevens, 2012).

Physically, stress-related alterations have been associated with dysfunction in every body system, secondary to increased allostatic load, causing prolonged "wear and tear" on the body. Imbalance of cortisol levels and inflammatory markers have serious negative effects, including the alteration of genes. Examples of adversity-related physical illnesses include increased cardiovascular disease, autoimmune conditions, chronic lung illness, headaches, obesity, smoking, generalized poor health, and early death. Structural changes of brain formation also include hyperactivation of the amygdala, loss of neural connections in the hippocampus, and overactivity of the orbitofrontal cortex, leading to impaired critical thinking capabilities, as well as increased probabilities of mental illness (Shonkoff et al., 2011). Psychological diseases with a proven connection to ACEs are depression, anxiety, attention deficit hyperactivity disorder, autism, binge-exploiting behaviors, and posttraumatic stress disorder; increased risk taking and violent behaviors have also been reported (Child Welfare Information Gateway, 2015).

■ CLINICAL INDICATIONS

Due to the impracticality of eradicating all poor parental and familial decision-making skills, complete elimination of ACEs in society is highly unlikely. However, with early detection and routine screening of every child, the likelihood of decreasing unfavorable health-related outcomes for children with adversities potentially could improve. Recent studies have identified that adversities tend to increase with age and accumulate over multiple years. By identifying high-risk children while they are still young, pediatric primary care providers (P-PCPs) can take advantage of brain plasticity by helping form a treatment plan that will match the needs of the children due to their adverse exposures. Well-child exams are the perfect opportunity for routine universal screening of ACEs. Identifying behaviorisms that could potentially be linked to adversity and toxic stress, such as regression, anger, developmental delays, and chronic inorganic causes of physical disablement, provides the P-PCP the chance to discuss the impact of ACEs on neurodevelopment, educate families about symptomatic treatment, and initiate early referrals for psychotherapy, psychiatry, biofeedback, and/or counseling if needed (Purewal et al., 2016). A detailed discussion of screening tools for ACEs is found in Chapter 32.

■ SUMMARY

Ineffective child-rearing practices and poor parental attachments in the early years of life have the possibility of impairing a child's physical, psychological, social, and emotional well-being. Without appropriate interactions, children's brains do not receive proper signals that allow for suitable neuronal development and connections, which can alter brain architecture. Therefore, early intervention is critical, as children and adolescents are more likely to develop negative psychological and physical symptoms in relation to toxic stress than adults, yet are less likely to seek help when they are feeling overwhelmed (American Academy of Pediatrics, 2017).

■ REFERENCES

Alberta Family Wellness Initiative. (2017). *Stress*. Retrieved from http://www.albertafamilywellness.org/what-we-know/stress
American Academy of Pediatrics. (2017). *Promoting resilience*. Retrieved from https://www.aap.org/en-us/advocacy-and-policy/aap-health-initiatives/resilience/Pages/Promoting-Resilience.aspx
Britto, P. (2014). How children's brains develop-New insights. *UNICEF*. Retrieved from https://blogs.unicef.org/blog/how-childrens-brains-develop-new-insights
Burgess-Chamberlin, L. (2008). *The amazing brain: What every parent and caregiver needs to know*. Retrieved from http://www.instituteforsafefamilies.org/sites/default/files/isfFiles/The_Amazing_Brain-1.pdf
Center on the Developing Child at Harvard University. (2017a). *Brain architecture*. Retrieved from http://developingchild.harvard.edu/science/key-concepts/brain-architecture
Center on the Developing Child at Harvard University. (2017b). *Five numbers to remember about early childhood development*. Retrieved from http://developingchild.harvard.edu/resources/five-numbers-to-remember-about-early-childhood-development

Centers for Disease Control and Prevention. 2014. *Violence prevention.* Retrieved from http://www.cdc. gov/violenceprevention/acestudy/index.html

Child Welfare Information Gateway. (2015). *Understanding the effects of maltreatment on brain development.* Retrieved from https://www.childwelfare.gov/pubPDFs/brain_development.pdf

Felitti, V. J., Anda, R. F., Nordenberg, D., Williamson, D. F., Spitz, A. M., Edwards, V., & Marks, J. S. (1998). Relationship of childhood abuse and household dysfunction to many of the leading causes of death in adults: The adverse childhood experiences (ACE) study. *American Journal of Preventive Medicine, 14*(4), 245–258. doi:10.1016/S0749-3797(98)00017-8

Harris, N., & Renschler, T. (2015). *ACE-Q user guide for health professionals.* Retrieved from http:// www.centerforyouthwellness.org/healthcare-professionals

Jefferis, P. G., & Oliver, C. (2006). Associations between maternal childrearing cognitions and conduct problems in young children. *Clinical Child Psychology and Psychiatry, 11*(1), 83–102. doi:10.1177/1359104506059125

Payne, P., Levine, P., & Crane-Godreau, M. (2015). Somatic experiencing: Using interoception and proprioception as core elements of trauma therapy. *Frontiers in Psychology, 6.* doi:10.3389/fpsyg.2015.00093

Purewal, S. K., Bucci, M., Guiterrez Wang, L., Koita, K., Silverio Margques, S., Oh, D., & Burke Harris, N. (2016). Screening for Adverse Childhood Experiences (ACEs) in an integrated pediatric care model. *Zero to Three Journal, 36*(3), 10–17.

Rossen, L., Hutchinson, D., Wilson, J., Burns, L., Allsop, S., Elliott, E. J., . . . Mattick, R. P. (2017). Maternal bonding through pregnancy and postnatal: Findings from an Australian longitudinal study. *American Journal of Perinatology, 34*(8), 808–817. doi:10.1055/s-0037-1599052

Shonkoff, J. P., Garner, A. S., Siegel, B. S., Dobbins, M. I., & Earls, M. F. (2011). The lifelong effects of early childhood adversity and toxic stress. *Pediatrics, 129*(1), 232–246. doi:10.1542/peds.2011-2663

Starecheski, L. (2015). *Take the ACE quiz and learn what it does and doesn't mean.* Retrieved from http://www.npr.org/sections/health-shots/2015/03/02/387007941/take-the-ace-quiz-and-learn-what-it-does-and-doesnt-mean

Stevens, J. (2012). *The adverse childhood experiences study—The largest public health study you never heard of.* Retrieved from http://www.huffingtonpost.com/jane-ellen-stevens/the-adverse-childhood-exp_7_b_1944199.html

Stevens, J. (2013). *Nearly 35 million U.S. children have experienced one or more types of childhood trauma.* Retrieved from http://acestoohigh.com/2013/05/13/nearly-35-million-u-s-children-have-experienced-one-or-more-types-of-childhood-trauma

CHAPTER 3

Psychotropic Medications for Children and Adolescents

ERICA D. KIERCE

The National Center for Health Statistics reported that 7.5% of U.S. children between the ages of 6 and 17 were prescribed medications for emotional or behavioral difficulties in 2011–2012 (Howie, Pastor, & Lukacs, 2014). Children under the age of 5 had a reported increase of 1.45% of psychotropic prescriptions in 2002–2005, but there was a decline to 1% from 2006–2009 (Chirdkiatgumchai et al., 2013). The Centers for Disease Control and Prevention reported a fivefold increase in the number of children under 18 on psychostimulants from 1988–1994 to 2007–2010, with the most recent percentage reported at 4.2 (National Center for Health Statistics, 2014).

While some stimulants and psychotropic medications are prescribed by pediatric primary care providers (P-PCPs) in primary care settings, and in particular those credentialed as pediatric primary care mental health specialists (PMHSs), many are prescribed by psychiatrists and psychiatric-mental health nurse practitioners (PMHNP). However, all P-PCPs are responsible for knowing when to prescribe, the anticipated outcomes, adverse side effects, and the best available evidence to medically manage the child or adolescent on stimulants or psychotropic medications. Thus, this chapter provides the most current information about simulant and psychotropic medications and other medications prescribed for children with emotional or behavioral and mental health problems, with a focus on safe prescribing for behavioral management, reduction in symptoms, and the knowledge needed to *intercept* adverse side effects of prescribed medications. In addition, this chapter provides P-PCPs with information about the safety and effectiveness of psychotropic medications for this population, with a focus on the privilege and responsibilities for safe prescribing practices.

■ PRIVILEGE OF PRESCRIBING

The privilege of prescriptive authority for all P-PCPs must be paired with selective, evidence-based, rational prescribing. This is especially important in the often controversial area of pediatric psychiatry. Before a decision to begin treatment with psychotropic medication is made, the P-PCP should determine if safer, non-psychotropic treatment options are appropriate in lieu of or in conjunction with psychotropic medications. Whenever clinically appropriate, psychotropic medication use should be avoided. "Above all, do no harm" (Hippocrates).

Rational Prescribing

The World Health Organization (WHO) defines rational prescribing as a pattern where "patients receive medications appropriate to their clinical needs, in doses that meet their own individual requirements for an adequate period of time, and at the lowest cost to them and their community" (WHO, 1985). In order to develop a habit of rational prescribing, the P-PCP is guided by a clear diagnosis, predetermined but amendable therapeutic goals, informed treatment process, and patient-centered education and follow-up. The process of rational prescribing begins by carefully defining the problem or target symptoms and making an appropriate diagnosis. With psychiatric diagnoses, the criteria in the *Diagnostic and Statistical Manual of Mental Disorders, Fifth Edition* (*DSM-5*; American Psychiatric Association [APA], 2013) should be met and particular attention given to ruling out exclusion criteria before making a diagnosis. Evidence to support medication use should be carefully evaluated. Therapeutic medication goals and target symptoms should be clearly identified. Expectations for the use of medication should be well-informed and reasonable. When providing medication management for pediatric patients, it's important to include the patient and family in decisions whenever appropriate. Potential risks and benefits should be presented before medication therapy is initiated. Education regarding risks and benefits should include why the medication was selected, potential benefits, and potential adverse reactions with long and short duration of use of psychotropic medications. Understanding of psychotropic medication risks and benefits is continuously evolving. For this reason, it's imperative that P-PCPs provide medication education using the best evidence-based information free of bias or falsehood.

Recent attention is given to decreasing irrational prescribing, especially pertaining to psychotropic use in children and adolescents. Indicators of irrational prescribing include the use of four or more psychotropic medications, two or more psychotropic medications from the same class, medications used in children younger than the age of 6, doses outside therapeutic ranges, and medications not indicated for the diagnosis. Prudent P-PCPs should be aware of patterns of irrational prescribing and minimize or eliminate irrational prescribing in the pediatric and adolescent patient populations.

■ PSYCHOTROPIC MEDICATIONS

For ease of locating information, psychotropic medications in this chapter are presented alphabetically by target diagnosis or symptomology.

Attention Deficit Hyperactivity Disorder (ADHD)

ADHD is the most commonly diagnosed behavioral psychiatric problems in pediatric patients. To meet *DSM-5* (APA, 2013) criteria, symptoms must be present in two or more settings, occur before the age of 12, and include persistent difficulty with inattention and/or hyperactivity. These symptoms must cause significant impairment in the child's development or role functioning. First-line treatment for preschool-age children includes behavioral interventions only. The 2015 American Academy of Pediatrics (AAP) ADHD practice guideline for preschool-age children supports using Dexedrine for those who do not improve with only behavioral management (American Academy of Pediatrics [AAP], 2011). For school-age children, first-line treatment includes behavioral and psychotropic interventions (AAP, 2011). The benefit and safety of long-term stimulant use in pediatric and adolescent populations has not been established; however, best outcomes are achieved with a combination of behavioral interventions and psychotropic medications.

CENTRAL NERVOUS SYSTEM STIMULANTS

Central nervous system (CNS) stimulants are the most commonly used drug class for the management of ADHD symptoms (AAP, 2011). Most CNS stimulants used for ADHD are formulations of either amphetamine or methylphenidate. Selection between agents is based upon the individual child or adolescent needs related to dosing formulation, duration, cost, and side effect profile or tolerability. The patient and family must be educated about the potential for stimulant abuse and dependency. P-PCPs can intercept the risk of abuse and dependency by using the lowest effective dose that produces therapeutic effects. A careful medical and psychiatric history and physical must be completed before prescribing CNS stimulants, giving careful attention to cardiovascular and neurological risk factors.

Side Effects

Commonly reported side effects include appetite suppression, sleep disturbance, headaches, dry mouth, gastrointestinal problems, and abdominal pain. Monitor for new or worsening anxiety, irritability, agitation, blurred vision, tremors, tics, heart palpitations, changes in blood pressure, and seizures (Cortese et al., 2013).

Intercept side effects by monitoring for new or worsening symptoms at each primary healthcare visit through SCARED (screen for child anxiety related disorders) screening for anxiety, history questions specific to subjective symptoms, and blood pressure readings on at least three extremities and in recumbent and sitting positions. In addition, question the child, adolescent, or parent about sleep patterns and determine appropriate interventions to improve sleep patterns, as adequate and restful sleep is an essential component for management of behavioral health.

Intercept adverse effects by documenting height, weight, and body mass index (BMI) prior to prescribing a stimulant and by monitoring changes in these anthropometric measurements at each primary care visit, as these may be negatively affected by stimulant use. Some stimulants, in particular methylphenidate, reduce appetite with a resultant loss in weight and body fat. Review nutritional status and daily caloric intake and make recommendations based on this information to assure a healthy diet for the child and adolescent. Offering a higher caloric intake at breakfast prior to administering the medications may help reduce weight loss from methylphenidate, especially Ritalin (Cortese et al., 2013).

Contraindications for the use of CNS stimulants include cardiovascular disease or structural heart abnormalities, severe hypertension, hyperthyroidism, agitation, history of drug abuse, within 14 days of administering monoamine oxidase inhibitors (MAOIs), glaucoma, or family history of Tourette's syndrome (Cortese et al., 2013).

Intercept contraindications by obtaining a detailed comprehensive personal and family history. Refer to cardiology prior to prescribing if the child or adolescent has a pertinent positive family history that is concerning or a pertinent positive personal history.

Warnings

Stimulants are associated with serious cardiovascular events including sudden death and myocardial infarction, even in children (Cortese et al., 2013). Stimulant use may exacerbate mood symptoms including aggression and hostility and cause manic or psychotic symptoms even in those with no history of these symptoms. These medications have a high potential for abuse. Monitor height and weight as these may be negatively affected by stimulant use (Table 3.1).

NONSTIMULANT MEDICATIONS FOR ADHD

Nonstimulant medications are indicated when symptoms are primarily hyperactivity or impulsivity or when stimulant options are not well-tolerated or are contraindicated. Best evidence suggests management with a low dose stimulant and an alpha-adrenergic agonist when clinically appropriate and when tics are present and distressing (American Academy of Child and Adolescent Psychiatry [AACAP], 2013).

ALPHA-2 ADRENERGIC AGONISTS AND ALPHA-2 AGONISTS

Medications such as Tenex, Clonidine, and Intuniv are helpful for physical manifestations of ADHD. These medications do not directly improve attention or concentration but rather work by decreasing response time, impulsivity, and hyperactivity. These drugs lower the heart rate and blood pressure; though the mechanism of action for ADHD management is not well-known (AACAP, 2013).

Side Effects

The most common side effects are dry mouth, dizziness, fatigue, headache, skin rash, and constipation. Orthostatic hypotension may also occur. Most cardiovascular side effects are dose dependent (Scahill, 2012).

Intercept side effects by advising the child, adolescent, or parent on measures for early recognition of xerostomia and measures for treatment. A reduction in salvia as side effect of psychotropic medications affects the oral mucosa and remineralization of tooth structure resulting in changes in oral health including an increase in dental cavities prior to experiencing the actual dry mouth (Swager & Morgan, 2011). Dental visits should be encouraged as well as good oral hygiene. The child or adolescent may have difficulty swallowing or speaking as the xerostomia increases and this may adversely affect their school performance as well as self-image. Sugarless gum, nonsticky candy, and foods such as

TABLE 3.1

CNS STIMULANT MEDICATIONS BY TYPE

ADHD Agents With Amphetamine/Dextroamphetamine*

Brand Name	Generic Name	Formulation
Adderall IR/XR	Amphetamine/dexmethamphetamine	Tablet/capsule
Adzenys XR-ODT	Brand name only	Oral disintegrating tablet
Dexedrine	Dextroamphetamine sulfate	Capsule
Evekeo	Brand name only	Tablet
ProCentra	Dextroamphetamine sulfate	Oral solution
Vyvanse	Brand name only lisdexamfetamine	Capsule
Zenzedi	Dextroamphetamine	Tablet

ADHD Agents With Methylphenidate/Dexmethylphenidate

Aptensio XR	Brand name only	Capsule
Concerta	Methylphenidate ER	Tablet
Daytrana	Brand name only	Transdermal patch
Focalin IR/XR	Dexmethylphenidate	Tablet/capsule
Metadate CD/ER	Methylphenidate ER	Capsule
Quillivant XR	Brand name only	Oral suspension
QuilliChew ER	Brand name only	Chewable tablet
Ritalin IR/SR/LA	Methylphenidate Methylphenidate ER	Tab/tab/capsule

*The most commonly prescribed CNS stimulants are listed alphabetically by active ingredient.

ADHD, attention deficit hyperactivity disorder; CD, controlled delivery; ER, extended release; IR, immediate release; LA, long acting; SR, sustained release; XR, extended release.

carrots and celery are recommended for individuals with xerostomia (Swager & Morgan, 2011). Appetite may change as tasting various flavors in foods is also altered by xerostomia. The P-PCP and psychiatric providers should always ask about symptoms of xerostomia and assess for evidence in both primary care and psychiatric practices.

Warnings

Avoid abrupt withdrawal or discontinuation to prevent rebound hypertension. These medications may be heavily sedating early in treatment. Avoid use in renal or cardiovascular disease. Assess for a family history of sudden cardiac arrest, especially in youth (Giovannitti, Thomas, & Crawford, 2015).

Intercept warning signs by advising adolescents and parents of younger children on this medication not to stop the medication, and if a problem is identified, to call the provider immediately. In addition, adolescents should be advised about safety related to possible drowsiness, with instructions to avoid driving and other activities that may be hazardous, such as working with machinery at school or during an after-school job.

Obtain an ECG and/or refer for a cardiac evaluation if there is a positive family history of sudden cardiac arrest or death.

STRATTERA

This nonstimulant option works more similarly to a serotonin–norepinephrine reuptake inhibitor (SNRI). The mechanism of action is selective inhibition of presynaptic norepinephrine reuptake. It may take several weeks to achieve therapeutic effect, and dosing is weight based. Strattera may be a good option for children who cannot tolerate stimulants or have an underlying mood disorder such as depression or anxiety (Biederman, Spencer, & Wilens, 2004).

Side Effects

The most common side effects include dry mouth, headache, abdominal pain, decreased appetite, insomnia, cough, somnolence, nausea, and vomiting (Biederman et al., 2004).

The *intercept* for side effects for Strattera are the same as listed in the general category of nonstimulant medications for ADHD. In addition, the interval history questions should include asking about unexplained cough and nausea and vomiting. If these complaints are acknowledged, routine evidence-based practices treating the complaints should be implemented.

Warnings

Strattera has a black box warning for increased suicidal behavior in children and adolescents as seen with SSRIs and SNRIs. Do not use within 14 days of an MAOI, with pheochromocytoma, cardiovascular disorders, or narrow-angle glaucoma. Strattera may cause sudden death in children with cardiovascular abnormalities. Monitor carefully for adverse psychiatric symptoms (Biederman et al., 2004).

Intercept warning signs of potential suicidal behaviors at each primary care visit through screenings with either the **h**ome, **e**ducation/**e**mployment, **a**ctivities, **d**rugs, **s**exuality, **s**uicide/depression, and **s**afety (HEEADSSS) or **S**trengths, **S**chool, **H**ome, **A**ctivities, **D**rugs/Substance Use, **E**motions/Eating/Depression, **S**exuality, and **S**afety (SHADESS) assessments and/or the Patient Health Questionnaire-Nine Item (PHQ-9).

Anxiety and Depressive Disorders

Antidepressant medications and anxiolytics are addressed together because many medications are indicated for the treatment of both disorders. Additionally, it can be difficult to differentiate between depressive and anxiety symptoms, and they often co-occur. However, it is critical to establish the correct diagnosis of anxiety or depression, since treatment for anxiety when the child actually has depression and vice versa results in no change in behavioral symptoms and the potential for worsening presentation. Selective serotonin reuptake inhibitors (SSRI) and SNRI are indicated for the treatment of depression and anxiety. Anxiolytics and other medications are mentioned specifically for the management of anxiety disorders and do not treat symptoms of depression. When treating children and adolescents, these medications should be used in conjunction with psychotherapy; treatment with medication alone is generally insufficient (American Academy of Child and Adolescent Psychiatry [AACAP], 2007).

SELECTIVE SEROTONIN REUPTAKE INHIBITORS (SSRIs)

SSRIs work by decreasing the reuptake of serotonin. Common examples include Prozac, Zoloft, Lexapro, and Celexa. Paxil should be avoided in children and adolescents. Benefits may take 4 to 6 weeks to establish. Some medications in this class are not approved for children younger than 12 years of age (Clark, Jansen, & Cloy, 2012).

The only Food and Drug Administration (FDA)-approved medication for treatment of depression in children and adolescents is fluoxetine. Benefits may take 4 to 6 weeks to establish. It is not advisable for a P-PCP to prescribe medications that are not FDA approved for children and adolescents; therefore, off-label prescribing should be avoided by P-PCPs unless prescribed in collaboration with a psychiatric specialist. In addition, children who are not responding to treatment should be referred by P-PCPs to psychiatric providers. Paxil (paroxetine) should *not* be prescribed for children or adolescents (National Institutes of Health: National Institute of Mental Health, n.d.).

Side Effects

The most common side effects include diarrhea, nausea, headaches, insomnia, sexual dysfunction, dizziness, dry mouth, sweating, tremor, and fatigue (Wernicke, 2004).

Intercepting side effects for SSRIs are the same interventions listed for non-stimulant medications for treatment of ADHD (listed previously). In addition, interval history questions about sweating, tremors, and fatigue should be asked. Fatigue can be addressed by establishing regular sleep patterns, with established times for sleep and wake periods. Daily multivitamins may be helpful.

Warnings

The black box warnings for SSRIs and SNRIs includes increased incidence of suicidal behavior in children and adolescents. SSRIs and SNRIs cannot be started prior to 14 days of stopping an MOAI. The parents must monitor for worsening mood or psychiatric symptoms. These drugs cannot be used if a bipolar disorder is suspected. Monitor for hyponatremia and for evidence of seizures (U.S. Food & Drug Administration, 2007).

Intercept warning signs of potential suicidal behaviors at each primary care visit through screenings with either the HEADSSS or SHADESS and/or the PHQ-9 assessment tools. If bipolar disorder is suspected, P-PCPs must refer to psychiatric providers for mental health management. The P-PCP should manage the medical conditions including review of comprehensive metabolic panels with specific attention to sodium levels, with immediate interventions if hyponatremia is identified.

FDA-APPROVED MEDICATIONS FOR ANXIETY

For the pediatric population, there are no medications that are FDA approved for treatment of anxiety disorders. FDA approval is only for treatment of obsessive-compulsive disorders (OCD). Some children may present with both an anxiety disorder and OCD, and often an improvement in symptoms is observed for both anxiety and with first-line treatments for OCD. Children with these co-morbid conditions should be referred by the P-PCP to a psychiatric specialist for evaluation and treatment.

SEROTONIN–NOREPINEPHRINE REUPTAKE INHIBITORS

SNRIs work by inhibiting the reuptake of serotonin and norepinephrine. Most SNRIs are not approved for use in children and adolescents. Two that are currently approved for children older than 7 years are Cymbalta and Effexor.

Side Effects

The most common side effects are similar to those for SSRIs and include dry mouth, headache, dizziness, tremor, changes in vision, abdominal pain, decreased appetite, insomnia, cough, somnolence, nausea, and vomiting (Schneeweiss et al., 2010).

Warnings

SNRIs have a black box warning for increased suicidal behavior in children and adolescents. Do not use an SNRI within 14 days of an MAOI. Other warnings include bone fractures, seizures, hyponatremia, Stevens–Johnson syndrome, and endocrine abnormalities (U. S. Food & Drug Administration, 2007).

Intercepting side effects and warnings for SNRIs are similar to those for SSRIs but also include early recognition of signs of Stevens–Johnson syndrome (Mayo Clinic, 2017) and endocrine abnormalities. Stevens–Johnson syndrome requires immediate medical attention as it is a Type IV hypersensitivity reaction with symptoms involving the skin and mucous membranes. Presenting symptoms include hyperthermia, a spreading red or purplish skin rash, and blisters on the skin and mucous membranes (Mayo Clinic, 2017).

Endocrine side effects must be monitored by the P-PCP through baseline testing of thyroid panel and the thyroid stimulating hormone (TSH) and repeated every 6 to 12 months based on the physical assessment findings and laboratory results. The thyroid gland is normally nonpalpable. Palpation of an enlarged thyroid gland requires a referral to endocrinology for further evaluation.

ANXIOLYTICS

Whenever possible, anxiolytics use should be avoided in children and adolescents. When these medications are clinically indicated, the lowest effective dose should be used and only for a limited amount of time. Behavioral modification and coping skills should be implemented along with medication for best-practice treatment (AACAP, 2007).

BENZODIAZEPINES

These medications work by depressing the CNS. Common examples include Ativan, Klonopin, and Valium. When possible, use weight-based dosing to determine a safe range (AACAP, 2007). Prescribe this medication to be administered on an as-needed basis when appropriate. Provide specific instructions to the parents on when the medication is to be administered to the particular child or adolescent.

Side Effects

The most common side effects are sedation, dizziness, weakness, confusion, coordination difficulties, upper respiratory infections, and depression (Uzun, Kozumplik, Jakovljević, & Sedić, 2010).

Intercepting these side effects is critical as there are safety concerns with unexpected sedation, weakness, and confusion. For example, children and adolescents traveling to school using public transportation may be at increased risk for injury or with confusion may not remember exactly where they were going. Confusion also plays a role in learning, as concentration needed for academic achievement is affected. These side effects may be intercepted by advising children, adolescents, and parents of the side effects and by notifying the P-PCP as soon as any of these symptoms are recognized. In addition, the P-PCP should be asking interval questions about these symptoms at each follow-up visit.

Warnings

Do not stop these medications abruptly. These medications may cause serious respiratory depression. Prolonged use may negatively affect neurodevelopment in a young child (Uzun at al., 2010).

Intercept warning signs by performing a complete neurological assessment in the primary care setting prior to starting the medications and at each follow-up visit. Assess respiratory status at each visit and recommend that the adolescent and/or parent assess respiratory status.

NON-BENZODIAZEPINES

Both Buspar and Vistaril are approved for management of anxiety symptoms in children and adolescents. Vistaril is an antihistamine with moderate anticholinergic properties. Buspar is administered on a scheduled basis and Vistaril is generally administered as needed (AACAP, 2007).

Side Effects

The most common side effect of Buspar is dizziness. Other side effects may include drowsiness, nausea, and headache. Vistaril commonly causes dry mouth and drowsiness. Both medications are fairly well-tolerated (Garcia, Logan, & Gonzalez-Heydrich, 2012).

Warnings

Avoid use of Buspar with MAOIs. Vistaril may cause a prolonged QT interval (Garcia et al., 2012). Intercept warning signs by asking if there is a family history of prolonged QT interval, which would be a reason to order a baseline ECG with follow-up annual ECGs. Cardiac referral may be indicated.

Autism Spectrum Disorder

Children with autism spectrum disorder (ASD) achieve best outcomes with structure, consistency, and predictability in their day. In some cases, use of psychotropic medications may improve functioning and help manage symptoms. This is more likely with co-occurring mood disorders. It is important to note the limited evidence to support the use of these medications in this population (Volkmar et al., 2014).

The most routinely prescribed drug classes for children with ASD include SSRIs, specifically Prozac, Lexapro, and Celexa, and second-generation antipsychotics, specifically risperidone and aripiprazole (Volkmar et al., 2014). Consider the use of second-generation antipsychotics for management of severe irritability or aggression. These drugs are discussed in greater detail in the relevant sections of this chapter.

Children and adolescents with a diagnosis of ASD may be more likely to experience adverse drug reactions. P-PCPs need to continually assess risks and benefits of treatment and discontinue medication if no clear benefit from treatment can be established. Anticipatory guidance includes providing education to the parents or guardians about indications and limits of medication use.

RISPERIDONE

Risperidone is FDA approved for children with a diagnosis of ASD to treat severe behaviors, temper tantrums, and self-injury behaviors (McCracken et al., 2002).

Side Effects

Two significant side effects for Risperidone are weight gain and elevated prolactin levels. Intercept side effects by educating the child, adolescents, and parents about possible weight gain and ways to avoid excess weight gain through healthy eating strategies. Obtain a detailed dietary history and make suggestions for healthy foods which will avoid excess weight gains. Prolactin levels should be obtained prior to beginning therapy and then every 6 months to monitor for elevated levels.

Warnings

Do not stop these medications abruptly. Intercept warning signs by performing a complete neurological assessment in the primary care setting prior to starting the medications and at each follow-up visit. The P-PCP should also question females about breast milk production and assess at each 6-month visit. Males should be observed for gynecomastia.

Pediatric Bipolar Disorder

Pediatric bipolar disorder is difficult to diagnose in children and adolescents and should be avoided until other mood disorders have been ruled out. P-PCPs who suspect a diagnosis of bipolar disorder should refer the child to a psychiatric mental health provider. The *DSM-5* (APA, 2013) introduced disruptive mood dysregulation disorder or DMDD; this term is intended to replace pediatric bipolar disorder whenever appropriate. DMDD includes episodes of mood disturbances and a persistently irritable mood. The diagnostic criteria for bipolar disorder in the *DMS-5* has not changed and includes episodes of mania and depression. A diagnostically significant episode of mania or hypomania must have occurred before a child can accurately be diagnosed as bipolar I or bipolar II. If no definitive episodes have occurred, DMDD is a more appropriate diagnosis in a child or adolescent. Medications for treatment of pediatric bipolar disorder are similar to those for adults with bipolar disorder. No medications are currently available for DMDD as this disorder is relatively new. Lithium, anticonvulsants, and second-generation antipsychotics are the most common agents for bipolar disorder in children and adolescents (Liu et al., 2011).

LITHIUM

Lithium is considered the "gold standard" treatment option for bipolar disorder. While it has noted efficacy, the side effects of lithium will prove to be intolerable for many people. A child or adolescent receiving lithium will need initial and ongoing lab work for lithium levels as well as thyroid panel and TSH levels. Lithium administration is weight based. It is approved for use off-label in children age 6 and older. Lithium also has a narrow therapeutic index. Blood levels for maintenance generally fall within 0.6 to 1.2 mmol/L. Lithium toxicity is generally related to high serum levels; however, toxicity may occur even at therapeutic levels (Seigel et al., 2014).

Side Effects

Most patients will experience leukocytosis. About half of patients taking lithium will experience polyuria and polydipsia, dry mouth, hand tremor, confusion, memory problems, and headaches. Muscle weakness and or twitching, electrocardiograph changes, nausea, vomiting, and diarrhea also commonly occur. Hypothyroidism and goiter may also develop (Siegel et al., 2014).

Intercept side effects with careful monitoring of complete blood count (CBC) and chemistry panel baseline and follow-up laboratory results for CBC and chemistry panel including thyroid panel, TSH, and lithium levels, blood urea nitrogen (BUN), and creatinine (AACC, 2017) are critical for safe management of children and adolescents who are prescribed lithium.

Warnings

As mentioned, lithium has a narrow therapeutic index and careful attention should be given to serum levels and signs of toxicity. Risk of toxicity is higher for patients who are dehydrated or have renal or cardiovascular disease. Though uncommon, lithium may cause nephrogenic diabetes insipidus (Siegel et al., 2014).

Intercept warning signs by recognizing the early warning signs of toxicity (see lithium side effects) and reducing the dose or stopping the drug until levels are within the therapeutic range, followed by treatment with a lower dose after 24 to 48 hours (Waring, 2006). Currently, there is no antidote for lithium toxicity (AACC, 2017).

ANTICONVULSANTS

Valproic acid (Depakote) and carbamazepine (Tegretol) are approved for treating epilepsy in children and are used as off-label bipolar agents. Both medications are prescribed with weight-based dosing. Carbamazepine is approved for children as young as 6 and valproic acid for use in children as young as 10. Both medications require initial and ongoing lab work to establish therapeutic serum concentrations. Both valproic acid and carbamazepine require liver function tests to monitor for liver damage (Wong and Lhatoo, 2000).

Side Effects

Common side effects of valproic acid include nausea, vomiting, diarrhea, headaches, asthenia, sedation, abdominal pain, tremor, flu syndrome, and visual disturbances. Common side effects of carbamazepine include ataxia, nausea, vomiting, sedation, and dizziness (Wong & Lhatoo, 2000).

Intercepting side effects includes initial and ongoing lab work to establish therapeutic serum concentrations. Both valproic acid (Depakote) and carbamazepine (Tegretol) require liver function tests to monitor for liver damage. Fever and neutropenia are symptoms of concern when a child or adolescent is on a psychotropic medication and need further investigation by infectious disease providers. In addition, at each primary care interval visit, history and review of systems (ROS) questions must focus on identification of known side effects previously listed.

Warnings

Valproic acid can cause fatal liver failure. Symptoms of toxicity generally occur within the first few months of treatment. Valproic acid may also cause fatal pancreatitis. Use cautiously in sexually active adolescent females as it may cause teratogenicity and neural tube defects. Carbamazepine has a black box warning for the risk of fatal dermatological reactions including toxic epidermal necrolysis and Stevens–Johnson syndrome, as well as warnings for aplastic anemia and agranulocytosis. Carbamazepine may decrease the efficacy of oral contraceptive agents (Munshi et al., 2010).

ATYPICAL OR SECOND-GENERATION ANTIPSYCHOTICS

Second-generation antipsychotics approved for use in pediatric bipolar disorder include aripiprazole (Abilify), risperidone (Risperdal), quetiapine (Seroquel), asenapine (Saphris), and olanzapine (Zyprexa) specifically for teenagers. These medications are frequently used for pediatric mood disorders as adjunctive therapy or as monotherapy even in the absence of psychotic features (Munshi et al., 2010). A few second-generation antipsychotics have indications for use in bipolar disorder; however, most are prescribed off label. The age of approval for use varies by each drug and should be considered before initiating treatment. For some patients, this drug class is preferable due to a decreased need for lab work. These medications are discussed in more detail in the psychotic disorders section.

Psychotic Disorders

Children and adolescents with psychotic disorders present similarly as do adults. The primary symptoms are delusions, or false fixed beliefs, and hallucinations or false sensory experiences. There may also be a recent history of isolating behavior and a flattened affect (Russell, 1994). It is important to rule out underlying medical issues or substance-induced psychotic symptoms prior to making a diagnosis of a psychotic disorder. There are two classes of antipsychotic medications, first and second generation. These classes are also referred to as typical or atypical antipsychotics. Both drug classes increase the risk of developing neuroleptic malignant syndrome (NMS). NMS is characterized by muscle rigidity, fever, altered mental status, and autonomic dysfunction (Wijdicks, 2014). NMS is uncommon but life threatening. Periods of medication initiation and increases present the greatest risk for developing NMS. Most cases begin within 1 to 2 weeks after the initiation of medication.

FIRST-GENERATION (TYPICAL) ANTIPSYCHOTICS

The first-generation (typical) antipsychotics were the first group of medications indicated for the treatment of psychotic disorders. While these medications are effective for treating positive symptoms of psychosis, they are not effective for treating the negative or affective symptoms of psychosis. Many first-generation antipsychotics are not indicated for use in children and adolescents. The primary side effects of concern with this group of medications focus on movement disorders or extrapyramidal symptoms. Extrapyramidal symptoms include akathisia, bradykinesia, dystonia, dyskinesia, parkinsonism, and tardive dyskinesia. These medications have a risk of an acute dystonic reaction. Benadryl and Cogentin are effective for immediate reversal of dystonia. Cogentin may be beneficial to prescribe with these medications to decrease akathisia. It is important to note there is currently no treatment for tardive dyskinesia and these symptoms may be permanent. Table 3.2 lists all first-generation antipsychotics approved for use in children and adolescents.

TABLE 3.2

FIRST-GENERATION ANTIPSYCHOTICS APPROVED FOR USE IN CHILDREN AND ADOLESCENTS

Medication	Approved Age for Use	Indication
Haloperidol (Haldol)	>3 >3 >3 >12	Schizophrenia/psychosis Tourette disorder Behavioral disorders Acute agitation
Thiothixene (Navane)	>12	Schizophrenia/psychosis
Pimozide (Orap)	>2	Tourette disorder
Perphenazine (Trilafon)	>12 >12	Intractable hiccups Schizophrenia
Trifluoperazine (Stelazine)	>6	Schizophrenia/psychosis

ATYPICAL SECOND-GENERATION ANTIPSYCHOTICS

This drug class was initially thought to treat both positive and negative symptoms of schizophrenia with little risk of developing extra pyramidal symptoms (EPS). We now understand negative symptoms are difficult to treat. Although there is less risk of developing EPS with second-generation antipsychotics, there is a greater risk for developing metabolic syndrome and other serious side effects. Significant weight gain, diabetes, and metabolic syndrome may occur. These medications also increase the risk of cardiovascular death, QTC prolongation, and arrhythmias (Riordan, Antonini, & Murphy, 2011). Table 3.3 lists all second-generation antipsychotics approved for use in children and adolescents.

To intercept the risk of significant metabolic symptoms, the following anthropometric and laboratory measures should be obtained: (a) baseline weight; (b) waist circumference; (c) hemoglobin A1c; and (d) lipid panels. The P-PCP must monitor laboratory results and weight frequently for each patient. P-PCPs and psychiatric providers must evaluate the prescribed dose on a regular basis. Some medications have a dose-dependent risk for the development of metabolic syndrome. For other medications, the risk for developing metabolic syndrome increases when the duration of treatment is prolonged (Riordan et al., 2011).

Unspecified Behavioral Disorders

It may be necessary to prescribe medication for the management of behavioral problems in children and adolescents who do not meet full criteria for other psychiatric disorders. Use caution and clinical judgment when using medications for this purpose. Alpha-2 agonists and some antipsychotic medications may be helpful for aggression by promoting sedation and decreased impulsivity. Avoid using CNS stimulants unless ADHD is suspected, as stimulants may increase aggressive

TABLE 3.3

SECOND-GENERATION ANTIPSYCHOTICS APPROVED FOR USE IN CHILDREN AND ADOLESCENTS		
Medication	Approved Age for Use	Indication
Aripiprazole (Abilify)	>6 >10 >13	Autism/Tourette disorder Bipolar mania Schizophrenia
Asenapine (Saphris)	>10	Bipolar disorder
Paliperidone (Invega)	>12	Schizophrenia
Lurasidone (Latuda)	>13	Schizophrenia
Olanzapine (Zyprexa)	>13 >13	Bipolar disorder Schizophrenia
Quetiapine (Seroquel)	>10 >12	Bipolar disorder Schizophrenia

behaviors. Use the lowest effective dose and reevaluate efficacy and risk/benefit frequently throughout therapy. If clear benefit cannot be established with a reasonable dose, discontinue the medication. Whenever possible, nonspecific behavioral disorders should be addressed with behavioral modifications recommended by a clinical psychologist or behavioral analyst.

■ SUMMARY

Prescribing medications for children and adolescents with behavioral and mental health disorders is challenging. P-PCPs must be knowledgeable concerning medications that are approved for use in the pediatric population as well as the potential risks and benefits of prescribing stimulants and psychotropic medications. Parents or guardians and age-appropriate adolescents must receive information on drug therapy and concurrent behavioral modification therapies before signing informed consent. Both the parent and adolescent must be informed and articulate understanding that there are no "safe" stimulant or psychotropic medications. P-PCPs must carefully consider all factors when prescribing medications for behavior management in children and adolescents, including the potential for adherence to the treatment and essential follow-up plans. The treatment plan must include monitoring laboratory values, biometrics, and assessment for mild and severe adverse reactions to the prescribed medications. There is still much unknown about the long-term effects of psychotropic medication use in the pediatric population. Therefore, it is imperative to exercise clinical judgment, prudence, and astute care management plans that include interventions that intercept adverse side effects and warning signs when prescribing medications for this vulnerable pediatric population.

■ REFERENCES

American Academy of Child and Adolescent Psychiatry. (2007). Practice parameter for the assessment and treatment of children and adolescents with anxiety disorders. *Journal of the American Academy of Child and Adolescent Psychiatry*, 46, 267–283. doi:10.1097/01.chi.0000246070.23695.06

American Academy of Child and Adolescent Psychiatry. (2013). Practice parameter for the assessment and treatment of children and adolescents with tic disorders. *Journal of the American Academy of Child and Adolescent Psychiatry*, 52, 1341–1359. doi:10.1016/j.jaac.2013.09.015

American Academy of Pediatrics. (2011). ADHD: Clinical practice guideline for the diagnosis, evaluation, and treatment of attention-deficit/hyperactivity disorder in children and adolescents. Subcommittee on attention-deficit/hyperactivity disorder, steering committee on quality improvement and management. *Pediatrics*, 128, 2011–2654. doi:10.1542/peds.2011-2654. doi:10.1542/peds.2011-2654

American Psychiatric Association. (2013). *Diagnostic and statistical manual of mental disorders* (5th ed.). Arlington, VA: American Psychiatric Publishing.

Biederman, J., Spencer, T., & Wilens, T. (2004). Evidence-based pharmacotherapy for attention-deficit hyperactivity disorder. *International Journal of Neuropsychopharmacology*, 7, 77–97. doi:10.1017/S1461145703003973

Chirdkiatgumchai, V., Xiao, H., Fredstrom, B. K., Adams, R. E., Epstein, J. N., Shah, S. S., . . . Froehlich, T. E. (2013). National trends in psychotropic medication use in young children: 1994–2009. *Pediatrics*, 132, 615–623. doi:10.1542/peds.2013-1546

Clark, M. S., Jansen, K. L., & Cloy, J. A. (2012). Treatment of childhood and adolescent depression. *American Family Physician*, 86, 442–448.

Cortese, S., Holtmann, M., Banaschewski, T., Buitelaar, J., Coghill, D., Danckaerts, M., . . . on behalf of the European ADHD Guidelines Group. (2013). Practitioner review: Current best practice in the management of adverse events during treatment with ADHD medications in children and adolescents. *Journal of Child Psychology and Psychiatry, 54,* 227–246. doi:10.1111/jcpp.12036

Garcia, G., Logan, G. E., & Gonzalez-Heydrich, J. (2012). Management of psychotropic medication side effects in children and adolescents. *Child and Adolescent Psychiatric Clinics of North America, 21,* 713–738. doi:10.1016/j.chc.2012.07.012

Giovannitti, J. A., Thomas, S. M., & Crawford, J. J. (2015). Alpha-2 adrenergic receptor agonists: A review of current clinical applications. *Anesthesia Progress, 62,* 31–38. doi:10.2344/0003-3006-62.1.31

Howie, L. D., Pastor, P. N., & Lukacs, S. L. (2014). Use of medication prescribed for emotional or behavioral difficulties among children aged 6–17 years in the United States, 2011–2012. *NCHS Data Brief, 148,* 1–8.

Mayo Clinic. (2017). *Patient care and health information: Diseases & conditions: Stevens-Johnson syndrome.* Retrieved from http://www.mayoclinic.org/diseases-conditions/stevens-johnson-syndrome/home/ovc-20317097

McCracken, J. T., McGough, J., Shah, B., Cronin, P., Hong, D., Aman, M. G., . . . McMahon, D. (2002). Risperidone in children with autism and serious behavioral problems. *New England Journal of Medicine, 347,* 314–321. doi:10.1056/NEJMoa013171

Munshi, K. R., Oken, T., Guild, D. J., Trivedi, H. K., Wang, B. C., Ducharme, P., & Gonzalez-Heydrich, J. (2010). The use of antiepileptic drugs (AEDs) for the treatment of pediatric aggression and mood disorders. *Pharmaceuticals, 3*(9), 2986–3004. http://doi.org/10.3390/ph3092986

National Center for Health Statistics. (2014). *Health, United States, 2013: With special feature on prescription drugs.* Hyattsville, MD. Retrieved from https://www.cdc.gov/nchs/data/hus/hus13.pdf

National Institutes of Health: National Institute of Mental Health. (n.d.). *Antidepressant medications for children and adolescents: Information for parents and caregivers.* Retrieved from https://www.nimh.nih.gov/health/topics/child-and-adolescent-mental-health/antidepressant-medications-for-children-and-adolescents-information-for-parents-and-caregivers.shtml

Riordan, H. J., Antonini, P., & Murphy, M. F. (2011). Atypical antipsychotics and metabolic syndrome in patients with schizophrenia: Risk factors, monitoring, and healthcare implications. *American Health & Drug Benefits, 4,* 292–302.

Russell, T. A. (1994). The clinical presentation of childhood-onset schizophrenia. *Schizophrenia Bulletin, 20,* 631–646. doi:10.1093/schbul/20.4.631

Scahill, L. (2012). Alpha-2 adrenergic agonists in children with inattention, hyperactivity, and impulsiveness. *CNS Drugs, 23,* 43–49. doi:10.2165/00023210-200923000-00006

Schneeweiss, S., Patrick, A. R., Solomon, D. H., Dormuth, C. R., Miller, M., Mehta, J., . . . Wang, P. S. (2010). Comparative safety of antidepressant agents for children and adolescents regarding suicidal acts. *Pediatrics, 125,* 876–888. doi:10.1542/peds.2009-2317

Siegel, M., Beresford, C. A., Bunker, M., Verdi, M., Vishnevetsky, D., Karlsson, C., . . . Smith, K. A. (2014). Preliminary investigation of lithium for mood disorder symptoms in children and adolescents with autism spectrum disorder. *Journal of Child Adolescent Psychopharmacology, 24*(7), 399–402. doi:10.1089/cap.2014.0019

Swager, W. M., & Morgan, S. K. (2011). Psychotropic-induced dry mouth: Don't' overlook this potentially serious side effect. *Current Psychiatry, 10,* 54–58.

U. S. Food & Drug Administration. (2007). *Antidepressant use in children, adolescents, and adults.* Retrieved from https://www.fda.gov/Drugs/DrugSafety/InformationbyDrugClass/ucm096273.htm

Uzun, S., Kozumplik, O., Jakovljević, M., & Sedić, B. (2010). Side effects of treatment with benzodiazepines. *Psychiatria Danubina, 22,* 90–93.

Volkmar, F., Siegel, M., Woodbury-Smith, M., King, B., McCracken, J., & State, M. (2014). American Academy of Child and Adolescent Psychiatry (AACAP) Committee on Quality Issues (CQI). Practice parameter for the assessment and treatment of children and adolescents with autism spectrum disorder. *Journal of the American Academy of Child & Adolescent Psychiatry, 53,* 237–257. doi:10.1016/j.jaac.2013.10.013

Waring, W. S. (2006). Management of lithium toxicity. *Toxicology Review, 25,* 221–230. doi:10.2165/00139709-200625040-00003

Wernicke, J. F. (2004). Safety and side effect profile of fluoxetine. *Journal of Clinical Psychiatry, 46,* 59–67. doi:10.1517/14740338.3.5.495

Wijdicks, E. (2014). Neuroleptic malignant syndrome. *Up to Date.* Retrieved from http://www.uptodate.com/contents/topic.do?topicKey=NEURO/4829

Wong, I. C. K., & Lhatoo, S. D. (2000). Adverse reactions to new anticonvulsant drugs. *Drug-Safety, 23*(1), 35–56. dooi:10.2165/00002018-200023010-00003

World Health Organization. (1985). The rational use of drugs. Report of the conference of experts. Nairobi, November 25–29, 1985.

CHAPTER 4

Social Determinants of Health and Effect on Behavioral Development

JULIE BALDYGA

In an era of globalization, healthcare has become overwhelmingly complex. In the United States and around the globe, health agendas continue to teeter between technology-based medical care, public health initiatives, and a new understanding of health as a social phenomenon (World Health Organization [WHO], 2017). Innovations in fields such as neuroscience, developmental psychology, sociology, and molecular biology have sparked a paradigm shift toward a multidisciplinary approach to health (Shonkoff & Garner, 2012). This paradigm shift is illustrated in the concept known as the social determinants of health (SDH).

This chapter provides an overview of concepts of SDH and their effects on child and adolescent development, focusing on behavioral, mental, and biological health. In addition, this chapter describes the role of pediatric primary care providers (P-PCPs) in addressing SDH at each healthcare visit with a goal of understanding the important role of SDH in achieving or in failure to achieve positive behavioral health outcomes.

■ UNDERSTANDING SDH

The World Health Organization's (WHO's) commission defined SDH as "the conditions in which people are born, grow, live, work, play and age" (WHO, 2017) that contribute to adverse health outcomes across the life span. The U.S. population continues to battle poor health outcomes, which include worsening mortality rates and increased rates of disease burden, although it spends the most money on healthcare when compared to other high-income nations (Commonwealth Fund, 2015).

Children are the most underserved and vulnerable population in the United States. Despite local, state, and national programs that have been created to address this population, many children continue to lack access to essential medical care and social services. SDH can lead to impairments in physical health, socioemotional development, behavioral health, and a level of educational attainment that provides opportunities to prosper as an adult (Duffee, Kuo, & Gitterman, 2016). Unfortunately, children who grow up poor tend to remain poor and are subject to the negative outcomes of SDH throughout adulthood (Fass, Dinan, & Aratani, 2009).

▓ WHAT ARE SDH?

Children, who account for the poorest segment of the population in the United States (Garg, Toy, Tripodis, Silverstein, & Freeman, 2015), are the most affected by SDH. Public health has played a significant role in the delivery of healthcare to the most vulnerable populations. Although factors specific to individuals, such as genetics, influence health, health outcomes can neither be confined to assessment of genetic factors alone nor can biomedical interventions be the only factor for improving health and health outcomes. Social and environmental factors have long been acknowledged as contributing factors to understanding health and providing treatment. Thus, it is the combination of the genetic, biomedical, social, environmental, and SDH that directly influences a child's overall health and, in particular, behavioral health. Furthermore, it is the assessment of the combination of these factors by the P-PCP that will best identify the most appropriate time to *intercept* potential adverse outcomes through interprofessional collaborations and the implementation of the best available evidence-based interventions.

SDH interact with each other and exert different levels of influence outside of the biological or genetic basis. Children who live and grow up in a culture of poverty face one of the most significant human stressors. Fifteen million children live in poverty in the United States (National Center for Children in Poverty, n.d.). Children living in poverty are subject to various SDH: a devastating experience is the inability of the parents to meet the child's daily needs, including safe housing and access to food due to a lack of personal and family resources. Many children and their families continue to lack healthcare insurance and may not have access to a healthcare provider outside of the emergency department (Kuo, Etzel, Chilton, Watson, & Gorski, 2012). In addition, many children reside in inadequate housing in neighborhoods where violence is present and overcrowding exists. Children living in inadequate housing are also at risk for exposure to many factors related to adverse healthcare outcomes, including but not limited to lead poisoning, second- or third-hand smoke, infestations with roaches and mites, and poor or no bedding. In one study, data revealed that African American children are twice as likely to have higher concentrations of lead present in their blood when compared with Caucasian children (Pascoe, Wood, Duffee, & Kuo, 2016). Poor socioeconomic circumstances and inadequate access to medical care and services are thought to contribute to 25% to 30% of early deaths (Shonkoff & Garner, 2012) that, in the United States, are most likely preventable. Table 4.1 provides examples of SDH.

▓ SDH AND HEALTH DISPARITIES

Health disparities are "preventable differences in the burden of disease, injury, violence, or opportunities to achieve optimal health that are experienced by socially disadvantaged populations" (Centers for Disease Control and Prevention [CDC], 2014). Data illustrate that SDH are the root cause of health disparities and the overall burden of disease (WHO, 2017). The distribution of money and resources at global, national, and local levels shapes SDH. The unequal burden of disease resulting from health disparities and exposure to SDH explains why some

TABLE 4.1

EXAMPLES OF SDH
Availability of resources to meet daily needs, including safe housing and access to food
Access to educational, economic, and job opportunities
Access to healthcare facilities and services
Availability of community-based resources
Language and literacy
Transportation options
Exposure to crime, violence, and social disorder

SDH, social determinants of health.

Source: Social Determinates of Health. (2017). *Healthy people 2020.* Retrieved from https://www.healthypeople.gov/2020/topics-objectives/topic/social-determinants-of-health

individuals are healthier than others in the United States. Thus, P-PCPs must consider not only children and adolescents' physical presentation and genetic factors but also the social and physical environments in which they live, play, and grow to provide optimal treatment plans, including for anticipated behavioral problems. *Intercepting* these problems requires P-PCPs to work collaboratively and interprofessionally to address the issues presented by pediatric/adolescent patients and their families.

■ SDH AND CHILD DEVELOPMENT

Child development is driven by interactions between genetic and environmental factors called epigenetic factors (see Chapter 35). The prior "nature versus nurture" debate has been replaced with a new framework: "nature dancing with nurture over time" (Shonkoff & Garner, 2012). SDH play an important role in physical, cognitive, and behavioral development throughout childhood and adolescence. Both social conditions and interpersonal experiences generate adversities that can lead to toxic stress (see Chapter 32) and affect brain development in early childhood. It can also alter longevity due to chronic illness. Adverse effects from exposure to prior SDH can be witnessed in the early stages of childhood. Thus, P-PCPs have the opportunity to develop treatment plans that can intercept adverse outcomes.

Prenatal Development

SDH can have negative outcomes on a developing fetus. Maternal inadequate access to healthy foods, intrauterine exposure to maternal smoking and/or substance use, and a lack of prenatal care and prenatal education can lead to premature birth and low birth weight (LBW; less than 2,500 g). LBW is the second

TABLE 4.2

NEGATIVE HEALTH OUTCOMES OF LBW
Delays in cognitive development, resulting in below-average IQ
Mental illness, including anxiety and depression
Behavioral and conduct disorders
Asthma and lung disease
Increased respiratory disorders and high blood pressure
Special healthcare needs and limitations on activity

LBW, low birth weight.

Source: The Urban Child Institute. (2012). *Prematurity and low birth weight*. Retrieved from http://www.urbanchildinstitute.org/articles/policy-briefs/prematurity-and-low-birth-weight

leading cause of infant death in the United States (Singh, Kenney, Ghandour, Kogan, & Lu, 2013). Infants born with LBWs can develop a wide range of negative health outcomes (see Table 4.2).

LBW is also associated with high infant mortality rates. Despite the medical advances and the decline in LBW infants in the United States, studies have found that rates of infant mortality for LBW infants (1,500–2,499 g) are six times higher than infants born at normal birth weights (2,500–4,000 g; Singh et al., 2013; Stanford Children's Health, n.d.). For children who do survive and live in lower socioeconomic status communities, and who experience nutritional deficiencies, can experience stunted growth. Polhamus, Dalenius, Mackintosh, Smith, and Grummer-Strawn (2011) found that 6% of children from birth to the ages of 4 to 6 years old, who qualified for nutritional assistance, had shorter stature. Same-age U.S. children who did not qualify for nutrition supplements had a reported 3.7% short stature (Pascoe et al., 2016).

Neurobiological Development

Brain development begins rapidly during early pregnancy and continues throughout the first few years of life. Prior to preschool-age years, between 4 and 5 years old, neuron-to-neuron connections are being sculpted (Maggi, Irwin, Siddiqi, & Hertzman, 2010). Some connections are reinforced and some die off. Brain sculpture is influenced by stimuli in the child's environment: verbal, visual, physical, emotional, touch, and smell. It is also influenced by preprogramed biological "critical periods." These periods occur when parts of the brain are activated and are ready to receive environmental stimuli. During this time of sculpture, cognitive, sensory, social and behavioral, and emotional developmental competencies are created (Maggi et al., 2010). Children who do not receive stimulation and are raised in an unsupportive emotional and physical environment are more likely to experience delays in cognitive, social, emotional, and behavioral development. These delays can be attributed to exposure to SDH such as poverty, limited community resources, and the lack of educational achievement. Although this relationship between SDH and early infant/child brain development has been established, it is very concerning that approximately 50% of developmental problems are not identified in children until they enter school (Kuo et al., 2012). Thus, failure to identify the social determinants of health is a missed opportunity for P-PCPs to intercept delays in physical, social–emotional, and behavioral health issues.

Brain development is also affected by toxic stress. Toxic stress is a response which occurs when a child is subject to frequent and/or persistent adversity, including burdens of socioeconomic hardship, chronic neglect, and mental illness (Shonkoff & Garner, 2012; see Chapter 32 in this book on toxic stress). Without adequate support from adults, toxic stress disrupts metabolic and circuitry response systems in the brain during critical times of development (Toxic Stress, n.d.). Toxic stress may permanently alter the brain's developing architecture. If toxic stress occurs frequently, an individual's physical, behavioral, and mental health can decline over the life span, thus increasing the risk for physical and behavioral health problems.

Chronic Conditions

Negative outcomes of SDH can cause a series of chronic health conditions and affect development during childhood and adolescence. Obesity and asthma are more prevalent in children from lower socioeconomic backgrounds (Pascoe et al., 2016). Children who are obese have an increased risk of developing asthma; however, the impact that obesity has on the risk of developing asthma is unknown (Lang, 2012). Obesity, asthma, and behavioral health problems affect an individual's quality of life and social–emotional and behavioral growth and development.

OBESITY

Childhood obesity has tripled since the 1970s (CDC, 2017). Data from the National Health and Nutrition Examination Survey (NHANES) from 2011–2014 revealed that obesity for children between the ages of 6 to 11 (17.5%) was higher than children ages 2 to 5 (8.9%). Adolescents between the ages of 12 to 19 had the highest rates of obesity (20.5%; Ogden, Carroll, Fryar, & Flegal, 2015). Minority children and adolescents are more likely to suffer from obesity, which can be attributed to cultural beliefs. Although body image development occurs across cultures, different ethnic/cultural groups value and disvalue body image differently. For example, the ideal body size of an African American woman is larger than that of a White woman (Caprio et al., 2008). Obesity in childhood can lead to diabetes, hypertension, and hypercholesterolemia, with expression in the childhood/adolescent years or in young, middle-aged adulthood. Obesity may also lead to childhood poor self-esteem, poor self-image, bullying, and, at times, aggressive behaviors in response to being bullied. SDH contributes to obesity in various ways. Poverty, poor access to healthy food, lack of playgrounds and recreational activities in communities, and neighborhoods prone to violence prevent children and their families from living a healthy lifestyle.

Psychological and Behavioral Problems Associated With Obesity

Obesity is not only associated with health-related problems. Poorer cognition, brain plasticity, and motor control are also associated with obesity across the life span

(Wang, Chan, Ren, & Yan, 2016). Obesity in childhood and adolescence may lead to psychological problems (Sahoo et al., 2015). Numerous evidence-based studies have found a higher prevalence of mental health problems, including depression and anxiety, in children and adolescents who are obese (Nemiary, Shim, Mattox, & Holden, 2012). However, other studies have concluded that the direct causal pathway from obesity to depression is not substantial (Nemiary et al., 2012). Obesity in childhood and adolescence can lead to experiences that indirectly cause depression. For example, individuals may experience bullying at school and/or cyberbullying online. Obese children are more likely to be bullied compared to non-obese children, regardless of academic achievement or socioeconomic status (Lumeng et al., 2010). Studies have found that obese children and adolescents have more specialty visits compared to healthy children, in which psychiatry was the most common specialty referral (Turer, Lin, & Flores, 2009). Lower self-esteem; extreme dieting behavior, including abusing laxatives, taking diet pills, and/or fasting; and symptoms of an eating disorder, such as bulimia nervosa or anorexia, are common psychological comorbidities of obesity (Rankin et al., 2016).

Obesity may also contribute to neurobehavioral problems during childhood and adolescence (Xanthopoulos et al., 2015). Obstructive sleep apnea (OSA) is a disorder characterized by extended airway obstruction and/or intermittent complete obstruction that interrupts regular ventilation during sleep (Chang & Chae, 2010). OSA is associated with sleep fragmentation, intermittent hypoxemia, and hypercapnia, in which afflicted individuals are subject to adverse effects on their health and quality of life (White, 2017). OSA has been linked to deficits in academic performance, emotion and behavior regulation, and cognition, including attention and executive functioning (Xanthopoulos et. al., 2015). Obese children and adolescents are four to five times more likely than non-obese children to develop OSA (Tripuraneni, Paruthi, Armbrecht, & Mitchell, 2013).

ASTHMA

Among children and adolescents in the United States, asthma is the leading chronic illness (Asher & Pearce, 2014). An estimated 6.2 million children and adolescents under the age of 18 have a diagnosis of asthma (Centers for Disease Control and Prevention [CDC], 2015). African American children experienced an approximate 50% increase in the rates of asthma from 2001 to 2009, accounting for the greatest increase among racial groups (CDC, 2015). In addition to a genetic predisposition to asthma, SDH are limited to risk factors for developing asthma (see Table 4.3).

Asthma attributes to disruptions in school attendance. Asthma accounted for the highest rate of absenteeism during the school year (Meng, Babey, & Wolstein, 2012). Poor school attendance can lead to school course failures which place the children at risk for failing a total grade level. Children of low socioeconomic status, minority children, and children living in urban cities visit the emergency department and are hospitalized at a greater rate than the general population due to asthma (Kuo, Etzel, Chilton, Watson, & Gorski, 2012). The ability to manage asthma may be significantly limited if children and their families lack or misunderstand asthma education, lack healthcare insurance, and/or do not have the accessibility of transportation to attend appointments at primary care practices or clinics.

TABLE 4.3

SDH AND ASTHMA
Second-hand smoke from tobacco
Third-hand smoke from tobacco
Air pollution
Indoor allergens including dust mites, pet dander, and cockroaches

SDH, social determinants of health.

Source: American Lung Association. (n.d.). *Cockroaches: Why are they an indoor air problem?* Retrieved from http://www.lung.org/our-initiatives/healthy-air/indoor/indoor-air-pollutants/cockroaches .html; World Health Organization. (2017). *About social determinants of health*. Retrieved from http:// www.who.int/social_determinants/sdh_definition/en

Psychological and Behavioral Problems Associated With Asthma

Children with asthma are more likely to develop psychological and behavioral problems compared to children without asthma (Chen, 2014). Uncontrolled asthma can contribute to a child's inability to engage in physical and/or social activities such as sports. This inability to associate with peers can lead to lower self-esteem, depression, and anxiety (Chen, 2014). Minority children with asthma are 60% more at risk compared to White children with asthma for developing psychological difficulties (Walker, 2012).

Asthma can also contribute to behavioral problems. School-age children between the ages of 6 and 12 are recommended 9 to 12 hours of sleep within a 24-hour period (CDC, 2017b). Children and adolescents suffering from asthma may experience nocturnal cough, especially if their asthma is not under control. Coughing can prevent them from getting the amount of sleep they need. Epidemiological literature demonstrates that impaired sleep can lead to problems in concentrating, lack of productivity, worsened mood, and difficulty with social interactions, prompting shy or anxious behavior (Kewalramani, Bollinger, & Postolache, 2008).

■ PRIMARY CARE PROVIDERS AND SDH

Traditional medical and nursing education focused on healthcare treatment, genetics, and biomedical interventions. Today, population healthcare and community-based training have been incorporated into medical, nursing, and healthcare providers' curricula. To render the best plan of care for individuals and their families from various populations that P-PCPs serve, primary care practices must collaborate with social services and other community agencies to meet the demands of families living with adversities. Collaboration within the healthcare macro system must be recognized as reciprocal and focused on addressing population health with the SDH framework. For example, the 2017 opioid crisis required all healthcare professionals to work together to critically analyze the components of the problem and then work interprofessionally to develop and implement a comprehensive plan to attack the opioid crisis.

The 2010 Patient Protection and Affordable Care Act (ACA; Adepoju, Preston, & Gonzales, 2015) has expanded opportunities in health by requiring that healthcare plans cover preventive care services to patients at no out-of-pocket expense. The ACA provides access to healthcare for every individual within the insurance marketplace. This extensive access to care also required a change from paper charts to electronic medical records (EMRs). The Institute of Medicine (Institute of Medicine [IOM], 2014) created measures to incorporate SDH within the EMRs. EMRs record crucial data that can enable providers to formulate an individualized and family healthcare plan. In addition, EMRs can be used to analyze population health and quality improvement initiatives to simultaneously improve individual and population health (Friedman, Parrish, & Ross, 2013). Twelve social and behavioral factors that affect health were identified, four of which were already routinely assessed during healthcare visits (e.g., race/ethnicity, tobacco use, alcohol use, and residential addresses [Capturing Social and Behavioral Domains and Measures in Electronic Health Records: Phase 2, 2014]). The additional eight factors include educational attainment, financial resource strain, stress, physical activity, neighborhood median household income, depression, social isolation, and intimate partner violence (Capturing Social and Behavioral Domains and Measures in Electronic Health Records: Phase 2, 2014). These domains help to address problem identification, clinical diagnoses, and treatment plans, as well as outcomes assessment.

The Role of P-PCPs

P-PCPs are strong advocates for promoting health for the pediatric population. They work with children, adolescents, and their families to develop the best plan of care through care coordination between medical and social services within their communities. An interprofessional approach to healthcare and population health has the potential to reduce the negative outcomes of SDH and improve positive health outcomes.

The medical home helps P-PCPs implement care that is family-centered, accessible, continuous, and culturally effective for children and adolescents (American Academy of Pediatrics, n.d.). A pediatric medical home is a partnership between families and community-based systems (Tonniges, Palfrey, & Mitchell, 2004). Table 4.4 highlights some community-based resources that promote child health and development.

■ BEHAVIORAL HEALTH PROBLEMS AND RELATION TO SDH

SDH can impact development during childhood and adolescence. Neural plasticity, defined as "the ability of the central nervous system to adapt in response to changes in the environment or lesions" (Sharma, Classen, & Cohen, 2013), and environmental influences impact brain development during childhood and adolescence (Perkins & Graham-Bermann, 2012). Prior to adolescence, a child's brain forms a series of connections between brain cells. Around the age of 11 or 12, the brain

TABLE 4.4

REFERRALS FOR COMMUNITY-BASED PROGRAMS

Women, Infants, and Children (WIC): A supplemental nutrition program for children who are at nutritional risk that provides states with funds for supplemental food, healthcare referrals, and education up to the age of 5.

Head Start: A federal program for children up to the age of 5 that helps prepare them for school, strengthening their cognitive, social, and emotional development and projecting the role of their parents as teachers.

Early Intervention Programs: Special support services for eligible infants and children with disabilities including psychological services, speech pathology and audiology, social work services, and physical and occupational therapy. *Consult the department of health in your state for all services offered in your area.*

Source: New York State Department of Health. (2017). *Early intervention programs.* Retrieved from https://www.health.ny.gov/community/infants_children/early_intervention; U.S. Department of Agriculture. (2018). *Women, infants, and children (WIC).* Retrieved from https://www.fns.usda.gov/wic/women-infants-and-children-wic

undergoes the process of pruning (Winters & Arria, 2011), in which approximately 50% of synaptic connections are pruned to make room for additional information processing (Spear, 2014). During this time, the prefrontal cortex (PFC), which is responsible for assessing situations, controlling emotions and impulses, and making rational decisions, is still in the process of maturing. Adolescents are likely to take risks and try new experiences. They are motivated to pursue rewards and avoid pain; however, they have limited judgment and decision-making skills, ultimately making them vulnerable to situations that might be harmful to their developing bodies (Winters & Arria, 2011). SDH that children and adolescents are exposed to, such as violence, the presence of gangs, and substance abuse, places them at a higher risk for developing behavioral health problems and/or mental disorders.

Psychological and Behavioral Problems Associated With Violence

Research on brain development has shown that exposure to violence influences normal development, causing deficits in brain volume related to cognition and processing emotions, dysfunction in dopamine-rich regions in the brain, and distorted lateralization of brain function (Perkins & Graham-Bermann, 2012). Children and adolescents exposed to violence in their home and/or community have a higher risk of developing an array of psychosocial problems including attachment issues, delays in emotional understanding, and social, behavioral, and intellectual difficulties. Research on cognitive neuroscience has shown that exposure to violence can cause neurobiological changes, which can lead to difficulties with cognition in memory and executive functioning, including organizing and synthesizing information, and language delays or disabilities (Perkins & Graham-Bermann, 2012). The risk of developing mental health problems such as anxiety, depression, and posttraumatic stress disorder is also associated with exposure to violence during this time of development (Forster, Grigsby, Unger, & Sussman, 2015).

Psychological and Behavioral Problems Associated With Gang Violence

The use of violence and the intent to use violence and aggression has been associated with violence exposure (Forster et al., 2015). Children and adolescents growing up in violence-prone areas where they feel unsafe, associate with youth involved with gangs, or engage in delinquent behavior are at a higher risk for gang initiation (Howell, 2010). A study by Pyrooz and Sweeten (2015) estimated that there were more than 1 million youth gang members who were disproportionately male, African American, Hispanic, and from single-parent households living in poverty in the United States in 2010. Adolescents involved in gangs are subject to adverse psychological and behavioral consequences. Gang activity has been related to difficulty in school, often leading to school dropout, engaging in criminal behavior that is both violent and nonviolent, and distributing and/or using narcotics. Studies have found that long-term gang participation during adolescence often continues into adulthood, in which poor health and mental health disorders are common (Gilman, Hill, & Hawkins, 2014).

Psychological and Behavioral Problems Associated With Substance Abuse

Children and adolescents living in poverty are more likely to be exposed to high-risk factors associated with substance abuse, including having a parent/caregiver who abuses drugs, has a mental illness, and/or engages in criminal behavior, and live in a chaotic home/community environment where gangs, criminal activity, and drug trafficking is present (CDC, 2017a). Vulnerability to substance abuse and addiction during adolescence is high. Alcohol, tobacco, and marijuana are the most common substances adolescents first try (National Institute of Health, 2014).

As previously mentioned, the PFC, which is responsible for assessing situations, controlling emotions and impulses, and making rational decisions, is still maturing, making situations that seem rewarding more enticing, regardless of the potential risks (Winters & Arria, 2011). Alterations in brain structure and function have been associated with substance and alcohol abuse during adolescence (Squeglia, Jacobus, & Tapert, 2009). Regions in the brain and processes that cause addiction overlap with those that are involved with fundamental cognitive functions such as learning, memory, reasoning, and impulse control (Gould, 2010). Cognitive deficits can have harmful implications on academic achievement and social functioning. Epidemiological research has shown that the earlier an individual uses drugs, the greater likelihood that they will develop a substance abuse problem (Winters & Arria, 2011).

Although alcohol, tobacco, and marijuana are the most commonly used drugs, the National Institute on Drug Abuse (2014) reports that younger adolescents also tend to use inhalant substances, such as breathing fumes emitted by household cleaning products, aerosol sprays, and/or gases. Inhalants can cause long-term consequences, such as delays in behavioral development and brain damage due to the lack of oxygen to the brain. The neurotoxic effects of continuous abuse can damage areas in the brain associated with controlling cognition (National Institute on Drug Abuse, 2012).

Older adolescents are likely to use, misuse, and/or abuse prescription medications, including opioid analgesics, such as oxycodone and hydrocodone (Young, McCabe, Cranford, Ross-Durow, & Boyd, 2012). Results from a survey conducted by National Survey on Drug Use and Health (2015) revealed that 276,000 adolescents between ages 12 and 17 used a prescription pain pill in 2015, 122,000 of which were addicted to prescription pain pills (Center for Behavioral Health Statistics and Quality, 2016). Adolescents may also turn to using heroin and synthetic heroin (fentanyl). Although illicit drug use has been declining, the rate of overdose from heroin among adolescents between ages 15 and 19 rose 19% in 2015 according the Centers for Disease Control and Prevention (Curtin, Tejada-Vera, & Warner, 2017). Heroin contributes to one fatality per 100,000 adolescents every year (Curtin et al., 2017). Studies on animals found that exposure to opioids during adolescence can negatively impact the sequencing of brain development (Thurstone, 2017). The chemical structures found in heroin mimic naturally occurring neurotransmitters in our bodies by tricking our receptors into locking and activating nerve cells, causing neurons to send abnormal messages throughout the brain and body. The effects of opioid abuse can be seen on brain scans of adolescent users when compared with adolescents who do not use opioids (Thurstone, 2017).

■ SUMMARY

As the paradigm shift continues within the healthcare arena incorporating the concept of SDH in primary care, P-PCPs have the opportunity to better serve the pediatric populations through family-centered care coordination with medical, behavioral, and social services. Combining these services can help alleviate the negative impacts that SDH have on childhood and adolescent growth and development and healthcare outcomes. By incorporating the ways environmental factors interact with biological and behavioral factors, healthcare delivery systems can deliver optimal comprehensive care to improve overall health outcomes for the U.S. pediatric population, thus leading to a medically and behaviorally healthy adult population.

■ REFERENCES

Adepoju, O. E., Preston, M. A., & Gonzales, G. (2015). Health care disparities in the post–affordable care act era. *American Journal of Public Health*, *105*(Suppl 5), S665–S667. doi:10.2105/AJPH.2015.302611

American Academy of Pediatrics. (n.d.). *AAP agenda for children: Medical home*. Retrieved from https://www.aap.org/en-us/about-the-aap/aap-facts/AAP-Agenda-for-Children-Strategic-Plan/pages/aap-agenda-for-children-strategic-plan-medical-home.aspx

American Lung Association. (2017). *Cockroaches: Why are they an indoor air problem?* Retrieved from http://www.lung.org/our-initiatives/healthy-air/indoor/indoor-air-pollutants/cockroaches.html?referrer=

Asher, I., & Pearce, N. (2014). Global burden of asthma among children. *International Journal of Tuberculosis and Lung Disease*, *18*(11), 1269–1278. doi:10.5588/ijtld.14.0170

Caprio, S., Daniels, S. R., Drewnowski, A., Kaufman, F. R., Palinkas, L. A., Rosenbloom, A. L., & Schwimmer, J. B. (2008). Influence of race, ethnicity, and culture on childhood obesity: Implications for prevention and treatment; A consensus statement of Shaping America's Health and the Obesity Society. *Diabetes Care*, *31*(11), 2211–2221. doi:10.2337/dc08-9024

Center for Behavioral Health Statistics and Quality. (2016). *Key substance use and mental health indicators in the United States: Results from the 2015 National Survey on Drug Use and Health* (HHS Publication No. SMA 16-4984, NSDUH Series H-51). Retrieved from http://www.samhsa.gov/data/

Center on the Developing Child Harvard University. (n.d.) *Toxic Stress.* Retrieved from http://developingchild.harvard.edu/science/key-concepts/toxic-stress/

Centers for Disease Control and Prevention. (2014). *Definitions.* The National Center for HIV/AIDS, Viral Hepatitis, STD, and TB Prevention. Retrieved from https://www.cdc.gov/nchhstp/socialdeterminants/definitions.html

Centers for Disease Control and Prevention. (2015). *Summary health statistics: National health interview survey.* Retrieved from https://ftp.cdc.gov/pub/Health_Statistics/NCHS/NHIS/SHS/2015_SHS_Table_C-1.pdf

Centers for Disease Control and Prevention. (2017a). *Childhood abuse and neglect: Risk and protective factors.* Retrieved from https://www.cdc.gov/violenceprevention/childmaltreatment/riskprotectivefactors.html

Centers for Disease Control and Prevention. (2017b). *Childhood obesity facts.* Retrieved from https://www.cdc.gov/healthyschools/obesity/facts.htm

Chang, S. J., & Chae, K. Y. (2010). Obstructive sleep apnea syndrome in children: Epidemiology, pathophysiology, diagnosis and sequelae. *Korean Journal of Pediatrics, 53*(10), 863–871. doi:10.3345/kjp.2010.53.10.863

Chen, J. (2014). Asthma and child behavioral skills: Does family socioeconomic status matter? *Social Science & Medicine, 115,* 38–48. doi:10.1016/j.socscimed.2014.05.048

Commonwealth Fund. (2015). *U.S. spends more on health care than other high-income nations but has lower life expectancy, worse health.* Retrieved from http://www.commonwealthfund.org/publications/press-releases/2015/oct/us-spends-more-on-health-care-than-other-nations

Curtin, S. C., Tejada-Vera, B., & Warner, M. (2017). *Drug Overdose Deaths Among Adolescents Aged 15–19 in the United States: 1999–2015.* NCHS Data Brief, (282), 1. Retrieved from https://www.cdc.gov/nchs/data/databriefs/db282.pdf

Duffee, J. H., Kuo, A. A., & Gitterman, B. A. (2016). Poverty and child health in the United States. *Pediatrics, 137*(4), 59–72. doi:10.1542/peds.2016-0339

Fass, S., Dinan, K., & Aratani, Y. (2009). *Child poverty and intergenerational mobility.* The National Center for Children in Poverty. Retrieved from http://www.nccp.org/publications/pdf/text_911.pdf

Forster, M., Grigsby, T., Unger, J., & Sussman, S. (2015) Associations between gun violence exposure, gang associations, and youth aggression: Implications for prevention and intervention programs. *Journal of Criminology, 2015,* 1–8. doi:10.1155/2015/963750

Friedman, D. J., Parrish, R. G., & Ross, D. A. (2013). Electronic health records and U.S. public health: Current realities and future promise. *American Journal of Public Health, 103*(9), 1560–1567. doi.org/10.2105/AJPH.2013.301220

Garg, A., Toy, S., Tripodis, Y., Silverstein, M., & Freeman, E. (2015). Addressing social determinants of health at well child care visits: A cluster RCT. *Pediatrics, 135*(2), e296–e304. doi:10.1542/peds.2014-2888

Gilman, A. B., Hill, K. G., & Hawkins, J. D. (2014). Long-term consequences of adolescent gang membership for adult functioning. *American Journal of Public Health, 104*(5), 938–945. doi:10.2105/AJPH.2013.301821

Gould, T. J. (2010). Addiction and cognition. *Addiction Science & Clinical Practice, 5*(2), 4–14. Retrieved from https://www.ncbi.nlm.nih.gov/pmc/articles/PMC3120118/pdf/ascp-05-2-4.pdf

Howell, J. (2010). *Gang prevention: An overview of research and programs.* Office of Juvenile Justice and Delinquency Prevention. Retrieved from https://www.ncjrs.gov/pdffiles1/ojjdp/231116.pdf

Institute of Medicine. (2014). Phase 2: Promoting domains and measures. In *Capturing social and behavioral domains and measures in electronic health records: Phase 2* (Summary). Retrieved from https://www.nap.edu/read/18951/chapter/1

Kewalramani, A., Bollinger, M. E., & Postolache, T. T. (2008). Asthma and mood disorders. *International Journal of Child Health and Human Development: IJCHD, 1*(2), 115–123. Retrieved from http://europepmc.org/backend/ptpmcrender.fcgi?accid=PMC2631932&blobtype=pdf

Kuo, A. A., Etzel, R. A., Chilton, L. A., Watson, C., & Gorski, P. A. (2012). Primary care pediatrics and public health: Meeting the needs of today's children. *American Journal of Public Health, 102*(12), e17–e23. doi:10.2105/AJPH.2012.301013

Lang, J. (2012). Obesity, nutrition, and asthma in children. *Pediatric Allergy Immunology and Pulmonology, 25,* 64–75. doi:10.1089/ped.2011.0137

Lumeng, J. C., Forrest, P., Appugliese, D. P., Kaciroti, N., Corwyn, R. F., & Bradley, R. H. (2010). Weight status as a predictor of being bullied in third through sixth grades. *Pediatrics*, *125*(6), e1301–e1307. doi.org/10.1542/peds.2009-0774

Maggi, S., Irwin, L. J., Siddiqi, A., & Hertzman, C. (2010). The social determinants of early child development: An overview. *Journal of Pediatrics and Child Health*, *46*(11), 627–635. doi:10.1111/j.1440-1754.2010.01817.x

Meng, Y., Babey, S., & Wolstein, J. (2012). Asthma-related school absenteeism and school concentration of low-income students in California. *Preventing Chronic Disease*, 9. doi:10.1016/j.amepre.2015.12.012

National Center for Children in Poverty. (n.d.). *Child Poverty*. Retrieved from http://www.nccp.org/topics/childpoverty.html

National Institute of Health. (2014). *Principles of adolescent substance use disorder treatment: A research-based guide*. Retrieved from https://www.drugabuse.gov/publications/principles-adolescent-substance-use-disorder-treatment-research-based-guide/introduction

National Institute on Drug Abuse. (2003). Risk factors and protective factors. *Preventing drug use among children and adolescents*. Retrieved from https://www.drugabuse.gov/sites/default/files/preventing-druguse_2.pdf

National Institute on Drug Abuse. (2012). *What are the other medical consequences of inhalant abuse?* Retrieved from https://www.drugabuse.gov/publications/research-reports/inhalants/what-are-other-medical-consequences-inhalant-abuse

Nemiary, D., Shim, R., Mattox, G., & Holden, K. (2012). The relationship between obesity and depression among adolescents. *Psychiatric Annals*, *42*(8), 305–308. doi:10.3928/00485713-20120806-09

New York State Department of Health. (2017). *Early intervention programs*. Retrieved from https://www.health.ny.gov/community/infants_children/early_intervention/

Ogden, C., Carroll, M., Fryar, C., & Flegal, K. (2015). Prevalence of obesity among adults and youth: United States, 2011–2014. *NCHS Data Brief*, (219), 1–8. Retrieved from https://www.cdc.gov/nchs/data/databriefs/db219.pdf

Pascoe, J. M., Wood, D. L., Duffee, J. H., & Kuo, A. (2016). Mediators and adverse effects of child poverty in the United States. *Pediatrics*, *137*(4), doi:10.1542/peds.2016-0340

Perkins, S., & Graham-Bermann, S. (2012). Violence exposure and the development of school-related functioning: Mental health, neurocognition, and learning. *Aggression & Violent Behavior*, *17*(1), 89–98. doi:10.1016/j.avb.2011.10.001

Polhamus, B., Dalenius, K., Mackintosh, H., Smith, B., & Grummer-Strawn, L. (2011). *Pediatric nutrition surveillance 2009 report*. Atlanta: U.S. Department of Health and Human Services, Centers for Disease Control and Prevention.

Pyrooz, D. C., & Sweeten, G. (2015). Gang membership between ages 5 and 17 years in the United States. *Journal of Adolescent Health*, 56, 414–419. doi:10.1016/j.jadohealth.2014.11.018

Rankin, J., Matthews, L., Cobley, S., Han, A., Sanders, R., Wiltshire, H., & Baker, J. (2016). Psychological consequences of childhood obesity: Psychiatric comorbidity and prevention. *Adolescent Health, Medicine and Therapeutics*, 7. Retrieved from https://www.ncbi.nlm.nih.gov/pmc/articles/PMC5115694/pdf/ahmt-7-125.pdf

Sahoo, K., Sahoo, B., Choudhury, A., Sofi, N., Kumar, R., & Bhadoria, A. (2015). Childhood obesity: Causes and consequences. *Journal of Family Medicine and Primary Care*, *4*(2), 187–192. doi:10.4103/2249-4863.154628

Sharma, N., Classen, J., & Cohen, L. G. (2013). Neural plasticity and its contribution to functional recovery. *Handbook of Clinical Neurology*, *110*, 3–12. doi:10.1016/B978-0-444-52901-5.00001-0

Shonkoff, J. P., & Garner, A. S. (2012). The lifelong effects of early childhood adversity and toxic stress. *Pediatrics*, *129*(1), 232–246. doi:10.1542/peds.2011-2663

Singh, G. K., Kenney, M. K., Ghandour, R. M., Kogan, M. D., & Lu, M. C. (2013). Mental health outcomes in U.S. children and adolescents born prematurely or with low birthweight. *Depression Research & Treatment*, *2013*, 1–13. doi:10.1155/2013/570743

Social Determinates of Health. (2017). *Healthy people 2020*. Retrieved from https://www.healthypeople.gov/2020/topics-objectives/topic/social-determinants-of-health

Spear, L. (2014). Adolescent neurodevelopment. *Journal of Adolescent Health*, *52*(2), S7–S13. Retrieved from http://ac.els-cdn.com/S1054139X12002078/1-s2.0-S1054139X12002078-main.pdf?_tid=221d35ca-9c95-11e7-b302-00000aab0f02&acdnat=1505755179_6a40d25d5d5530fca1d804d75ca6ae4e

Squeglia, L. M., Jacobus, J., & Tapert, S. F. (2009). The influence of substance use on adolescent brain development. *Clinical EEG and Neuroscience: Official Journal of the EEG and Clinical Neuroscience Society (ENCS), 40*(1), 31–38. Retrieved from https://www.ncbi.nlm.nih.gov/pmc/articles/PMC2827693/pdf/nihms177745.pdf

Stanford Children's Hospital. (n.d.). *Low birth weight*. Retrieved from http://www.stanfordchildrens.org/en/topic/default?id=low-birthweight-90-P02382

Thurstone, C. (2017). *A precious natural resource: The developing adolescent brain*. Retrieved from http://www.heritage.org/sites/default/files/2017-07/05%202017_IndexofCultureandOpportunity_Teen%20Drug%20Use.pdf

Tonniges, T., Palfrey, J., & Mitchell, M. (2004). Introduction to the medical home. *Pediatrics, 113*, 1472. Retrieved from http://pediatrics.aappublications.org/content/pediatrics/113/Supplement_4/1472.full.pdf

Tripuraneni, M., Paruthi, S., Armbrecht, E. S., & Mitchell, R. B. (2013). Obstructive sleep apnea in children. *Laryngoscope, 123*(5), 1289–1293. Retrieved from https://www.ncbi.nlm.nih.gov/labs/articles/23288669/

Turer, C. B., Lin, H., & Flores, G. (2013). Health status, emotional/behavioral problems, health care use, and expenditures in overweight/obese US children/adolescents. *Academic Pediatrics, 13*(3), 251–258. doi:10.1016/j.acap.2013.02.005

Urban Child Institute. (2012). *Prematurity and low birth weight*. Retrieved from http://www.urbanchildinstitute.org/articles/policy-briefs/prematurity-and-low-birth-weight

U.S. Department of Agriculture. (2017). *Women, infants, and children (WIC)*. Retrieved from https://www.fns.usda.gov/wic/women-infants-and-children-wic

Walker, V. G. (2012). Factors related to emotional responses in school-aged children who have asthma. *Issues in Mental Health Nursing, 33*(7), 406–429. doi:10.3109/01612840.2012.682327

Wang, C., Chan, J. Y., Ren, L., & Yan, J. H. (2016). Obesity reduces cognitive and motor functions across the lifespan. *Neural Plasticity, 2016*, 1–13. doi:10.1155/2016/2473081

White, D. P. (2017). Advanced concepts in the pathophysiology of obstructive sleep apnea. *Advances in Oto-Rhino-Laryngology, 80*, 7–16. doi:10.1159/000470522

Winters, K. C., & Arria, A. (2011). Adolescent brain development and drugs. *Prevention Researcher, 18*(2), 21–24. Retrieved from https://www.ncbi.nlm.nih.gov/pmc/articles/PMC3399589/pdf/nihms386812.pdf

World Health Organization. (n.d.). *About social determinants of health*. Retrieved from http://www.who.int/social_determinants/sdh_definition/en

Xanthopoulos, M., Gallagher, P., Berkowitz, R., Radcliffe, J., Bradford, R., & Marcus, C. (2015). Neurobehavioral functioning in adolescents with and without obesity and obstructive sleep apnea. *Sleep, 38*(3), 401–410. Retrieved from https://academic.oup.com/sleep/article/38/3/401/2416905/Neurobehavioral-Functioning-in-Adolescents-With

Young, A., McCabe, S., Cranford, J., Ross-Durow, P., & Boyd, C. (2012). Nonmedical use of prescription opioids among adolescents: Subtypes based on motivation for use. *Journal of Addictive Diseases, 31*(4), 332–341. doi:10.1080/10550887.2012.735564

Intercepting Stress and Behavioral Health Issues: Building Resiliency in Children

MARY WEGLARZ, EILEEN CORCORAN, DEBORAH GUTTER, AND NINA B. COLABELLI

For more than 20 years, resiliency has been described as a coping mechanism to adversity; however, recently many questions have emerged—what does it mean to be resilient, who is resilient, how do children and adolescents build resiliency, and why is resiliency essential for success? We know that today's children are exposed to war, guns, violence, crime, natural disasters, and everyday stress. Despite exposures to one or more of these hardships, resilient children have good physical and mental health, and their resilience or capacity to cope with difficulties protects them from the long-term adverse effects of trauma (National Scientific Council on the Developing Child [NSCDC], 2004). Pediatric primary care providers (P-PCPs), who are educated about resiliency, are in the unique position to assess child and family strengths, identify behaviors indicative of stress, and offer guidance and recommend services to help build child, adolescent, and family resilience. This chapter presents the evidence for building resiliency in children and the role of P-PCPs, which includes attention to the office environment and structure, comprehensive assessment, ongoing support, and community referrals. Building resiliency in children *intercepts* the impact of adversity on a child's emotional, social, and behavioral health.

■ RESILIENCE

Survivor reports from terrorist attacks, natural disasters, and other crises reveal that resilience is not extraordinary but common among people (American Psychological Association [APA], 2011). Everyone encounters difficulties, as the adverse childhood experience (ACE) study demonstrated; over 60% of us have faced a trauma of some kind in childhood (Centers for Disease Control and Prevention [CDC], 2013; see Chapter 32 on toxic stress). Resilience is a process of adaptation and growth in children and adolescents that helps them address stress and threats in their life. The primary factor necessary to develop resilience is a loving, supportive family relationship bolstered by caring outside relationships (APA, 2011). Children build resiliency throughout the developmental years when they respond to challenges in a manner that leads to positive outcomes in their health and well-being (NSCDC, 2004). A resilient child or adolescent is confident and has a positive self-image. The self-assured child has the ability to (a) develop realistic plans and implement them; (b) manage emotions; (c) problem-solve; and (d) communicate successfully (APA, 2011).

■ CHRONIC ILLNESSES, CULTURE, AND RESILIENCE

A child's health and development affect resilient behaviors (NSCDC, 2004). Children with chronic health conditions, such as asthma, diabetes, and bowel disease, or families with special needs children experience stress while attempting to balance their life and home environment. During a crisis, chronically ill children and their families may have difficulty keeping the illness and behaviors in control. A lack of control creates additional challenges on the family structure when attempting to build resilient behaviors (Cousino & Hazen, 2013). In addition, the context of the child's family, community, and culture influences the family's ability to cope when stressed (Luthar, 2003; Masten & Powell, 2003). Examples of stressors include disruption of the family unit when there is death of a family member or friend, separation, or divorce. Communities with high crime and/or violence rates place additional stressors on the family unit and dynamics. Developing resilient behaviors may be difficult for these children and families, as limited protective resources are available in communities with high crime and violence rates. The children and families may live in fear and in an environment that lacks prevention resources. In addition, adolescents may be attracted to individuals who commit crimes and display violent behaviors, thwarting the development of resilient behaviors.

Family culture influences parenting values and styles (Lubell, Lofton, & Singer, 2008). There are differences across cultures, and supportive P-PCPs understand how a family's culture influences their parenting choices. Family culture might have brought them to the United States for a better life and care, and they reside here as undocumented citizens. These families are part of a culture that is worried about deportation and living in fear. Some factors in a child's family, community, and culture can be modified and strengthened to support the child's development of resiliency. A P-PCP has a responsibility to the children and families served to understand their culture, community, strengths, and challenges and locate appropriate community and cultural resources for the family unit.

■ A "STRENGTHENING FAMILIES" APPROACH TO IMPROVE OUTCOMES

"Strengthening Families" is an approach created by the Center for the Study of Social Policy (Harper Browne, 2014) to assist professionals working with families with the aim of preventing a major trauma to a child: abuse and neglect. They identify five interrelated factors in a child's life that can strengthen family resilience, prevent the long-term effect of stress, and help children grow into healthy adults. Every family has strengths and a P-PCP's knowledge and awareness of the five protective factors can assist him or her with identifying strengths and supporting the vision of optimal growth and development for every child (Center for the Study of Social Policy/American Academy of Pediatrics [CSSP/AAP], 2014; Moore, Chalk, Scarpa, & Vandivere, 2002).

Parental Resilience

Everyone experiences stress. Resilient parents are competent during times of stress. When parents feel successful meeting challenges and making healthy choices for themselves and their family, they feel accomplished and it increases their resiliency (Raikes & Thompson, 2005). They are in control of situations and choices, and better able to provide their child with nurturing attention and form positive parent–child relationships. In turn, a strong attachment and bond with their child helps development of their child's resilience (Harper Browne, 2014).

Social Connections

Parents need a connection to other individuals and groups to feel a sense of belonging. Individuals or groups can be extended family members, friends, neighbors, or community members or leaders. These relationships provide the parent with companionship, information, encouragement, and emotional support that validates the parent's choices. Participation in religious communities, their child's school, or other social institutions allows the parent to give to others and develop a stronger sense of self-worth. Children benefit from their parent's positive social connections. These supports can relieve the parent of some of their parenting demands and teach positive parenting that can nurture their attachment with their child (Harper Browne, 2014; Jordan, 2006).

Concrete Help in Times of Need

Interrelated with social connections is a family's need for concrete help. Positive connections with extended family, friends, and community can provide logistical assistance with child care, respite, and transportation. A parent's ability to identify need and ask for help is a parental strength (Moore, Chalk, Scarpa, & Vandivere, 2002). Connections to community institutions such as the Red Cross, food banks, and local social services offer supplies when finances are short, guidance with finances and insurance, and job fairs. Concrete assistance relieves some stress and is critical to helping parents feel that they can provide for their children (Harper Browne, 2014).

Parent Knowledge of Child Development

Best practices for parenting are not traditionally taught in high school courses or college to all who attend. Rather, parenting is cyclical: New parents need to evaluate their experiences while growing up with their parents to determine how they want to parent their children. Regular routines have always been recommended and are useful; however, research has influenced current parenting practices, for example, placing an infant on their tummy to sleep is not safe, or sitting an infant in front of a television screen is not recommended and does not present opportunities for interactive play. Social media, smartphones, instant access to information on the Internet are uncharted in relation to parenting styles and offer new challenges to successful parenting (see Chapter 22 on social media and behavioral health). Children benefit if their parents understand their infant's, child's, and/or adolescent's developmental needs, can identify when their infant, child, and/or adolescent needs help, and have the skills to positively parent (Harper Browne, 2014; NSCDC, 2004).

Social and Emotional Competence of Children

A child's social and emotional competence is developed in the early years of life. It gives a child the capacity to attach with their parent, form relationships first with their parent and then with others, regulate their emotions, and grow. This competency impacts their health, well-being, and development and prepares the child to be a competent, resilient adult. Development of this factor is enhanced when parents are resilient and have social connections, concrete support, and knowledge of child development (Harper Browne, 2014; Shonkoff & Garner, 2012).

■ RESILIENCY ASSESSMENT

Resiliency develops within the context of a child's family, community, and culture and is strengthened by the presence of the five protective factors (Harper Browne, 2014). Parenting and raising a resilient child is not easy. A P-PCP is an additional support for the family. In their supportive role, the P-PCP has a responsibility to learn about the communities and cultures of families in their practice. Also with knowledge and understanding of the protective factors, the P-PCP can use them within their assessment to identify family strengths and needs. P-PCPs use screening tools and an assessment to guide recommendations that build resilience (CSSP/AAP, 2014). The P-PCP's assessment might refer a family to social services for financial assistance, to suggest parenting classes or a book to a struggling adolescent parent, or, to those who lack family or friends, upcoming events to meet others and learn about their community.

Screening

P-PCPs work with a variety of families: some who have well children and others with children with chronic illness, specials healthcare needs, behavioral health problems, or mental illness. All these families have strengths (Moore et al., 2002). One strength is simply that they are seeking care for the child. However, even those with well children experience stressors and require additional support and resources. P-PCPs gather information about the child's health and development and anticipate upcoming behavior challenges parents might confront as the child ages (CSSP/AAP, 2014). To assist with assessing the child, ask parents to complete screening tools that screen the child's development, behavior, and for such

TABLE 5.1

SCREENING TOOLS

Eliciting Parental Strengths and Needs: https://brightfutures.aap.org/Bright%20 Futures%20Documents/AAP_BF_ElicitingParentalStrength_Tipsheet_FINAL.pdf

Edinburgh Postnatal Depression Scale: http://www.fresno.ucsf.edu/pediatrics/downloads/ edinburghscale.pdf

Depression Screening: The Patient Health Questionaire-2: http://www.cqaimh.org/pdf/ tool_phq2.pdf

The Patient Health Questionaire-9: http://www.integration.samhsa.gov/images/res/ PHQ%20-%20Questions.pdf

Safe Environment for Every Kid (SEEK) Parent Questionaire-R (PQ-R): https://docs. wixstatic.com/ugd/77e10d_c5ec3492b03d4540b20874d622ef3557.pdf

Developmental Screening: Learn the Signs. Act Early: https://www.cdc.gov/ncbddd/ actearly

Pediatric Symptom Checklist: https://www.brightfutures.org/mentalhealth/pdf/ professionals/ped_sympton_chklst.pdf

Autism-Specific Screening: Checklist for Autism in Toddlers (CHAT): http://www. helpautismnow.com/CHAT_Checklist_English.pdf

Modified Checklist for Autism in Toddlers (CHAT): https://www.autismspeaks.org/ what-autism/diagnosis/screen-your-child

Substance Use Screening: CRAFFT (Car, Relax, Alone, Forget, Friends, Trouble) Screening Questionnaire: http://www.integration.samhsa.gov/clinical-practice/sbirt/ CRAFFT_Screening_interview.pdf

Alcohol Screening: CAGE Questionnaire: http://www.integration.samhsa.gov/clinical-practice/sbirt/CAGE_questionaire.pdf

diagnoses such as autism, attention deficit hyperactivity disorder (ADHD), and others. To assess the home environment, use tools that screen for parental depression, major stress, substance use, domestic violence, discipline, and food insecurity (Dubowitz et al., 2011; Flynn et al., 2015; Hornor, 2015). Each of these screens can be completed while waiting to be seen (Table 5.1).

Assessment

The P-PCP reviews the results of screening tools during each well-child healthcare visit and as appropriate during episodic visits. It is important for P-PCPs to observe and listen to both the child and parent. What is their affect? Children learn from their parents and pick up cues from them. Just as a parent's calm can assure his or her child, parental fears can make the child uneasy. How do the parent and child interact? Is the parent attuned to the child's needs? What is the parent's mood, and how does the parent describe their child's mood and temperament?

Verify any parental concerns about the child's physical health and development and consider whether the parents' knowledge aligns with what the P-PCP observes (CSSP/AAP, 2014). The ability to ask questions is a strength (Moore et al., 2002). Acknowledge that parenting a child is stressful and additionally hard when a child has a chronic illness, special needs, or behavioral health issues (Cousino & Hazen, 2013). What parenting stresses are they experiencing? If it is related to their child's condition, what is their understanding of the child's health, the child's care needs? Are they prepared to care for their child's special needs? Or are they finding that the child's care is too demanding? Do they have the support of a spouse, extended family, or friends? A parental strength is having friends and family support. It is also one for the child; does the child have friends? Does the parent know these friends and invite them into their home?

Parenting stress can also be related to daily routines and challenges, as parents and children juggle home, work, school, and play. What is the family routine throughout the day? Regular routines help children feel secure, give a sense of predictability, and teach children about the need to transition from meals to daycare or school, or to play. Transitions are examples of change. How well does the child adapt to change? Are there any significant changes happening at home? If the child or parent answers yes, then ask how the parent and child are coping.

Children living within a healthy household have a sense of security and can focus on their own development. Healthy households have structure, rules, reasonable expectations, and open communication (Moore et al., 2002). Questions which illicit information about the child and parent's communication with each other enable the P-PCP to evaluate whether the child and parent are listening to each other.

P-PCPs, caring for children, must also take the time to ask about parental health. Does the parent have a chronic illness, mental illness, or a substance use disorder? If yes, are they receiving appropriate care? If they are not in care, the P-PCP can make recommendations for referral to care. Healthy parents are better able to cope with the day-to-day parenting challenges (Moore et al., 2002). Parents also have unmet personal, emotional, or mental health needs and cannot be expected to adequately parent a child with behavioral health problems.

Red Flags

The P-PCP looks, listens, and learns. Red flags can be observed or heard during the office visit by the P-PCP or their staff. The P-PCP models attentive behavior by keeping office interruptions to a minimum. Children left unattended in the waiting room or office or parents who ignore the children while on their cellphones during the visit are red flag behaviors that need to be addressed by the P-PCP. Tense communication between the parent and child is also a red flag; an angry, fatigued, or overwhelmed parent provides the P-PCP with evidence that the parents need assistance.

During the examination of the child, the P-PCP may document developmental regression or a withdrawn child. Other signs of stress in the child may include parental report of new onset of enuresis, behavior changes, mood changes, separation anxiety, unusual fear of the dark, excessive tantrums, aggressive behavior, headaches, stomach aches, eating and sleeping difficulty, appetite changes,

changes in school performance, and high-risk behaviors (CSSP/AAP, 2014). The child's school might have referred the child to the P-PCP because of a high absenteeism rate, which could be a sign of a school phobia or bullying. An identified red flag is an opportunity for the P-PCP to intercept the problem by offering appropriate assistance to the family.

■ BUILDING RESILIENCE

The goal of the P-PCP's interventions is aimed at building resiliency, which intercepts behavioral problems. Goals are established by assessing and evaluating the office's mission and environment. Care provided in family-centered medical homes support resilience (Bethell, Newacheck, Hawes, & Halfon, 2014). The completed screenings and assessment will direct the P-PCP toward the appropriate referrals and relevant anticipatory guidance. The P-PCP's approach and interventions are individualized to the needs of the child and family. Some advice to recommend to families and children that assists with building resilience is identified in Table 5.2.

The Office Environment

Within the family-centered medical home, waiting rooms welcome the child and family to the P-PCP's practice. P-PCPs can use the office space as a venue for building protective factors (CSSP/AAP, 2014). A family-friendly room has books and

TABLE 5.2

RECOMMENDATIONS TO BUILD RESILIENCE
Help the child to establish good relationships with friends and family
Change the reaction to stressful events—response matters
Change is everywhere—put energy where it can help
Take frequent, consistent, small steps toward realizing goals
Don't detach—be proactive in adverse situations
Learn from events—self-reflection and self-discovery breed strength
Trust your instincts—develop confidence
See the big picture—don't blow things out of proportion
Be optimistic—instead of worrying about fears, visualize what you want
Self-care is key—exercise, enjoy, relax
Journal, meditate, or be in touch with your spiritual side

Source: Adapted from American Psychological Association. (2011). *The road to resilience.* Retrieved from http://www.apa.org/helpcenter/search

interactive family games. Health education materials for children and parents within the waiting room educate and may open dialogue to a concern during the visit.

PEDIATRIC INTEGRATED CARE COLLABORATIVE

Some P-PCP practices have behavioral health services available in the office. The Substance Abuse and Mental Health Services Administration (SAMHSA) funded the National Child Traumatic Stress Network (NCTSN) to establish the Pediatric Integrated Care Collaborative (PICC). The collaborative assists with the integration of mental/behavioral health services with pediatric primary care (Asarnow, Rozenman, Wiblin, & Zeltzer, 2015). One of PICC's goals is to promote resilience and assist in the prevention of trauma (Dayton et al., 2016). The threats, adversities, or trauma of one family member affects all family members, and the PCP practicing within a PICC is connected to services that support healthy caregiving and child development and enhance the building of child, adolescent, and family resilience (see Chapter 33 on trauma-informed care).

Referrals

Preparation on the part of the P-PCP is needed to support families. A list of programs in the community that support families (Flynn et al., 2015) should be prepared as a resource for the parents, child, and adolescent. Provide phone numbers to the parents and adolescents for the local public health department; health insurance and public assistance access; and domestic violence shelters, abuse hotlines, and other crisis centers. Identify local support groups for parents dealing with the child's health, development, or behavioral issues. Many states have 2-1-1 hotlines to help families find resources for housing, utilities, food, health, jobs, shelters, and assistance in an emergency. Parents who need these types of assistance may have a difficult time parenting a child, especially one with behavioral health problems. Additional hotline numbers that a P-PCP should know about are listed in Table 5.3. It is best to manage the referral on an individual basis with direct contact with the new agency. The P-PCP's knowledge of the family's strengths and vulnerabilities is essential for meaningful collaboration with supporting programs (Dayton et al., 2016). Consideration can also be given to referrals for prevention that will help build resilient families and children, such as evidence-based home visiting or parenting programs (Hornor, 2015). The P-PCP collaborates with the family, specialists, and community providers to develop a health plan, and is prepared and aware which specialists and community resources can best meet the needs of the child and family. Parents who use the resources are better able to develop their own resiliency skills and to help their child build resiliency.

Anticipatory Guidance

Prior to discharge from the P-PCP's office, the P-PCP should review health information and provide anticipatory guidance focused on the child's behavioral health problems. Evidence-based materials support a healthy family and build resiliency (Coker et al., 2016). Educational materials that build resilience include but are not limited to responding to infant cues, positive parenting, positive peer relationships, and information about impact of stress on health.

TABLE 5.3

HELPLINES AND WEBSITES
Help lines such as 2-1-1 Help Line Center: dial 211; http://www.211.org
National Domestic Violence Hotline: 1–800–799–7233; http://www.thehotline.org
Help Me Grow: https://helpmegrownational.org/affiliates
Learning Disabilities: http://ldnavigator.ncld.org
National Suicide Prevention Lifeline: 1–800–273–8255; https://suicidepreventionlifeline.org
Bullying Prevention: https://www.stopbullying.gov/index.html
Youth Violence Prevention: https://www.cdc.gov/violenceprevention/youthviolence
National Human Trafficking Hotline: 1–888–373–7888; https://humantraffickinghotline.org

■ RESILIENT YOUTH

The supportive P-PCP aims to help the family raise resilient youth. Developmentally, individual factors can promote resilience. An affectionate, responsive infant who maintains a regular schedule, a preschooler who is friendly with a higher frustration level, a school-age child who is well liked and flexible in their coping abilities, and an adolescent who is responsible, perceptive, and independent are most likely to develop resiliency skills more easily. Family factors such as a nurturing bond with the caregiver or religious beliefs contribute to the development of resilience. Children with strong community factors such as a supportive peer group, a positive school experience, or other larger community support have another strong basis for resilience (Blaustein & Kinniburgh, 2010).

Ginsburg (2015) has identified the "seven Cs" of a resilient youth: competence, confidence, connection, character, contribution, coping, and control. The competent youth can handle challenging situations, has confidence in his/her ability, is connected with family and community, has a character that is based upon strong morals and values, and makes personal contributions to help make the world a better place. The resilient youth has learned to cope with stress and does not choose high-risk behaviors as a coping strategy. Resilient youth are in control of their future.

■ SUMMARY

While resilience is normative, many factors in today's world can affect the ability of a child or family to become resilient. P-PCPs contribute to resilient youth by anticipating possible challenges faced by parents, children, and/or families; supporting prevention programs for families; recognizing the influence of culture and family customs on behavior patterns; and integrating a strength-based focus in their assessment of families. The use of screening tools and asking the appropriate questions assists P-PCPs in their critical role in this aspect of child development. Analysis of the results of screening tools completed by the parents and the child, appropriate assessment questions, office-based interventions, and timely referrals to therapy in community resources are critical components of the behavioral health assessment to enable the P-PCPs to intercept problems and build child, adolescent, and family resiliency.

■ REFERENCES

American Psychological Association. (2011). *The road to resilience.* Retrieved from http://www.apa.org/helpcenter/search

Asarnow, J. R., Rozenman, M., Wiblin, J., & Zeltzer, L. (2015). Integrated medical-behavioral care compared with usual primary care for child and adolescent behavioral health: A Meta-analysis. *JAMA Pediatrics*, 169, 929–937. doi:10.1001/jamapediatrics.2015.1141

Bethell, C. D., Newacheck, P., Hawes, E., & Halfon, N. (2014). Adverse childhood experiences: Assessing the impact on health and school engagement and the mitigating role of resilience. *Health Affairs*, 33, 2106–2115. doi:10.1377/hlthaff.2014.0914

Blaustein, M., & Kinniburgh, K. (2010). *Treating traumatic stress in children and adolescents.* New York, NY: The Guilford Press.

Center for the Study of Social Policy/American Academy of Pediatrics. (2014). *Promoting children's health and resiliency: A Strengthening families approach.* Retrieved from http://www.cssp.org/reform/strengthening-families/messaging-at-the-intersection/Messaging-at-the-Intersections_Primary-Health.pdf

Centers for Disease Control and Prevention. (2013). *Adverse childhood experiences (ACE) study.* Retrieved from http://www.cdc.gov/ace/

Coker, T. R., Chacon, S., Elliott, M. N., Bruno, Y., Chavis, T., Biely, C., . . . Chung, P. J. (2016). A parent coach model for well-child care among low-income children: A Randomized controlled trial. *Pediatrics*, 137, e20153013. doi:10.1542/peds.2015-3013

Cousino, M. K., & Hazen, R. A. (2013). Parenting stress among caregivers of children with chronic illness: A systematic review. *Journal of Pediatric Psychology*, 38, 809–828. doi:10.1093/jpepsy/jst049

Dayton, L., Agosti, J., Bernard-Pearl, D., Earls, M., Farinholt, K., McAlister Groves, B., & Wissow, L. (2016). Integrating mental and physical health services using a socio-emotional trauma lens. *Current Problems in Pediatric and Adolescent Health Care*, 46, 391–401. doi:10.1016/j.cppeds.2016.11.004

Dubowitz, H., Lane, W. G., Semiatin, J. N., Magder, L. S., Venepally, M., & Jans, M. (2011). The safe environment for every kid model: Impact on pediatric primary care professionals. *Pediatrics*, 127, e962–e970. doi:10.1542/peds.2010-1845

Flynn, A. B., Fothergill, K. E., Wilcox, H. C., Coleclough, E., Horwitz, R., Ruble, A., . . . Wissow, L. S. (2015). Primary care interventions to prevent or treat traumatic stress in childhood: A systematic review. *Academic Pediatrics*, 15, 480–492. doi:10.1016/j.acap.2015.06.012

Ginsburg, K. R. (2015). *Building resilience in children and teens: Giving kids roots and wings* (3rd ed.). Elk Grove Village, IL: American Academy of Pediatrics.

Harper Browne, C. (2014). *The strengthening families approach and protective factors framework: Branching out and reaching deeper.* Washington, DC: Center for the Study of Social Policy.

Hornor, G. (2015). Childhood trauma exposure and toxic stress: What the PNP needs to know. *Journal of Pediatric Health Care*, 29, 191–198. doi:10.1016/j.pedhc.2014.09.006

Jordan, A. (2006). *Tapping the power of social networks: Understanding the role of social networks in strengthening families and transforming communities.* Retrieved from the Annie E. Casey Foundation: http://www.aecf.org/m/resourcedoc/AECF-TappingthePowerofSocialNetworks-2006.pdf

Lubell, K. M., Lofton, T., & Singer, H. H. (2008), *Promoting healthy parenting practices across cultural groups: A CDC research brief.* Retrieved from Centers for Disease Control and Prevention, National Center for Injury Prevention and Control: https://stacks.cdc.gov/view/cdc/5273

Luthar, S. S. (Ed.). (2003). *Resilience and vulnerability: Adaptation in the context of childhood adversities.* New York, NY: Cambridge University Press. doi:10.1017/CBO9780511615788

Masten, A. S., & Powell, J. L. (2003). A resilience framework for research, policy, and practice. In S. S. Luthar (Ed.), *Resilience and vulnerability: Adaptation in the context of childhood adversities* (pp. 1–25). New York, NY: Cambridge University Press. doi:10.1017/CBO9780511615788.003

Moore, K. A., Chalk, R., Scarpa, J., & Vandivere, S. (2002). *Family strengths: Often overlooked, but real.* Retrieved from Child Trends: https://www.childtrends.org/publications/family-strengths-often-overlooked-but-real

National Scientific Council on the Developing Child. (2004). *Young children develop in an environment of relationships. Working paper no. 1.* Retrieved from www.developingchild.harvard.edu

Raikes, A. H., & Thompson, R. A. (2005). Efficacy and social support as predictors of parenting stress among families in poverty. *Infant Mental Health Journal, 26,* 177–190. doi:10.1002/imhj.20044

Shonkoff, J. P., & Garner, A. S. (2012). The lifelong effects of early childhood adversity and toxic stress. *Pediatrics, 129,* 232–246. doi:10.1542/peds.2011-2663

SECTION II

Infant Population

CHAPTER 6

Identifying and Intercepting Behavioral Health Problems in Infancy

DONNA HALLAS

Pediatric primary care providers (P-PCPs) must acknowledge the paradigm shift to attain behavioral health for all by viewing behavioral health as beginning at the moment of conception and existing on a continuum throughout the life span, delicately balancing between behavioral/mental health and well-being versus behavioral health disorders/mental illness and malady. In this view, the intrauterine experience plays a critical role in behavioral health and the question: Is the fetus, who is exposed to a positive intrauterine environment, and receives essential nutrients for best organ development, and grows in a safe intrauterine environment free from undue external traumas, more likely to have healthy behavioral/mental health experiences throughout the life span than fetuses who grow in challenging intrauterine environments? Thus, the question becomes: Is the fetus, who is exposed to intrauterine insults—for example, prescribed medications that may potentially harm the infant (Class C, D, and/or X drugs), intrauterine malnutrition, maternal obesity, maternal metabolic disorders or other diseases, maternal or familial mental health disorders, illicit drugs, and/or alcohol—more likely to experience behavioral/mental illness and malady throughout the life span? The question for evaluation of these infants is a primary focus of this chapter, as we examine, analyze, and evaluate the best available evidence to *identify* and *intercept* behavioral health problems prior to conception, post-delivery, and during the first year of life.

■ THE INTRAUTERINE EXPERIENCE: WHEN INSULTS OCCUR

Jacobsen et al. (1994) conducted a prospective, longitudinal study to compare the effects of prenatal exposure to alcohol, smoking, and illicit drugs (opiates and cocaine) to the birth size of the infant. Birth weight was influenced by combined exposure to alcohol and smoking behaviors, alcohol alone to reduced length, and reduced head circumference to opiate exposure. Mwaniki, Atieno,

Lawn, and Newton (2012) reported the results of a systematic review examining the effect on neurodevelopmental outcomes after intrauterine and neonatal insults. The systematic review included the analysis of 153 articles. The included studies analyzed 2,815 individuals with 37% (1,048 individuals) experiencing neurodevelopmental impairments including learning difficulties, cognitive or developmental delay, cerebral palsy, and hearing and visual impairments. These articles representing just a few examples of intrauterine insults provide significant insight into problems that can be intercepted by obstetric providers by obtaining a comprehensive history and providing appropriate anticipatory guidance during the prenatal period.

■ THE INTRAUTERINE EXPERIENCE: INTERCEPTING THE INSULT

While some intrauterine insults and the adverse effects are unavoidable (e.g., maternal unintended exposure to non-vaccine preventable viral or bacterial organisms; genetic disorders; unintended external trauma such as a motor vehicle accident), there are specific intrauterine insults such as smoking, alcohol, specific prescribed medications, and/or illicit drug use prior to and during the prenatal period that can be intercepted by the P-PCPs, and, in particular, by prenatal and P-PCPs. Prenatal providers are on the front lines for early identification of women who are smoking, use alcohol and/or illicit drugs during the prenatal period, or who have untreated mental health disorders, such as anxiety, depression, or eating disorders, which may adversely impact fetal growth, development, and in particular neurodevelopment. The standard of care now calls for obstetric providers to routinely screen *all* prenatal women for behaviors that are known to adversely impact fetal development and neurodevelopment.

Pediatric and family providers also have the potential to positively impact the health and well-being of the fetus. These professionals should identify mothers in their practices who are pregnant and struggling raising their infant, toddler, or older child. Office-based screening for maternal depression during the first 6 months of the postpartum period and for adverse childhood experiences (ACEs; see Chapter 32) may reveal a positive screen, and the pediatric provider can refer the mother for further assessment, evaluation, and early treatment to improve the family dynamics for herself, her spouse or significant other, the fetus, and the children living in the household.

■ PREMATURE INFANTS AND BEHAVIORAL HEALTH ASSESSMENT

In 2015, the preterm birth rate, identified as infants born less than 37 weeks' gestational age, was reported as 9.63% of the total number of registered births in the United States (3,978,497), with increases in preterm birth rates among non-Hispanic Black and Hispanic women (Martin, Hamilton, Osterman, Driscoll, & Matthew, 2017). Neurobehavioral impairments, including cognitive and attention deficits, and behavioral problems remain a persistent health problem for premature infants (Anderson & Doyle, 2003; Noble & Boyd, 2012). Worldwide, 52% of infants born less than 28 weeks' gestational age were estimated to have some degree of neurodevelopmental impairment, of which 7% suffer long-term neurodevelopmental impairments (Blencove et al., 2013). Noble and Boyd conducted a systematic review of neonatal assessment tools with the goal of determining which tools provided the most relevant data for clinicians to clinically predict neonates who were most likely to have neurobehavioral impairments. Based on the results of the neonatal assessments, early intervention (EI) services should be initiated as early as clinically possible to reduce untoward neurodevelopmental outcomes. The authors concluded that three neonatal assessments have strong psychometric qualities for use in clinical settings (Table 6.1). The following three tests were identified: Prechtl's Assessment of General Movements (GMs) that documents spontaneous movements that identify infants with early central nervous system (CNS) dysfunction—the authors concluded had the GMs had the best prediction of future outcomes for cerebral palsy; Test of Infant Motor Performance (TIMP) that evaluates motor control, organization of posture, and movement for functional activities—the authors concluded that the TIMP had the best evaluative validity because the test is supported by evidence from two randomized controlled trials; and the Neurobehavioral Assessment of the Preterm Infant (NAPI), which measures the progression of neurobehavioral performance and has strong psychometric properties and is useful for clinical evaluation of the preterm infant.

Since the infants are in the neonatal intensive care unit (NICU) when these tests are initially performed, P-PCPs need to be advised of which testing was performed in the NICU and the results of the testing. The GMs and the TIMP can be used to assess the premature infant until the infant is 4 months old. Therefore, NICU providers and community-based private pediatric practices and clinics that routinely care for the NICU graduates should collaborate to select one of these reliable noninvasive tests to perform while the infant is in the NICU and then as a follow-up reevaluation with the same test in the pediatric office. Repeating tests will enable the P-PCP to initiate EI services at the earliest time frame to attempt to intercept some of the neurodevelopmental adverse outcomes seen in the premature population.

TABLE 6.1

RECOMMENDED NEONATAL ASSESSMENT TOOLS

Tool	Source	Availability
Brazelton Neonatal Screening	Retrieve from https://www.brazeltontouchpoints.org/offerings/nbo-and-nbas	Assessor must be trained
Prechtl's Assessment of General Movements (GMs)	Retrieve from http://general-movements-trust.info/content/46/41/invitation	Assessor must be trained
Test of Infant Motor Performance (TIMP)	Retrieve from http://thetimp.com	Assessor must be trained
Neurobehavioral Assessment of the Preterm Infant (NAPI)	Retrieve from http://med.stanford.edu/NAPI/training.html	Assessor must be trained

■ MATERNAL AND FAMILY ASSESSMENT

Assessing for depression in adolescent, young adult females, and all females caring for infants is the first critical step to identify women who may have problems parenting an infant and may be the first step in the pediatric or family practice primary care office to intercept maternal–infant relationship problems and the infant's potential for adverse exposures which may lead to infant behavioral health problems. Either Edinburgh's (Cox, Holden, & Sagovsky, 1987) or Beck's postnatal depression scales (Beck & Gable, 2005) are reliable and valid screening tools that can be easily administered in primary care settings, including obstetric and pediatric practices. Early identification of depression with either treatment in the primary care office or referral for treatment is one strategy that may intercept potential maternal–infant bonding and relationship problems, including signs of abnormal infant behavioral growth and development. The Centers for Disease Control and Prevention (CDC) estimates that between 11% and 20% of the women who give birth each year have postpartum depression. This estimate is based on the self-report of postpartum depression symptoms that are gathered on the Pregnancy Risk Assessment Monitoring System (PRAMS) tool reported by 27 states each year (Ko, Rockhill, Tong, Morrow, & Farr, 2017). Data further reveal that women younger than 19 years old and those between 20 and 24 years old reported higher rates of postpartum depression. In addition, women who delivered full-term infants with low birth weights, women who smoked during pregnancy, and women whose babies were in the NICU also reported a higher incidence of postpartum depression (Ko et al., 2017).

In 2017, the American Academy of Pediatrics reaffirmed their earlier recommendations for screening all pregnant women (Earls and The Committee on Psychological Aspects of Child and Family Health, 2010) and recommended screening all pregnant women, mothers of newborns, and mothers of infants at consecutive visits when the infants present for the first office visit shortly after birth, and then when the infant is 2, 4, and 6 months old, to identify and refer for treatment any woman who screens positive for maternal depression. Intercepting potential problems early in the maternal–infant relationship is critical to establishing healthy behavioral developmental patterns in infancy. Specific details for the assessment, diagnosis, and treatment of infantile depression are discussed in Chapter 7.

INFANT ATTACHMENT THEORIES

Psychoanalytical theorists pioneered the development of the first infant social–emotional psychoanalytic theory based upon the infant's emotional development within the maternal relationship focusing on the emergence of the infant's sense of self (Erikson, 1964; Freud, 1938). The significance of the infant–maternal dyad relationship influences growth throughout the life span. A strong, emotional, satisfying, and comforting relationship establishes the foundation for social–emotional development throughout the life span. In contrast, an ineffective early relationship may lead to relationship struggles throughout each stage of the life cycle.

Theoretical frameworks for maternal–infant attachment and bonding have been developed by numerous researchers (Ainsworth, 1973; Bowlby, 1969, 1982; Brazelton, Koslowski, & Main, 1974; Klaus & Kennell, 1976). In these theoretical frameworks, early attachment relationships are viewed as critical to the infants' development throughout infancy and early childhood, and determines the progression of secure and trusting relationships. Failure of infant–maternal bonding and the establishment of secure, trusting relationships may result in lifelong social–emotional conflicts. Consistent with these theorists' beliefs on the significance of attachment and bonding, Erikson's developmental theory (1964) stressed the development of infant trust within the early maternal–infant relationship. Failure of the infant to develop trusting relationships encumbers trust and impedes relationship building throughout childhood, adolescence, and adult life.

Based upon these theoretical frameworks and application to clinical practice, P-PCPs who appropriately screen the maternal–infant relationship and the infant's emotional state of trust and security may have the opportunity to intercept signs of mistrust and insecurity by providing guidance to obviate trends and factors that are negatively influencing the development of maternal–infant trusting relationships.

■ NORMAL NEWBORN SOCIAL–EMOTIONAL DEVELOPMENT

Infant mental health was initially researched by Ainsworth (1973), Bowlby (1951, 1969), and Brazelton (1963) as they individually developed mother–infant attachment theories. Bowlby defined infant mental health as "the infant and young child should experience a warm, intimate, and continuous relationship with his mother (or permanent mother substitute) in which both find satisfaction and enjoyment" (1951, p. 13). Based on these theorists and their theories, successful mental health development is based on attachment and bonding for infants and children to age 3 that permits infants to regulate and express their emotions and form close and secure relationships with their mother and caregivers (Bowlby, 1983).

Thus, the patterns for normal infant social–emotional development begin at birth. Birthing centers that encourage the mother to breastfeed the newborn immediately after birth are supporting initial bonding patterns. Skin-to-skin contact and kangaroo care while comforting the infant and during feedings support bonding in the early postpartum period and during early infancy (Carfoot, Williamson, & Dickson, 2003; Moore, Andersen, & Bergman, 2007). A randomized controlled trial conducted by Dumas et al. (2012) supported the need for the nurse to interact with parents in the early postpartum period. The researchers studied the influence of birth routines on mother–infant interactions at day 4 of life. The results of their investigation revealed evidence of a sensitive period for separation after birth. Thus, the researchers concluded that immediate and uninterrupted skin-to-skin contact at birth and rooming-in should be the standard of care to support the establishment of the mother–infant relationship (Dumas et al., 2012).

Postpartum nurses should assess bonding patterns throughout the 48 hours the mother and infant remain hospitalized post-delivery. Nurses should support the new, as well as the experienced, mother as she cradles, comforts, and responds to the infant in the first 48 hours of life as these first few days lay the foundation for a healthy mother–infant relationship. Nurses are role models and advocates for mothers who need assistance, assurance, and continuous reassurance that they are displaying good parenting skills while caring for their newborns.

Upon discharge from the hospital, the office nurse and P-PCP must assess bonding patterns and provide support and guidance as needed to the mother. A behaviorally healthy newborn/infant who is stressed during an examination should respond to the mother's comfort measures, such as holding the infant closely to the chest, rocking the infant, and/or talking quietly to the infant. An infant who does not respond should first be assessed for possible physical problems such as visual or hearing impairment. If vision and hearing are evaluated as normal for age, then the P-PCP must consider other reasons for the infant's behavior. Was there an intrauterine exposure that was not previously identified? What is the infant's behavior at home? Ask the mother to describe how she responds to the infant at home. How long does the infant cry before the mother or another family member responds to the infant's needs? Ask the mother to describe a typical day with the infant: feeding, sleeping, interaction patterns. Answers to these questions will provide the P-PCP with a snapshot of relationship of the mother and infant upon which to make decisions about the state of the social–emotional development of the infant and whether interventions are needed to intercept the potential for inadequate mother–infant attachment and bonding patterns.

■ BREASTFEEDING AND BEHAVIORAL HEALTH

Breastfeeding offers a unique opportunity for the mother to establish a strong bonding and attachment relationship with the newborn. Mothers should be encouraged to breastfeed the newborn immediately after birth with support and guidance from the professional staff and family member(s) present in the birthing center. Mothers who are HIV positive cannot breastfeed their infant; however, they can hold their newborn immediately after delivery to establish the initial step for a positive mother–infant bonding and attachment relationship. Breastfed infants experience more frequent contact with their mother and undivided attention from the mother while breastfeeding. Breastfeeding along with these close mother–infant interactions sustained for 1 year have been shown to correlate to improved mental health for the child up to 14 years of age (Oddy et al., 2010).

Baby-friendly hospitals (World Health Organization [WHO], 1990) offer the most comprehensive breastfeeding services for mothers during the postpartum period, with support from lactation consultants and nurses who are educated in evidence-based breastfeeding practices, as well as breastfeeding classes during the postpartum hospital stay. Referrals should be made to community support groups as the mother will continue to need support for successful breastfeeding after discharge from the brief postpartum hospital stay. Baby-friendly hospitals discourage the use of pacifiers and do not discharge the newborns with a supply of formula, since encouraging exclusive breastfeeding but providing formula to "take home" provides mixed messages to the mother whose milk supply may take up to 2 weeks to be established.

A relationship between breastfeeding and positive outcomes for behavioral and/or mental health in both the mother and the baby, and even throughout growth of children into adulthood, has been scientifically researched with evidence showing a reduction in adverse behavioral health outcomes for the child/adolescent and improved mental health for the mother (Oddy et al., 2010). In 2017, the World

Alliance for Breastfeeding Action and the La Leche League International (WABA/ LLLI, 2017) sponsored a joint statement supporting the benefits of breastfeeding and the reduction in mental health problems for the mother and the infant. In addition, studies have shown that mothers who breastfeed their infants have better sleep patterns and longer sleep periods than mothers who formula-feed their infants, which is correlated to better maternal well-being (Doan, Gardiner, Gay, & Lee, 2007; Kendall-Tackett, Cong, & Hale, 2011).

The *intercept* for prevention of maternal–infant depression and infant long-term behavioral health problems is for P-PCPs to include assessment of maternal breastfeeding and infant responses to breastfeeding in every primary care office visit. The P-PCP should observe the mother breastfeeding in the office so that any problems can be identified and appropriate anticipatory guidance can be provided to the mother. Follow-up phone calls to the mother by office staff and/or texting the mother to provide support are also helpful strategies to support the continuation of breastfeeding throughout the first year of life.

■ FULL-TERM NEWBORN AND INFANT BEHAVIORAL HEALTH ASSESSMENTS

There are a limited number of valid and reliable screening tools to assess the social–emotional development of infants. Screening tools that can easily be incorporated in primary care settings are listed in Table 6.2. It is the responsibility of the P-PCP to select one or more of the available social–emotional screening tools that best fit the office dynamics, and then evaluate the effectiveness of the tool for the early identification of infants at risk for abnormal social, emotional, and/or behavioral health development in the populations that the P-PCP serves. Office personnel can be trained to administer the screening tools, although clarifying parental responses on the tool and the analysis and evaluation of the results

TABLE 6.2

INFANT SOCIAL–EMOTIONAL HEALTH SCREENING TOOLS

Tool	Source	Availability
The Ages and Stages Questionnaire: Social–Emotional-2 (ASQ:SE-2)	Brookes Publishing, Baltimore, MD Retrieve from http://www.redleafpress.org/ cw_Search.aspx?k=asq	Must be purchased
Parents' Evaluation of Developmental Status (PEDS)	Retrieve from http://www.pedstest.com/ default.aspx	Must be purchased
Denver Developmental Screening Test II (DDST II)	Retrieve from http://denverii.com	Download free copy

are the responsibility of the P-PCP. The P-PCP also determines the necessary interventions to intercept identified problems and makes appropriate referrals.

Screening Tools

Parent report measures are an extremely useful method for screening and assessing the social–emotional development of infants. Parent reports are considered more reliable than professional observation alone for screening infants for social–emotional developmental and potential problems (Pontoppidan, Niss, Pejtersen, Julian, & Vaever (2017). The Ages and Stages Questionnaire: Social–Emotional-2 (ASQ:SE-2; Squires, Bricker, & Twombly, 2015) is used to screen infants at 2, 6, and 12 months old. The ASQ:SE-2 is also used to screen children up to 60 months old at routine healthcare visits: 18, 24, 30, 36, 48, and 60 months old. The ASQ:SE-2 screens on seven key social–emotional key issues: self-regulation, compliance, adaptive functioning, autonomy, affect, self-communication, and interaction with people. Another tool is the Parents' Evaluation of Developmental Status (PEDS). The PEDS is a valid and reliable tool for screening social–emotional development in infants that can be used in primary care settings. Both of these tools are completed by the mother or primary caregiver prior to the primary care office visit, either at home or while she is in the waiting area. It takes about 10 minutes to complete each of these forms. Ideally, the PCP should review the parental responses and the score for the ASQ:SE-2 or the PEDS before entering the examination room. This review provides an opportunity for the PCP to identify questions that may clarify the parent's answers and ask additional questions about the parent–infant attachment relationship and the infant's social–emotional development. Based on the parent's responses, the PCP can determine appropriate actions to improve and intercept problem behaviors. *Interception* includes: (a) providing anticipatory guidance to initiate a change in infant or parenting behaviors; (b) referring the infant to EI services; (c) referring the parent to community-based parenting classes or parenting classes offered in the primary care office; and (d) referring the infant–mother (parent) dyad for an evaluation by a psychiatric specialist for diagnosis and treatment of problems that cannot be managed in the primary care center.

The Denver Developmental Screening Test, second edition (DDST II) is a developmental screening tool for infants to children up to 7 years old. The DDST II screens for four major categories of growth and development, one of which is the social–emotional development. Since the DDST II can be used for monthly assessments of infants, the P-PCP has numerous opportunities to assess the social–emotional development of the infant. When a potential problem is identified on the DDST II, the P-PCP may then use one of the specific tools to screen for social–emotional development, as previously discussed (ASQ-SE-2 or the PEDS).

P-PCPs who serve at-risk populations of infants, children, and adolescents (e.g., children in foster care; parents with a history of inadequate parenting skills; parents, who themselves, were raised by alcoholic or substance abusing parents; mothers with a history of depression, etc.) may choose to purchase one of the specific social–emotional developmental tools for regular use in office screenings for early identification of affected infants, with the goal of intercepting parenting behaviors that do not support positive infant social–emotional development. In addition, the P-PCP may refer the parent for counseling for their behaviors and for parenting classes.

■ IDENTIFYING NORMAL INFANT BEHAVIORAL DEVELOPMENT

Growth patterns for the identification of healthy and happy infants are well-established (Erikson, 1964; McLeod, 2008/2017). Anticipated patterns for healthy and happy social and emotional development for infants are also well-established (Erikson, 1964). P-PCPs assess these developmental patterns throughout infancy during each well-infant health maintenance visit. Between 1 and 3 months old, infants recognize their parents' voices, follow their parents' movements, and are responsive to their environment by smiling and vocalizing through cooing sounds. Throughout infancy, social and emotional development continues as the infant continues to interact with parents, siblings, and other individuals who enter their world. Infants laugh, play interactive games (e.g., peek-a-boo), and display inquisitive behaviors recognized as the development of object permanence (e.g., the infant searches for a toy placed under a blanket). Around 9 months, infants demonstrate their need to be in the presence of their mother, father, or another daily caregiver when evidence of stranger anxiety emerges.

Self-comforting behaviors are also a part of normal infant social and emotional development. Infants whose social and emotional development is being guided by healthy parental responses will demonstrate self-comforting behaviors when infant stressors, such as disappearance of an object or stranger anxiety, are experienced by the infant, and the infant reacts (e.g., cries, refuses to play or eat), and then soon adjusts to the new situation (e.g., stops crying and begins to respond) without undue evidence of distress (e.g., continuous non-comforting crying). Infants develop normal social and emotional attributes when they receive appropriate recognition of their accomplishments (e.g., displaying affection, laughing, babbling) from their parents or daily caregivers. P-PCPs who assess the social and emotional development of infants and recognize, at the earliest time point, an infant who is outside the norm, have the potential to intercept the development of abnormal behaviors and reestablish normal social–emotional infant development by providing anticipatory guidance to the parents and/or referrals for further assessment and treatment for problematic mother–infant behaviors.

■ INTERCEPTING INFANT BEHAVIORAL HEALTH PROBLEMS

How often do P-PCPs assess the social–emotional development of infants? P-PCPs who routinely use screening tools during each office visit have the potential for early identification of infants who display social–emotional developmental problems. However, with limited time for full infant assessments, the focus of many well-infant visits is on analysis of anthropometric measurements, motor development, paternal concerns, and immunizations, thus allowing little time for discussion or assessment of the infant's social–emotional development. In addition, diagnosis of infants with behavioral disorders is challenging. Even when infants display clinically significant emotional or behavioral problems, the characteristics of the presenting problem may not be recognized (van Zeijl et al., 2006). Lack of recognition of symptoms leads to underdiagnosed and missed opportunities to intercept these early onset behaviors through primary care behavioral health strategies to improve the maternal–infant interactions, attachment and bonding experiences, and the infant social–emotional behavioral development. P-PCPs should reinforce positive attachment behaviors such as mother–infant kissing, hugging, cuddling, softly talking to the infant, gently massaging the infant's extremities, and prolonged quiet time with gazing and direct eye contact between mother and infant.

■ DIAGNOSIS OF PHYSICAL, SOCIAL, AND EMOTIONAL PROBLEMS

There are compelling links among the physical growth and development parameters, the infant's physical appearance, and social–emotional behavioral problems during infancy. Early recognition of the problem(s) is critical to the health and well-being of the infant. Recognition of the evidence that social–emotional development is below the expected norm is a major step toward intercepting abnormal social–emotional infant development, with the goal of providing interventions that reverse abnormal development.

Physical evidence is generally recognizable by P-PCPs as the infants present with a variety of signs including but not limited to unexplained bruising, inadequate weight gain, and edema of extremities secondary to infliction of injury resulting in a fracture. Infants who have been exposed to trauma, maltreatment, abuse, and neglect are less likely to be interactive with the P-PCP, display fear by crying and turning away from the examiner, and may show little to no interest in a toy; thus, the differential diagnosis of impaired social–emotional development must be considered (see Chapter 33).

Physical acts that result in a disruption in the attachment and bonding relationship for the mother–infant dyad include mother–infant separation, either temporary or permanent, and maternal abandonment. While the P-PCP may know that the infant is experiencing this loss, there are times that the P-PCP will not be informed of the loss; thus, the P-PCP must recognize the subtle signs that the infant may display, such as reduced appetite, disruption in sleep pattern, excessive crying without evidence of self-comforting efforts, and refusal to "go to" or acknowledge another caregiver.

Other exposures that place the infant at risk for abnormal social–emotional development include dysfunctional family dynamics, such as family violence, maternal anxiety or depression, and paternal mental illness. Additional factors include infants with challenging temperament and affect, infants who cry without the ability to cease crying through self-comforting measures, high levels of stranger anxiety, and infants who fail to interact with the mother or primary caregiver. The P-PCP must recognize these signs that provide evidence of abnormal trends in social–emotional developmental behaviors.

▧ TREATMENT STRATEGIES

For infants who are thriving in their social–emotional development, P-PCPs can easily provide anticipatory guidance for the mother and family members to maintain the infant's behavioral and mental health and well-being. Normally occurring behaviors, such as stranger anxiety and displays of frustration, can be managed with strategies in which the mother gently and confidently introduces a new person to the infant, with comforting hugs from the mother, and with the mother speaking in a soft, reassuring tone to the infant. Knowing that the infant takes cues from the mother (father or a significant other caregiver) and responds to the cues is an important part of educating the parent on typical infant responses to new encounters.

However, there are atypical responses that an infant may display that raise red flags (Fitzgerald, Weatherston, & Mann, 2011) and P-PCPs must intercept these behaviors by providing either more direct interventions in the primary care setting or referring the mother–infant dyad to psychiatric providers who specialize in infant behavioral and mental health. A lack of clear attachment and bonding behaviors between the mother and infant is a major concern; lack of maternal nurturing responses is also a concern. The P-PCP must consider maternal depression as a possible cause for the mothers affect and refer the mother for an evaluation. Even if the mother alone or the mother–infant dyad are followed by a psychiatric provider, the P-PCP continues providing primary care for the infant and should obtain follow-up history on the mother and infant's behaviors, offering supportive guidance in primary care settings to enable the infant to develop a normal social–emotional skill set. Communicating acceptance of the mother's behaviors to improve the mother–infant relationship is an important component of the primary care visit. The P-PCP must assess for infant safety in all encounters with the mother by asking critical questions that may be red flags for adverse infant outcomes. If problematic behaviors are detected, the P-PCP must act immediately and appropriately to assure the infant's safety. See Table 6.3 for sample questions.

TABLE 6.3

QUESTIONS TO ILLICIT MATERNAL–INFANT BEHAVIORAL PROBLEMS

1. How are you feeling while caring for your infant?
2. Is there anything that happens during the day or night that concerns you about your baby?
3. How do you feel when your baby cries for a long period of time?
4. What do you do when your baby cries?
5. When your baby is crying, how long do you wait to pick up your infant?
6. How do you feel when the baby cries?
7. Tell me about your baby's temperament?
8. How do you feel about yourself as a mother?
9. Do you have support from your spouse, significant other, family members?
10. Have you had any feelings or impulses to hurt your baby?

SUMMARY

Infancy is a wonderful time for healthy parents and healthy infants to grow together within healthy home and community environments that support the social–emotional development of infants, thus establishing the foundation for lifelong behavioral and mental health. P-PCPs must assess the mother–infant bonding and attachment relationship, maternal nurturing behaviors, and maternal responses to the infant, as well as the infant's social–emotional developmental patterns, at every primary care encounter. If observations or testing are not within the anticipated norms for the maternal responses to the infant, such as the mother has evidence of depression or the infant is not responding to the mother or the provider as expected for the age of the infant, interventions appropriate for the primary care setting should be instituted. If the mother's and/or infant's behavioral and mental health needs exceed the capacity of the primary care setting, then they should be referred to psychiatric providers who specialize in the care of mothers with behavioral or mental health disorders and/or infants whose social–emotional development is below the anticipated norms.

REFERENCES

Ainsworth, M. D. (1973). The development of infant-mother attachment. In B. M. Caldwell & H. N. Riccuiti (Eds.), *Review of child development research* (pp. 1–94). Chicago, IL: University of Chicago Press.

Anderson, P., Doyle, L. W., Victorian Infant Collaborative Study Group. (2003). Neurobehavioral outcomes of school-age children born extremely low birth weight or very premature in the 1990's. *Journal of American Medical Association, 289,* 3264–3272.

Beck, C. T., & Gable, R. K. (2005). *The postpartum depression screening scale: Postpartum mood and anxiety disorders.* 5. Retrieved from https://scholarsarchive.jwu.edu/disorders/5

Blencowe, H., Lee, A. C. C., Cousens, S., Bahalim, A., Narwal, R., Zhong, N., . . . Lawn, J. E. (2013). Preterm birth-associated neurodevelopmental impairment estimates at regional and global levels for 2010. *Pediatric Research, 74,* 17–34. doi:10.1038/pr.2013.204

Bowlby, J. (1951). *Maternal care and mental health.* Geneva, Switzerland: World Health Organization Monograph (Serial no. 2).

Bowlby, J. (1969). *Attachment & loss: Vol. 1: Attachment* (2nd ed.). New York, NY: Basic Books.

Bowlby, J. (1982). *Attachment & loss. Vol. I: Attachment.* New York, NY: Basic Books.

Bowlby, J. (1983). *Attachment* (2nd ed.). New York, NY: Basic Books.

Brazelton, T. B. (1963). The early mother-infant adjustment. *Pediatrics, 32,* 931–937.

Brazelton, T. B., Koslowski, B., & Main, M. (1974). The origins of reciprocity in mother–infant interaction. In M. Lewis & L. A. Rosenblum (Eds.), *The effect of the infant on its caregiver.* New York, NY: Wiley-Interscience.

Carfoot, S., Williamson, P. R., & Dickson, R. (2003). A systematic review of randomized controlled trials evaluating the effect of mother/baby skin-to-skin care on successful breastfeeding. *Midwifery, 19,* 148–155. doi:10.1054/midw.2002.0338

Cox, J. L., Holden, J. M., & Sagovsky, R. (1987). Detection of postnatal depression: Development of the 10-item Edinburgh postnatal depression scale. *British Journal of Psychiatry, 150,* 782–786. doi:10.1192/bjp.150.6.782

Doan, T., Gardiner, A., Gay, C. L., & Lee, K. A. (2007). Breastfeeding increases sleep duration of new parents. *Journal of Perinatal and Neonatal Nursing, 21,* 200–206. doi:10.1097/01.JPN.0000285809.36398

Dumas, L., Lepage, M., Bystrova, K., Matthiesen, A.-S., Welles-Nystrom, B., & Widstrom, A-M. (2012). Influence of skin-to-skin contact and rooming-in on early mother-infant interaction: A Randomized controlled trial. *Clinical Nursing Research, 22,* 301–336.

Earls, M. F., and The Committee on psychological aspects of child and family health. (2010). Incorporating recognition and management of perinatal and postpartum depression into pediatric practice. *Pediatrics, 126,* 1032–1039. doi: 10.1542/peds.2010-2348

Erikson, E. (1964). *Insights and responsibilities.* New York, NY: Norton.

Fitzgerald, H. E., Weatherston, D., & Mann, T. L. (2011). Infant mental health: An interdisciplinary framework for early social and emotional development. *Current Problems in Pediatric Adolescent Health Care, 41,* 178–182. doi:10.1016/j.cppeds.2011.02.001

Freud, S. (1938). *An outline of psychoanalysis.* London: Hograth.

Jacobson, J. L., Jacobson, S. W., Sokol, R. J., Martier, S. S., Ager, J. W., & Shankarana, S. (1994). Effects of alcohol use, smoking, and illicit drug use on fetal growth in black infants. *The Journal of Pediatrics, 124*(5), 757–764. doi:10.1016/S0022-3476(05)81371-X

Kendall-Tackett, K. A., Cong, Z., & Hale, T. W. (2011). The effect of feeding method on sleep duration, maternal well-being, and postpartum depression. *Clinical Lactation, 2,* 22–26. Retrieved from http://www.uppitysciencechick.com/kendall-tackett_CL_2-2.pdf

Klaus, M. H., & Kennell, J. H. (1976). *Maernal-infant bonding.* St. Louis, MO: Mosby.

Ko, J. Y., Rockhill, K. M., Tong, V. T., Morrow, B., & Farr, S. L. (2017). Trends in postpartum depression symptoms – 27 States 2004, 2008, 2012. *Morbidity and Mortality Weekly Report, 66,* 153–158. doi:10.15585/mmwr.mm6606a1

Martin, J. A., Hamilton, B. E., Osterman, M. J. K., Driscoll, A. K., & Matthew, T. J. (2017). Births: Final data for 2015. *National Vital Statistics Reports, 66,* 1–70. Retrieved from https://www.cdc.gov

McLeod, S. (2008/2017). Erik Erikson. *Simple Psychology.* Retrieved from https://www.simplypsychology.org/Erik-Erikson.html

Moore, E. R., Andersen, G. C., & Bergman, N. (2007). Early skin-to-skin contact for mother and their healthy newborn infants. *Cochrane Database of Systematic Reviews,* (3), CD003519. doi:10.1002/14651858.CD003519.pub2

Mwaniki, M. K., Atieno, M., Lawn, J. E., & Newton, C. R. J. C. (2012). Long-term neurodevelopmental outcomes after intrauterine and neonatal insults: A systematic review. *The Lancet, 379,* (9814), 455–452. doi:10.1016/S0140-6736(11)61577-8

Noble, Y., & Boyd, R. (2012). Neonatal assessments for the preterm infant up to 4 months corrected age: A systematic review. *Developmental Medicine & Child Neurology, 54,* 129–139. doi:10.1111/j.1469-8749.2010.03903.x

Oddy, W. H., Kendall, G. E., Li, J., Jacoby, P., Robinson, M., de Klerk, N. H., . . . Stanley, F. J. (2010). The long-term effects of breastfeeding on child and adolescent mental health: A pregnancy cohort study followed for 14 years. *Journal of Pediatrics, 156,* 568–574. doi:10.1016/j.jpeds.2009.10.020

Pontoppidan, M., Niss, N. K., Pejtersen, J. H., Julian, M. M., & Vaever, M. S. (2017). Parent report measures of infant and toddler social-emotional development: A systematic review. *Family Practice, 34,* 127–137. doi:10.1093/fampra/cmx003

Squires, J., Bricker, D., & Twombly, M. S. (2015). *Ages & stages questionnaires: Social–emotional (ASQ:SE-2): A parent completed child monitoring system for social–emotional behaviors* (2nd ed.). Baltimore, MD: Brookes Publishing. Retrieved from http://products.brookespublishing.com/Ages-Stages-Questionnaires-Social-Emotional-Second-Edition-ASQSE-2-P849.aspx

World Alliance for Breastfeeding Action and the La Leche League International. (2017). *Breastfeeding and mental health: Joint statement from WABA and LLLI in celebration of World Health Day.* Retrieved from http://waba.org.my/breastfeeding-and-mental-health/

World Health Organization. (1990). *Baby-friendly hospital initiative.* Retrieved from http://www.who.int/nutrition/topics/bfhi/en/

van Zeijl, J., Mesman, J., Stolk, M. N., Alink, L. R., van Ijzendoorn, M. H., & Bakermans-Kranenburg, M. J., et al. (2006). Terrible twos? Assessment of externalizing behaviors in infancy with the child behavior checklist. *Journal of Child Psychology and Psychiatric, 47,* 801–810. doi:10.1111/j.1469-7610.2006.01616.x

CHAPTER 7

Infant Depression

DONNA HALLAS

Infant depression has been studied as a phenomenon within psychology and psychiatry since the early 1970s. The *Diagnostic and Statistical Manual of Mental Disorders, Fifth Edition* (*DSM-5*; American Psychiatric Association [APA], 2013) eliminated the terminology "disorders usually classified in infancy, childhood, and adolescence" and classified them as neurodevelopmental disorders removing infantile depression as a discrete condition. Pediatric primary care providers (P-PCPs) who provide care to infants need to be familiar with the best available evidence for recognizing signs of infantile depression to avoid missing the opportunity for early recognition of this problem. Recognizing the signs of infant and/or maternal depression affords the opportunity for P-PCPs to implement strategies to *intercept* negative emotional infant development to positive emotional outcomes. Research has shown that infants exposed to stress have lasting effects on the developing brain, and these infants have a greater risk of depression and anxiety in later childhood and adulthood (Murgatroyd, Wu, Bockmuhl, & Spengler, 2010). This chapter discusses research on infant depression, signs and symptoms of infantile depression, and provides strategies to enable mothers and other caregivers to actively engage the emotional development of infants throughout the first year of life.

■ INFANT EMOTIONS

Infants express emotional feelings as early as 2 months old, for example, by showing interest in the mother, father, or siblings or other immediate family members and family pets through eye contact or smiling at the individual and following the activities as the individual moves about in the "baby's world." Two-month-old infants also show signs of contentment, often after breastfeeding or bottle feeding, as well as signs of distress when experiencing discomfort, pain, or hunger (Izard, Huebner, Risser, McGinnes, & Dougherty, 1980). Izard et al. (1980) demonstrated that 8-month-old infants were capable of seven discrete emotions: joy, contentment, anger, disgust, surprise, interest, and sadness. The emotions that remain a concern from this early work with young infants are anger, disgust, and sadness. These powerful negative emotions in an infant, whose normal growth pattern supports rapid brain growth and development, is problematic when left unchecked and without relief, since the latest neuroscientific research reveals that the brain imprints negative emotions into the developing brain architecture (Lipina & Colombo, 2009; The Urban Child Institute, n.d.), which may have life-long adverse effects.

Granat, Gadassi, Gilboa-Schechtman, and Feldman (2017) reported the results of a study with 100 women with symptoms of depression and anxiety following childbirth. Participants were grouped, for study purposes, into an observational group of mothers with a clinical diagnosis of postpartum depression or anxiety and a healthy control group of postpartum women. The mothers in the observational group had no prior history of anxiety or depression. Mother–infant interactions were micro-coded using video analysis for maternal and infant's social behaviors. Infant negative and positive emotions were analyzed using four emotional paradigms: anger with mother, anger with stranger, joy with mother, and joy with stranger. Study results revealed that infants of depressed mothers looked less at their mothers, which the researchers identified as consistent with the characteristics of social withdrawal (Granat et al., 2017). Furthermore, the researchers reported that infants of mothers with a diagnosis of depression and anxiety had problems with self-regulation. In the researchers'/clinicians' clinical work following the study, they reported that depressed mothers who participated in interaction-focused therapy (Feldman, 2016) showed improvement in their interaction behaviors with their infants.

It is well known that an infant's initial environmental interactions are with the mother or consistent primary caregiver and that these interactions play a major role in the infant's early emotional and social experiences. Cohen and Tronick (1983) demonstrated that infants as young as 3 months old were sensitive and reactive to negative maternal facial expressions. Field (1984) found that infants of mothers with a diagnosis of depression became accustomed to the mother's flat or negative emotions, thus expressing personal deficits in emotional development, and in interactions with unfamiliar adults, generalized these flat emotions with these adults as well (Field et al., 1988). Thus, it is imperative for P-PCPs to identify infants of all ages who are not interacting with the mother, other adults, and/or the provider and perform an assessment using one of the standardized assessment tools that measure the social–emotional development of the infant and tools to assess the mother for evidence of depression (Table 7.1), thus potentially intercepting problems via appropriate maternal and infant interventions.

■ INFANT EMOTIONAL DEVELOPMENT AND MATERNAL DEPRESSION

Mason, Briggs, and Silver (2011) conducted a study with 232 postpartum mothers investigating whether a positive maternal postpartum depression screen (Edinburgh Postnatal Depression Scale) was correlated with maternal report of

TABLE 7.1

SOCIAL–EMOTIONAL ASSESSMENT TOOLS

Instrument	Measures	Scoring
Ages and Stages Questionnaire	Infant social–emotional development	High total score = High risk
Social–Emotional (ASQ: SE)	Parental responses screens: seven key social–emotional areas Age of use: 6 to 60 months old	For poor social–emotional development
Edinburgh Postnatal Depression Scale (EPDS)	Postpartum women 10-item, 5-point Likert scale	Score of 10 or greater = Depression
Maternal Postnatal Attachment Scale (MPAS)	Maternal feelings of attachment	High or low attachment total score

poorer infant social–emotional development and more negative reports of maternal feelings of attachment to the infant. The results revealed that infants of mothers with a positive postpartum depression screen 2 months after delivery were at risk for deficits in social–emotional development, and at 6 months postpartum, the mother–infant interactions were dysfunctional. Thus, maternal postpartum depression was the critical link between inadequate maternal attachment feelings toward the infant and the adverse effects on the infant's social–emotional development.

Gress-Smith, Luecken, Lemery-Chalfant, and Howe (2011) investigated the prevalence of maternal depression at 5 and 9 months postpartum in Latina women and compared these results to infant outcomes, specifically, infant weight gain, physical health, and sleeping pattern at 9 months old. Results revealed that postpartum depression in these women led to significantly negative effects in the infant with overall lower weight gains, more minor health problems, and more nighttime awakenings at 9 months old.

Hayes, Goodman, and Carlson (2013) investigated the associations of maternal antenatal depression on infant disorganized attachment at 12 months. Study participants were 79 women who met the *DSM-IV* criteria for major depressive disorder before their pregnancy. Results revealed that the mothers of infants, who were classified as disorganized at 12 months, had a higher level of antepartum depressive symptoms as compared to infants classified as organized. The researchers further report that disorganized infants who are exposed to warm, positive parenting early in infancy were less likely to show evidence of negative attachment outcomes at 12 months old.

■ INFANT ATTACHMENT

Infant attachment and bonding has been studied for many years by psychologists Freud (1949), Bowlby (1969), Ainsworth (1973), and Klaus and Kennell (1976), with all researchers purporting the significance of maternal–infant attachment and bonding to positive outcomes for the infant throughout infancy, childhood, and later adult years. The links between maternal–infant bonding and attachment and the relationship to infant development is now well recognized as just as important as infant nutrition (Miklush & Commelly, 2013).

To prevent adverse effects on infant growth and development, maternal–infant bonding and negative outcomes for infant social–emotional development, maternal affect, mood, and possible depression must be assessed by obstetric providers prior to delivery and by P-PCPs in the postpartum period (see Table 7.1). Mothers who screen positive for depression must be referred for treatment to prevent adverse maternal outcomes as well as to prevent the adverse effects on the infant, which can affect the infant throughout their life span.

■ RECOGNIZING THE EMOTIONALLY TROUBLED INFANT

Keren and Tyano (2006) described cases of infants and toddlers who were exposed to early traumatic maternal–infant interactions. They concluded that poor quality of the interpersonal relationship between the mother and infant led to aggressive and withdrawal behaviors toward peers and a lack of pleasure and interest with outbursts of crying in the infant and toddler. Infants who experience poor-quality maternal–infant social–emotional interactions present with a sad affect, such as lack of a spontaneous smile with the mother and other adults, minimal interest in the environment, and hesitancy to interact with unfamiliar adults.

The infant may have longer episodes of crying, and often inconsolable episodes of crying. The infant may show little or no pleasure in feeding since the infant has not experienced attachment, bonding, and comfort during feedings. Sleep patterns may not be established or the sleep pattern may be disrupted with periods of waking and crying, in which the infant is not comforted. Infants may learn to self-comfort, which may be evident when the infant is stressed in a pediatric office procedure, such as an injection, and the infant reaction is one of some crying followed by self-comfort rather than seeking security and comfort from the mother.

Assessing and Evaluating the Emotionally Troubled Infant

A detailed history from the mother, father, and other caregivers is essential for the P-PCP to effectively evaluate social and emotional developmental problems that are challenging to detect in an infant. Observing, assessing, and evaluating the interactions between the mother and infant during the office visit is a critical part of each well and episodic infant examination. One or more standardized assessment tools should be administered (see Table 7.1) and a complete physical examination should be performed to rule out other causes of the infant's presenting affect.

Infants with mental health problems can be identified when the history reveals an infant who cries more than normally expected for age, has altered sleeping and feeding patterns, and in later infancy has a tendency toward aggressive behaviors (Bolten, 2012). In addition, infants with persistent crying, sleeping, and eating problems were shown to be at higher risk for developing behavioral health problems (Hemmi, Wolke, & Schneider, 2011).

Astute evaluations of these mother–infant dyad interactions provide the opportunity for the P-PCPs to intercept problematic social and emotional development through appropriate anticipatory guidance, and in circumstances where the mother's screening is positive for depression, make a referral for the mother to receive individual therapy and family therapy to improve mother–infant interactions. The overarching behavioral health outcomes for all infants are to live in a safe environment and to grow and develop in a secure maternal–infant (caregiver) relationship in which the infant has opportunities to develop within the normal range of social–emotional development, thus establishing the foundation for social–emotional development throughout child and adolescent years.

▪ INTERVENTIONS FOR THE EMOTIONALLY TROUBLED INFANT

P-PCPs must consider the family unit, including the mother–infant dyad, paternal support, and family support available to help the mother–infant establish a strong maternal–infant attachment relationship. Brief office-based interventions may be one way to help develop the maternal–infant bonding relationship. Instructions on effective feeding strategies and ways to establish sleep patterns are essential if the infant is to achieve normal growth and developmental milestones. Encouraging maternal–infant play and contact activities each day for a specific time frame in which the mother reports back to the P-PCP may be an effective strategy. Office-based interventions in which the mother is asked to observe her infant and comment on "what she sees" may provide an opportunity to provide insight into the mother's perspective of the infant. Asking the mother to videotape her infant on a smartphone and bring the video to the office for review is also a strategy that can be used during a brief office-based intervention. Encouraging the mother to hug, cuddle, and speak softly to the infant also builds the mother's sense of worth while interacting with the infant. Hallas, Koslap-Petraco, and Fletcher (2017) showed that brief office-based intervention for the social–emotional development of toddlers was an effective strategy to build maternal confidence and infant social–emotional development. These same principles can be applied to brief office-based interventions for mothers of infants.

▪ SUMMARY

Infantile depression, while no longer classified in the *DSM-5* (APA, 2013), must be recognized as a potential problem for the infant who is being raised by a mother who has experienced antenatal depression or is experiencing postpartum depression while raising the infant. The research evidence is clear. Infants who are deprived of nurturing, caring, warm maternal interactions are victims of negative outcomes in the area of social–emotional development, often showing evidence of infantile depression: sad affect, little to no eye contact, excessive crying behaviors, altered sleep patterns, poor feeding patterns with a resultant poor weight gain, and alterations in bonding and attachment behaviors. Such negative infant outcomes most often lead to adverse behavioral health outcomes for the infant as they grow and develop throughout childhood and into adulthood. P-PCPs have the unique opportunity to identify these infants and mothers and to intercept the adverse outcomes by referring the mother for treatment, providing specific anticipatory guidance to achieve infant normal developmental patterns, and/or referring the infant with the mother for family therapy.

■ REFERENCES

Ainsworth, M. D. (1973). The development of infant-mother attachment. In B. M. Caldwell & N. H. Riccuitu (Eds), *Review of child development research* (pp. 1–94). Chicago, IL: University of Chicago Press.

American Psychiatric Association. (2013). *Diagnostic and statistical manual for mental health disorders* (5th ed.). Arlington, VA: Author. doi:10.1176/appi.books.9780890425596

Bolten, M. I. (2012). Infant psychiatric disorders. *Early Child Adolescent Psychiatry*, 22(Suppl. 1), S69–S74. doi:10.1007/s00787-012-0364-8

Bowlby, J. (1969). *Attachment and loss: Vol. 1: Attachment*. New York, NY: Basic Books.

Cohen, J. F., & Tronick, E. Z. (1983). Three-month-old infants' reaction to simulated maternal depression. *Child Development*, 54, 334–335.

Feldman, R. (2016). The neurobiology of mammalian parenting and the biosocial context of human caregiving. *Hormones and Behavior*, 77, 3–17. doi:10.1016/j.yhbeh.2015.10.001

Field, T. M. (1984). Early interactions between infants and their postpartum depressed mothers. *Infant Behavioral Development*, 7, 1998–2004. doi:10.1016/S0163-6383(84)80012-0

Field, T. M., Healy B., Goldstein, S., Perry, S., Bendell, D., Schanberg, S., . . . Kuhn, C. (1988). Infants of depressed mothers show "depressed" behavior even with non-depressed adults. *Child Development*, 59, 1569–1579. doi:10.2307/1130671

Freud, S. (1949). *An outline of psychoanalysis*. New York, NY: Norton.

Granat, A., Gadassi, R., Gilboa-Schechtman, E., & Feldman, R. (2017). Maternal depression and anxiety, social synchrony, and infant regulation of negative and positive emotions. *Emotion*, 1, 11–27. doi:10.1037/emo0000204

Gress-Smith, J. L., Luecken, L. J., Lemery-Chalfant, K., & Howe, R. (2011). Postpartum depression prevalence and impact on infant health, weight, and sleep in low-income and ethnic minority women and infants. *Maternal Child Health Journal*, 16, 887–893. doi:10.1007/s10995-011-0812-y

Hallas, D., Koslap-Petraco, M., & Fletcher, J. (2017). Socia–emotional development of toddlers: Randomized controlled trial of an office-based intervention. *Journal of Pediatric Nursing*, 33, 33–40. doi:10.1016/j.pedn.2016.11.004

Hayes, L. J., Goodman, S. H., & Carlson, E. (2013). Maternal antenatal depression and infant disorganized attachment at 12 months. *Attachment & Human Development*, 15, 133–153. doi:10.1080/14616 734.2013.743456

Hemmi, M. H., Wolke, D., & Schneider, S. (2011). Associations between problems with crying, sleeping and/or feeding in infancy and long-term behavioural outcomes in childhood: A meta-analysis. *Archives of Diseases in Childhood*, 96, 622–629. doi:10.1136/adc.2010.191312

Izard, C. E., Huebner, R. R., Risser, D., McGinnes, G., & Dougherty, L. (1980). The young infant's ability to produce discrete emotional expressions. *Developmental Psychology*, 16, 132–140. doi:10 .1037/0012-1649.16.2.132

Keren, M., & Tyano, S. (2006). Depression in infancy. *Child Adolescent Psychiatric Clinics of North America*, 15, 883–897. doi:10.1016/j.chc.2006.05.004

Klaus, M. H., & Kennell, J. H. (1976). *Maternal–infant bonding*. St. Louis, MO: Mosby.

Lipina, S. J., & Colombo, J. A. (2009). *Poverty and brain development during childhood: An approach from cognitive psychology and neuroscience*. Washington, DC: American Psychology Association.

Mason, Z. S., Briggs, R. D., & Silver, E. J. (2011). Maternal attachment feelings mediate between maternal reports of depression, infant social–emotional development, and parenting stress. *Journal of Reproductive and Infant Psychology, 29*, 328–394. doi:10.1080/02646838.2011.629994

Miklush, L., & Commelly, C. D. (2013). Maternal depression and infant development: Theory and current evidence. *MCN: The American Journal of Maternal/Child Nursing, 38*, 369–374. doi:10.1097/NMC.0b013e3182a1fc4b

Murgatroyd, C., Wu, Y., Bockmuhl, Y., & Spengler, D. (2010). Genes learn from stress. *Epigenetics, 5*, 194–199. doi:10.4161/epi.5.3.11375

Urban Child Institute. (n.d.). *Baby's brain begins now: Conception to age 3*. Retrieved from http://www.urbanchildinstitute.org/why-0-3/baby-and-brain

CHAPTER 8

Fetal Alcohol Spectrum Disorder

LEANNE ELIZABETH ROHLF

Fetal alcohol spectrum disorder (FASD) is a group of disorders that can occur when the fetus experiences intrauterine exposure to alcohol. Alcohol present in a developing fetus's bloodstream can interfere with the development of the brain and other critical organs, structures, and physiological systems (National Institute of Alcohol Abuse and Alcoholism [NIAAA], 2017). Prenatal exposure to alcohol can permanently damage the developing fetus and is the leading *preventable* cause of birth defects as well as intellectual and neurodevelopmental disabilities (Williams, Smith, & Committee on Substance Abuse, 2015). Often a person with FASD has a combination of physical, mental, behavioral, and learning difficulties throughout their life span. This chapter discusses FASDs, and includes strategies for prevention including early identification of maternal alcohol use during pregnancy, appropriate screenings for both the mother and child, and interventions and treatments for the child throughout adolescence. *Intercepting* alcohol use during pregnancy should be a major goal for *all* healthcare professionals, including but not limited to adult primary healthcare providers, obstetricians, dentists, and pediatric primary care providers (P-PCPs), which includes pediatricians, pediatric and family nurse practitioners, and physician assistants. Primary prevention is key to eliminating the devastating effects on the developing fetus and the adverse outcomes the child experiences throughout their lifetime.

■ STATISTICAL DATA

The exact numbers of how many children and adults living with FASD is not known because often the biological mother refuses to admit consumption of alcohol during pregnancy. The Centers for Disease Control and Prevention (CDC, 2017) reports that among pregnant women one in 10 reported some alcohol use and one in 33 reported binge drinking in the past 30 days (Figure 8.1). The highest prevalence of use in pregnancy were that of 35- to 44-year-olds, college graduates, and unmarried women. Additionally, FASDs are commonly undetected or misdiagnosed. Many symptoms of FASD can mirror other disorders

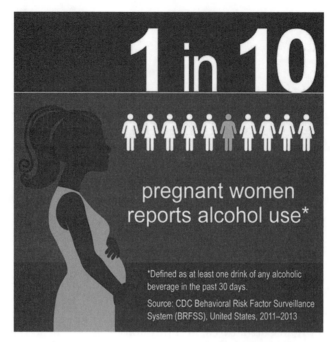

FIGURE 8.1 Alcohol use by pregnant women.

including attention deficit disorders, depression, anxiety, conduct, and impulse disturbance disorders.

There are minimal estimates available for the full range of people living with FASD. Based on community studies using physical examinations, experts estimate that the full range of FASDs in the United States and some Western European countries might number as high as two to five per 100 school children (CDC, 2017).

■ FETAL ALCOHOL SPECTRUM DISORDERS

The following medical disorders are identified under the term FASD in the *Diagnostic and Statistical Manual of Mental Disorders, Fifth Edition* ([DSM-5]; American Psychiatric Association [APA], 2013).

Fetal Alcohol Syndrome (FAS)

FAS resides on the most complex end of the spectrum of FASD and has strict diagnostic criteria. Children diagnosed with FAS must meet three specific criteria: facial abnormalities, growth deficits, and display central nervous system (CNS) abnormalities.

Alcohol-Related Neurodevelopmental Disorders (ARNDs)

Individuals with ARND do not have the FAS facial abnormalities, but may have developmental disabilities, including structural and/or functional CNS dysfunction (brain damage) with behavioral and learning problems (National Organization on Fetal Alcohol Syndrome [NOFAS], 2017).

Alcohol-Related Birth Defects (ARBD)

ARBD describes the physical defects linked to prenatal alcohol exposure, including heart, skeletal, kidney, ear, and eye malformations in the absence of apparent neurobehavioral or brain disorders (NOFAS, 2017).

Partial Fetal Alcohol Syndrome (pFAS)

The child with a diagnosis of pFAS does not meet full criteria for FAS. However, most often, a history of maternal alcohol consumption during pregnancy is elicited postnatally, and the child displays some facial, growth, or CNS abnormalities (NOFAS, 2017).

Neurobehavioral Disorder Associated With Prenatal Alcohol Exposure (ND-PAE)

A new criterion for FASD was published in the *DSM-5* (APA, 2013) that indicates a new psychiatric diagnosis under the name Neurobehavioral Disorder Associated with Prenatal Alcohol Exposure (ND-PAE). This disorder is associated with evidence of prenatal alcohol exposure and CNS involvement, as indicated by impairments in the following three areas: cognition, self-regulation, and adaptive functioning (NIAAA, 2017).

Pathophysiological Affects of Intrauterine Alcohol Exposure

FASD is considered a disorder of brain development. Alcohol is a teratogen that results in dysmorphia of the growing fetus through interference with nerve cell development and functioning. Alterations are seen in the ability of cells to grow and survive with an increased formation of cell-damaging free radicals. These cellular alterations can lead to altered pathways of biochemical signals within the cell and altered expression of certain genes and genetic information (CDC, 2017).

The developing fetus lacks the ability to process or metabolize alcohol through the liver and other organs. When a pregnant woman drinks alcohol, it easily passes across the placenta to the fetus and disrupts normal patterns of fetal development. The CNS develops in the first weeks of pregnancy. Alcohol intake during the first 3 to 8 weeks of pregnancy has the potential to cause damage to the developing brain. The impairments associated with FASD are often related to underlying structural changes in the brain. Brain imaging might reveal decreases in brain size, damage to the basal ganglia, and reduced size of the cerebellum (Tsang, Lucas, Olson, Pinto, & Elliott, 2016).

■ PREVENTION OF FASD

P-PCPs have the responsibility to educate women of childbearing age on the risks of alcohol consumption during pregnancy (Fetal Alcohol Spectrum

Disorders, 2016). There are many misconceptions about the safety of alcohol in pregnancy. Women should be informed that there are no known safe amounts of alcohol to consume at any time during pregnancy. To fully prevent FASD, a woman should not drink alcohol at any time during the pregnancy, or when she is planning or trying to start a family. The P-PCP should provide this information to women of child-bearing age and conduct routine alcohol screenings, using the Audit-C tool (smasha.gov) that quickly assesses alcohol use and abuse with a three-item questionnaire, as well as suggest immediate interventions and referrals for counseling. Cognitive behavioral therapy (CBT), and/or referral for other psychotherapeutic interventions are measures that may *intercept* the transmission of alcohol to the fetus, since the mother would be identified early and receive treatment to stop alcohol use during pregnancy. It is critical for all healthcare providers to realize that no one person can be excluded from testing, as women who drink are from all socioeconomic backgrounds and educational levels. Failure to screen every pregnant woman represents a missed opportunity to identify women who are secretly using alcohol, which subsequently results in adverse effects on her unborn baby.

Furthermore, women must be informed that the effect of alcohol can include physical, behavioral, and learning problems for the child throughout the life span. Neural cell growth takes place on a continuum throughout gestation and the presence of alcohol at any time during pregnancy creates the risk of permanent changes in neural development (Clarren, Salmon, & Johnson, 2011; Walker, Edwards, & Herrington, 2016). The message must be strong and presented in a meaningful way. Every woman of childbearing age must clearly understand the adverse consequences of alcohol consumption on the growing fetus. How that message is delivered is very important. Quiet nonintrusive history-taking is step one. Using the skill set of motivational interviewing is an effective strategy to enable women to participate in understanding the adverse outcomes for their child. Motivational interviewing permits women to be active participants in the decision-making process to avoid alcohol throughout pregnancy or to seek assistance to stop alcohol intake if there is a history of alcohol use or abuse. Based on the conversation, primary care providers can intercept intrauterine alcohol exposure by referring women for counseling and to alcohol anonymous (AA) meetings. Referrals are most effective when made prior to pregnancy; however, referrals should be made during pregnancy as soon as an alcohol problem is identified.

FASD is strongly associated with higher levels of alcohol consumption but even a single occurrence of alcohol use may lead to changes in fetal brain cell development (Wattendorf & Muenke, 2005). Nearly half of all pregnancies in the United States are unplanned, and many women do not know they are pregnant until 4 to 6 weeks after conception. This leaves time in which a woman may unknowingly expose the unborn fetus to alcohol, causing potential permanent damage to the fetus's brain development. The pattern of alcohol consumption—higher amount, faster rate, and/or greater frequency—is the key teratogenic factor (Walker et al., 2016). According to the Institute of Medicine (1996), of all the substances of abuse (including cocaine, heroin, and marijuana), alcohol produces by far the most serious neurobehavioral effects in the fetus.

■ SCREENING FOR ALCOHOL IN PRIMARY CARE PRACTICES

The effects of alcohol exposure in the infant and young child can be difficult to detect due to significantly varying signs and symptoms. Early identification of prenatal alcohol exposure can lead to earlier interventions. This early recognition can create opportunities for additional assessments, monitoring of developmental delays, and referrals to help find services and supports for both the child and family. Two screening tools that can be used in primary care settings are the CRAFFT tool (which represents an acronym for specific questions asked of a teenager [car, relax, alone, forgot, friends, trouble] related to drug and alcohol use) (American Academy of Pediatrics [AAP], 2018; Children's Hospital Boston, 2009), which is recommended for adolescents, and the Audit C (Bradley et al., 2003; Bush, Kivlahan, McDonell, Fihn, & Bradley, 1998), which is recommended for use in adults but may also be used in the adolescent population.

In the newborn, a common way to identify prenatal alcohol exposure is the analysis of meconium for the presence of fatty acid ethyl esters (The Problems of Making a Diagnosis of FAS/FASD in the Neonatal Period, 2015). This method helps detect any alcohol exposures during the second and third trimesters. The reported levels of fatty acid ethyl esters may help interpret the amount of intrauterine alcohol exposure. Using the information obtained through analysis of the meconium, the infant and young child can be screened and tested at an earlier age to evaluate their development and plan early intervention services. Another screening method is to obtain a urine or blood sample from the newborn immediately or soon after birth to determine the presence or absence of alcohol in the newborn's system.

It is critical to remember that the role of the P-PCP in screening for FASD is to be knowledgeable and aware of ways to prevent fetal exposure to alcohol throughout the pregnancy. In addition, the P-PCP must have the skill set to identify signs and symptoms of possible FASD in the young pediatric patient. Providers are responsible to provide nonjudgmental education for the family and make appropriate and timely referrals.

In addition, a new recommendation from the American Academy of Pediatrics is to screen parents who may have been raised in a home with an alcoholic parent (Williams, Smith, & Committee on Substance Abuse, 2015). The literature on toxic stress shows that parents who have been raised by alcoholic parents may experience parenting problems. For more detailed information on screening parents and the effects on parenting, please refer to Chapter 32 on toxic stress and Chapter 33 on trauma-informed care.

■ DIAGNOSIS OF FASD

P-PCPs should consider the diagnosis of FASD when assessing any child who presents with developmental, behavioral, or school difficulties (Table 8.1). In comparison to the general population, individuals with FASD have a higher incidence of concurrent psychiatric, emotional, and behavioral problems (Williams, et al., 2016). Other comorbid conditions include mood disorders, attention deficit

TABLE 8.1

SYMPTOMS IN CHILDREN WITH FASD

- Facial abnormalities including small eye openings, smooth, wide philtrum, and thin upper lip
- Delayed development and problems with speech, coordination, or social skills
- Poor intrauterine growth
- Poor growth after birth
- Decreased muscle tone and coordination
- Poor reasoning, impaired judgment, and inability to understand consequences
- Hyperactive, impulsive, and aggressive behavior
- Vision and hearing abnormalities
- Poor sucking and feeding in infancy
- Difficulties in school and low IQ

FASD, fetal alcohol spectrum disorder.

hyperactivity disorders (ADHD), substance use disorders, and suicide. Delayed diagnosis and treatment often correspond to higher levels of one or more of these comorbid conditions.

Currently, a confirmed diagnosis of FASD is made by medical providers and psychologists with specific training in the evaluation and diagnosis of FASD. There are several methods in which these experts evaluate a child for a diagnosis of FASD. Research continues to explore diagnostic techniques with the goal of creating a standard for the diagnosis. Each of the current methods used in clinical practice today supports obtaining information through history, physical examination, and neurodevelopment within four health parameters: (a) prenatal and postnatal growth, (b) facial features, (c) brain development and cognitive function, (d) and exposure to alcohol in utero (Benz, Rasmussen, & Andrew, 2009).

A child who is screened and thought to have a differential diagnosis of FASD should be referred to a developmental pediatrician or agency specialized in the assessment, diagnosis, and treatment of children with presentations suggestive of FASD. The specialists can then confirm or rule out the diagnosis of FASD. Having a formal diagnosis of FASD helps to guide families to available resources and to establish appropriate treatment goals and expectations for the child.

Children with FASD often have specific facial features that are characteristic of intrauterine exposure to alcohol (Wilhoit, Edwards, & Herrington, 2017). For example, the P-PCP should measure the palpebral fissure length in children with facial features suggestive of FASD. The palpebral length will be short in children with FASD. The measurement can be obtained by using a small plastic ruler to measure the distance between the inner canthi and medial canthi and then the measurement is compared with an established canthi distance chart. In addition, children have a thin upper lip, and a smooth philtrum. Children may have low set ears, and frontal bossing. In addition to the facial features, the children experience cognitive delays that become more evident during the early school years when these children have difficulties learning to read, perform math problems, and often fail to achieve passing grades in their grade level.

Publicly available photos of infants and children with facial features of alcohol syndrome are available on the web at https://www.google.com/search?source=hp&ei=BqwGW8_nD4Ha5gKwgarwDg&q=photos+of+fetal+alcohol+syndrome&oq=photos+of+fetal+&gs_l=psy-ab.1.0.0l4j0i22i30k1l6.1612.5423.0.8038.18.11.0.1.1.0.244.437.0j1j1.3.0....0...1c.1.64.psy-ab..14.3.445.0...92.PTefvINkNCY.

■ TREATMENT OF FASD

There is no cure for children who have a diagnosis of FASD. The disorder affects the child throughout his or her life span. Treatment for a child with FASD depends on the severity of exposure and symptom presentation. The treatment plan for the child is designed to meet the individual needs of the particular child and is revised based on the child's progress in physical growth, social–emotional, intellectual, behavioral, and mental health development (Carpenter, Blackburn, & Egerton, 2014).

Although there is no cure for the abnormal brain development or negative effects due to fetal alcohol exposure, research shows that early intervention and treatment services can improve a child's cognitive and social development (CDC, 2017). It is important for children diagnosed with FASD to be identified as early as possible to establish services to meet their needs and facilitate success going forward. Each child's treatment will be individualized and may include modifications to medical care, school environment, family structures, and social relationships.

Medical Treatment

Medical treatment for a child diagnosed with FASD may include varying specialists based on their individual presentation and needs. Families of children with FASD commonly seek psychiatric services in order to manage behavior, mood, and learning difficulties (Carpenter et al., 2014). Medications commonly used in the treatment of children are varying ADHD medications, antidepressants, anxiety medications, neuroleptics, and mood stabilizers (Ozsarfati & Koren, 2015). Not all children require medications and some are helped best with individualized therapy. Some children respond to treatment with a combination of medications and therapy. For further information on these medications, please see Chapter 3.

The Role of the School District

School districts play a key role in identification and interception of difficulties with learning and behaviors. Often schools have the abilities to provide a range of support services for children with FASD, including special education programs, school counselors, psychologists, and occupational or other therapists. Children without access to special education programs early in life (early intervention services) are at an increased risk of developing long-term learning problems and often fall behind their peers.

Parenting

Often, the mother who abused alcohol during pregnancy is not responsible for the care of the newborn and infant immediately after birth. The caregiver may be the father, a grandparent, another relative, or the infant may be placed in out-of-home care. Regardless of who is parenting the newborn, infant, and later the child, the primary caregiver plays an important role in the treatment of the child with FASD. Often, children with FASD do not respond to typical styles of parenting and require modifications in the home (Brown, 2015). Suggestions for interacting with a child with FASD is summarized in Table 8.2. Specialized therapists are trained in parenting a child affected by alcohol and can assist in creating a home environment that works for the child and the family. P-PCPs should know their catchment area and the specific services available within the child's community that can provide these specialized services to the child and family.

■ SUMMARY

The CDC (2017) reports that among pregnant women one in 10 reported any alcohol use and one in 33 reported binge drinking in the past 30 days. Alcohol is a teratogen for every fetus who experiences intrauterine exposure to alcohol. FASD is completely preventable! The message "Do not drink alcohol while pregnant" is everywhere: posters in public venues and public transportation; liquor bottles; social media; and medical offices. So how do P-PCPs *intercept* this major problem and assure that women of childbearing age and, in particular, pregnant women embrace this message? First, talk about the relationship between alcohol and adverse consequences, including drinking and driving, to adolescents during routine visits. Let adolescents know the relationship between alcohol and the adverse consequences of alcohol intrauterine exposure. Volunteer to speak at high schools within your community. Advocate for children at every opportunity. Make opportunities happen in your community and in your office setting.

TABLE 8.2
SUGGESTIONS FOR INTERACTING WITH CHILDREN WITH FASD
• Create visual schedules • Maintain consistent structure and routine • Provide clear, simple directions • Review expectations • Use visual reminders when available • Utilize timers for chores and tasks • Provide consistent rewards and punishments • Maintain consistency among involved caregivers • Provide frequent positive reinforcement • Parents and all caregivers must practice patience and acceptance of limitations

FASD, fetal alcohol spectrum disorder.

In addition to public advocacy, the role of the P-PCPs is to screen and identify infants, children, and/or adolescents with suspected FASD. The P-PCP should refer the child to a provider who can conduct a full evaluation to confirm diagnosis as soon as possible. The P-PCP can lead the "medical home" care management for the child and family by remaining actively involved in the ongoing assessment and management of the changing needs of the child and family. Leading initiatives to improve the outcomes for the child with a diagnosis is a significant role for P-PCPs.

P-PCPs also have the knowledge, skills, and ability to screen women of reproductive age and initiate referrals by making the appointment with the woman for a substance use evaluation. Follow-up for these referrals is essential, as many women may not recognize the need for care and fail to keep the medical appointments, counseling, or attendance at AA meetings.

■ REFERENCES

American Academy of Pediatrics. (2018). The CRAFFT Screening Questions. Retrieved from https://brightfutures.aap.org/Bright%20Futures%20Documents/CRAFFT.pdf

American Psychiatric Association. (2013). *Diagnostic and statistical manual of mental disorders* (5th ed., pp. 86, 798–801). Washington, DC: Author. doi:10.1176/appi.books.9780890425596

Benz, J., Rasmussen, C., & Andrew, G. (2009). Diagnosis of fetal alcohol spectrum disorder: History, challenges, and future directions. *Paediatric Child Health*, 14, 213–237. doi:10.1093/pch/14.4.231

Bradley, K. A., Bush, K. R., Epler, A. J., Dobie, D. J., Davis, T. M., Sporleder, J. L., . . . Kivlahan, D. R. (2003). Two brief alcohol-screening tests form the alcohol use disorders identification test (AUDIT-C): Validation in a female veteran affairs patient population. *Archives of Internal Medicine*, 163, 821–829. Retrieved from https://www.integration.samhsa.gov/images/res/tool_auditc.pdf

Brown, J. (2015). The challenges of caring for a child with FASD. *Adoption & Fostering*, 39(3), 247–255. doi:10.1177/0308575915599096

Bush, K., Kivlahan, D. R., McDonell, M. B., Fihn, S. D., & Bradley K. A. (1998). The AUDIT alcohol consumption questions (AUDIT-C): An effective brief screening test for problem drinking. *Archives of Internal Medicine*, 3, 1789–1795. Retrieved from https://www.integration.samhsa.gov/images/res/tool_auditc.pdf

Carpenter, B., Blackburn, C., & Egerton, J. (2014). *Fetal alcohol spectrum disorders: Interdisciplinary perspectives*. New York, London: Routledge.

Centers for Disease Control and Prevention. (2017). *FASD*. Retrieved from https://www.cdc.gov/ncbddd/fasd/

Children's Hospital Boston. (2009). *The CRAFFT screening interview*. Retrieved from http://www.ceasar-boston.org/CRAFFT/pdf/CRAFFT_English.pdf

Clarren, S., Salmon, A., & Jonsson, E. (2011). *Prevention of fetal alcohol spectrum disorder FASD: Who is responsible?* Weinheim, Germany: Wiley-Blackwell. doi:10.1002/9783527635481

Fetal alcohol spectrum disorders: Prevention, identification, and intervention. (2016). *The Nurse Practitioner*, 41(8), 34–35. doi:10.1097/01.NPR.0000490194.34920.90

Institute of Medicine. (1996). *Fetal alcohol syndrome: Diagnosis, epidemiology, prevention, and treatment*. Washington, DC: National Academies Press. Retrieved from http://www.come-over.to/FAS/IOMsummary.htm

National Institute of Alcohol Abuse and Alcoholism. (2017). *Fetal Alcohol Exposure*. Retrieved from https://www.niaaa.nih.gov/alcohol-health/fetal-alcohol-exposure

National Organization on Fetal Alcohol Syndrome. (2017). *FASD*. Retrieved from https://www.nofas.org/about-fasd/

Ozsarfati, J., & Koren, G. (2015). Medications used in the treatment of disruptive behavior in children with FASD--a guide. *Journal De La Thérapeutique Des Populations Et De La Pharamcologie Clinique* [Journal of Population Therapeutics and Clinical Pharmacology], 22(1), e59.

Photos of children with fetal alcohol syndrome. (2018). Retrieved from: https://www.google.com/search?source=hp&ei=BqwGW8_nD4Ha5gKwgarwDg&q=photos+of+fetal+alcohol+syndrome&o

q=photos+of+fetal+&gs_l=psy-ab.1.0.0l4j0i22i30k1l6.1612.5423.0.8038.18.11.0.1.1.0.244.437.0j1j1.
3.0....0...1c.1.64.psy-ab..14.3.445.0...92.PTefvINkNCY

Substance Abuse and Mental Health Services Administration. (2018). The Audit-C. Retrieved from https://www.integration.samhsa.gov/images/res/tool_auditc.pdf

The problems of making a diagnosis of FAS/FASD in the neonatal period. (2015). *Adoption & Fostering, 39*(3), 270–274. doi:10.1177/0308575915598939

Tsang, T., Lucas, B., Olson, H., Pinto, R., & Elliott, E. (2016). Prenatal alcohol exposure, FASD, and child behavior: A meta-analysis. *Pediatrics, 137*(3), e20152542–e20152542. doi:10.1542/peds.2015-2542

Walker, D. S., Edwards, W. E. R., & Herrington, C. (2016). Fetal alcohol spectrum disorders: Prevention, identification, and intervention. *The Nurse Practitioner, 41*(8), 28–34. doi:10.1097/01. NPR.0000488709.67444.92

Wattendorf, D. J., & Muenke, M. (2005). Fetal alcohol spectrum disorders. *American Family Physician, 72*(2), 279.

Wilhoit, L. F., Scott, D. A., & Simecka, B. A. (2017). Fetal alcohol spectrum disorders: Characteristics, complications, and treatment. *Community Mental Health Journal, 53*, 711–718. doi:10.1007/s10597-017-0104-0. [Epub 2017 Feb 6].

Williams, J. F., Smith, V. C., & Committee on Substance Abuse. (2015). Fetal alcohol spectrum disorders. *Pediatrics, 136*, e1395–e1406, e1395–e1406. doi:10.1542/peds.2015-3113

CHAPTER 9

Case Study: Failure to Thrive or Child Abuse

JAMES T. MULHOLLAND, STEPHANIE BROWN, AND PAULA BARBEL

CASE PRESENTATION

Chief Complaint

An 8-month-old female infant was seen in her home 2 days ago, by a Child Protective Service (CPS) worker who was making a visit for another child, when she noticed that the infant looked thin and had concerning markings on her face and arms. She instructed the mother to bring the infant to the pediatric primary care office.

◼ COMPREHENSIVE HISTORY

Case Worker Report

An 8-month-old female presented to the pediatric primary care office for an evaluation based on concerns raised by a CPS worker who had visited the home 2 days prior to the infant coming into the office. The infant was accompanied by her biological mother and three siblings. The infant lived with her mother, three siblings aged 2, 5, and 7, and the mother's boyfriend. The biological mother was the primary caregiver for the infant. The CPS worker had been at the infant's home for an unrelated issue and noticed the infant looked thin and had concerning markings on her body that the CPS worker felt may be consistent with possible physical abuse, neglect, and undernourishment. The CPS worker instructed the mother to bring her baby to the clinic for further evaluation.

◼ HISTORY OF PRESENT ILLNESS (HPI)

During the history, the mother stated, "My baby's bruises are mostly accidental, but sometimes, the infant just hurts herself." The mother reported the infant is always trying to sit up from a lying position and she fell forward and a little later, the mother saw the bruises on the baby's face. The mother explained the multiple scratch marks on the infant by stating, "My infant scratches her scalp all the time." She also reported that her rings accidently scratch the infant on her back during bathing the infant and/or changing the diaper. Furthermore, the mother reported that within the past few days, the infant's arm was stuck in a laundry basket and the arm was bruised when she pulled the arm too hard to remove it from the basket.

The mother reported that she discontinued the formula because she felt formula was unnatural and preferred feeding the baby whole milk and table food. The mother also reported a diaper rash for the past 4 days which she felt was caused by some loose stools. Some of the new table foods do not seem to agree with the baby, but said, "The baby will adjust...I fed my other three children the same way with home-made foods and they are just fine."

■ BIRTH AND PERTINENT INFANT HISTORY

The infant was born prematurely at 32 weeks' gestational age at a community hospital. The newborn experienced respiratory distress and was transferred to a pediatric hospital with a neonatal intensive care unit (NICU). At the onset of labor, the mother was unaware that she was pregnant; therefore, she did not receive any prenatal care. She admitted to using alcohol a few times a week and smoking half a pack of cigarettes a day. The infant's parents were not involved in her care in the NICU and did not return to the hospital when she was ready for discharge; thus she was placed in foster care.

The infant remained in foster care until she was 5 months old. She was initially described as a "colicky baby," and suffered from gastroesophageal reflux disease (GERD). It was reported that the infant did not smile, coo, or babble during the first 5 months of life. The infant was returned back to her biological mother when she was 5 up to 8 months of age. She presented to her primary care office at age 8 months in accordance with CPS instructions.

Allergies: No known allergies
Medications: No prescribed medications; no vitamins or supplements

■ FAMILY HISTORY

Mother: 32 years old, with a history of alcohol use on a weekly basis, and daily tobacco use; negative medical history
Father: 39 years old, but the infant's mother does not know his location and has not had any contact with him since the baby was born.
Siblings: Three siblings, ages 7, 5, and 2; children are healthy

■ PHYSICAL EXAMINATION: PERTINENT FINDINGS

General: The physical examination revealed a decline in body weight from the 53rd percentile down to the 1st percentile. Her height velocity was stable. She appeared thin and undernourished.

Skin: Bruises were present on the face in several locations and in various stages of healing. There was a circular area of bruising to her left upper arm. There was a linear abrasion to the posterior scalp. There were two small, circular areas of bruising to the midline of the lower back. No bruising was visible on the abdomen. There was a significant diaper rash, without evidence of vaginal or anal trauma.

Head: The anterior fontanel was soft and flat. The scalp was negative for scalp hematomas, Battle's sign, or raccoon eyes.

Eyes: Her pupils were reactive to light; equal, and visual tracking was normal.

Ears: The tympanic membrane had no evidence of hemotympanum.

Musculoskeletal: There was full range of motion and no tenderness to palpation on any extremity. She was not able to sit on her own without support except for about 2 seconds. She was not observed falling forward while sitting, and she was not observed attempting to sit while lying prone.

■ SCREENINGS

The Denver Developmental Screening Test II (DDST II) was performed on this child. The results showed delays in all areas, including personal–social, fine motor, language, and gross motor development, even with chronological age correction of 8 weeks for prematurity, which requires a referral for early intervention services. The mother was asked to complete the Ages and Stages Infant Questionnaire. The mother's responses on this questionnaire were not consistent with the findings on the DDST II, which demonstrated the mother's lack of awareness of the infant's delayed development.

■ DIFFERENTIAL DIAGNOSES

Failure to Thrive

The most concerning finding with this infant is the failure to thrive (FTT). FTT is not a diagnosis; thus a pediatric primary care provider (P-PCP) must investigate the causes of the infant's FTT and treat the underlying causes.

UNDERLYING CAUSES OF FTT TO CONSIDER IN THIS CASE

Numerous conditions as causes of FTT should be considered as differential diagnoses, including organic disorders, food refusal, idiopathic low intake, dysfunctional feeding, illness, neglect, and fetal alcohol syndrome. Organic disorders include such disorders as milk allergy, GERD, and celiac disease and result in mostly malabsorption of needed nutrients (Levine et al., 2011; Levy et al., 2009; Nangia & Tiwari, 2013). Thirty-five percent of children with FTT have some type of organic disorder (Levy et al., 2009).

Food aversion or food refusal tends to peak around 5.6 months of age (Levy et al., 2009). Dysfunctional feeding includes the over- or under-dilution of formula, inadequate food availability, poor breastfeeding, and neglect (Nangia &

Tiwari, 2013). Chronic infections or malignancy may increase the child's caloric demands, which may not be matched by the caloric intake (Nangia & Tiwari, 2013). Genetic disorders such as Trisomy 21 and metabolic disorders like inborn errors of metabolism results in a poor utilization of nutrients required to maintain an adequate bodyweight (Nangia & Tiwari, 2013).

Neglect and *child abuse* are the leading differential in this case especially when FTT is coupled with developmental delays and the presenting physical injuries, for example, bruising to the face, forehead, ears, extremities, or trunk of the body (Nangia & Tiwari, 2013; Sheets et al., 2013). These injuries are not consistent with the history provided by the mother.

■ DIAGNOSTIC TESTS AND CRITERIA

Diagnostic testing to evaluate FTT requires blood, urine, stool, and additional testing to rule out infections, chronic diseases, inflammatory conditions, immunodeficiency, and malabsorption. Additional specialized testing can be done to rule out rarer disorders (Nangia & Tiwari, 2013). Specific testing that may be considered for this infant is listed in Table 9.1.

TABLE 9.1

DIAGNOSTIC TESTING
• Complete blood count
• Comprehensive metabolic panel
• Phosphorus and magnesium
• Thyroid stimulating hormone
• Free thyroxine
• HIV (results can be obtained from the newborn screen)
• C-reactive protein or erythrocyte sedimentation rate
• Celiac serologies
• Allergy testing (allergy testing was not needed in this case as there was no evidence of allergies affecting the infant's development)
• Hemoglobin A1C
• Urinalysis and culture
• Stool fecal elastase
• Sweat chloride testing
• Genetic testing (based on presentation, it was not needed in this case)
• Additional testing may include plain radiographs, ultrasound, and CT scan

Sources: Blood testing: Harper, N. S. (2014). Neglect: Failure to thrive and obesity. *Pediatric Clinics of North America*, *61*(5), 937–957. doi:10.1016/j.pcl.2014.06.006; Nangia, S., & Tiwari, S. (2013). Failure to thrive. *Indian Journal of Pediatrics*, *80*(7), 585–589. doi:10.1007/s12098-013-1003-1; Rabago, J., Marra, K., Allmendinger, N., & Shur, N. (2015). The clinical geneticist and the evaluation of failure to thrive versus failure to feed. *American Journal of Medical Genetics. Part C, Seminars in Medical Genetics*, *169*(4), 337–348. doi:10.1002/ajmg.c.31465

Additional testing: Christian, C. W., Block, R., Committee on Child Abuse and Neglect, & American Academy of Pediatrics. (2009). Abusive head trauma in infants and children. *Pediatrics*, *123*(5), 1409–1411. doi:10.1542/peds.2009-0408

The blood work revealed iron deficiency anemia, which is consistent with early introduction of cow's milk before 12 months of age. All other serology testing was within normal limits.

A radiology consult was made to determine if the injuries the infant experienced were consistent with nonaccidental trauma (NAT). Radiographs to assess for fractures in various stages of healing were performed; ultrasounds to assess for soft tissue injuries, especially to abdominal organs, or more advanced imaging (Christian, Block, Committee on Child Abuse and Neglect, & American Academy of Pediatrics, 2009; Sheets et al., 2013) may be conducted. In this case, there was evidence of three healing fractures to the upper extremities sustained at different times; no skull fractures or other fractures were identified.

With all cases of suspected child abuse, and this case specifically due to the injuries to the head, one must consider different types of head injuries. Concerning head injuries include subdural hematomas, localized brain contusions or shearing injuries, skull fracture, epidural hemorrhages, and retinal hemorrhage (Christian et al., 2009; Jenny, Hymel, Ritzen, Reinart, & Hay, 1999). If any of these injuries were present, a neurosurgical and ophthalmology consult would have been made (Christian et al., 2009).

Medical providers are mandated reporters of suspected child abuse and neglect, and a referral to CPS and law enforcement must be made (Christian et al., 2009). The referral was made to CPS for this infant, and the infant was removed from her home, and her siblings were removed as well.

■ RED FLAGS

Red flags are defined as the recognition of signs and symptoms that lead to the formulation of differential diagnoses that must be investigated to rule in or out the possibility or presence of medical or surgical conditions that, if undiagnosed, placed the individual at increased risk for adverse healthcare outcomes and/or death (Anzaldua, 2010). There are numerous red flags present throughout this case. The initial red flag is the presentation of the infant's mother to the hospital at the time of delivery without any prenatal care, even though this is her fourth pregnancy. The next red flag is the mother's admission of using alcohol on a weekly basis throughout the pregnancy, even though she "did not know she was pregnant." In addition, the information presented that the mother was not involved in the care of her premature infant after delivery and the infant was placed in foster care is also a red flag for potential child maltreatment and neglect, when the infant was returned to the biological mother at 5 months.

The CPS worker identified red flags, such as "the infant looked thin and had concerning markings on her body," which the CPS worker felt may be consistent with possible physical abuse, neglect, and undernourishment at the home, and informed the mother to take the infant to the pediatric office. The mother did not arrive at the office for 48 hours. In retrospect, the CPS worker should have called in her concerns about the infant, and the infant should have been brought to the office or hospital on that day. The CPS worker should not have left the home, as she believed that the infant was not in a safe environment.

For fairness in evaluating any pediatric or adolescent of suspected or child maltreatment or neglect, the diagnostic workup by all P-PCPS must be objective and nonaccusatory. In this case, the mother's report on the history of the injuries was *not consistent* with the findings on the infant and the developmental abilities of the infant. Therefore, red flags were raised during the interview process.

Another red flag, in this case, is the information that the infant, while in foster care for the first 5 months of life, and prior to returning to the biological mother, did not smile, coo, or babble. Based on the history of maternal alcohol intake throughout the pregnancy, the infant's behavior in the first 5 months of life warrants a thorough evaluation for possible fetal alcohol syndrome. See Chapter 8 for a detailed discussion of fetal alcohol syndrome.

■ TREATMENT

The final diagnosis for this infant was FTT secondary to neglect with concern for NAT. CPS was notified and the infant was hospitalized for further evaluation. She was treated for iron deficiency anemia (IDA), placed on formula and infant foods, an iron supplement, multivitamin, and she began to gain weight in the hospital. The infant was removed from the care of her biological mother and placed in foster care. See Chapter 30 for discussion on child abuse and maltreatment including neglect.

■ SUMMARY

This infant presented to the primary care office with clinical evidence of FTT and possible physical abuse and neglect. A comprehensive history, physical examination, and diagnostic testing, including serology and radiology testing based on presentation, are the standard of care for infants and children presenting with similar symptoms and concerns of child maltreatment or neglect. The P-PCP must intercept any possibility for further injury to any infant, child, or adolescent presenting to care by notifying CPS of the findings and the infant/child must be removed from the home, if the home environment is determined to be unsafe.

In this case, the infant was returned to foster care due to neglect and physical abuse in the biological home that had manifested in her FTT and physical injuries. Approximately 37% of children return to foster care following reunification with their biological families (Lee, Jonson-Reid, & Drake, 2012). As is consistent with this case, children placed into foster care are more likely to be in fair to poor health, have learning disabilities, developmental delays, and speech delays (Turney & Wildeman, 2016). This infant had significant weight gain after re-entering foster care. She received speech therapy and physical therapy services to help her attain developmental milestones in all areas of delayed development. The parental rights of the biological parents were terminated and plans were made for the foster care parents to adopt the infant. It is the responsibility of the P-PCPs to protect the infant, provide supportive care to the foster parents, monitor the growth and development of the infant, and refer the infant promptly for any early intervention services that are needed to enable the infant to achieve optimal health.

■ REFERENCES

Anzaldua, D. A. (2010).Medical red flags. Chapter 1. *An acupuncturist's guide to medical red flags and referrals*. Boulder, CO: Blue Poppy Enterprises.

Christian, C. W., Block, R., Committee on Child Abuse and Neglect, & American Academy of Pediatrics. (2009). Abusive head trauma in infants and children. *Pediatrics, 123*(5), 1409–1411. doi:10.1542/peds.2009-0408

Harper, N. S. (2014). Neglect: Failure to thrive and obesity. *Pediatric Clinics of North America, 61*(5), 937–957. doi:10.1016/j.pcl.2014.06.006

Jenny, C., Hymel, K. P., Ritzen, A., Reinert, S. E., & Hay, T. C. (1999). Analysis of missed cases of abusive head trauma. *JAMA, 281*(7), 621–626. doi:10.1001/jama.281.7.621

Lee, S., Jonson-Reid, M., & Drake, B. (2012). Foster care re-entry: Exploring the role of foster care characteristics, in-home child welfare services and cross-sector services. *Children and Youth Services Review, 34*(9), 1825–1833. doi:10.1016/j.childyouth.2012.05.007

Levine, A., Bachar, L., Tsangen, Z., Mizrachi, A., Levy, A., Dalal, I., . . . Boaz, M. (2011). Screening criteria for diagnosis of infantile feeding disorders as a cause of poor feeding or food refusal. *Journal of Pediatric Gastroenterology and Nutrition, 52*(5), 563–568. doi:10.1097/MPG.0b013e3181ff72d2

Levy, Y., Levy, A., Zangen, T., Kornfeld, L., Dalal, I., Samuel, E., . . . Levine, A. (2009). Diagnostic clues for identification of nonorganic vs organic causes of food refusal and poor feeding. *Journal of Pediatric Gastroenterology and Nutrition, 48*(3), 355–362. doi:00005176-200903000-00021

Nangia, S., & Tiwari, S. (2013). Failure to thrive. *Indian Journal of Pediatrics, 80*(7), 585–589. doi:10.1007/s12098-013-1003-1

Rabago, J., Marra, K., Allmendinger, N., & Shur, N. (2015). The clinical geneticist and the evaluation of failure to thrive versus failure to feed. *American Journal of Medical Genetics. Part C, Seminars in Medical Genetics, 169*(4), 337–348. doi:10.1002/ajmg.c.31465

Sheets, L. K., Leach, M. E., Koszewski, I. J., Lessmeier, A. M., Nugent, M., & Simpson, P. (2013). Sentinel injuries in infants evaluated for child physical abuse. *Pediatrics, 131*(4), 701–707. doi:10.1542/peds.2012-2780

Turney, K., & Wildeman, C. (2016). Mental and physical health of children in foster care. *Pediatrics, 138*(5), e20161118. Epub 2016 Oct 17. doi:10.1542/peds.2016-1118

Identifying and Intercepting Behavioral Health Problems in Children With Inborn Errors of Metabolism

BOBBIE SALVESON

Inborn errors of metabolism (IEM) are comprised of single gene defects that result in a decrease in function or absence of a specific enzyme leading to an accumulation of toxic compounds. Many disorders are autosomal recessive inheritance, and the incidence is increased in communities with high levels of consanguinity. These disorders may present in severe forms in the neonatal period or less severe forms later in life (Ahrens-Nicklas, Slap, & Ficicioglu, 2015). All of the IEM have a spectrum of severity, from neonatal death to multiple nonspecific symptoms occurring later in life. Some of these symptoms are behavioral/psychiatric in nature and may include speech disorders, learning disabilities, behavioral issues, attention deficit hyperactivity disorder (ADHD), depression, anxiety, and psychosis. These psychiatric symptoms may be the reason families initially seek help from a behavioral health specialist. While these disorders are rare, patients born in areas without newborn screening, older patients with atypical psychotic features, or treatment resistance in patients with mood disorders should be referred to a metabolic geneticist for a diagnostic workup, as delays in diagnosis can result in irreversible damage (Walterfang, Bonnot, Mocellin, & Velakoulis, 2013).

A comprehensive medical review was done by Giannitelli et al. (2017) on the 160 patients in their child psychiatric unit, and it was found that 10% of the patients had an IEM, genetic disorder, or autoimmune disease. Patients with known IEM diagnosis may also display behavioral/psychiatric symptoms if unable to adhere to prescribed treatment. These patients may need referral to social work or other agencies to help procure treatment. This chapter presents assessment, diagnosis, and treatments for children with a diagnosis of IEM as well as insights into the comorbid behavioral health problems that may occur in these children. Early identification of potential comorbid behavioral health problems with the implementation of treatment plans in primary care settings may help *intercept* the display of symptoms of comorbid behavioral health problems for children with IEM.

■ NEWBORN SCREENING FOR IEM

In the United States, newborn screening has allowed for early detection and treatment for many IEM disorders. Over the past two decades, with the advent of expanded newborn screening, many disorders are diagnosed in the newborn period and treatment may be initiated early. The Recommended Uniform Newborn Screening Panel (RUSP) was established in 2006 by the Advisory Committee on Heritable Disorders and Genetic Diseases in Newborns and Children (ACHDGDNC) in the Department of Health and Human Services of the United States. The first panel had 29 core conditions and 25 secondary conditions; as of November 2016, the panel has 34 core conditions and 26 secondary conditions (ACHDGDNC, 2016). Once a condition is recommended for induction on the newborn screen panel, it may take several years to be included on a state panel. Since each state decides which conditions to include, there is no uniform time frame to assure all conditions are tested as newborns. For example, New York State began testing for maple syrup urine disease (MSUD) in 1975, but in Washington State, this test was not added to the panel until 2004 (Wadsworth Laboratory, 2017; Washington State Department of Health, 2017). States differ on policies for parental decision to opt out of the newborn screen, with only three states having mandatory screening (Kilakkathi, 2012). Medical providers differ on their opinions concerning mandatory inclusion of specific IEM on the newborn screen in their particular states. However, if the goal to diagnose as early as possible for any and all conditions in which interventions to intercept adverse outcomes is to be realized, then all medical providers should support mandatory newborn screening in every state (Hallas, 2016). Additionally, there are known IEM that are not yet included in newborn screening in the United States (IEMBase, 2017). Thus, many of the IEM that can be identified early in the newborn period to avoid adverse outcomes are not identified or treated at the earliest possible time frame. Worldwide, newborn screening is not uniform, often dependent on the ability to pay for screening, and may not be available to all newborns (Therrell et al., 2015).

■ GENETIC MUTATION ANALYSIS

As newborn screening has expanded, the ability to identify specific genetic mutations has also developed. Genetic mutation analysis has revealed many different mutations of the specific gene defect for each disorder, and scientists are learning which mutations correlate with more severe disease and which have a later onset, less severe phenotype. The combination of mutations creates a spectrum of disease severity. Some mutations present in the newborn period as severe disease; some are known to present in later childhood, adolescence, and even adulthood, with milder presentation. There are also mutations of unknown clinical significance as well as the unknown contribution of severe heterozygous mutations to disease (Pan & Vockley, 2013). Even with known mutations, the phenotypic presentation can differ between family members with the same mutation. This variability and the yet unknown contribution of novel mutations may result in symptomatic presentation outside of the newborn period, with behavioral/mental health symptoms being the initial presentation of an IEM (Argmann, Houten, Zhu, & Schadt, 2016).

Failure to adhere to treatment plans is a major factor in the potential development of behavioral and mental health problems in patients with confirmed IEM. Adherence to treatment is challenging, in particular, in light of the individual's and family's desire or ability to remain on the recommended diet or treatment plan. Pediatric primary care providers (P-PCPs) who are knowledgeable about the challenges may be better prepared to intercept the challenging behaviors, which may prevent some adverse effects associated with noncompliance to treatment plans. Special formulas used for amino acid supplementation have strong tastes and the limited protein diets (ranging from 0 to 20 g of natural protein/day) are very restrictive. In addition, these special formulas and foods required for treatment of many disorders are expensive and state mandates for insurance coverage vary per state law. A state review of insurance coverage for these formulas and foods found that 18 states required no coverage for adults and eight states required coverage for formula only, but not low protein foods (Berry et al., 2013). As children enter adolescence, compliance with their prescribed diet becomes even more challenging, resulting in emergence and exacerbation of behavioral and mental health problems and diagnoses.

■ PROHIBITIVE COSTS FOR TREATMENT

While pharmaceutical treatments are available for some of the disorders, the cost is prohibitive for many patients and families, even those with insurance. The cost of the oral drug Kuvan (sapropterin), a partial treatment for some patients with phenylketonuria (PKU), can range from $57,000 a year for a child to $200,000 a year for a large adult (Pollack, 2007). For the enzyme replacement drugs, delivered by monthly infusion, cost for the drug alone exceeds $50,000/year (Herper, 2012). Children and their families must also travel to infusion centers, which typically operate during regular business hours on weekdays, with some limited Saturday hours—requiring parents to be absent from their place of employment. Infusion centers also care for patients receiving all types of infusion therapy, including cancer chemotherapy, creating other scheduling issues. These drugs are delivered intravenously, and IV access can be painful, and difficult, resulting in patient's discontinuation of therapy (U.S. Food and Drug Administration, 2015).

■ IEM ASSOCIATED WITH MENTAL HEALTH PRESENTATIONS

A list of the IEM disorders with potential behavioral and mental health symptoms is presented in order of prevalence in Table 10.1. Each disorder is briefly described in this section including treatment considerations, typical mental health symptoms, and other presenting symptoms as applicable.

TABLE 10.1

INBORN ERRORS OF METABOLISM AND COMMON NEUROPSYCHIATRIC PRESENTATIONS

Name of Disorder	Prevalence*	Recommended Uniform Newborn Screening Panel (USA)	Treatment	Common Neuropsychiatric Symptoms
Phenylketonuria (PKU)	1:10,000 1:5,000 (Middle East)	Yes (1960s)	Dietary restriction of protein Sapropterin (Kuvan) Large neutral amino acids	Executive function concerns (attention deficits, memory problems, lack of impulse control) Depression Anxiety
Galactosemia	1:10,000	Yes (1960s)	Strict avoidance of galactose and lactose	Speech apraxia, dysarthria Learning disabilities Anxiety Depression
Congenital Adrenal Hyperplasia (CAH)	1:15,000	Yes (1970s)	Glucocorticoid therapy Mineralocorticoid therapy Sodium replacement	Depression Anxiety Substance abuse
X-Linked Adrenoleukodystrophy	1:20,000	Yes (2016)	Stem-cell transplant Lorenzo's oil Corticosteroid therapy	Mania Affective psychosis Cognitive impairment
Wilson Disease	1:30,000	No	Chelation therapy (penicillamine) Zinc Liver transplant (for liver failure)	Emotional lability Impulsiveness Disinhibition Self-injury

(continued)

TABLE 10.1   (CONTINUED)

INBORN ERRORS OF METABOLISM AND COMMON NEUROPSYCHIATRIC PRESENTATIONS

Name of Disorder	Prevalence*	Recommended Uniform Newborn Screening Panel (USA)	Treatment	Common Neuropsychiatric Symptoms
Urea Cycle Disorders (UCD)	1:35,000	Yes (2000s)	Dietary restriction of protein Avoidance of metabolic stress Nitrogen scavenging drugs	Eating disorders Hallucinations Acute psychosis Behavioral disorders
Cobalamin C Disorder (cblC)	1:37,000–1:100,000	Yes (2000s)	IM supplementation of hydroxycobalamin	Autism Intellectual disability Feeding disorder Depression (adolescence) Aggressive behavior (adolescence)
Gaucher Disease	1:50,000	No	Enzyme replacement Miglustat Avoidance of NSAIDs	Hypochondriasis Depression Neurosis
Fabry Disease	1:50,000–1:117,000	No	Pain medications (gabapentin) ACE inhibitor Enzyme replacement	Depression Anxiety Psychosis
Propionic Aciduria (PA)	1:105,000	Yes (2000s)	Dietary restriction of protein Avoidance of catabolic state L-carnitine supplementation Liver transplant	Autism Intellectual disability

(continued)

TABLE 10.1 (CONTINUED)

INBORN ERRORS OF METABOLISM AND COMMON NEUROPSYCHIATRIC PRESENTATIONS

Name of Disorder	Prevalence*	Recommended Uniform Newborn Screening Panel (USA)	Treatment	Common Neuropsychiatric Symptoms
Niemann–Pick type C Disease	1:150,000	No	None	Psychosis, cognitive decline (adolescent and adult)
Maple Syrup Urine Disease (MSUD)	1:185,000 1:380 (Mennonite)	Yes (2000s)	Liver transplant Dietary restriction of protein Isoleucine and leucine supplementation	ADHD Depression Anxiety
Homocystinuria (CBS) Methylenetetrahydrofolate Reductase (MTHFR)	1:200,000– 1:350,000 (much higher in some countries)	Yes (2000s)	Low protein diet Vitamin B$_{12}$ Folate Betaine (CbS) Pyroxene (MTHFR)	Intellectual disability (children) Psychosis (adolescents) Anxiety (adolescents) Obsessive-compulsive disorder (adolescents) (CbS type)
Porphyria	0.13:100,000 (Europe)	No	Symptomatic during attacks Avoid substance abuse Good nutritional intake	Anxiety Depression Altered mental status Psychosis

Note: *Prevalence data obtained from GeneReviews (GeneReviews®, 2017) online.
ACE, angiotensin converting enzyme; ADHD, attention deficit hyperactivity disorder; NSAIDs, nonsteroidal anti-inflammatory drugs.

Phenylketonuria

PKU is an autosomal recessive disorder causing a deficiency of the enzyme phenylalanine hydroxylase or cofactor tetrahydrobiopterin. In the United States, newborn screening identifies patients with PKU or other defects of tetrahydrobiopterin. If untreated, this disorder causes irreversible mental retardation with severe aggressive and self-injurious behavior.

Treatment is directed by a metabolic geneticist and consists of lifetime restriction of phenylalanine (Phe) using a protein-restricted diet. Diet is adjusted based on Phe levels in the blood. Supplementation of essential amino acids is accomplished using special formulas. Some individuals may be responsive to sapropterin (Kuvan), which allows for a greater intake of natural protein (Berry et al., 2013).

Results from a review by Gentile, Ten Hoedt, and Bosch (2010) revealed a 50% increased risk of moderate to severe symptoms of depression and anxiety, as well as deficits in executive function (attention, short-term memory, planning, organization, behavioral inhibition, and social interaction) in individuals with a diagnosis of PKU. These issues occur even in patients who have been on treatment all their lives, but are worse in those with less control of the Phe levels. Another study found the depressive symptoms were worse in those subjects with a higher degree of executive function impairment (Clacy, Sharman, & McGill, 2014).

Galactosemia

Galactosemia is an autosomal recessive disorder causing a deficiency of the enzyme galactose-1-phosphate uridyltransferase (Zschocke & Hoffmann, 2004). This disorder is identified on newborn screening. There is a spectrum of presentation, with the severe form presenting at birth and less severe forms at school age.

Treatment is directed by a metabolic geneticist and consists of lifetime elimination of lactose (all dairy products and human milk) and replacement with soy formula (Van Karnebeek & Stockler, 2012). Recommendations include ongoing neuropsychiatric testing for developmental delay, speech concerns, and learning disabilities.

In classical galactosemia, symptoms present in the newborn period, with poor feeding, lethargy, liver failure, and Escherichia coli sepsis; untreated symptoms and failure to diagnose leads to an increase in mortality rates. Older patients may experience central nervous system (CNS) issues, including learning disabilities, executive function deficits, speech and language disorders, and premature ovarian failure (Waisbren et al., 2012).

Unfortunately, literature suggests that even with treatment, patients may develop tremor, nutritional deficits, reduced bone density, diminished cognitive functioning, speech abnormalities, depression, and anxiety (Simons et al., 2006). A study of 33 adults with a diagnosis of galactosemia demonstrated that each 10-year increment of age was associated with a threefold increase in the odds of depression (Waisbren et al., 2012). Waisbren et al. (2012) suggested that the study results indicated a need for ongoing psychosocial evaluation with attention to depression and anxiety. Furthermore, they suggest that establishing social relationships may help decrease the negative impact galactosemia has on the individual.

Congenital Adrenal Hyperplasia

Congenital adrenal hyperplasia (CAH) is an autosomal recessive disorder that results in deficient cortisol and mineral corticoid production, which results in accumulation of steroid precursors that are converted to adrenal androgens. Exposure to androgens, starting in-utero, contributes to virilization, both physically and behaviorally (Engberg et al., 2015). CAH is identified via newborn screening.

Treatment is managed by an endocrinologist and includes lifetime replacement of glucocorticoids and mineralocorticoids as well as salt replacement during periods of metabolic stress. Unfortunately, exogenous replacement of steroids can result in overtreatment, resulting in issues with weight gain and mood disturbances (Brand et al., 2000).

Engberg et al. (2015) conducted an age-matched cohort study in Sweden and reviewed the medical records of 335 girls and women with a diagnosis of CAH. Study results revealed that women with CAH were twice as likely, compared with unaffected females, to be diagnosed with a mental and behavioral disorder due to psychoactive substance use, with an almost threefold increased risk of alcohol misuse. They also had twice the risk of being diagnosed with adjustment disorder. A small case review by Brand et al. (2000) described four young women with CAH who developed anorexia nervosa secondary to disturbed body image, suggesting a need for further studies in this area.

X-Linked Adrenoleukodystrophy

X-linked adrenoleukodystrophy (X-ALD) is an x-linked autosomal recessive disorder caused by a deficiency of enzymes or a problem with importing certain peroxisomal proteins, resulting in the buildup of very long chain fatty acids (Zschocke & Hoffmann, 2004). X-ALD was added to the recommended uniform screening panel in the United States in November 2016. Diagnosis is made by enzyme studies and mutation analysis. Measurement of serum organic acids will show elevations in very long chain fatty acids, and liver function studies may be abnormal (Giannitelli et al., 2017).

Treatment involves collaboration between a metabolic geneticist and neurologist and consists of bone marrow transplantation as soon as diagnosis is established, prior to onset of symptoms. Otherwise, treatment is only symptomatic. Lorenzo's oil may help symptomatically, but does not improve long-term outcomes. Adrenal steroid replacement therapy is necessary if Addison's disease is present, but has no effect on the cerebral manifestations of the disorder (Engelen et al., 2012).

Affecting more males than females, the earlier onset form of X-ALD presents between the ages of 4 and 10 years with behavioral problems, including increased aggression, intellectual regression, adrenal insufficiency, and leukodystrophy, progressing to decerebration and death within 2 to 4 years after diagnosis of X-ALD. In the later onset forms of the disorder, mania and affective psychosis are often presenting symptoms and can be treatment-resistant (Walterfang et al., 2013). Later onset forms of the disorder also may affect adult heterozygous women, but these women generally only present with myelopathy.

Wilson Disease

Wilson disease is an autosomal recessive disorder causing a defect in copper ATPase, which results in the inability to break down copper in the body, leading to an accumulation of copper in the liver, basal ganglia, and kidneys. Diagnosis is made by measuring serum ceruloplasmin, copper in the urine, and a liver biopsy to determine degree of hepatic damage (Nia, 2014).

Treatment is generally directed by a metabolic geneticist or neurologist. Chelation therapy using penicillamine is helpful, but must be initiated in early stages of the disease to avoid permanent brain damage (Nia, 2014). Dietary avoidance of copper (fish, liver) and zinc supplementation are also part of the treatment plan. Liver transplant may be recommended if cirrhosis is present on liver biopsy. Unfortunately, treating the psychiatric issues can be difficult, as antipsychotics can actually worsen the psychiatric symptoms for patients with Wilson disease. These patients also have an increased risk of developing neurological side effects from the antipsychotic medications (Bonnot, Herrera, Tordjman, & Walterfang, 2015).

There is a range of presentation in Wilson disease; however, 30% to 60% of patients may present with psychiatric symptoms as the first manifestation (Bonnot et al., 2015; Srinivas et al., 2008). Behavioral abnormalities range from mood disorders to personality changes, including aggressive behavior to schizophrenia with treatment resistance, and often extreme sensitivity to neuroleptic drugs (Bonnot et al., 2015; Srinivas et al., 2008). Other symptoms include Kayser–Fleischer rings, which present as a dark, brownish yellow ring around the iris, jaundice, and tremor (Zschocke & Hoffmann, 2004).

Urea Cycle Disorders

Urea cycle disorders result from a deficiency in one of the enzymes in the urea cycle (Zschocke & Hoffmann, 2004). Severity of the disease and presentation depend on which enzyme is deficient, as well as sex, with boys more severely affected than girls. The level of consciousness and long-term damage to the brain is determined by the toxic levels of ammonia and specific amino acids accumulated in the body. An absence or deficiency in the first four enzymes of the cycle results in a severe hyperammonemia when the newborn is 3 to 5 days old. Unfortunately, not all the urea cycle defects are detected on the newborn screen. Thus, the recommendation for any pediatric patient presenting with encephalopathy or unexplained confusion at any age is to obtain an ammonia level (Serrano et al., 2010).

Treatment consists of aggressive detoxification of ammonia. Long-term management includes avoiding metabolic stress, protein-restricted diet, and supplementation of arginine or citrulline depending on the missing enzyme. Sodium benzoate or sodium phenylbutyrate to keep ammonia levels low, vitamin and trace element supplementation, and carnitine supplementation are necessary in some patients (Zschocke & Hoffmann, 2004). It is imperative that a specialist manages these patients for ongoing laboratory testing and dietary adjustment.

Ornithine transcarbamylase deficiency is the most common defect (1:14,000) and will severely affect newborn males, but has an extremely variable presentation in females, even those who are carriers of the disorder. For the later onset forms of ornithine transcarbamylase deficiency, presenting symptoms may be attention deficits, learning difficulties, behavioral problems, or psychosis (Serrano et al., 2010; Tsai et al., 2007).

In urea cycle disorders, history may reveal unexplained vomiting, particularly after a meal high in protein, "picky" eating (avoidance of protein), and unexplained episodes of confusion. The only urea cycle disorder with physical findings is Argininosuccinic aciduria, which may present with lower extremity spasticity (Enns, 2008).

Cobalamin C Disorder

Cobalamin C (cblC) disorder is an autosomal recessive disorder that causes defects in the intracellular cobalamin pathway. This defect does not allow syntheses of methylcobalamin and adenosylcobalamin, resulting in a buildup of homocysteine and low plasma methionine levels. This disorder is identified on the newborn screening panel (Zschocke & Hoffmann, 2004). In older patients, total plasma homocysteine is elevated, plasma methionine is decreased, and urinary methylmalonic acid (MMA) is elevated. There is a variable presentation in patients with this disease: 90% present with the severe, early onset infantile form, while the other 10% of the children present after 12 months of age (Tsai et al., 2007). In infants with the severe form of the disease, presentation is hypotonia, poor feeding, failure to thrive, developmental delay, and decreased visual acuity. Even with treatment, many of these children have neurocognitive deficits. Children with later onset forms of cblC disorder may present with cognitive decline, ataxia, seizures, hemolytic uremic syndrome, and pulmonary arterial hypotension. Adolescents and adults present with symptoms of attention deficits, aggressive behavior, schizophrenic symptoms, and cognitive deficits. Physical symptoms may include neuropathy, ataxia, thromboembolism, and glomerulonephropathy (Tsai et al., 2007).

A systematic comprehensive case review was performed by Huemer et al. (2014) with the goal of obtaining a better perspective on patients with late onset cblC disorder. Fifty-eight cases were reviewed, with age of onset of symptoms from 1 to 44 years. Huemer et al. (2014) reported that presenting symptoms in adolescents were psychiatric symptoms, ataxia, and cognitive decline. Unfortunately, time to diagnosis ranged from 3 months to more than 20 years. In patients with later onset forms of the disease, symptoms improved and some even resolved with treatment (Huemer et al., 2014), thus supporting early identification as an important means of intercepting the adverse outcomes of this disorder.

Treatment is managed by a metabolic geneticist and consists of intramuscular injection of hydroxycobalamin, betaine to decrease plasma homocysteine, folate, and sometimes supplementation with carnitine and methionine (van Karnebeek & Stockler, 2012).

Gaucher Disease

Gaucher disease (GD) is an autosomal recessive disease, caused by a deficiency in the enzyme of glucocerebrosidase, causing an accumulation of glucosylceramide in the body. There are three types of this disease diagnosed using symptoms, age of onset, and genetic mutation analysis. The diagnosis of GD is the assay of glucocerebrosidase enzyme activity in peripheral blood leukocytes or other nucleated cells. In affected individuals, this will be elevated. A genetic analysis is also performed to further define the type of disease (Staretz-Chacham, Choi, Wakabayashi, Lopez, & Sidransky, 2010). Treatment is enzyme replacement therapy; however, the medication does not cross the blood–brain barrier. Thus, enzyme replacement therapy does not alter the neurologic progression or psychiatric manifestations of the disease (Staretz-Chacham et al., 2010).

Ninety-nine percent of the cases of GD are type 1 disease. Symptoms of type 1 disease include hepatosplenomegaly, thrombocytopenia, and anemia, as well as bone abnormalities such as avascular necrosis, osteopenia, and osteosclerosis (Packman, Wilson Crosbie, Riesner, Fairley, & Packman, 2006).

GD type 2 presents with severe CNS involvement and results in death within the first 2 years of life. GD type 3 presents with neurologic and psychiatric symptoms and may have some of the visceral physical symptoms and the addition of slowed horizontal saccadic eye movements (a quick simultaneous movement between two or more phases of fixation in the same direction). Psychosis and mood disorders can be presenting symptoms of GD type 3. Early onset dementia has also been documented in individuals with type 1 disease (Perez-Calvo et al., 2000).

Packman et al. (2006) compared the Minnesota Multiphasic 2 survey results of 71 patients with type I GD to results of patients with chronic heart disease and pain. The results showed that patients with GD were more likely to experience depression, hypochondriasis, and hysteria—more likely to be overwhelmed and defensive. These results suggest that even in the form of the disease without neurologic symptoms, patients experience mental health issues.

Fabry Disease

Fabry disease is a deficiency in the enzyme alpha galactosidase A (alpha Gal A), resulting in an accumulation of globotriaosylceramide (Zschocke & Hoffmann, 2004). There are many variants of this disease, including later onset forms. Definitive diagnosis is confirmed by low enzyme activity in the blood or in cultured fibroblasts from a tissue biopsy. However, in women affected by the disease, the enzyme activity may fall within the normal range, so genetic testing for the mutated alpha-Gal A allele must be performed (Schiffmann, 2009).

The classical form of the disease presents in early childhood with episodes of severe pain and paresthesias of the extremities. Disease progression may result in angiokeratomas (benign skin lesions of capillaries that are seen as small marks of red to blue color), corneal and lenticular opacities, vessel ectasia (dilation) in skin and mucous membranes, and hypohidrosis (decreased sweating). As patients age, proteinuria, hyposthenuria, and lymphedema develop. Progressive renal and cardiac deterioration may occur in patients with Fabry disease. In addition, there is a high propensity for the individual to experience an ischemic stroke (Staretz-Chacham et al., 2010).

Treatment with enzyme replacement therapy reduces the level of pain associated with the disease, with improved outcomes when started early in the course of disease. Treatment with angiotensin converting enzyme (ACE) inhibitors to reduce proteinuria, and gabapentin to decrease paresthesia is also standard (Staretz-Chacham et al., 2010).

Due to the episodes of severe, debilitating pain, patients with Fabry disease are at a high risk of major depression, substance abuse, and suicide. These behavioral and mental health issues are often overlooked as a complicating factor in the disease (Staretz-Chacham et al., 2010). Thus, ongoing screening evaluations for depression, substance abuse, and suicidal ideation are essential to identify and *intercept* patients with evidence or symptoms of these known risks.

Niemann–Pick Type C Disease

Niemann–Pick type C disease (NPC) results from an error in cellular trafficking of exogenous cholesterol leading to lysosomal accumulation of unesterified cholesterol. Definitive diagnosis is biochemical analysis of skin biopsy (Zschocke & Hofmann, 2004).

There is great variability in presentation, depending on the type of mutation: a rapidly progressive neonatal phenotype to a neurodegenerative adult onset form. All forms of the disease demonstrate cognitive decline; however, the onset may range from subtle defects in executive functioning to rapidly progressive dementia with mutism and apathy. Children often present with difficulties at school and behavioral problems, while teenagers may present with apathy and mutism and may receive a diagnosis of schizophrenia rather than NPC. In a review by Sevin et al. (2007), 45% of the patients with NPC presented with symptoms that were consistent with schizophrenia. Another significant presenting physical finding is that nearly 90% of these patients also presented with splenomegaly (Sevin et al. 2007). Some patients also present with vertical gaze palsy, but most often, the vertical gaze palsy presents after the onset of psychiatric symptoms. About 30% of patients experience seizures that are difficult to control (Sevin et al., 2007).

Treatment for NPC is supportive and is focused on symptom control. Miglustat may also be used to treat the neurological manifestations of the disease; however, its use remains off-label in the United States (van Karnebeek & Stockler, 2012).

Propionic Acidemia

Propionic acidemia (PA) is an autosomal recessive disorder that causes a deficiency of propionyl-Coenzyme A carboxylase. Symptoms include frequent metabolic crises, which may be accompanied by hyperammonemia. This disorder is included on the newborn screening panel (Zschocke & Hoffmann, 2004).

Treatment of PA is directed by a metabolic geneticist and includes a lifetime dietary restriction of protein with supplementation of deficient amino acids in a special formula, carnitine supplementation, biotin supplementation, and intermittent metronidazole to decrease enteral propionic acid. Sick-day protocols are important, as severe metabolic aciduria can occur in periods of catabolism (van Karnebeek & Stockler, 2012).

Even in patients who are compliant with treatment, there is growth delay, developmental and speech delays, and intellectual disability. Psychiatric symptoms include behavioral changes and expressive autistic-like behaviors, such as repetitive movements, abnormal social interactions, communication difficulties, ritualistic behaviors, and inflexibility in planning (Witters et al., 2016). A case study of eight patients with PA reported by Witters et al. (2016) revealed that five of the patients also had a diagnosis of autism. Ongoing neuropsychiatric evaluation is important for patients with PA to intercept potential problems as soon as possible through appropriate interventions based on the neuropsychiatric symptom presentation.

Maple Syrup Urine Disease

MSUD is an autosomal recessive disorder that causes a deficiency in the branched chain alpha-oxoacid dehydrogenase complex resulting in buildup of toxic metabolites. This disorder is detected by newborn screening (Zschocke & Hoffmann, 2004).

The milder forms of the disease may present with psychomotor retardation, fluctuating and progressive neurologic disease, and ketoacidotic decompensation (keto anemic vomiting). The psychiatric symptoms in patients with diagnosed MSUD include ADHD, depression, and anxiety. In an age-matched control study of 26 patients with MSUD (11 treated with liver transplantation, 15 with diet control), ADHD, lower IQ, and depression were significantly higher in patients with MSUD compared to controls. These behaviors were present in individuals with MSUD regardless of whether they had a liver transplant or were managed by strict dietary control (Muelly et al., 2013). Patients with MSUD require ongoing close follow-up care including frequent assessments and evaluations for these concerns.

Treatment is directed by a metabolic geneticist and includes orthotropic liver transplant or lifetime restriction of dietary protein with supplementation of essential amino acids in a special formula (Van Karnebeek & Stockler, 2012). Behavioral, cognitive, and psychiatric evaluations are also a critical part of the treatment plans.

Homocystinuria

Homocystinuria is an autosomal recessive disorder that causes a deficiency of cystathione beta synthase (CbS) or methylenetetrahydrofolate reductase (MTHFR) deficiency. CbS deficiency results in a buildup of homocysteine due to the body's inability to break down homocysteine. MTHFR enzyme deficiency interferes with the body's ability to process methionine, causing a buildup of homocysteine in the body. This disorder is detected on routine newborn screening in the United States (Zschocke & Hoffmann, 2004).

Homocystinuria (CbS type) can present with a spectrum of severity with symptoms usually beginning around school age. Psychiatric symptoms include intellectual disabilities, mood disorders, obsessive-compulsive disorder, and schizophrenia-like symptoms. Obsessive-compulsive disorder has been reported in 50% of the patients with the CbS type of homocystinuria (Abbott, Folstein, Abbey, & Pyeritz, 1987). Other symptoms may include a marfanoid appearance, epilepsy, progressive myopia, lens dislocation, osteoporosis, and thromboembolism.

In the MTHFR type, patients may have up to a 70% greater risk of developing schizophrenic symptoms (Muntjewerff et al., 2008). In the later onset forms of the disease, schizophrenia may be the presenting symptom. Occasionally, there will also be ataxia and insidious intellectual disability. Treatment will often improve the psychiatric symptoms, thus avoiding the use of antipsychotic medications (Muntjewerff et al., 2008).

Treatment is managed by a metabolic geneticist, with the goal of keeping plasma homocysteine <30 micromoles/l. This is accomplished by lifetime adherence to a diet low in protein, supplementation with pyridoxine, folic acid, betaine, and vitamin C (Van Karnebeek & Stockler, 2012).

Porphyria

Porphyria is a group of eight diseases, which are caused by enzyme deficits in the heme metabolism, leading to accumulation of porphyrin or one of its precursors. The inheritance pattern is autosomal dominant. Diagnosis is made by measuring the urine and blood for porphyrin precursors during an acute attack, and DNA analysis for specific mutations to type the disease (Nia, 2014).

Psychiatric symptoms during attacks may present as hallucinations, delusions, thought disorders, and depression. Hallucinations may affect as many as 40% of patients with porphyria (Bonnot et al., 2015). The hepatic forms of this disease may also present with severe abdominal pain, nausea, and vomiting; however, if the patient is also presenting with severe psychiatric symptoms, these symptoms may be considered part of the psychosis. Urine may be red or brown during attacks in the early onset of the disease. Extreme photosensitivity with skin blistering may also be present (Nia, 2014).

Treatment involves avoidance of attack triggers, such as drugs that are known enzyme inducers, hunger, stress, alcohol, hormones, and menstruation. Other acute therapy is geared to the type of porphyria diagnosed (Nia, 2014).

■ DIAGNOSTIC CONSIDERATIONS FOR IEM

When considering psychiatric symptoms secondary to a diagnosis of IEM, the detection of the underlying disorder is of primary importance, as treatment is most effective at preventing permanent damage when started early in the disease process (Walterfang et al., 2013). For any patient presenting with behavioral problems or psychiatric symptoms for the first time, a referral to genetics and a metabolic workup should be performed if any of the following are included in the patient's history:

1. There is a family history of metabolic or other neurological disorder, or unexplained childhood deaths.
2. The patient was born in an area where newborn screening was not performed, or the current uniform guidelines had not been adopted in the state of birth.
3. The presentation of psychiatric symptoms occurs with other symptoms: neurologic, cognitive, or other more systemic symptoms.
4. The symptoms are episodic and triggered by specific events that may cause metabolic stress, like surgery, increased protein intake, illness, prescription of new medications, or menstruation (Pan et al., 2017).

Additional History

Patients may have a history of vomiting, selective eating patterns, seizures, or periods of altered consciousness. A three-generation family history should be obtained, with attention to any deaths, mental health issues, seizures, or intellectual disabilities.

Physical Examination Findings

A careful physical examination may reveal changes in muscle tone, gaze abnormalities, dysmorphic features, splenomegaly, or mental status changes.

Diagnostic Testing

Basic laboratory tests should be ordered, including metabolic panel, complete blood count, C-reactive protein and erythrocyte sedimentation rate, TSH, free T4, vitamin D, and blood/urine toxicology. Other laboratory tests can be considered depending on symptoms, including ammonia, homocysteine, plasma amino acids, and urine organic acids (Giannitelli et al., 2017).

■ LONG-TERM MANAGEMENT CONSIDERATIONS

All patients with diagnosed IEM should have treatment directed by a metabolic geneticist or endocrinologist. For the majority of individuals with a diagnosis of IEM, laboratory evaluations and ongoing dietary adjustments are a significant component of an effective treatment plan. Ongoing communication with the subspecialists should also include sickness protocols, as many of the IEM worsen when the body is under additional metabolic stress. For patients receiving supplements and medications, dosage changes should be updated regularly in the patient's electronic medical record.

All patients with IEM should receive a baseline neuropsychiatric evaluation, and close monitoring for neuropsychiatric symptoms should continue during all primary care visits. Intercepting potential behavioral and mental health problems is critical to achieving the best possible healthcare outcomes for the child. Intercept can be accomplished through close attention to academic progress, social interaction, and frank discussions with parents and patients regarding prompt reporting of new behavioral or psychiatric symptoms in between and during all healthcare visits.

■ SUMMARY

P-PCPs are the leaders in the medical home for children with a diagnosis of IEM. Thus, all P-PCPs should be aware of the importance of reviewing the newborn screen results and making appropriate referrals as soon as any evidence of a problem emerges. This chapter describes numerous IEM and the various behavioral and mental health problems that are related to the individual IEM. P-PCPs have the opportunity to intercept outcomes through early identification of signs and symptoms of behavioral problems, assessment and screening of the child, and referral for treatment.

■ REFERENCES

Abbott, M. H., Folstein, S. E., Abbey, H., & Pyeritz, R. E. (1987). Psychiatric manifestations of homo-cystinuria due to cystathionine beta-synthase deficiency: Prevalence, natural history, and relationship to neurologic impairment and vitamin B6-responsiveness. *American Journal of Medical Genetics, 26,* 959–969. doi:10.1002/ajmg.1320260427

Advisory Committee on Heritable Disorders and Genetic Diseases in Newborns and Children. (2016). *Recommended uniform screening panel.* Retrieved from https://www.hrsa.gov/advisorycommittees/mchbadvisory/heritabledisorders/recommendedpanel/index.html

Ahrens-Nicklas, R. C., Slap, G., & Ficicioglu, C. (2015). Adolescent presentations of inborn errors of metabolism. *Journal of Adolescent Health, 56,* 477–482. doi:10.1016/j.jadohealth.2015.01.008

Argmann, C. A., Houten, S. M., Zhu, J., & Schadt, E. E. (2016). A next generation multiscale view of inborn errors of metabolism. *Cell Metabolism, 23,* 13–26. doi:10.1016/j.cmet.2015.11.012

Berry, S. A., Brown, C., Grant, M., Greene, C. L., Jurecki, E., Koch, J., . . . Cederbaum, S. (2013). Newborn screening 50 years later: Access issues faced by adults with PKU. *Genetics in Medicine: Official Journal of the American College of Medical Genetics, 15*(8), 591–599. doi:10.1038/gim.2013.10

Bonnot, O., Herrera, P. M., Tordjman, S., & Walterfang, M. (2015). Secondary psychosis induced by metabolic disorders. *Frontiers in Neuroscience, 9,* 177. doi:10.3389/fnins.2015.00177

Brand, M., Schoof, E., Partsch, C.-J. N., Peter, M., Hoepffner, W., Dörr, H. G., & Sippell, W. G. (2000). Anorexia nervosa in congenital adrenal hyperplasia: Long-term follow-up of 4 cases. *Experimental and Clinical Endocrinology & Diabetes: Official Journal, German Society of Endocrinology [and] German Diabetes Association, 108*(6), 430–435. doi:10.1055/s-2000-8139

Clacy, A., Sharman, R., & McGill, J. (2014). Depression, anxiety, and stress in young adults with phe-nylketonuria: Associations with biochemistry. *Journal of Developmental and Behavioral Pediatrics: JDBP, 35*(6), 388–391. doi:10.1097/DBP.0000000000000072

Engberg, H., Butwicka, A., Nordenström, A., Hirschberg, A. L., Falhammar, H., Lichtenstein, P., . . . Landén, M. (2015). Congenital adrenal hyperplasia and risk for psychiatric disorders in girls and women born between 1915 and 2010: A total population study. *Psychoneuroendocrinology, 60,* 195–205. doi:10.1016/j.psyneuen.2015.06.017

Engelen, M., Kemp, S., de Visser, M., van Geel, B. M., Wanders, R. J. A., Auborg, P., & Poll-The, B. T. (2012). X-linked adrenoleukodystrophy (X-ALD): Clinical presentation and guidelines for diagnosis, follow-up and management. *Orphanet Journal of Rare Diseases, 7,* 51. doi:10.1186/1750-1172-7-51

Enns, G. M. (2008). Neurologic damage and neurocognitive dysfunction in urea cycle disorders. *Seminars in Pediatric Neurology, 15,* 132–139. doi:10.1016/j.spen.2008.05.007

GeneReviews®. (2017). In Pagon R. A., Adam M. P., Ardinger H. H., Wallace S. E., Amemiya A., Bean L. J., . . . Stephens K. (Eds.). Seattle, WA: University of Washington. Retrieved from http://www.ncbi.nlm.nih.gov/books/NBK1116

Gentile, J. K., Ten Hoedt, A. E., & Bosch, A. M. (2010). Psychosocial aspects of PKU: Hidden disabilities–A review. *Molecular Genetics and Metabolism, 99*(Suppl 1), 64. doi:10.1016/j.ymgme.2009.10.183

Giannitelli, M., Consoli, A., Raffin, M., Jardri, R., Levinson, D. F., Cohen, D., & Laurent-Levinson, C. (2017). An overview of medical risk factors for childhood psychosis: Implications for research and treatment. *Schizophrenia Research, 192,* doi:10.1016/j.schres.2017.05.011

Hallas, D. (2016). Let's prevent parents from becoming newborn screen refusers! *Contemporary Pediatrics.* Retrieved from contemporarypediatrics.modernmedicine.com.

Herper, M. (2012). *The first drug with a $1 million price tag may already be on the market.* Retrieved from https://www.forbes.com/sites/matthewherper/2012/05/01/the-first-drug-with-a-1-million-price-tag-is-already-on-the-market/

Huemer, M., Scholl-Bürgi, S., Hadaya, K., Kern, I., Beer, R., Seppi, K., . . . Karall, D. (2014). Three new cases of late-onset cblC defect and review of the literature illustrating when to consider inborn errors of metabolism beyond infancy. *Orphanet Journal of Rare Diseases, 9,* 161. doi:10.1186/s13023-014-0161-1

IEMBase. (2017). *Inherited errors of metabolism knowledgebase.* Retrieved from http://iembase.org/index.asp

Kilakkathi, V. (2012). *Newborn screening in America: Problems and policies.* Cambridge, MA: Council for Responsible Genetics.

Muelly, E. R., Moore, G. J., Bunce, S. C., Mack, J., Bigler, D. C., Morton, D. H., & Strauss, K. A. (2013). Biochemical correlates of neuropsychiatric illness in maple syrup urine disease. *The Journal of Clinical Investigation, 123*(4), 1809–1820. doi:10.1172/JCI67217

Muntjewerff, J., Gellekink, H., den Heijer, M., Hoogendoorn, M. L. C., Kahn, R. S., Sinke, R. J., & Blom, H. J. (2008). Polymorphisms in catechol- O-methyltransferase and methylenetetrahydrofolate reductase in relation to the risk of schizophrenia. *European Neuropsychopharmacology*, *18*(2), 99–106. doi:10.1016/j.euroneuro.2007.06.005

Nia, S. (2014). Psychiatric signs and symptoms in treatable inborn errors of metabolism. *Journal of Neurology*, *261*(Suppl 2), 559. doi:10.1007/s00415-014-7396-6

Packman, W., Wilson Crosbie, T., Riesner, A., Fairley, C., & Packman, S. (2006). Psychological complications of patients with Gaucher disease. *Journal of Inherited Metabolic Disease*, *29*(1), 99–105. doi:10.1007/s10545-006-0154-x

Pan, L. A., Martin, P., Zimmer, T., Segreti, A. M., Kassiff, S., McKain, B. W., . . . Vockley, J. (2017). Neurometabolic disorders: Potentially treatable abnormalities in patients with treatment-refractory depression and suicidal behavior. *American Journal of Psychiatry*, *174*(1), 42–50. doi:10.1176/appi.ajp.2016.15111500

Pan, L., & Vockley, J. (2013). Neuropsychiatric symptoms in inborn errors of metabolism: Incorporation of genomic and metabolomic analysis into therapeutics and prevention. *Current Genetic Medicine Reports*, *1*(1), 65–70. doi: 10.1007/s40142-012-0004-0

Perez-Calvo, J., Bernal, M., Giraldo, P., Torralba, M. A., Civeira, F., Giralt, M., & Pocovi, M. (2000). Co-morbidity in Gaucher's disease results of a nation-wide enquiry in Spain. *European Journal of Medical Research*, *5*(6), 231–235.

Pollack, A. (2007, December 14). Agency approves drug to treat genetic disorder that can lead to retardation. *The New York Times*. Retrieved from https://www.nytimes.com/2007/12/14/health/14genetic.html

Schiffmann, R. (2009). Fabry disease. *Pharmacol Therapy*, *122*(1):65–77. doi:10.1016/j.pharmthera.2009.01.003

Serrano, M., Martins, C., Pérez-Dueñas, B., Gómez-López, L., Murgui, E., Fons, C., . . . Vilaseca, M. A. (2010). Neuropsychiatric manifestations in late-onset urea cycle disorder patients. *Journal of Child Neurology*, *25*(3), 352–358. doi:10.1177/0883073809340696

Sevin, M., Lesca, G., Baumann, N., Millat, G., Lyon-Caen, O., Vanier, M. T., & Sedel, F. (2007). The adult form of Niemann-Pick disease type C. *Brain: A Journal of Neurology*, *130*(1), 120–133. doi:10.1093/brain/awl260

Simons, A., Eyskens, F., De Groof, A., Van Diest, E., Deboutte, D., & Vermeiren, R. (2006). Cognitive functioning and psychiatric disorders in children with a metabolic disease. *European Child & Adolescent Psychiatry*, *15*(4), 207–213. doi:10.1007/s00787-006-0524-9

Srinivas, K., Sinha, S., Taly, A. B., Prashanth, L. K., Arunodaya, G. R., Janardhana Reddy, Y. C., & Khanna, S. (2008). Dominant psychiatric manifestations in Wilson's disease: A diagnostic and therapeutic challenge! *Journal of the Neurological Sciences*, *266*(1–2), 104–108. doi:10.1016/j.jns.2007.09.009

Staretz-Chacham, O., Choi, J. H., Wakabayashi, K., Lopez, G., & Sidransky, E. (2010). Psychiatric and behavioral manifestations of lysosomal storage disorders. *American Journal of Medical Genetics. Part B, Neuropsychiatric Genetics: The Official Publication of the International Society of Psychiatric Genetics*, *153B*(7), 1253–1265. doi:10.1002/ajmg.b.31097

Therrell, B. L., Padilla, C. D., Loeber, J. G., Kneisser, I., Saadallah, A., Borrajo, G. J. C., & Adams, J. (2015). Current status of newborn screening worldwide: 2015. *Seminars in Perinatology*, *39*(3), 171–187. doi:10.1053/j.semperi.2015.03.002

Tsai, A. C., Morel, C. F., Scharer, G., Yang, M., Lerner-Ellis, J. P., Rosenblatt, D. S., & Thomas, J. A. (2007). Late-onset combined homocystinuria and methylmalonic aciduria (cblC) and neuropsychiatric disturbance. *American Journal of Medical Genetics. Part A*, *143A*(20), 2430–2434. doi:10.1002/ajmg.a.31932

U.S. Food and Drug Administration. (2015). *The voice of the patient: Neurological manifestations of inborn errors of metabolism*. Retrieved from https://www.fda.gov/ForIndustry/UserFees/PrescriptionDrugUserFee/ucm368342.htm

van Karnebeek, C. D., & Stockler, S. (2012). Treatable inborn errors of metabolism causing intellectual disability: A systematic literature review. *Metabolic Genetics and Metabolism*, *105*, 368–381. doi:10.1016/j.ymgme.2011.11.191

Wadsworth Laboratory. (2017). *Newborn screening milestones*. Retrieved from https://www.wadsworth.org/programs/newborn/screening/history

Waisbren, S. E., Potter, N. L., Gordon, C. M., Green, R. C., Greenstein, P., Gubbels, C. S., . . . Berry, G. T. (2012). The adult galactosemic phenotype. *Journal of Inherited Metabolic Disease*, *35*(2), 279–286. doi:10.1007/s10545-011-9372-y

Walterfang, M., Bonnot, O., Mocellin, R., & Velakoulis, D. (2013). The neuropsychiatry of inborn errors of metabolism. *Journal of Inherited Metabolic Disease*, 36(4), 687–702. doi:10.1007/s10545-013-9618-y

Washington State Department of Health. (2017). *Table of newborn screening history in Washington state*. Retrieved from https://www.doh.wa.gov/YouandYourFamily/InfantsandChildren/NewbornScreening/AboutUs

Witters, P., Debbold, E., Crivelly, K., Vande Kerckhove, K., Corthouts, K., Debbold, B., . . . Morava, E. (2016). Autism in patients with propionic acidemia. *Molecular Genetics and Metabolism*, 119(4), 317–321. doi:10.1016/j.ymgme.2016.10.009

Zschocke, J., & Hoffmann, G. F. (Eds.). (2004). *Vademecum metabolicum: Manual of metabolic pediatrics* (2nd ed.). Friedrichsdorf, Germany: Milupa GmbH.

CHAPTER 11

Case Study: Infant Colic

KIMBERLY CIFELLI, CAROLINE BOURASSA,
AMANDA NEILAN, KELSEY HEINER, AND
KRISTEN HAY

CASE PRESENTATION

Chief Complaint

A 7-week-old female presents to the office for intermittent, uncontrollable, evening-time fussiness for the past 2 weeks.

Over the course of several weeks, the parents of the 7-week-old infant become increasingly concerned regarding intermittent periods of fussiness, crying, irritability, and frequent contact with the pediatric primary care office seeking medical advice to calm their infant.

Day 1

The mother of a 7-week-old full-term infant calls the office to report the infant has been crying intermittently for the past week. The mother describes the episodes as occurring during the evenings with a duration of 3 to 4 hours. The mother reports that the infant's face becomes beet red with her legs drawn up toward her chest while she is screaming. The mother has tried interventions such as rocking, darkening the room, music, patting her back, and using a pacifier with little effect. She has also been giving the infant simethicone gas drops and probiotics. Eventually, the infant settles without the mother knowing which intervention helped. The mother is worried, but seems to be coping well and asks if there is anything further she should do to help her daughter. The mother states, "I do not remember having such a difficult time consoling my first daughter."

The infant is formula-fed and consumes 5 ounces every 3 hours. The infant has a small amount of reflux after each feed, without vomiting or respiratory difficulty. The mother reports seven wet diapers each day and one bowel movement. The nurse recommends continuing to console the infant and to reduce the quantity of the feeds to 4 ounces every 2 to 3 hours in case of overfeeding. The nurse also recommends trying gripe water to soothe the infant.

Day 2

The mother calls the office again in the evening to inform about the infant's fussiness. The mother has increased the frequency of feeds and reduced the quantity of formula with little

(continued)

change in the infant's behavior. At the time of the call, the infant is not crying. The nurse recommends switching to hydrolyzed formula in case the infant has a feeding intolerance.

Day 3
The parents call the office during a crying episode. The parents are very worried and the infant is inconsolable by their report. The infant is coughing and has some difficulty breathing. The nurse practitioner advises the parents to bring the infant to the emergency department (ED) to rule out any emergent conditions. By the time the parents arrive at the ED, the infant is no longer crying and the workup is normal.

Day 4
The parents visit the office for a follow-up visit the next morning. Since leaving the ED, the infant has not had an episode of inconsolable crying. The infant is taking approximately 4 ounces of hydrolyzed formula every 2 to 3 hours. The parents are using simethicone gas drops, probiotics, and gripe water as directed.

■ COMPREHENSIVE HISTORY

History of Present Illness

This is an otherwise healthy 7-week-old female, presenting to office with complaints of intermittent fussiness for 2 weeks. The crying episodes usually occur for a few hours each evening, with a high-pitched cry, appears flushed, has legs often drawn up, and is difficult to console. The infant's mother has called the office each day for the past 3 days speaking with the nurse, and visited the ED last night for same symptoms without significant findings. The infant eventually calms with quieting of environment, darkening of room, slow movements, and gentle back massage. There were initial concerns for overfeeding the infant; at this visit, the infant consumes 5 to 6 ounces of formula every 3 hours with some spit up. The mother reduced feedings to 4 ounces every 2 to 3 hours without change in symptoms. The infant was changed to a completely hydrolyzed formula 3 days ago. The infant is receiving probiotic drops once daily, infant gas relief drops twice daily, and gripe water most nights with some improvement in symptoms. The infant usually stays awake during the episodes of crying for about 3 hours and then sleeps for approximately 2 hours, averaging 14 hours of sleep spaced out throughout the per day and night. The mother denies fever, vomiting, blood in stool, rash, apnea, or cyanosis.

Past Medical History

BIRTH HISTORY
The infant was delivered via repeat cesarean section at 39 weeks' gestation to 32-year-old, gravida 2, para 2 mother; Apgar score of 9 at 1 and 5 minutes, respectively, after delivery, and discharged from hospital on day 2 of life. Mother received prenatal care beginning at 8 weeks' gestation, denies alcohol or drug use during pregnancy, denies illness during pregnancy, denies history of sexually transmitted infections, her group B Streptococcus (GBS) screen was negative. Her congenital

heart disease (CHD) screen was negative, she passed her hearing test, and her newborn screen was negative.

Allergies: No known allergies.

MEDICATIONS

The following medications were ordered and administered by the mother per instructions: Gripe water 2.5 mL four times a day as needed; Lactobacillus reuteri DSM 17938, five drops by mouth daily; simethicone infant gas drops 0.5 mL by mouth, twice a day, as needed

Medical and surgical: Noncontributory

Immunizations: Hepatitis B vaccine on day 1 of life

Family History

Mother: 32-year-old female with history of asthma

Father: 35-year-old male with history of lactose intolerance

Sibling: 2-year-old female with history of atopic dermatitis

Screening Tools

Although colic was first documented in English literature as early as the 16th century, little standardization has developed in terms of screening processes for diagnosis. A recent systematic review recognized the lack of standardized screening tools for infantile colic (Garcia Marqués, Chillón Martinez, González Zapata, Rebollo Salas, & Jiménez Rejano, 2017). Most tools focus on the variables of crying and irritability. These tools often rely on symptoms reported by parents. The systematic review investigated the reliability and validity of four existing screening tools. One tool investigated was a 24-hour crying diary reported by parents, with validity confirmed using audiotapes of negative vocalization by infants, which parents characterized as crying (Garcia Marqués et al., 2017). This screening tool lacked further description of patient's presentation and reliability was not tested. This tool could be helpful for obtaining further information from the parents early on in symptoms of colic, but might be redundant given this point in the infant's duration of presenting symptoms.

Colic is a diagnosis of exclusion. Colic is characterized by a variety of symptoms including fussiness, difficulty to console, excessive crying, facial flushing, abdominal discomfort including reflux, extensor positioning, and change in sleeping pattern (Garcia Marqués et al., 2017). For this case, symptoms of colic aligned well with one of the most recognized criteria of colic known as Wessel's "rule of threes" (Wessel, Cobb, Jackson, Harris, & Detwiler, 1954). The rule of threes characterizes colic by at least 3 hours of crying per day, 3 or more days a week, and lasting at least 3 weeks in duration (Johnson, Cocker, & Chang, 2015). The crying usually peaks around 6 weeks of age and resolves between 3 and 6 months of age (Johnson et al., 2015).

This infant was brought to the ED and to the pediatric primary care office to ensure that no other emergent conditions coexist. A comprehensive history and physical examination must be performed, as it is a way of screening to rule out other possible causes of the presenting symptoms (Johnson et al., 2015). Once the differential diagnoses have been excluded, a diagnosis of colic can be based upon clinical presentation and history.

Review of Systems

General: Well infant with periods of fussiness usually in the evenings as described in the history of present illness (HPI)

Head: Denies trauma, denies swelling or bulging of fontanelles, denies seizures, denies tremors

Eyes: Denies itching, swelling, redness, or discharge

Ear: Denies signs of pain or drainage

Nose: Denies congestion or drainage, denies frequent sneezing

Mouth: Denies difficulty latching or swallowing, denies lesions

Neck: Denies decreased range of motion

Chest: Denies history of murmur or cyanosis, denies shortness of breath

Abdomen: Reports drawing legs up to chest during each sustained nighttime crying episode, denies visible blood in the stool, denies abdominal distention, denies emesis

Genitourinary: Reports seven wet diapers in past 24 hours and three soft, yellow stools

Musculoskeletal: Denies hypotonia, denies trauma or swelling, denies hair tourniquet

Skin: Denies rash, denies pruritus, reports face appears red when crying

Endocrinology: Denies weight loss or lethargy

Physical Examination

General: Well appearing infant sleeping in prone position on exam table

Cardiovascular: Apical rate and rhythm regular, heart rate 140, S1S2, no murmurs/rubs/gallops, no bruits, taps, heaves, or thrills

Pulmonary/vascular: Femoral and brachial pulses equal, +2 bilateral, cap refill less than 2 seconds, no edema

Respiratory: Respiratory rate 40, pattern regular, respirations quiet. No retractions or use of accessory muscles. Good aeration on auscultation of all lung fields. No wheezes, stridor, rhonchi, or rales. Symmetrical chest excursion, inspiration:expiration 2:1, anterior–posterior to transverse ratio 1:2.

Gastrointestinal: Abdomen flat, nondistended. Bowel sounds present and active all four quadrants. Abdomen soft and nontender to palpation all four quadrants. No bruits or palpable masses. No organomegaly.

▪ DIFFERENTIAL DIAGNOSES: BEHAVIORAL HEALTH

Colic

Colic is a benign process in which an infant has bursts of inconsolable crying for more than 3 hours per day, more than 3 days per week, and for longer than 3 weeks (Johnson et al., 2015). The paroxysms typically occur in the evening and are unprovoked (Johnson et al., 2015). A distended abdomen, fever, and lethargy are considered red flags and must be investigated further before diagnosing an infant with colic (Johnson et al., 2015).

PATHOPHYSIOLOGY OF COLIC

The cause of colic is unknown (Johnson et al., 2015). Potential causes include alterations in fecal microflora, intolerance to cow's milk protein or lactose, gastrointestinal immaturity or inflammation, increased serotonin secretion, poor feeding techniques, and maternal smoking or nicotine replacement therapy (Johnson et al., 2015).

BEHAVIORAL CONSIDERATIONS FOR COLIC

Parental reassurance and support is the main aspect of treatment (Johnson et al., 2015). The parents or caregivers should be educated on the benign and self-limited nature of colic. Resources for support should be offered (Johnson et al., 2015).

■ GASTROESOPHAGEAL REFLUX

Gastroesophageal reflux (GER) is a common, self-limited process in infants (Jung, 2001). The term GER refers to a functional or physiologic process in a healthy infant with no underlying systemic abnormalities (Jung, 2001). It involves regurgitation, or "spitting up" (Jung, 2001). This is the passive return of gastric contents retrograde into the esophagus (Jung, 2001).

Infants with GER typically regurgitate with normal weight gain, without signs or symptoms of esophagitis, without significant respiratory symptoms, and without neurobehavioral symptoms (Jung, 2001).

Pathophysiology of GER

In the gastrointestinal tract, the lower esophageal sphincter is located at the distal end of the esophagus and is under tonic smooth muscle control (Jung, 2001). Gastric refluxate may return into the esophagus when the transient lower esophageal sphincter relaxes without swallowing (Jung, 2001). Delayed gastric emptying is another cause of GER. It usually resolves by 6 to 12 months of age (Jung, 2001).

Behavioral Considerations for GER

Gravitational and positional factors may exacerbate GER (Jung, 2001). Upright and prone positioning of the infant during feedings is beneficial (Jung, 2001). Parents may be very concerned about the amount of "spit-up," or what they may term as vomiting, that the infant is experiencing and present on phone calls to the office and in person as anxious about the infant, with feelings of ineffective parenting, blaming themselves for their infant's physical symptoms. Reassurance through anticipatory guidance is an effective means for *intercepting* the parents' feelings and encouraging bonding and attachment with their infant.

■ MILK PROTEIN ALLERGY

Symptoms of food protein allergy include those commonly associated with immunoglobulin E-associated reactions (Hypoallergenic Infant Formulas, 2000). These include angioedema, urticaria, wheezing, rhinitis, vomiting, eczema, and anaphylaxis (Hypoallergenic Infant Formulas, 2000). However, some infants may experience irritability or colic as the only symptom of food protein allergy (Hypoallergenic Infant Formulas, 2000).

■ DISCUSSION OF COLIC

Crying is a physiologically and socially useful tool for newborns and infants. Differentiated crying begins soon after birth and serves as means of communication (Brazelton, 1962). The infant cries in response to environmental changes and physiologic needs, including changes in temperature, hunger, pain, dissatisfaction, and loneliness (Harrison, 2008). As parents respond to these cries, the infant also learns to expect that her needs will be met (Brazelton, 1962). However, some infants experience persistent crying that is unrelieved by meeting their needs (Figure 11.1).

Infantile colic typically develops in healthy infants and peaks around 6 to 8 weeks of age and spontaneously resolves by 3 to 4 months (Cohen & Albertini, 2012). Infantile colic is characterized by the "rule of threes": periods of crying that last for 3 or more hours per day, for 3 or more days per week, and for a minimum of 3 weeks (Wessel et al., 1954). Periods of fussiness are frequently reported to occur between 6 p.m. and 10 p.m., with less frequent surges between 4 a.m. to 7 a.m. and between 9 a.m. and 11 a.m. (Brazelton, 1962). The incidence of colic varies depending on methodology, and is reported to be anywhere from 10% to 40% of infants younger than 3 months old (Lucassen et al., 2001). However, prospective studies have narrowed the range from 5% to 19% (Canivet, Hagander, Jakobsson & Lanke, 1996; Høgdall, Vestermark, Birch, Plenov, & Toftager-Larsen, 1991).

It is important to note that infantile colic is not associated with any morbidity or mortality (Weissbluth, Christoffel, & Davis, 1984). However, colic accounts for 10% to 20% of all pediatric visits in the first 4 months of life (Iacovou, Ralston, Muir, Walker, & Truby, 2012). While colic itself is benign, the *stress of caring for a colicky baby can negatively impact the family*. Mothers of colicky babies report feelings of frustration, incompetence, helplessness, and anxiety (Stifter & Bono, 1998). Colic is associated with higher maternal depression scores (Vik et al., 2009) and less face-to-face interaction time between mothers and infants (Papousek & von Hofacker, 1998). "Crying and irritability" are also frequently cited by caregivers as the cause of shaken baby syndrome (Barr, Trent, & Cross, 2006). Thus, pediatric primary care providers (P-PCPs) must be knowledgeable of the course of infantile colic and provide anticipatory guidance that intercepts the negative feelings the parents are feeling and guides them into comfort measures for the infant.

There is little high-quality data that suggests a correlation with age of the mother, sex of the infant, allergies, type of feeding, severity of gas, or elimination patterns (Hewson, Oberklaid, & Menahem, 1987). There are a few modern

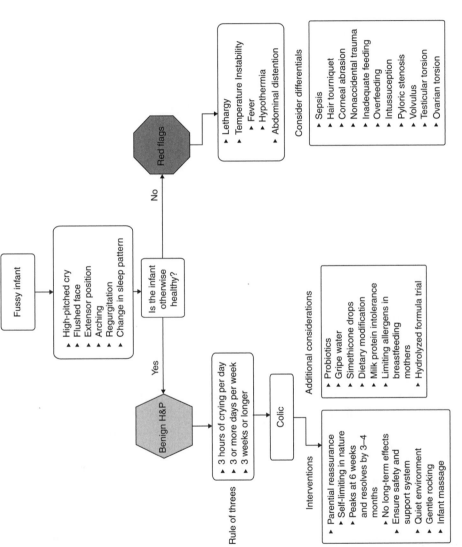

FIGURE 11.1 Formulating the differential diagnosis for the fussy infant. H&P, history and physical (exam).

theories to explain colic in infants, including gastrointestinal disorders (Savino et al., 2004), maternal anxiety, difficult temperament (Raiha, Lehtonen, Huhtula, Saleva, & Korvenrata, 2002), and neurologic immaturity (Wessel et al., 1954). However, the evidence to support such theories is limited in quality and quantity and is often contradictory. Given that colic crying tends to be cyclical and occurs around the same time each day, studies have demonstrated that unexplained crying in the infant is to be expected and may serve to discharge tension and restore homeostasis (Lester & Boukydis, 1985).

While the cause of colic remains unknown, crying in infancy is normal and occurs in most babies. In a study of 80 healthy infants, the median duration of daily crying at 6 weeks of age was 2.75 hours, only 15 minutes less than what is considered to be colic (Brazelton, 1962). Similarly, two other studies revealed that healthy infants aged 1 to 3 months cried for about 2 hours per day (Lehtonen & Korvenranta, 1995; St. James-Roberts & Halil, 1991).

■ TREATMENT

The cause of infantile colic is unknown and it is a diagnosis of exclusion (Johnson et al., 2015). While this may lead treatment management to be difficult, there is significant research on various modalities that have shown success. The treatment management plan should be family focused since there is no real solution to infantile colic (Johnson et al., 2015). Medical professionals play a key role in providing families with evidence-based interventions and reassurance.

Parental Reassurance

Parental reassurance is a top priority after diagnosis of colic. Despite the benign nature of the condition, it can elicit a significant amount of stress, low self-esteem, and frustration for parents (Vik et al., 2009). Several studies have identified the association between infantile colic and maternal postpartum depression. Using the Edinburgh Postnatal Depression Score, Vik et al. (2009) identified infantile colic as being a significant risk factor for maternal depression 6 months after birth, despite the resolution of prolonged crying. One inductive qualitative interview study that aimed to highlight the parental life of a baby with colic identified the major feelings of powerlessness and sense of worry that parents endure (Landgren & Hallström, 2011). It is of great value for providers to empower parents during this difficult period with strategies and support. Reminding parents of the self-limiting nature of this condition, and that infants typically grow out of it by 3 to 4 months of age, may bring significant reassurance and comfort (Johnson et al., 2015).

Dietary Modifications

While the etiology of colic remains unknown, the effects of nutrition on infantile colic have been closely examined. For some infants, associated symptoms of infantile colic are thought to be secondary to cow's milk protein (Johnson et al., 2015). Dietary modifications may result in an improvement of symptoms. Infantile colic affects breastfed and bottle-fed infants equally; however, there are different recommendations for dietary changes. Mothers who are breastfeeding are recommended to continue, but to consume a low allergen diet. Eliminating foods such as cow's milk, bovine protein, soy, egg, wheat, nuts, and seafood has shown to improve symptoms for some cases (Johnson et al., 2015). A randomized controlled trial identified 137 minutes less crying per day in mothers who excluded cow's milk, eggs, peanuts, tree nuts, wheat, soy, and fish (Johnson et al., 2015). A systematic review additionally identified the benefits of relieving colic symptoms with a hypoallergenic maternal diet (Iacovou et al., 2012). It is also recommended to eliminate other irritating foods such as caffeine, onions, cabbage, and legumes (Iacovou et al., 2012). Providers should recommend mothers to seek out expert nutritional guidance as a restricted diet may cause gaps in a mother's nutrition.

Recommendations for formula-fed infants with colic include changing formulas. The different formula options vary from partially hydrolyzed, extensively hydrolyzed, and completely hydrolyzed. Hydrolyzed formulas contain milk protein but are more broken down and less likely to cause gastrointestinal upset thought to evoke colic symptoms (Iacovou et al., 2012). A review of 13 studies identified a statistically significant decrease in crying time with hydrolyzed formulas (Iacovou et al., 2012). It is recommended that infants should be given new formula over a 2-week period. Since the taste may be not as palatable in more hydrolyzed formula, mixing the new formula with the old formula in increasing ratios over 4 days helps with the adjustment (Johnson et al., 2015). The cost implication of changing to hydrolyzed formula is significant, as it is expensive and may not be covered by assistance programs such Women, Infants, and Children (Johnson et al., 2015). However, if parents do wish to try a new formula, a hydrolyzed composition has shown to be effective for some infants. It is recommended that regular formula be restarted around 3 to 6 months of age.

Probiotics

The use of Lactobacillus reuteri (L. reuteri) strain DSM 17938 for breastfed infants has shown positive effects on colic symptoms (Johnson et al., 2015). A review on management of infantile colic identified four out of five clinical trials using L. reuteri reduced symptoms of colic and reported no adverse effects. Five drops of L. reuteri per day reported 61 minutes of less crying in one systematic review and two meta-analyses (Johnson et al., 2015). While one study identified increasing fussiness of L. reuteri use in bottle-fed infants, for breastfed infants this is a safe treatment option (Johnson et al., 2015).

Medications

Different medications have been studied to identify effective treatment for reducing infantile colic symptoms. Deemed as a safe over-the-counter drug for gas, simethicone has been discussed as an agent to decrease colic symptoms (Roberts, Ostapchuk, & O'Brien, 2004). However, a randomized placebo-controlled multicenter trial, in addition to two RCTs, has shown no benefit to this drug in relieving symptoms (Metcalf, Irons, Sher, & Young, 1994). Other medications that have been investigated for management of infantile colic include dicyclomine and proton pump inhibitors. The use of dicyclomine was found to have side effects, specifically in infants younger than 6 months, which consist of apnea, constipation, diarrhea, and drowsiness (Johnson et al., 2015). Proton pump inhibitors were identified to be no more effective than the placebo in helping reduce fussiness and crying time (Johnson et al., 2015).

Complementary and Alternative Therapies

In addition to medications and diet changes, there are also alternative therapies for the management of colic that parents and medical professionals may consider as options. Recent research has studied the effectiveness of massage therapy on colic symptoms. A randomized controlled trial studied the effects of massage and rocking therapy on 100 infants with colic symptoms (Sheidaei et al., 2016). One group received a massage for 15 to 20 minutes once during the day and once before bedtime. In the other group, the infants were rocked for 5 to 25 minutes when the colic symptoms appeared. Sheidaei et al. (2016) concluded that massage therapy significantly improved colic symptoms, reducing the amount of cries from 8.34 in a day to 4.26 a day. A study conducted by Nahidi, Gazerani, Yousefi, and Abadi (2017) also investigated the effects of massaging and rocking on infantile colic. The authors concluded that infant massage therapy was more effective than rocking for symptom management. While massage therapy is not a cure for infant colic, this research evidence supports offering this as a comfort measure for the infant by the parents and should be recommended by the P-PCP. Massage therapy is a complementary treatment modality, with no side effects, that also promotes positive contact between parent and child and parent–infant attachment and bonding.

There have also been several studies that examined the use of herbs and nutraceuticals as ways to help with infant colic symptoms. The use of fennel extract and peppermint has been examined. However, many of these trials are with significant limitations and small research studies. One study examined the effect of mentha piperita (peppermint oil) to help control infantile colic compared to simethicone. The study determined that there was little difference in the effect of the mentha piperita and simethicone, and further studies were recommended (Alves, de Brito, & Cavalcanti, 2012). Another RCT examined 125 infants with colic and the effects of foeniculum vulgare (fennel seed oil) on symptoms. The results revealed that fennel seed oil is helpful in reducing intestinal spasms and helps increase motility of the small intestine (Alexandrovich, Rakovitskava, Kolmo, Sidorova, & Shushunov, 2003). Compared to the placebo control group, the treatment group showed an improvement of colic symptoms and no observed side effects (Alexandrovich et al., 2003). Similar to peppermint oil studies, more research studies on fennel seed oil must be conducted to establish a benefit for infants with colic.

■ FOLLOW-UP CARE

Management of children with colic presenting with excessive or prolonged crying is determined on a case-by-case basis, dependent upon the history, examination, and family dynamics; some parents tolerate and cope with the crying infant better than others. Additionally, the lack of strong supporting evidence for any one strategy, combined with the number of proposed etiologies, may lead P-PCPs to recommend a variety of interventions, alone or in combination (Parker & Magee, 2011).

The frequency of follow-up for infants with colic is also individualized. Some families may require more frequent follow-up (via phone or in person) and re-examination for reassurance that the infant is continuing to do well and growing normally (Parker & Magee, 2011). Other infants, whose parents are coping well and have strong support networks, can be seen less frequently, for example, at the next regularly scheduled well visit. In all cases, parents should be encouraged to return to the office if the infant develops symptoms that were not present during the initial evaluation, such as vomiting or a rash.

Outcomes

Parents often worry about the long-term effects of colic on their children. At their 1-year follow-up, a group of colicky infants compared with non-colicky infants showed no differences in behavior on the nine dimensions assessed using the Toddler Temperament Scale (Raiha, Lehtonen, Korhonen, & Korvenranta, 1996). An association between infant colic and later development of asthma or allergic disease has also not been shown (Castro-Rodriguez et al., 2001). Colic does not appear to influence long-term cognitive development. In a prospective study in which approximately 15% of the children had a history of colic, average IQ scores at 5 years of age were similar among children with and without a history of colic (Rao, Brenner, Schisterman, Vik, & Mills, 2004). Hemmi, Wolke, and Schneider (2011) conducted a meta-analysis of longitudinal studies looking at the risk of behavior problems in later childhood. They found that this risk was increased when colic persisted later into infancy at 5 months of age. Other studies showed the risk was greatest when colic was seen in conjunction with psychosocial factors and other regulatory problems (e.g., feeding, sleeping), thus making it challenging to establish a causal relationship (Douglas & Hill, 2011). Overall, the literature is conflicting on the subject of behavioral sequelae and shows multiple confounding factors, making it challenging to pinpoint colic as the cause of behavioral problems.

Generally, once colic resolves there is little lasting effect on levels of maternal anxiety or depression (Clifford, Campbell, Speechley, & Gorodzinsky, 2003). However, when added to an already existing routine of poor communication and poor coping within the family, colic may negatively impact family dynamics. P-PCPs must assess for signs of family dysfunction, distress, and coping resources.

Until the exact cause of colic is known, the best recommendation for the discouraged family is to give them time, resources, and support. Often an empathic understanding shown by the P-PCPs, despite multiple failed attempts to remedy the baby's discomfort, will help the family through a trying time.

■ SUMMARY

In summary, colic is a diagnosis by exclusion. Even the most experienced parents question their parenting abilities when confronted with an infant with colic.

The persistent crying frustrates the parents, especially when efforts to comfort the infant fail. P-PCPs play a significant role in ruling out organic causes for the persistent crying and in intercepting potential adverse outcomes through anticipatory guidance and implementation of the currently best available evidence for treatment management of colic. Assessing for possible maternal depression is an important part of the treatment plan, with appropriate referrals for mothers of infants who may be struggling while caring for the infants in the first few months of life prior to the naturally anticipated alleviation of colic symptoms.

Overall, further research is needed regarding the validity and reliability of colic screening tools and the effectiveness of treatment plans.

■ REFERENCES

Alexandrovich, I., Rakovitskava, O., Kolmo, E., Sidorova, T., & Shushunov, S. (2003). The effect of fennel (foeniculum vulgare) seed oil emulsion in infantile colic: A randomized, placebo-controlled study. *Alternative Therapy Health Medicine*, 9(4), 58–61. Retrieved from https://www.ncbi.nlm.nih.gov/pubmed/12868253

Alves, J., de Brito, R. de. C., & Cavalcanti, T. (2012). Effectiveness of Mentha piperita in the treatment of infantile colic: A crossover study. *Evidence-Based Complementary and Alternative Medicine*, 2012, 1–4. doi:10.1155/2012/981352

Barr, R. G., Trent, R. B., & Cross, J. (2006). Age-related incidence curve of hospitalized shaken baby syndrome cases: Convergent evidence for crying as a trigger to shaking. *Child Abuse & Neglect*, 30(1), 7–16. doi:10.1016/j.chiabu.2005.06.009

Brazelton, T. B. (1962). Crying in infancy. *Pediatrics*, 29, 57–588. Retrieved from http://pediatrics.aappublications.org/content/29/4/579.full.pdf

Canivet, C., Hagander, B., Jakobsson, I., & Lanke, J. (1996). Infantile colic—less common than previously estimated? *Acta Paediatrica*, 85, 454–458. doi:10.1111/j.1651-2227.1996.tb14060.x

Castro-Rodriguez, J., Stern, D., Halonen, M., Wright, A., Holberg, C., Taussig, L., & Martinez F. (2001). Relation between infantile colic and asthma/atopy: A prospective study in an unselected population. *Pediatrics*, 108, 878–882. doi:10.1542/peds.108.4.878

Clifford, T., Campbell, M., Speechley, K., & Gorodzinsky, F. (2003). Sequelae of infant colic: Evidence of transient infant distress and absence of lasting effects on maternal mental health. *Archives of Pediatric & Adolescent Medicine*, 157, 486. doi:10.1001/archpedi.157.5.486

Cohen, G. M., & Albertini, L. W. (2012). Colic. *Pediatrics in Review*, 33(7), 332–333. doi:10.1542/pir.33-7-332

Douglas, P., & Hill, P. (2011). Managing infants who cry excessively in the first few months of life. *BMJ*, 343, d7772. doi:10.1136/bmj.d7772

García Marqués, S., Chillón Martínez, R., González Zapata, S., Rebollo Salas, M., & Jiménez Rejano, J. J. (2017). Tools assessment and diagnosis to infant colic: A systematic review. *Child: Care, Health and Development*, 43, 481–488. doi:10.1111/cch.12454

Harrison, V. (2008). *The newborn baby*. Cape Town, South Africa: Juta & Company Ltd.

Hemmi, M., Wolke, D., & Schneider, S. (2011). Associations between problems with crying, sleeping and/or feeding in infancy and long-term behavioural outcomes in childhood: A meta-analysis. *Archives of Disease in Childhood*, 96, 622. doi:10.1136/adc.2010.191312

Hewson, P., Oberklaid, F., & Menahem, S. (1987). Infant colic, distress, and crying. *Clinical Pediatrics*, 26(2), 69–76. doi:10.1177/000992288702600203

Høgdall, C. K., Vestermark, V., Birch, M., Plenov, G., & Toftager-Larsen, K. (1991). The significance of pregnancy, delivery and postpartum factors for the development of infantile colic. *Journal of Perinatal Medicine*, 19(4), 251–257. doi:10.3748/wjg.14.4662

Hypoallergenic infant formulas. (2000). *American Academy of Pediatrics*, 106(2). Retrieved from http://pediatrics.aappublications.org/content/106/2/346

Iacovou, M., Ralston, R. A., Muir, J., Walker, K. Z., & Truby, H. (2012). Dietary management of infantile colic: A systematic review. *Maternal Child Health*, 16(6), 1319–1331. doi:10.1007/s10995-011-0842-5

Johnson, J. D., Cocker, K., & Chang, E. (2015). Infantile colic: Recognition and treatment. *American Family Physician, 92*(7), 577–582. Retrieved from http://www.aafp.org/afp/2015/1001/p577.html

Jung, A. (2001). Gastroesophageal reflux in infants and children. *American Family Physician, 64*(11), 1853–1861. Retrieved from http://www.aafp.org/afp/2001/1201/p1853.html

Landgren, K., & Hallström, I. (2011). Parents' experience of living with a baby with infantile colic— A phenomenological hermeneutic study. *Scandinavian Journal of Caring Sciences, 25*(2), 317–324. doi:10.1111/j.1471-6712.2010.00829.x

Lehtonen, L., & Korvenranta, H. (1995). Infantile colic: Seasonal incidence and crying profiles. *Archives of Pediatrics & Adolescent Medicine, 149*(5), 533–536. doi:10.1001/archpedi.1995.02170180063009

Lester, B. M., & Boukydis, C. F. Z. (Eds.). (1985). *Infant crying: Theoretical and research perspectives.* New York, NY: Plenum Press.

Lucassen, P. L. B. J., Assendelft, W. J. J., van Eijk, J. Th. M., Gubbels, J. W., Douwes, A. C, & van Geldrop, W. J. (2001). Systematic review of the occurrence of infantile colic in the community. *Archives of Disease in Childhood, 84*, 398–403. doi:10.1136/adc.84.5.398

Metcalf, T. J., Irons, T. G., Sher, L. D., & Young, P. C. (1994). Simethicone in the treatment of infant colic: A randomized, placebo controlled, multicenter trial. *Pediatrics, 94*(1), 29–34. Retrieved from http://pediatrics.aappublications.org/content/pediatrics/94/1/29.full.pdf

Nahidi, F., Gazerani, N., Yousefi, P., & Abadi, A. R. (2017). The comparison of the effects of massaging and rocking on infantile colic. *Iranian Journal of Nursing and Midwifery Research, 22*(1), 67–71. doi:10.4103/ijnmr.IJNMR_31_13

Papousek, M., & von Hofaker, N. (1998). Persistent crying in early infancy: A non-trivial condition of risk for the developing mother–infant relationship. *Child: Care, Health, and Development, 24*(5), 395–424. doi:10.1046/j.1365-2214.2002.00091.x

Parker, S., & Magee, T. (2011) *The Zuckerman Parker handbook of developmental and behavioral pediatrics for primary care* (3rd ed.). Philadelphia, PA: Lippincott Williams & Wilkins.

Raiha, H., Lehtonen, L., Huhtala, V., Saleva, K., & Korvenrata, H. (2002). Excessively crying infant in the family: Mother–infant, father–infant and mother–father interaction. *Child: Care, Health, & Development, 28*(5), 419–429. doi:10.1046/j.1365-2214.2002.00292.x

Raiha, H., Lehtonen, L., Korhonen, T., & Korvenranta, H. (1996). Family life 1 year after infantile colic. *Archives of Pediatric & Adolescent Medicine, 150*, 1032–1036. doi10.1001/archpedi.1996.02170350034005

Rao, M., Brenner, R., Schisterman, E., Vik, T., & Mills, J. (2004). Long-term cognitive development in children with prolonged crying. *Archives of Disease in Childhood, 89*, 989. doi:10.1136/adc.2003.039198

Roberts, D. M., Ostapchuk, M., & O'Brien, J. G. (2004). Infantile colic. *American Family Physician, 70*(4), 735–740. Retrieved from http://www.aafp.org/afp/2015/1001/p577.html

Savino, F., Cresi, F., Pautasso, S., Palumeri, E., Tullio, V., Roana, J., . . . Oggero, R. (2004). Intestinal microflora in breastfed colicky and non-colicky infants. *Acta Paediatrica, 93*(6), 825–829. doi:10.1111/j.1651-2227.2004.tb03025.x

Sheidaei, A., Abadi, A., Zayeri, F., Nahidi, F., Gazerani, N., & Mansouri, A. (2016). The effectiveness of massage therapy in the treatment of infantile colic symptoms: A randomized controlled trial. *Medical Journal of the Islamic Republic of Iran, 30*, 351. Retrieved from https://www.ncbi.nlm.nih.gov/pmc/articles/PMC4934450/

St. James-Roberts, I., & Halil, T. (1991). Infant crying patterns in the first year: Normal community and clinical findings. *Journal of Child Psychology and Psychiatry, 32*(6), 915–968. doi:10.1111/j.1469-7610.1991.tb01922.x

Stifter, C. A., & Bono, M. A. (1998). The effect of infant colic on maternal self-perceptions and mother–infant attachment. *Child: Care, Health and Development, 24*(5), 339–351. doi:10.1046/j.1365-2214.2002.00088.x

Vik, T., Grote, V., Escribano, J., Socha, J., Verduci, E., Fritsch, M., . . . European Childhood Obesity Trial Study Group. (2009). Infantile colic, prolonged crying and maternal postnatal depression. *Acta Pædiatrica, 98*(8), 1344–1348. doi:10.1111/j.1651-2227.2009.01317.x

Weissbluth, M., Christoffel, K. K., & Davis, T. (1984). Treatment of infantile colic with dicyclomine hydrochloride. *The Journal of Pediatrics, 104*(6), 951–955. Retrieved from https://www.ncbi.nlm.nih.gov/pubmed/6374085

Wessel, M., Cobb, J., Jackson, E., Harris, G., & Detwiler, A. (1954). Paroxysmal fussing in infancy, sometimes called "colic." *American Academy of Pediatrics, 14*(5), 421–434. Retrieved from http://pediatrics.aappublications.org/content/pediatrics/14/5/421.full.pdf

SECTION III
Toddler Population

CHAPTER 12

Physical, Emotional, Social, and Behavioral Development of Toddlers

MARY KOSLAP-PETRACO

Toddlers are unique individuals and appropriate developmental assessment is essential to their physical growth and well-being. Their social–emotional developmental issues can be the cause of behavior problems. Evaluation presents the opportunity to ensure that any developmental delays are evaluated at the earliest possible age, which provides the ability to initiate interventions to *intercept* any identified delays. When interventions are initiated early, the toddler has the best opportunity to improve or resolve the delay. Toddler behaviors are naturally impulsive and having temper tantrums is a hallmark of this age group. These behaviors can be a challenge for both first-time and seasoned parents. Parenting the always busy toddler requires understanding, patience, love, and attention from the caregivers on a daily basis. Toddlers can quickly vacillate between normal behaviors and abnormal behaviors. When parents are not prepared to manage these behaviors, the pediatric primary care provider (P-PCP) must often intercept the behaviors and provide workable interventions to the parents. This chapter offers support to parents and guardians, especially the mothers, to intercept potential parenting issues.

■ NORMAL BEHAVIORS AND INITIAL EVIDENCE OF BEHAVIORAL HEALTH PROBLEMS

Receptive and Expressive Language Development

Receptive and expressive language development is a critical cognitive and emotional skill learned during the toddler years. Development not only occurs on a continuum with expectations that overlap age ranges but language is also integrated across multiple developmental domains. Language development requires intact cognitive skills to construct conceptual frameworks and physical development to coordinate the necessary oral–motor response (Briggs-Gowan & Carter, 1998, 2006; Briggs-Gowan, Carter, Irwin, Wachtel, & Cicchetti, 2004; U.S. Department of Health & Human Services, 2010). Language consists of articulation, receptive and expressive language skills, and the use of nonverbal symbols arising from the interaction between innate communication abilities and environmental influences. Any significant delay in language or speech skills without a delay in other developmental domains is categorized as a developmental language disorder, developmental dysphasia, or specific language impairment (Hagan, Shaw, & Duncan, 2017).

Cognitive Development

Cognitive development is a measure of the child's ability to problem-solve through intuition, perception, and verbal and nonverbal reasoning. It encompasses the ability not only to learn and understand but also to retain this information and apply it as needed (Hagan et al., 2017).

Cognitive development does not result from neurobiological development alone, although neural connections are necessary to allow sensory inputs to reach the brain (U.S. Department of Health & Human Services, 2010). A developmental disability or delay identified in any one area will affect other developmental domains as well (U.S. Department of Health & Human Services, 2010). For example, a child with hearing impairment would not be able to listen to what is occurring in their surroundings, which will affect the child's ability to speak and respond to commands. Any sensory or motor deficit can limit the toddler's level of experience for cognitive and language development because of limited opportunities to explore the environment (U.S. Department of Health & Human Services, 2010). In addition, language is connected to interactions and relationships that are meaningful and include significant language exchanges.

Developmental delays put added stress on the parent–child relationship. Parents of toddlers with speech language delay reported themselves as being significantly less nurturing and more punitive in their discipline than parents of children who were developing typically. Parental accounts also revealed that children with speech language delay were more detached and less reactive than children without a delay (Carson, Carson, Klee, & Jackman-Brown, 2007).

Physical or motor development encompasses gross and fine motor ability. Gross motor ability includes the control of large groups of muscle involved in walking, sitting, or transferring from one position to another. Fine motor abilities involve the skills to manipulate objects with the hands in order to eat, draw, and play. Children progress through motor milestones in an orderly fashion, attaining these functions in a clear and sequential process. Motor delay is defined as a significant delay in motor abilities without a delay in other developmental categories (Hagan et al., 2017).

■ SOCIAL–EMOTIONAL DEVELOPMENT

Social and emotional development includes the child's interactions, as evidenced by the formation and maintenance of relationships and responsiveness to the presence of others. Social and emotional delay ultimately presents as behavioral abnormalities that differ from normal behavioral responses by their quantity, severity, nature, and duration (U.S. Department of Health & Human Services,

2010). Parents do not understand how deeply babies' and toddlers' social–emotional development is affected by their early experiences (Parenting infants and toddlers today, 2010).

Fostering healthy social and emotional development provides the foundation for school readiness in programs serving infants, toddlers, and their families. Cognitive and social–emotional development are interrelated (From Research to Practice, 2012). Physical, language, cognitive, social, emotional, and psychological development all need to be assessed to determine appropriate toddler development. Delays in any or all of these areas can cause lifelong issues for both the toddler and the parent if not intercepted with appropriate interventions.

A study by Bocknek, Brophy-Herb, Fitzgerald, Burns-Jager, and Carolan (2012) tested a novel latent construct which reflected psychological absence and examined its relations with maternal depression, mother–toddler interactions, and toddlers' social–emotional outcomes in a low-income sample. Structural equation modeling confirmed a psychological absence construct and revealed that psychological absence, measured at the child's 36-month-birthday-related assessment, is a significant predictor of children's social–emotional development at 36 months, mediated by mother–child interaction (Bocknek et al., 2012).

Another study examined the effectiveness of an office-based educational program to improve maternal confidence and the social–emotional development of toddlers. The Toddler Care Questionnaire (TCQ) was administered to all mothers as a pre- and postintervention test. The treatment intervention was a video recorded (DVD) parenting skills intervention on the social–emotional development of toddlers and on maternal confidence in caring for toddlers (Hallas, Koslap-Petraco, & Fletcher, 2017). Pairwise comparisons of adjusted means showed significant improvements for both toddler groups on the Brigance toddler screen and no statistically significant difference in gains between the groups. The mixed-model results for the TCQ showed an overall significant improvement from pre- to posttest and a nonsignificant interaction between group and time, indicting no significant difference in gains seen by treatment groups (Hallas et al., 2017). P-PCPs who encounter mothers who struggle with caring for their toddlers may find brief office-based interventions a valuable tool for educating parents and intercepting unacceptable behaviors.

■ TODDLER TEMPERAMENT

Temperament can be defined as the biologically based core of individual differences in style of approach and response to the environment that is stable across time and situations (Shiner & Caspi, 2003). Thomas and Chess's temperament theory (Chess & Thomas, 1985; Strelau & Angleitner, 2013), in addition to describing several temperament dimensions, classified children as belonging to three types: "easy," "slow to warm up," or "difficult." Toddlers' temperament trait configurations were best described by three profiles: a typical, well-adjusted profile; an expressive profile, prone to externalizing problems; and a fearful profile, prone to internalizing problems (Akker, Dekovic, Prinzie, & Asscher, 2010; Buss & Plomin, 1984). Negative and positive parenting styles influence the development of temperament profiles over time (Akker et al., 2010). Parents who constantly yell or continually say "no" to every behavior send negative messages to their toddlers. Redirecting an unwanted behavior to a more positive one guides the toddler in a manner that promotes self-esteem.

Lickenbrock et al. (2013) indicated that temperament and attachment predicted toddler behavior. Toddlers who were secure with mothers and low in temperamental negative reactivity showed more committed compliance than those who were insecure and low in negative reactivity or secure and high in negative reactivity. In addition, interactions revealed that relations between infant–mother attachment and defiance depended on infant–father attachment security, temperament, and context. Findings highlight the differential and complex roles of temperament and attachment as potential precursors of later social competence.

P-PCPs should consider whether the behavior is part of a normal developmental phase or temperament style before labeling that child with a behavior disorder (Tomlin, 2004). Specific behaviors that have received considerable research investigation include negative emotionality; behaviors related to impulsivity; persistence with undesirable behaviors, lack of compliance, or resistance to control; and short attention span and low effort control (Tomlin, 2004). Appropriate assessment affords the opportunity to intercept abnormal behaviors. P-PCPs can observe the behavior of the toddler during the encounter and *intercept* those behaviors by demonstrating positive, nurturing parenting skills that set appropriate limits. It is also important to ask how the parent disciplines the child. Observing the interaction between the parent and child also offers the P-PCP insight into the relationship between the parent and child. If the answers to any of these questions in Table 12.1 raise red flags, then the P-PCP can offer interventions to intercept the issues that are cause for concern (Hagan et al., 2017).

Temperament in toddlers can be affected by the parenting styles of their mothers. Maternal encouragement can range from protective, gentle encouragement, or intrusive. As mothers demonstrated behavior toward either extreme end of this continuum, thus engaging in either more protective or more intrusive behavior, they reported that their toddlers' separation anxiety increased (Kiel et al., 2016). P-PCPs can intercept these parenting behaviors and offer advice to the mothers by modeling appropriate parenting skills.

In a theoretical framework developed by Bocknek, Brophy-Herb, Fitzgerald, Burns-Jager, and Carolan (2012), a novel latent construct reflecting psychological absence was tested and its relations with maternal depression, mother–toddler interactions, and toddlers' social–emotional outcomes were examined. Structural equation modeling confirmed a psychological absence construct and revealed that psychological absence, measured at the child's 36-month-birthday-related assessment, is a significant predictor of children's social–emotional development at 36 months, mediated by mother–child interaction. An insecure mother–toddler relationship sets the toddler up for a life of less than secure relationships. Toddlers at highest risk, those with earlier behavioral problems from higher demographic-risk families, benefit the most from mothers' emotional talk. Informing parents about the use of emotional talk may be a cost-effective, simple strategy to support at-risk toddlers' social–emotional development and reduce behavioral problems (Brophy-Herb et al., 2015). Toddlers who are able to build trusting, secure, loving relationships with their mothers have the underpinning for lifelong social emotional health. P-PCPs need to assess the relationship between the mother or

TABLE 12.1

SAMPLE QUESTIONS FOR ELICITING TODDLER SOCIAL–EMOTIONAL HISTORY

How do you describe your child's personality?
What do you find difficult about parenting your child?
What about your child makes you most proud?
Have there been any stresses in your family?
How do you, the parent, offer emotional support to your toddler?
Does the toddler look to the parent for reassurance during the encounter?
Does the parent ensure that the toddler is safe?
Does the parent provide positive reinforcement to the toddler's behaviors?

primary caregiver and the toddler and intercept any issues in the relationship. P-PCPs need to be prepared to provide immediate intervention as soon as parenting issues are identified.

■ TODDLER ASSESSMENT FOR BEHAVIORAL PROBLEMS

Assessment should include a health history about the accomplishments of the child, family dynamics, and questions and/or concerns the parent or guardian has about the toddler. Assessment of developmental history should include previous results of Denver Developmental Screening Test II (DDSTII), achievement of developmental milestones, and any results from other standardized evaluations such as Ages and Stages (Briggs-Gowan & Carter, 2006; Gartstein, & Rothbart, 2003; Glascoe, 1992; Squires, Bricker, & Twombly, 2015). If any delays are noted, ask the status of services such as early intervention, speech, occupational and/or physical therapy, and special education the toddler has received. If the toddler has delays and is not receiving early intervention (EI) services, then an EI referral should be made by the P-PCP. Parents or guardians should be asked if there is any new family history, such as a new medical condition or death of a close family member, as this may be related to a toddler's abnormal social–emotional behaviors (Hallas, 2011). Assessment of social history should include any noted behavioral issues and a review of family structure and support systems. If any evidence of a dysfunctional family is identified, ask about family structure and function.

The P-PCP should assess for speech and language development, such as clarity of words, number of words in vocabulary, and development of social skills (Hallas, 2011). Initially, toddlers will point or gesture to objects that he or she would like to explore. A toddler whose caregiver does not correctly interpret the toddler's gesturing language may see first signs of the toddler's temper or frustration via acting out behaviors or temper tantrums. Parental/caregiver recognition of a toddler's initial expressive gesture language may be a critical component of the toddler's healthy development and may be the first intercept in prevention of adverse social–emotional development patterns. Use the Modified Checklist for Autism in Toddlers Surveillance and Screening Algorithm: Autistic Spectrum Disorders (ASD) for Toddlers (M-CHAT; Robbins, & Dumont-Mathiew, 2006; Robbins,

Fein, Martin, & Green, 2001) at 18- and 21- and/or 24-month-old episodic visits (Hallas, 2011). See Chapters 14 and 25 for discussions on ASD. Interaction between the parent and/or guardian and toddler should also be closely observed during each healthcare visit. Observe for visual contact between parent and toddler and parental interactions such as comforting the child and positive verbal communication (Hagan et al, 2017).

Various screening tools are available to evaluate toddlers to determine normal from abnormal behaviors. Any abnormalities identified emphasize the need for timely referrals to intercept potential problems through early intervention speech, occupational, or physical therapy services. Screening tools provide objective assessments of toddler behavior and abilities. Multi-domain screening tests which are administered by healthcare professionals or by families or caregivers cover all of the domains. A number of screening tools are easy to use in primary care settings. The most comprehensive and psychometrically sound screening tools are found in Table 12.2.

TABLE 12.2

EFFECTIVE TODDLER SCREENING TOOLS

Tool and Explanation
- Ages and Stages Questionnaires: Social–Emotional-2, Infant–Toddler Social and Emotional Assessment Ages and Stages Questionnaire, 3rd ed. (ASQ-3)
  - Designed to be implemented in a range of settings and can easily be tailored to fit the needs of many families
  - Clear drawings and simple directions help parents indicate children's skills in language, personal–social, fine and gross motor, and problem solving
  - First-level screening tool to determine which children need further evaluation to determine their eligibility for early intervention or preschool services (Ringwalt, 2008)
  - Age range is birth to 60 months and takes 15–20 minutes to complete
- Brief Infant–Toddler Social and Emotional Assessment and Child Behavior Checklist 1½-5
  - 42-item parent-report questionnaire used to screen for social–emotional and behavioral problems and developmental delay in 12- to 36-month-olds (Briggs-Gowan & Carter, 2002)
- BRIGANCE® Early Childhood Screens
  - Identifies potential developmental delays and giftedness in language, motor, self-help, social–emotional, and cognitive skills—all in 10–15 minutes per child
  - Three different testing levels, including ages 0–35 months, and takes 10 minutes to administer (Curriculum Associates, 2013)
- Denver Developmental Screening Test II
  - Assesses children for possible developmental problems
  - An objective measure must be used to confirm suspected problems
  - Can also be used to monitor children at risk for developmental problems
  - Screens children's development in four areas of functioning: fine motor–adaptive, gross motor, personal–social, and language skills
  - Test had limited specificity (43%) and a high over-referral rate
Authors of the DDST II need to engage in further development of the instrument, including revising scoring criteria and item placement in relation to children's ages (Frankenburg, Dodds, Archer, Shapiro, & Bresnick, 1992).

■ EFFECTIVE TODDLER SCREENING TOOLS

Although all measures show acceptable reliability, a systematic review by Pontoppidan, Niss, Pejtersen, Julian, and Væver (2017) revealed the most comprehensive and psychometrically sound measures are the Ages and Stages Questionnaires: Social–Emotional-2; Infant–Toddler Social and Emotional Assessment; Brief Infant–Toddler Social and Emotional Assessment; and Child Behavior Checklist 1–1/5–5.

■ TREATMENT OF EMOTIONAL, SOCIAL, AND BEHAVIORAL HEALTH PROBLEMS

The development of emotional, social, and behavioral health in toddlers is primarily the responsibility of the parents. Working parents do send their toddlers to day care, but for the most part, toddlers are with one or both parents for the majority of their days and nights. The toddler years are a critical time for development of emotional, social, and behavioral health. Parents must themselves have personal control of their feelings and emotions, and must be able to "go-with-the-flow" when caring for their toddler. Toddlers are impulsive and parents must recognize the difference between impulsive behaviors that are normal and those behaviors that need interventions to assure normal development.

Primary care visits with the P-PCP provides an opportunity for parents to discuss toddler behaviors and to learn about the normal and expected behaviors. Brief educational programs on DVDs are an efficient way to offer information to mothers while in the office waiting area. Mothers who struggle with caring for their toddlers may find brief office-based interventions a valuable educational tool to improve their confidence in their parenting skills (Hallas et al., 2017). If office-based interventions do not resolve parenting issues, the P-PCP must be prepared to make the appropriate referral (i.e., mental health or parenting classes).

Anticipatory Guidance

Anticipatory guidance is the cornerstone for treating toddlers and their families to both intercept aberrant behaviors as well as reinforce appropriate behaviors. Advise parents to develop strategies to consistently manage the power struggles that result from the toddler's need to control the environment. Allowing the toddler to choose between two sets of clothes to be worn for the day is an example. Ask the parent to acknowledge the behaviors that the parent likes and try to ignore the ones he or she does not like. Have the parent set limits for the toddler by using distraction, gentle restraint, and when necessary a brief time-out. The toddler can be separated from the cause of the problem. Structure and routine are important for toddlers. In today's world, structure and routine can be difficult for parents who are both often working outside the home and are stressed themselves. Advise parents that to discipline is to teach. Appropriate discipline teaches the toddler how to get along in the world and with others.

TIME-OUT FOR TODDLERS

Time-out is an effective technique to avoid paying negative attention. The goal is to not communicate with the toddler during a time-out to allow time to calm down. Time-outs should be brief and last between 60 to 90 seconds. Effective time-out has three elements: Do not raise the voice, be calm, and speak softly; as few words as possible should be used. An example is "children who throw things at others must do a time-out." The time-out should be ended by looking to the future such as "let's have a hug and go outdoors." Recalling the bad behavior reminds the toddler that if that behavior is repeated, it is a good way to get attention. Never criticize the child, only the behavior. An example would be "I do not like it at all when you run away from me but I love you very much." Intercept aggressive behaviors by advising parents to teach toddlers not to hit, bite, or use other aggressive behaviors. The parent can model this for the child by never hitting or spanking the child and always speaking in a respectful manner to the parent's partner (Hagan et al., 2017).

COMMUNICATING WITH TODDLERS

Encourage parents to sing and read to their toddlers. If parents are overheard to be using baby talk, intercept and advise them to speak normally to the toddler. Two-year-olds should be able to use two-word sentences such as "go out" or "want water" and be able to follow simple two-step commands. An example is "go to your room and bring me back a book." Encourage parents to talk to their toddlers. Advise them to keep the toddler near and tell the toddler exactly what the parent is doing. Toddlers usually love to work with their parents. Suggest parents describe in words exactly what they are doing when preparing a meal or completing other physical work. Toddlers often respond slowly to verbal information at this age. Intercept parent frustration and let them know that the toddler will be slow to answer. The parent should also be advised to speak and answer questions slowly and repeat what the toddler says in a positive way.

HEARING AND VISION

Hearing and vision problems may be misinterpreted by the parent as behavioral problems. Hearing can be an issue for children; explain to parents that if the toddler must look at the parent to understand what is being said, the toddler needs a hearing test. If the toddler sits too close to the television or holds books close to the face, the toddler may be having difficulty seeing. Advise the parent to ask for vision testing for the toddler. Accidents are best avoided; therefore advise the parent to ensure that the home is safe and make sure to include street safety.

BEGIN BUILDING A POSITIVE SELF-IMAGE EARLY

Intercept potential problems with overweight by discussing healthy eating with parents. Having toddlers assist with food preparation teaches a toddler what is healthy to eat and sets the toddler on a path of lifelong positive relationships with food. Children who are overweight when they enter school may be subjected to teasing, leading to a poor self-image. Children with poor oral hygiene when they enter school may also be teased by classmates leading to a poor self-image. Intercept potential dental caries by limiting juice and advising the parent about proper tooth brushing. Dental caries are 100% preventable.

SAFE MEASURES AVOID BEHAVIORAL PROBLEMS

Assess car seat safety by reviewing the need to strap the toddler into an appropriately sized car seat for every ride no matter how short. The safest seat for all children until age 13 years is the back seat. Advise parents to role-model safe behavior in cars by wearing seat belts themselves.

ESTABLISHING BEDTIME ROUTINES

Have parents establish sleep routines such as teeth brushing and reading a story before bed. Reading to toddlers establishes a lifelong love of reading. One way to encourage the independence of the toddler is to allow the child to choose what story to read each evening. Parents should not be surprised if the toddler chooses the same book each and every night. This pattern is a normal part of toddler routines in which they feel safe. While toddlers fight to assert their independence, they love structure and routine.

TOILET TRAINING

Review with parent cues for toilet training readiness, such as the diaper staying dry for several hours or by asking the toddler if he or she wants to wear big boy or big girl underwear. See Chapter 13 for details on toilet training.

KEEPING THE TODDLER SAFE

Intercept deadly accidents by asking parents where they store guns and ensure that all guns are safely locked away. Home fires are an ever-present danger. Ask parents if they have smoke detectors in the home and that they are in working order with fresh batteries. A good way to remember when to change the batteries is to remind parents to change the batteries when changing the time on clocks in the spring and fall. Intercept burn injuries by advising parents to keep all matches locked up and to teach toddlers about the danger of hot surfaces such as stoves (Hagan et al., 2017).

■ TREATING TEMPER TANTRUMS

Temper tantrums are an expected developmental event in the lives of most toddlers. They occur when the toddler is angry or frustrated and is unable to control feelings. Temper tantrums can range from whining and crying to the toddler throwing himself or herself on the floor kicking and screaming. Toddlers resort to temper tantrums when they feel a loss of control. Developmentally they have few options to express their loss of control so they resort to temper tantrums which are most often very trying for parents who also experience a sense of loss of control (Green, Whitney, & Potegal, 2011). The loss of control creates a situation that can only escalate when parents, mostly the mothers, do not have coping skills to manage their unhappy toddlers (Whalley & Hyland, 2013). Over time as toddlers mature, they learn to manage their frustrations and the temper tantrums will cease. Parents need to have effective strategies at their fingertips to assist the toddler in resolving the temper tantrums. A parent who has effective interventions to intercept the tantrum feels in control while assisting the toddler in managing frustrations. Interventions to stop or limit temper tantrums consist of the following: ignoring the child's behavior, ensuring that the situation is safe, getting down to the child's level and speaking softly to the child, and using positive reinforcement once the toddler regains control of himself or herself (Gault-Caviness, 2000). An example is to simply ignore the behavior and speak softly to tell the toddler that mom will speak to him or her when the toddler regains control. If the tantrum is occurring in a public place, the parent may want to leave with the child and just sit quietly with the child somewhere safe until the child regains control. Another example is a mother who gets down on the floor close to her child and reminds the child in a soft voice that mommy knows he or she is having a very hard time and that she will resume speaking to the toddler once the toddler regains control. The parent would then ignore the behavior until the temper tantrum is over. P-PCPs can review these strategies with parents and practice the interventions during regular visits to intercept parental frustration and give them tools to assist their toddlers through this normal developmental stage (Hallas et al., 2017).

■ SUMMARY

Toddlers are terrific. They are curious, inquisitive, and they want to be noticed. They are learning what it means to be a member of the family and how to get along with their family members, all the while feeling good about themselves. Learning to be part of the family prepares toddlers to be part of a much larger world as they grow and approach school attendance, and then move on to an even larger world later as school-age children and teens and ultimately into adulthood. It is an amazing experience to watch toddlers grow and develop into happy, successful, well-adjusted human persons. The P-PCP can be the key to helping parents or caregivers successfully navigate this exhilarating but challenging time in their toddlers' lives.

■ REFERENCES

Akker, A., Dekovic, M., Prinzie, P., & Asscher, J. (2010). Toddlers' temperament profiles: Stability and relations to negative and positive parenting. *Journal of Abnormal Child Psychology*, 38(4), 485–495. doi:10.1007/s10802-009-9379-0

American Psychiatric Association. (2013). *Diagnostic and statistical manual of mental disorders* (5th ed.). Washington, DC: Author.

Bocknek, E. L., Brophy-Herb, H. E., Fitzgerald, H., Burns-Jager, K., & Carolan, M. T. (2012). Maternal psychological absence and toddlers' social–emotional development: Interpretations from the perspective of boundary ambiguity theory. *Family Process*, 51(4), 527–541. doi:10.1111/j.1545-5300.2012.01411.x

Briggs-Gowan, M. J., & Carter, A. S. (1998). Preliminary acceptability and psychometrics of the infant–toddler social and emotional assessment ITSEA: A new adult-report questionnaire. *Infant Mental Health*, *19*, 422–455. Retrieved from https://scholar.google.com/scholar?hl=en&as_sdt=0%2C33&as_vis=1&q=Briggs-Gowan%2C+M.J.%2C+%26+Carter%2C+A.S.+%281998%29.+Preliminary+acceptability+and+psychometrics+of+the+infant-toddler+social+and+emotional+assessment+ITSEA%3A+A+new+adult-report+questionnaire.+Infant+Mental+Health%2C+19%2C+422%E2%80%934 55.+&btnG=

Briggs-Gowan, M. J., & Carter, A. S. (2002). *Brief infant-toddler social and emotional assessment (BITSEA) manual, Version 2.0*. New Haven, CT: Yale University. Retrieved from https://scholar.google.com/scholar?q=Briggs-Gowan+M.J.,+%26+Carter,+A.S.+(2002).Brief+Infant-Toddler+Social+and+Emotional+Assessment+(BITSEA)&hl=en&as_sdt=0&as_vis=1&oi=scholart&sa=X&ved=0ahUKEwionJWG7KHXAhUE5iYKHSzUDqsQgQMIJzAA

Briggs-Gowan, M. J., & Carter, A. S. (2006). *Manual for the brief infant-toddler social & emotional assessment BITSEA – Version 2*. San Antonio, TX: Psychological Corporation, Harcourt Press. Retrieved from https://academic.oup.com/jpepsy/article/29/2/143/926026

Briggs-Gowan, M. J., Carter, A. S., Irwin, J., Wachtel, K., & Cicchetti, D. (2004). The brief infant toddler social and emotional assessment: Screening for social-emotional problems and delays in competence. *Journal of Pediatric Psychology*, (29), 143–155. Retrieved from https://www-ncbi-nlm-nih-gov.proxy.library.stonybrook.edu/pubmed/?term=Briggs-Gowan%2C+M.J.%2C+Carter%2C+A.S.%2C+Irwin%2C+J.%2C+Wachtel%2C+K.%2C+%26+Cicchetti%2C+D.

Brophy-Herb, H. E., Bocknek, E. L., Vallotton, C. D., Stansbury, K. E., Senehi, N., Dalimonte-Merckling, D., & Lee, Y. (2015). Toddlers with early behavioral problems at higher family demographic risk benefit the most from maternal emotion talk. *Journal of Developmental & Behavioral Pediatrics*, *36*(7), 512–520. doi:10.1097/DBP.0000000000000196

Buss, A. H., & Plomin, R. (1984).*Temperament: Early developing personality traits*. Hillsdale, MI: Erlbaum.

Carson, C., Carson, D., Klee, T., & Jackman-Brown, J. (2007). Self-reported parenting behavior and child temperament in families of toddlers with and without speech-language delay. *Communication Disorders Quarterly*, *28*(3), 155–165. doi:10.1177/15257401070280030501

Carter, A. S., & Briggs-Gowan, M. J. (2006). *Manual for the infant-toddler social & emotional assessment ITSEA – Version 2*. San Antonio, TX: Psychological Corporation, Harcourt Press. Retrieved from www.pearsonclinical.com/childhood/products/100000652/infant-toddler-social-emotional-assessment-itsea.html

Chess, S., & Thomas, A. (1985). *Temperament in clinical practice*. New York, NY: Guilford.

Curriculum Associates. (2013). *Brigance Early Childhood Screen III*. Retrieved from http://www.curriculumassociates.com/products/detail.aspx?title=brigec-screens

Frankenburg, W. K., Dodds, J., Archer, P., Shapiro, H., & Bresnick, B. (1992). The Denver II: A major revision and restandardization of the Denver developmental screening test. *Pediatrics*, *89*(1). Retrieved from http://pediatrics.aappublications.org/content/89/1/91

From Research to Practice. (2012). *Zero to Three*, *33*(1), 37–43. Retrieved from Journal Archive Zero to Three.,https://www.zerotothree.org/resources/series/journal-archive

Gartstein, M. A., & Rothbart, M. K. (2003). Studying infant temperament via the revised infant behavior questionnaire. *Infant Behavior and Development*, *26*, 64–86. Retrieved from https://www.researchgate.net/.../222579297_Gartstein_MA_Rothbart_MK_Studying_inf

Gault-Caviness, Y. (2000). Temper tantrums. *Essence (Essence)*, *30*(12), 154. Retrieved from http://eds.a.ebscohost.com.proxy.library.stonybrook.edu/ehost/detail/detail?vid=7&sid=f0d602e1-7d4a-4aff-a183-4cce62f12d43%40sessionmgr4010&bdata=JnNpdGU9ZWhvc3QtbGl2ZSZzY29wZT1zaXRl#AN=2941356&db=pbh

Glascoe, F. P., Byrne, K. E., Ashford, L. G., Johnson, K. L., Chang, B., & Strickland, B. (1992). Accuracy of the Denver-II in developmental screening. *Pediatrics*, *89*(6). Retrieved from http://pediatrics.aappublications.org/content/89/6/1221

Goldsmith, H. H. (1996). Studying temperament via construction of the toddler behavior assessment questionnaire. *Child Development*, *67*, 218–235. doi:10.2307/1131697

Green, J. A., Whitney, P. G., & Potegal, M. (2011). Screaming, yelling, whining, and crying: Categorical and intensity differences in vocal expressions of anger and sadness in children's tantrums. *Emotion*, *11*(5), 1124–1133. doi:10.1037/a0024173

Hagan, J. F., Shaw, J. S., & Duncan, P. (Eds.). (2017). *Bright futures: Guidelines for health supervision of infants, children, and adolescents* (4th ed.). Elk Grove, IL: American Academy of Pediatrics.

Hallas, D. (2011). Obtaining an interval history. *Pediatric Primary Care*, 9. Retrieved from http://samples.jbpub.com/9781449600433/00433_ch02_009_016.pdf

Hallas, D., Koslap-Petraco, M., & Fletcher, J. (2017). Social–emotional development of toddlers: Randomized controlled trial of an office-based intervention. *Journal of Pediatric Nursing*, 33, 33–40. doi:10.1016/j.pedn.2016.11.004.

Kiel, E., Premo, J., Buss, K., Kiel, E. J., Premo, J. E., & Buss, K. A. (2016). Maternal encouragement to approach novelty: A curvilinear relation to change in anxiety for inhibited toddlers. *Journal Of Abnormal Child Psychology*, 44(3), 433–444. doi:10.1007/s10802-015-0038-3

Lickenbrock, D. M., Braungart-Rieker, J. M., Ekas, N. V., Zentall, S. R., Oshio, T., & Planalp, E. M. (2013). Early temperament and attachment security with mothers and fathers as predictors of toddler compliance and noncompliance. *Infant & Child Development*, 22(6), 580–602. doi:10.1002/icd.1808

Parenting Infants and Toddlers Today. (2010). Young children's social–emotional development: Key finds from a 2009 national parent survey. *Zero to Three*, 30(4), 43–44. Retrieved from http://www.pyramidmodel.org/wpcontent/uploads/2016/10/key_findings_from_zt3_2009_national_parent_survey.pdf

Pontoppidan, M., Niss, N. K., Pejtersen, J. H., Julian, M. M., & Væver, M. S. (2017). Parent report measures of infant and toddler social–emotional development: A systematic review. *Family Practice*, 34(2), 127–137. doi:10.1093/fampra/cmx003

Ringwalt, S. (2008). *Developmental screening and assessment instruments with an emphasis on social and emotional development for young children ages birth through five*. Chapel Hill, NC: The University of North Carolina, FPG Child Development Institute, National Early Childhood Technical Assistance Center. Retrieved from http://www.nectac.org/~pdfs/pubs/screening.pdf

Robbins, D., & Dumont-Mathiew, T. M. (2006). Early screening for autism spectrum disorders: Update on the modified checklist for autism in toddlers and other measures. *Journal of Developmental Pediatrics*, 27(2 Suppl.), S111–S119. Retrieved from https://www-ncbi-nlm-nih-gov.proxy.library.stonybrook.edu/pubmed/16161090

Robbins, D., Fein, D., Martin, M., & Green, J. (2001). The modified checklist for autism in toddlers: An initial study investigating the early detection of autism and pervasive developmental disorders. *Journal of Autism and Developmental Disorders*, 31, 131–144. Retrieved from https://www.m-chat.org/_references/Robins_JADD01.pdf

Shiner, R., & Caspi, A. (2003). Personality differences in childhood and adolescence: Measurement, development, and consequences. *Journal of Child Psychology and Psychiatry*, 44, 2–32.

Squires, J., Bricker, D, & Twombly, E. (2015). *Ages & Stages Questionnaires: Social-Emotional* (2nd ed.). Baltimore, MD: Brooks Publishing. Retrieved from http://products.brookespublishing.com/Ages-Stages-Questionnaires-Social-Emotional-Second-Edition-ASQSE-2-P849.aspx

Strelau, J., & Angleitner, A. (2013). *Explorations in temperament: International perspectives on theory*. Retrieved from https://books.google.com/books?isbn=1489906436

Tomlin, A. (2004). Thinking about challenging behavior in toddlers: Temperament style or behavior disorder? *Zero To Three*, 24(4), 29–36.

U.S. Department of Health & Human Services. (2010). Infant toddler development screening and assessment. *National Infant and Toddler Child Care Initiative Zero to Three*. Retrieved from http://www.pyramidmodel.org/wp-content/uploads/2016/10/key_findings_from_zt3_2009_national_parent_survey.pdf

Whalley, B., & Hyland, M. (2013). Placebo by proxy: The effect of parents' beliefs on therapy for children's temper tantrums. *Journal Of Behavioral Medicine*, 36(4), 341–346. doi:10.1007/s10865-012-9429-x

CHAPTER 13

Recognizing and Intercepting Problems During Toilet Training

AUDRA N. RANKIN

The topic of toilet training is an issue that causes many caregivers to seek advice from clinicians. When is the optimal time? What is the optimal method? What happens when a child shows no interest? These questions are often discussed at preventative care visits and are an important part of anticipatory guidance for parents and caregivers. This chapter discusses factors that should be considered when assessing toilet training readiness, common methods used in Western culture, and difficulties that may be encountered during the training process. Interventions to *intercept* potential and identified problems are presented throughout the chapter.

■ TOILET TRAINING READINESS

When assessing toilet training readiness, clinicians should think about physiological and psychological factors. Physiological milestones that should be reached prior to training include reflex sphincter control which may occur as early as 9 months and myelinization of pyramidal tracts which typically occurs around 12 to 18 months. Psychological readiness includes understanding verbal cues and demonstrating positive relationships with caregivers (Christopherson, 1991). Some experts recommend waiting 3 months after the achievement of these milestones to begin training as attempting to toilet train before these milestones have been met may lead to difficulties. For many parents, the time frame of training may not be as important as the ease of the training process. Discussing normal developmental milestones and encouraging parents to wait until the child is ready will facilitate toilet training success (Christopherson, 1991).

Timing of Training

Although there is no universal timeline for toilet training readiness, many clinicians agree that most healthy children reach necessary physiological and psychological milestones around 18 months of age and may be completely trained by 2 to 3 years of age (Brazelton et al., 1999). Current guidelines in North America from the American Academy of Pediatrics (AAP) and the Canadian Pediatric Society suggest avoiding training prior to 18 months of age due to physical readiness (Kiddoo et al., 2006). The AAP also stresses the importance of parents not beginning toilet training until the child is behaviorally, developmentally, and emotionally ready. Clinicians should plan on discussing toilet training methods and expectations at the 12- to 18-month visit and at the 2-year health maintenance visit (Kiddoo et al., 2006).

In the United States, 26% of toddlers achieve daytime continence by 24 months, 88% by 30 months, and 98% by 36 months (Kimball, 2016). The age of initiation of toilet training has risen in the United States. Schum et al. (2002) found children toilet trained in the late 1990s achieved bowel and bladder control 12 to 15 months later than children trained in the 1950s (Kiddoo et al., 2006). Many factors may have impacted this delay, including a push for using a child-centered approach, an increased understanding of pediatric physiological development, the use of effective disposable diapers, and more parents working outside the home (Nunen, Kaerts, Wyndaele, Vermandel, & Hal, 2015). Negative consequences of delayed potty training may include higher financial expense because of prolonged diaper use and an increased risk of acute infectious diarrhea in child care centers (Vermandel, Weyler, Wachter, & Wyndaele, 2008).

▪ FACTORS IMPACTING TOILET TRAINING

Toilet training should be viewed as a complex operant and social learning process (Vermandel et al., 2008). Clinicians should consider social, cultural, and economic influences as well as child, parent, and caregiver perspectives (Brazelton et al., 1999). Factors such as a child being away from a parent for several hours a day, day-care attendance, health conditions, and developmental delays may impact toilet training readiness and success (Brazelton et al., 1999).

Gender

The age of toilet training readiness is similar in girls and boys, but girls consistently tend to complete toilet training before boys. This may be due to several factors. Girls are often more motivated by socialization (Brazelton et al., 1999) and are often more physically mature with advanced language skills (Kiddoo et al., 2006). Alternatively, male success may be more dependent on physiologic maturation (Brazelton et al., 1999) and they may experience difficulties with learning separate postures for voiding and defecating (Kiddoo et al., 2006).

Cultural Considerations

There are often variances in toilet training initiation. Past studies have found that African American children typically began toilet training around 21 months of age and were successfully trained by 30 months, while Caucasian children began toilet training around 30 months of age and were trained by 39 months. European American mothers stated children were able to be toilet trained at 28.1 months, while Puerto

Rican, African American, and West Indian–Caribbean mothers felt children were ready to begin toilet training between 20.2 and 22.2 months (Kiddoo et al., 2006).

Behavioral and Developmental Differences

Special considerations should be made for children with physical, mental, behavioral, and developmental handicaps. These children may have impaired communication, sensory process difficulties, and compromised motor skills making the toilet training process difficult (Kiddoo et al., 2006). While many children who present with delays may just need additional reassurance and support (Jacob, Grodzinski, & Fertleman, 2016), they should not be expected to toilet train at the same rate as other children (Kiddoo et al., 2006)

Chronic Illness

Children with chronic illness may also need additional time with the toilet training process. Frequent medications like diuretics and antibiotics may cause increased urination and diarrhea, respectively, complicating toilet training. In addition, it is important to consider anomalies that may result in the inability to feel bladder fullness (Brazelton et al., 1999).

Environmental Factors

Variances in the home and school environment may encourage or delay the toilet training process. Children may be more likely to respond to peers who are displaying toileting skills and this peer pressure may override maturational factors, resulting in more rapid toilet training. Conversely, caregivers should be cautious of varying toileting practices at home and day care. For example, wearing a diaper at day care but toilet training at home may cause a delay in training (Brazelton et al., 1999).

■ TOILET TRAINING METHODS

There are two commonly used toilet training methods in Western society: Brazelton's child-oriented theory (Brazelton et al., 1999) and Azrin and Foxx's (1973) structured behavioral theory. Brazelton's theory is a child-centered approach where caregivers respond to a child's signals, while Azrin and Foxx's (1973) method is a structured behavioral method where caregivers elicit specific toilet training behaviors (Brazelton et al., 1999). There is insufficient evidence to recommend one training method over the other (Kiddoo et al., 2006). The decision should be made on an individual basis considering the timing of training and environmental factors (Brazelton et al., 1999).

Brazelton's Child-Oriented Theory

Developed in 1962, Brazelton's method encourages parents to have minimal involvement in the toilet training process while children experiment with toileting at their own pace. Brazelton's approach asks that training is delayed until at least 18 months of age and initiation is dependent on reaching several milestones including voluntary bowel and bladder control, cooperation with training, and achievement of gross motor skills (such as walking) that indicate complete myelinization of pyramidal tracts (Brazelton et al., 1999).

The method is comprised of several steps:

1. Place potty chair in bathroom most frequently used by the child.
2. Child sits on potty chair with clothes on.
3. Child sits on potty chair without clothes/diaper immediately after having a dirty diaper. (The dirty diaper is placed in potty chair to show the purpose of the chair.)
4. Child is taken to potty chair several times without a diaper.
5. Child is encouraged to approach the potty chair alone. (Christopherson, 1991)

Azrin and Foxx's Structured Behavioral Theory

Developed in the early 1970s, Azrin and Foxx (1973) use a parent-oriented method that is based on the belief that most healthy children can be potty trained within a few hours (Christopherson, 1991). Similar to the Brazelton et al. (1999) child-centered approach, Azrin and Foxx's (1973) method is also dependent on reaching several milestones before initiation. These include being able to stay dry for several hours, having sufficient muscle tone, having the ability to follow simple instructions, and being motivated to use toileting skills (Brazelton et al., 1999).

Four principles in this toilet training method include increased fluid intake, regularly scheduled toilet times, positive reinforcement for correct elimination, and overcorrection for accidents (Brazelton et al., 1999). Due to the more intense nature of this program, clinicians may advise caregivers that reinforcement should not be done too quickly or strongly, as it may lead to regression. Additionally, there is a risk of inadvertently encouraging the child to perform incorrect behaviors, such as accidents, because these behaviors may occur more than correct elimination. Special consideration should be given for children with cardiac or renal disease that may not be able to tolerate increased fluid intake and for children with mental disabilities or behavior problems (Brazelton et al., 1999).

There is no clear evidence that one method is better than the other. Clinical practice guidelines from the American Academy of Family Physicians and the AAP provide recommendations on toilet training timing and approach. Both the American Academy of Family Physicians and the AAP suggest starting training when the parent and child are ready, usually around 2 years of age. They also suggest using a child-oriented approach, with caregivers encouraging successes and avoiding punishment or shaming (Kiddoo et al., 2006). Additional evidence on the efficacy of toilet training programs that can be adapted for cultural or environmental factors or that may be modified for children who are diagnosed with physical disabilities or behavioral disorders is needed (Kiddoo et al., 2006).

■ TOILETING CHALLENGES, REGRESSION, AND REFUSAL

There is no universal definition of being successfully toilet trained (Kiddoo et al., 2006). Although many may define toilet training as a child's ability to avoid accidents, Western culture typically defines successful toilet training as the ability to also eliminate in socially acceptable sites, dress and undress, close the bathroom door, and wash hands. As a result, there may be discrepancies between the definition of initial toilet training success and mastery (Brazelton et al., 1999).

Training Challenges

Children may express fears related to using the toilet. Noises from standard and auto toilet flushing or using the bathroom in public may cause distress in some children. Additionally, children may be afraid they will fall in the toilet bowl or be "sucked" in the toilet when it is flushed. Explaining flushing, using a potty seat, and encouraging toilet use at a familiar friend's or caregiver's home may help to alleviate some of these concerns (Kimball, 2016). Although often a completely normal toileting challenge, children with toilet fears may also have problems with other behaviors such as panic disorder, separation anxiety, fear of physical injury, obsessive compulsive disorder, and social phobia (Defenderfer, Davies, Raicu, Brei, & Klein-Tasman, 2016). Special consideration of persistent fears by the clinician is necessary.

It is very normal for children to be toilet trained with urine first and then stool. In these instances, some children may opt to have regular bowel movements in their pants or ask for a diaper to have a bowel movement. This is often related to a child's fear that having a bowel movement may cause pain. A history of hard stools has been shown to have a correlation to toileting refusal due to discomfort (Christopherson, 1991). The following steps may help alleviate bowel movement fears, thus, *intercepting* potential behavioral health problems:

1. Allow the child to use a diaper for a bowel movement.
2. Bring the child into the bathroom and allow him or her to have a bowel movement in a diaper near the toilet.
3. Have the child sit on the toilet to have a bowel movement while wearing a diaper.
4. Have the child sit on the toilet to have a bowel movement without a diaper.
5. Have the child keep feet flat on the floor or keep feet flat on a small step stool to help the child feel secure and facilitate the stooling process (Kimball, 2016).

Intercepting Toilet Training Accidents

Many caregivers are discouraged by their children having accidents. It is important to remember that accidents happen! Often accidents are a result of a variety of factors including limited access to a toilet, clothing that is difficult to remove, or acute illness or stress (Brazelton et al., 1999). Encourage caregivers to stay positive when accidents occur and avoid shaming. In addition, P-PCPs may be able to assist parents to intercept accidents by planning timed bathroom breaks.

Intercepting Toilet Training Resistance: Avoiding Power Struggles

Toilet training regression is also a common occurrence in children. Regression is often seen with the birth of a new sibling or a major transition such as with a new caregiver, new house, moving from a crib to a bed, or death of a loved one. If a child is experiencing regression, caregivers may allow a child to use a diaper for a few days (Kimball, 2016). During these times it is important to avoid intense toilet training. (Brazelton et al., 1999).

When facing potty training resistance, either initially or due to regression, caregivers should carefully consider the child's readiness. Additionally, caregivers may consider modeling the toileting process as well as reading books about toilet training to foster interest in the child (Kimball, 2016). If a child is consistently refusing toilet training, encourage the parents to allow a training break for 3 months to eliminate possible caregiver–child power struggles (Brazelton et al., 1999; Kiddoo, et al. 2006).

■ SUMMARY

In summary, there is no clear definition of what defines successful toilet training or a roadmap to achieve these results. Although evidence related to working with special populations is limited, it is clear that determining toilet training readiness and the appropriate method should be based on the individual child in conjunction with the P-PCPs and caregiver. P-PCPs play a unique role in helping parents achieve successful toilet training by providing education and guidance to the parents and by intercepting potential problems with evidence-based interventions (Arzin & Foxx, 1973; Brazelton et al., 1999).

■ REFERENCES

Azrin, R. M., & Foxx, N. H. (1973). Dry pants: A rapid method of toilet training children. *Behaviour Research and Therapy, 11*, 435–442. Retrieved from https://www.ncbi.nlm.nih.gov/pubmed/4777640

Brazelton, T., Christopherson, E., Frauman, A., Gorski, P., Poole, J., Stadtler, A., & Wright, C. (1999). Instruction, timeliness, and medical influences affecting toilet training. *Pediatrics, 103*(6), 1353–1358. Retrieved from https://www.ncbi.nlm.nih.gov/pubmed/10353953

Christopherson, E. (1991). Toileting problems in children. *Pediatric Annals, 20*, 240–244. Retrieved from doi:10.3928/0090-4881-19910501-07

Defenderfer, E., Davies, W., Raicu, A., Brei, N., & Klein-Tasman, B. (2016). Childhood toilet fears as an early behavioral indicator of anxiety. *Children's Health Care, 46*, 366–378. doi:10.1080.02739615.2016.1193808. Published online May 26, 2016.

Jacob, H., Grodzinski, B., & Fertleman, C. (2016). Fifteen-minute consultation: Problems in the healthy child—Toilet training. *Archives of Disease in Childhood Education & Practice Edition, 101*, 119–123. doi:10.1136/archdischild-2015-308973

Kiddoo, D., Klassen, T. P., Lang, M. E., Friesen, C., Russel, K., Spponer, C., & Vandermeer, B. (2006). The effectiveness of different methods of toilet training for bowel and bladder control. Evidence Report/Technology Assessment No. 147. *AHRQ Publication NO. 07-E003.* Rockville, MD: Agency for Healthcare Research and Quality. Retrieved from https://www.ncbi.nlm.nih.gov/pubmedhealth/PMH0022937

Kimball, V. (2016). The perils and pitfalls of potty training. *Pediatric Annals, 45*(6), e199–e201. doi:10.3928/00904481-20160512-01

Nunen, K., Kaerts, N., Wyndaele, J., Vermandel, A., & Hal, G. (2015). Parents' view on toilet training (TT): A quantitative study to identify the beliefs and attitudes of parents concerning TT. *Journal of Child Health Care, 19*, 265–274. doi:10.1177/1367493513508232

Schum, T., Kolb, T., McAuliffe, T., Simms, M., Underhill, R., & Lewis, M. (2002). Sequential acquisition of toilet-training skills: A descriptive study of gender and age differences in normal children. *Pediatrics, 109*(3), 1–7. Retrieved from http://pediatrics.aappublications.org/content/109/3/e48

Vermandel, A., Weyler, J., Wachter, S., & Wyndaele, J. (2008). Toilet training of healthy young toddlers: A randomized trial between a daytime wetting alarm and timed potty training. *Journal of Developmental and Behavioral Pediatrics, 29*, 191–196. doi:10.1097/DBP.0b013e31816c433a

CHAPTER 14

Autism, Global Developmental Delays, and Genetic Syndromes

NANCY KRAMER

The Agency for Healthcare Research and Quality (AHRQ) of the U.S. Department of Health & Human Services (2016) estimated the incidence of autism spectrum disorder (ASD) occurs in one in every 68 children or 14.7 cases per 1,000, with most children diagnosed at age 4 or later. Parental concern or early developmental surveillance allows for earlier diagnosis and interventions, though it is estimated that only 42% to 55% of pediatricians regularly screen toddlers for ASD (McPheeters et al., 2016). ASD is more common in males (1:42) than in females (1:189), with inheritability estimated to be between 40% and 90% (McPheeters et al., 2011).

According to the *Diagnostic and Statistical Manual of Mental Disorders, Fifth Edition* (*DSM-5*; American Psychiatric Association [APA], 2013a), both ASD and global developmental delays (GDDs) are categorized as neurodevelopmental disorders. Changes in the diagnostic criteria for ASD based on the revisions between the *DSM-IV-TR* and the *DSM-5* for ASD now combine the subcategories of ASD, Asperger's disorder, childhood disintegrative disorder, and pervasive developmental disorder (PDD) under the category Autism Spectrum Disorder (American Psychiatric Association [APA], 2013b). The PDD category also includes the subcategories of PDD-NOS (not otherwise specified) and Rett's disorder. These changes are based on evidence from clinical field trials. According to the *DSM-5* (APA, 2013a), autism is now identified according to severity levels, which includes a range of support needed for intervention related to social deficits and repetitive behaviors. A core feature of ASD includes marked impairment in social functioning with a marked difficulty in developing meaningful relationships.

The *DSM-5* also defines GDD. In the *DSM-IV*, GDD was known as Mental Retardation, Severity Unspecified. According to the *DSM-5*, "this diagnosis is reserved for individuals younger than age 5 when the clinical severity cannot be reliably assessed during early childhood" (APA, 2013a, p. 41). Key to diagnosing this category is the child's failure in accomplishing developmental milestones in two or more areas, which may include intellectual functioning (American Academy of Neurology [AAN], 2011). Delays or deficits may occur in multiple areas, such as fine and gross motor skills, social development, language development, reasoning, and adaptive skills (Zero to Three, 2016). It is typical for children with this diagnosis to score 1.5 to 2 standard deviations below the mean for their age and cultural context (Zero to Three). Causes of GDD include but are not limited to social neglect, fetal alcohol syndrome (FAS), metabolic disorders such as PKU and storage diseases, and genetic disorders such as Fragile X syndrome, Rett's syndrome, 22q11 deletion syndrome, and Down syndrome (AAN, 2011; APA, 2013a; Zero to Three, 2016).

▦ OVERVIEW OF DEVELOPMENTAL PRESENTATION

Caring for and treating children is caring for families. Health promotion should be the foundation of heath supervision with children and adolescents. Promotion focuses on well-being rather than prevention of illness and disorders. The focus of promotion in mental health is on obtaining healthy outcomes and includes efforts to improve the child's ability to accomplish age-appropriate milestones, develop a positive self-esteem, and strengthen his or her ability to cope. Mental health is critical to a child's physical, psychosocial, and emotional health as well as his/her ability to learn. Health promotion is an important approach to reducing mental, emotional, and behavioral disorders and associated problems. Pediatric primary care providers (P-PCPs) should take every opportunity to promote health with each contact regardless of the setting. If possible, observations should be over time. Health supervision should also include interview questions and anticipatory guidance.

Early recognition of developmental disorders and intervention are the key in providing every child the opportunity to accomplish developmentally appropriate tasks, develop a positive sense of self-esteem, strengthen his/her ability to cope with adversity, and lead a productive life (Cangialose & Allen, 2014; Crais et al., 2014; Lowry, 2012). Though ASD is not easily diagnosed at a young age, there are characteristics that may lead the nurse practitioner to become suspicious and vigilant in his/her attention to each child. GDD has many possible causes, some of which are treatable; hence early recognition and diagnosis are essential in helping the child and family lead a more productive life (AAN, n.d.). Knowledge of individual differences and variations in growth and achieving developmental milestones enables the nurse practitioner to detect manifestations of delays and red flags. The nurse practitioner needs an understanding of not only physical development but also psychosocial, language, and cognitive development, with special attention to behaviors associated with attachment, communication, coping, and play. This knowledge provides an opportunity for early recognition of mental health disorders; enables the nurse practitioner to provide age-appropriate parental guidance; facilitates improved prognosis and quality of life; and provides for early collaboration, referral, and treatment as appropriate. Though most children accomplish the milestones within a predictable period of time, some demonstrate mild to severe developmental delays, which can lead to developmental disabilities. According to the Centers for Disease Control and Prevention (CDC, 2014) *Morbidity and Mortality Weekly Report* on screening for developmental delays, it is estimated that 15% of children ages 3 to 17 have developmental disabilities. Many children do not receive early screening, diagnosis, and interventions.

According to the CDC, approximately 2% to 3% of the 15% of children estimated to have developmental delays actually receive intervention by the age of 3. The key for early intervention and *intercepting* problems as early as possible is routine screening, which also includes attention to parent's or caregiver's report or concern.

■ ASSESSMENT

Developmental Presentation—Early Signs and Onset

AUTISM SPECTRUM DISORDER

Curiosity and exploration are common characteristics of the social development of infants and toddlers. As the child develops, play becomes characterized by symbolism and the young child begins to learn the use of objects as a means to an end. The presence or absence of behaviors associated with the development of social and communication skills may assist the nurse practitioner in early recognition of evidence that may predispose to a diagnosis of ASD. Significant evidence of ASD in a child younger than 12 months of age may include limited eye contact with the caregiver, lack of social smiling and vocalization with caregiver, lack of symbolic play, lack of social imitative play (peek-a-boo, pat-a-cake), and limited or no use of speech and social gestures (Cangialose & Allen, 2014; Chiu, 2011; Lowry, 2012; Soares & Patel, 2012). The nurse practitioner may note difficulty in keeping the infant engaged in social behavior or observe the infant withdrawing or pulling away from social interaction. In older infants or toddlers (ages 16–24 months), the parents may report that the infant is no longer exhibiting or has regressed from a previously learned social response that he or she demonstrated at an earlier age (Lowry, 2012; National Institute of Neurological Disorders and Stroke [NINDS], 2015). Responses demonstrating under or over reactivity may become more evident during the second year of life. It is not uncommon for parents to describe their child as irritable though others may be described as "easy." In addition, reduced muscle tone and difficulty with auditory and visual–spatial processing may be noted. Though none of these behaviors is diagnostic on their own, the nurse practitioner needs to be vigilant and cognizant of parents' reports and of changes in the child's development over time.

As the child moves into the toddler and preschool ages, an aura of detachment or isolation may be noted. Children of this age may demonstrate difficulty in communicating a need for closeness and comfort (Cangialose & Allen, 2014; Lowry, 2012; NINDS, 2015). Facial and vocal expressions as well as social gestures may be limited. The child has difficulty with give and take behavior. Normal development at this age would include interest in pretend play as well as an interest in interacting and playing with other children, which may be lacking in children with social interaction disorders. An increase in repetitive motor and verbal behaviors may also be noted. For example, the child may fixate on an inanimate item, such as a piece of paper, a stick, or a light switch and subsequently engage in repetitive action or an attachment to that object. Repetitive motor behaviors may include repetitive arm or leg movement, such as arm flapping. Any attempts to reduce the repetitive motion or remove the object of attachment may lead to marked anxiety and agitation in response to change (Cangialose & Allen, 2014; Lowry, 2012). Minor changes to a routine or something in the environment, such as bedtime rituals or changing the child's dinner dishes, may also lead to agitation. Repetitive verbal behaviors may be displayed such as echolalia, which is parroting the words of others.

School-age children appear aloof and have limited social interactions and few if any friends (NINDS, 2015). Social discomfort is further demonstrated by limited understanding or interest in group activities, games, or play. Conversation is limited and may be characterized by echolalia, perseveration (continued repetition of a meaningless word or phrase), and unusual speech tone and rhythm. Behavioral patterns may include unusual interests, ritualistic or compulsive behaviors, as well as motor stereotypy (persistent repetition of words, posture, or movement without meaning).

Characteristic behaviors in an adolescent may include limited understanding of social rules and expectations and limited friendships. Speech patterns continue to be characterized by limited reciprocal conversations, perseveration, echolalia, and unusual expression of affect, such as laughing inappropriately. As with the school-age child, behavioral patterns continue to be ritualistic or compulsive with elements of aggression leading to parenting challenges.

Many authors and organizations have identified key red flags associated with ASD (Crais et al., 2014; Lowry, 2012; Wetherby et al., 2004/2012). Being aware of the red flags, which correspond to early developmental signs, may better facilitate early recognition and interventions. Key red flags at 6 months may include lack of appropriate eye gaze and fixation on faces, lack of turning toward sounds, and no smiles. Key red flags at 9 months may include no smiles or facial expressions, and no exchange of vocalization between the infant and parent. Key red flags at 12 months may include not turning head in response to his/her name, no babbling, lack of gestures, poor eye contact, limited play, lack of shared enjoyment, and presence of repetitive actions or movements. Key red flags at 18 months may include loss of word skills, no social connection, and speech may be limited to parroting what is heard. Key red flags at 24 months may include no shared pleasure when playing, no two-word meaningful phrases, and lack of social interest in other children.

GLOBAL DEVELOPMENTAL DELAY

According to the *DSM-5* (APA, 2013a), the diagnosis of GDD is reserved for children no younger than 6 months and younger than 5 years as demonstrated by failure to meet expected developmental milestones. Developmental delays may be evident in several areas of intellectual functioning. This diagnosis may be used for children who are too young to participate in standardized testing or unable to be assessed because of limited intellectual functioning. Further assessment is required at a later time. Delays must be evident in two or more areas of development (AAN, 2011). According to Zero to Three (2016), diagnosis must include deficits in intellectual functioning and adaptive behaviors. Intellectual functioning may include "verbal and nonverbal problems solving, planning, symbolic reasoning, motor skills, social judgment, and learning" (p. 36). Delays may include vision, hearing, speech, fine and gross motor skill, activities of daily living, social development, and emotional development (AAN, 2011; Moeschler, Shevell, & Committee on Genetics, 2014). GDD may also predict future intellectual disabilities (ID), which may be applied to older children who have undergone IQ testing (Moeschler, Shevell, & Committee on Genetics, 2006). Adaptive behavior refers to "performance of age-expected communication, social, and daily living skills required for independent day-to-day adaptive functioning" (Zero to Three, 2016, p. 36).

Early signs of GDD include delays in at least two developmental domains, which may include fine/gross motor skills, speech/language, cognitive, social/personal, and activities of daily living. GDD needs to be further evaluated in relation to observable abnormalities, such as cardiac defects, abnormal skin findings, and unusual appearance.

■ SCREENING

Autism Spectrum Disorder

The key to early intervention is early screening, monitoring, and referral (Lewis, 2017). The American Academy of Pediatrics (AAP) recommends that P-PCPs routinely screen children at ages 18 and 24 months using an autism specific screening tool (AAP] 2016; Dreyer, 2016; Soares & Patel, 2012). Cangialose and Allen (2014) contend that although most recommendations suggest ASD screening at ages 18 and 24 months, P-PCPs can assess for key developmental behaviors, such as lack of eye contact, poor response to name, lack of interest in other children, and lack of attention, at 9, 12, and 15 months well-child checks. According to the *DSM-5* (APA, 2013a), a primary diagnostic feature of ASD is impaired communication. Preverbal communication and vocalization deficits as well as stereotyped behavior may be evident through observations as well as parent/caregiver report (Cangialose & Allen, 2014; Crais et al., 2014; McPheeters et al., 2016; Plum & Wetherby, 2013). In a comparison of ASD-specific screening tools for infants and toddlers, Cangialose and Allen (2014) evaluated their value in identifying early developmental patterns indicative of ASD in children younger than age 18 months. In a review of relevant literature, they compared the utility and validity among the Modified Checklist for Autism in Toddlers (M-CHAT), the Early Screening of Autism Traits questionnaire (ESAT), and the Infant–Toddler Checklist (ITC). They concluded that the identification of children at risk for developing ASD could be assessed for children as young as 16 months with the M-CHAT and with the ESAT in children as young as 14 months. Communication delays in children as early as 9 months can be detected by the ITC.

Global Developmental Delay

Screening for GDD should be part of developmental screening that occurs with the use of a norm-referenced, age-appropriate screening tool at 9, 18, and 30 months of age (Lewis, 2017; Soares & Patel, 2012). Developmental delays, evidence of risk factors, presence of dysmorphic features or features suggestive of a syndrome, and family history may prompt the nurse practitioner to refer the child for additional diagnostic evaluation. Mackrides and Ryherd (2011) recommended screening at regular intervals with a validated screening tool. The use of parent-completed tools is also supported by the literature, which recommends the Ages and Stages Questionnaire (Ages and Stages) and the Parents' Evaluation of Developmental Status (PEDS; Mackrides & Ryherd, 2011).

■ DIAGNOSIS

Autism Spectrum Disorder

Keys to avoiding ASD behaviors that disrupt normal growth and family functioning include early identification and planning. Families should participate as full partners in the health diagnosis. Open and informed communication between the nurse practitioner and family is an important part of diagnosis, treatment, and in establishing an intervention plan. A thorough medical history of the child and his or her family should be conducted. Evaluation should include a developmental history, past medical history, review of systems, communication patterns, play/leisure activities, and social and family history. The incidence of gastrointestinal, sleep, and neurological disorders should also be assessed as they are more likely to be present in a child with ASD. Family and homelife information should include the composition of the household, family members' health, employment status of parents, and recent major changes in the family. A complete physical examination should be conducted with special consideration for common comorbidities, which may be present with ASD.

Medical testing is not routinely done unless the child presents with features or symptoms which suggest a disorder that warrants additional testing. There is no specific laboratory, neuroimaging, or pathology diagnostic test to determine ASD. EEG may be considered if the child is demonstrating behaviors suggestive of seizures (Howe, Palumbo, & Neumeyer, 2016). Baseline testing may be ordered in order to differentiate among disorders that present with behaviors similar to those found in ASD. According to Howe et al. (2016), genetic abnormalities may be detected in 10% to 20% of cases with ASD. Though genetic testing may not alter the plan of care for the child, it may be helpful in providing guidance to the family regarding future testing and comorbidities. The American College of Medical Genetics and the AAP currently recommend moving "CMA to a first-tier test in place of a karyotype" as was previously recommended in the 2008 guidelines (Schaefer & Mendelsohn, 2013, p. 3). Chromosomal microarray analysis (CMA) or comparative genomic hybridization (CGH) testing replaces conventional cytogenetic studies unless there is a specific suspected syndrome, such as Down, Turner, or Klinefelter syndromes, or a family reproductive history suggestive of specific chromosomal abnormalities (Cameron, Xu, Jung, & Prasad, 2013; Schaefer & Mendelsohn, 2013). In cases where children present with a history of lethargy, regression, dysmorphic features, recurrent vomiting, seizures, or mental disabilities, the American College of Medical Genetics recommends testing for inborn errors of metabolism (Lingen et al., 2015; Schaefer & Mendelsohn, 2013).

According to the *DSM-5*, key clinical features of ASD include "deficits in communication and social interaction across multiple contexts" and "restricted, repetitive patterns of behavior" (APA, p. 50, 2013a). Severity is further defined and broken down into more specific examples in the *DSM-5* (2013). The *DSM-5* notes that patterns of behavior are present from an early age and cause significant impairment in major areas of functioning. Patterns of behavior are often depicted as repetitive or stereotyped and may include vocalizations as well as body movements. Descriptions of deficits and patterns of behavior are further delineated and rated in severity by *DSM-5* under the diagnostic criteria for ASD. Zero to Three (2016) suggests that diagnosis of children younger than 18 months can be considered with caution. The AAP recommends that all children be screened for ASD at ages 18 and 24 months (2016).

Given the complexity of ASD features, there may be a tendency to overlook the diagnosis of comorbidity. In a review of evidence-based practice parameters, Volkmar et al. (2014) found that approximately 50% of children diagnosed with ASD demonstrate severe or profound intellectual disability. Thirty-five percent are found to have mild to moderate intellectual disability with remaining children falling within the normal range for IQ. Other comorbidities include hyperactivity, obsessive-compulsive disorder (OCD), aggression, stereotypes, tics, and affective disorders. Given the complexity of neurodevelopmental disorders, it is important for the nurse practitioner to assess for the presence of unusual features and a history of developmental regression, which need to be evaluated along with potential biological causes, such as infections, metabolic disorders, trauma, toxicity, endocrine, and genetic disorders (Volkmar et al., 2014). Concerns about neurological or genetic disorders should promote a referral along with additional neuroimaging and laboratory tests as appropriate for the practice setting.

According to Zero to Three (2016), key clinical features of ASD include impaired difficulty relating to others, atypical communication, repetitious behavior, and abnormal sensory and motor processing. The diagnostic classification system for young children (Zero to Three) can be a useful resource for the nurse practitioner as it provides more details related to the young child. Zero to Three recognizes mental and developmental health challenges in young children, which provides a better understanding of how relationships and environmental factors contribute to these disorders. In addition, it uses diagnostic criteria in a manner which allows for a more effective intervention plan and subsequently provides guidance for parents and other professionals who may be involved in multimodal care.

Zero to Three further delineates ASD by providing an early atypical autism spectrum disorder (EAASD) classification. EAASD uses the same symptom criteria as ASD but with more attention to expression of the behavioral manifestations of social communication as demonstrated by the infants and young children between the ages of 9 and 36 months. The diagnostic algorithm requires the presence of at least two social communication symptoms and at least one of the restrictive and repetitive symptoms (Zero to Three, 2016). When considering this diagnosis, the P-PCP needs to rule out other language or intellectual delays or disabilities that may demonstrate similar symptoms. The importance of considering EAASD includes the need for ongoing surveillance and screening over time because of the likelihood that the infant or young child is at higher risk for developing ASD.

The nurse practitioner should be attentive to parental reports of a child who shows no eye contact or social smile as well as lack of interest in social relatedness with family and peers. The parents may express concern over the child's ability to make friends as well as his or her desire to play alone rather than become engaged in age-appropriate activities such as those involved in cooperative or parallel play. Sometimes the child is described as easy or not demanding attention, or they may be prone to temper tantrums triggered by common auditory or visual stimuli. Lack of progression or regression of language skills may be evident. Expressive language may be absent or delayed or may include scripted speech, such as excerpts from songs or TV programs and echolalia or parroting, which is the repetition of words made by another person. Activities are often repetitive, self-stimulatory, ritualistic, and nonfunctional in nature. Anxiety and excitement may provoke the onset of these behaviors, examples of which include head banging, arm flapping, preoccupation with an object, or perseverative preoccupation with a game or TV show.

Global Developmental Delay

Zero to Three suggests that diagnostic criteria for GDD include deficits in adaptive behavior and cognitive functioning. Cognitive functioning includes communication, problem-solving, symbolic reasoning, motor skills as well as learning skills. Delays are documented as "2 standard deviations below the mean on a test of developmental/intellectual functioning" (Zero to Three, 2016, p. 36). Adaptive behavior refers to age-appropriate communication, social activities, and activities of daily living, and is defined by Zero to Three as "functioning that is 2 standard deviations below the mean in at least two areas of adaptive functioning" (Zero to Three, 2016, p. 36). Furthermore, the diagnosis of GDD may involve more extensive clinical evaluation, imaging studies, and laboratory evaluation in the presence of family history, suspected risk factors, and observable abnormalities. No one guideline is comprehensive for all developmental delays though the American Academy of Neurology provides a practice parameter for evaluation which was originally published in 2003 and has subsequently been reprinted in several other AAN publications (AAN, n.d.; Burns, 2013; Michelson et al., 2011; Shevell et al., 2003; Srour, Mazer, & Shevell, 2006) (see Figure 14.1).

The most commonly diagnosed GDDs include Down syndrome, FAS, Fragile X, Rett syndrome, and 22q11.2 deletion syndrome (DeGeorge syndrome), in addition to ASD and those demonstrated by medical problems, along with hearing, vision, and language disorders (AAN, n.d.). Many genetic disorders, such as Down syndrome, FAS, and neurofibromatosis, can be identified based on the presence of dysmorphic features, skin abnormalities, and abnormal behavioral responses to the environment, such as hypersensitivity to sound, sleep problems, and hyperactivity. Refer to Table 14.1 for key features of common global developmental delays. Dysmorphism refers to the presence of facial or body deformities, such as the size and shape of facial features, digits, and genitalia (Satya-Murti, Cohen, & Michelson, 2013). Growth deficiencies, along with major malformations or minor anomalies, assist with making the diagnosis. Most large-scale studies note that clinical features have been found to be predictive in the identification of etiology 40% to 60% of the time (Srour et al, 2006). In addition to clinical evaluation, diagnostic studies may include imaging and laboratory evaluation. As with ASD, Schaefer and Mendelsohn (2013) recommend CMA testing for GDD to replace conventional cytogenetic studies unless there is a specific suspected syndrome, such as Down,

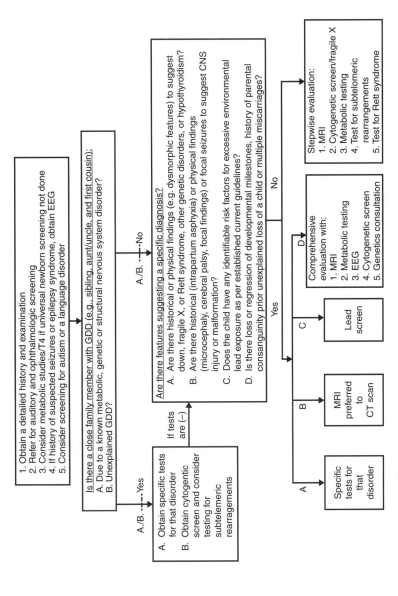

FIGURE 14.1 Evaluation of the child with GDD.

CNS, central nervous system; EEG, electroencephalogram; GDD, global developmental delays.

Source: From Shevell, M., Ashwal, S., Donley, D., Flint, J., Gingolg, M., Hirtz, D., . . . Sheth, R. D. (2003). Practice parameter: Evaluation of the child with global developmental delay. Report of the Quality Standards Subcommittee of the American Academy of Neurology and the Practice Committee of the Child Neurology Society. *Neurology, 60*(3), 367–380. Retrieved from http://n.neurology.org/content/60/3/367. doi:10.1212/01.WNL.0000031431.81555.16. Reprinted with permission.

TABLE 14.1

KEY FEATURES OF COMMON GLOBAL DEVELOPMENTAL DELAYS

Syndrome/Etiology	Key Features	Diagnostic Considerations
Down Syndrome (Trisomy 21) Abnormal cell division involving chromosome 21 occurs resulting in extra genetic material from chromosome 21	Abnormal hair whorls Low nasal bridge Brushfield spots Epicanthal folds with palpebral fissures that slant down Small mandible Myopia Midface hypoplasia Short, broad hands, feet, and digits Clinodactyly Transverse palmar crease Short stature Brachycephaly Congenital heart disease Developmental delays	If the expectant parents choose to forgo prenatal tests, most cases of Down syndrome will be diagnosed after the baby is born. Down syndrome may be suspected in the presence of certain physical characteristics. Diagnostic procedures available for prenatal diagnosis of Down syndrome are chorionic villus sampling (CVS) and amniocentesis, which are nearly 100% accurate in diagnosing Down syndrome. Amniocentesis and CVS may also be able to distinguish between the genetic types of Down syndrome: Trisomy 21, translocation Down syndrome, and mosaic Down syndrome.
Fetal Alcohol Syndrome (FAS) Disruption of fetal development caused by high levels of maternal intake of alcohol during pregnancy, which passes across the placenta to the fetus. The developing fetus doesn't process alcohol the same way as an adult leading to an increased concentration of alcohol, hence preventing enough nutrition and oxygen from getting to the fetus's vital organs	Low philtrum Midface hypoplasia Nail hypoplasia or dysplasia Short palpebral fissures Thin upper lip Microcephaly Growth deficiencies Small for gestational age Mental retardation Infant irritability/child hyperactivity Poor coordination Hypotonia	Diagnosing FAS can be a challenge because there is no medical test, like a blood test, to provide a definitive diagnosis and some other disorders, such as ADHD (attention deficit hyperactivity disorder), have symptoms like FAS. Diagnosis includes a careful history of maternal drinking during the pregnancy; physical appearance and distinguishing features of the child; patterns of physical, cognitive, and psychosocial growth; and development and meeting developmental milestones.

(continued)

TABLE 14.1   (CONTINUED)

KEY FEATURES OF COMMON GLOBAL DEVELOPMENTAL DELAYS

Syndrome/Etiology	Key Features	Diagnostic Considerations
Fragile X X-linked inherited syndrome caused by a defect in the FMR1 gene located on the X chromosome	Long jaw High forehead Large or protuberant ears Hyper extensible joints Large testicles Initial shyness followed by extreme verbosity Broad nasal bridge Prominent chin and nose Mental retardation Autistic-like behavior	Targeted mutation analysis (methylation-sensitive PDR, Southern blot)
Rett Syndrome Gene mutation (change in DNA) in the MECP2 gene, which is found on the X chromosome	Females with unexplained moderate to severe mental retardation Truncal ataxia Autistic features Cessation and regression of development Acquired microcephaly	Sequence analysis/mutation screening
Tuberous Sclerosis Autosomal dominant neurocutaneous disorder Present in 1%–4% of persons with ASD	Adenoma sebaceum Hypopigmented skin lesions (as leaf spots) Benign growth or tubers, which can impact brain, skin, and major organs Mild to moderate intellectual disability Delayed development Seizures Renal lesions Eye involvement	Evidence of skin lesions; MRI or CT which will show evidence or tuberous growths on various organs

(continued)

TABLE 14.1 (CONTINUED)

KEY FEATURES OF COMMON GLOBAL DEVELOPMENTAL DELAYS

Syndrome/Etiology	Key Features	Diagnostic Considerations
22q11.2 Deletion Syndrome (DeGeorge syndrome, Velocardiofacial syndrome) Deletion of part of chromosome 22; Autosomal dominant syndrome usually inherited from mother	Developmental delay Hypotonia Speech and language delay Cleft palate Congenital heart defects Mild microcephaly Hypospadias Umbilical hernia Normal growth or somatic overgrowth	Microarray comparative genomic hybridization or subtelomere FISH

Sources: American Academy of Neurology. (n.d.). *AAN guideline summary for clinicians: Evaluation of the child with global developmental delay.* Retrieved from http://tools.aan.com/professionals/practice/guidelines/guideline_summaries/Global_Devlopmental_Delay_Clinicians.pdf; Bassett, A. A., McDonald-McGinn, D. M., Devriendt, K., Digilio, M. C., Goldenberg, P., Habel, A., . . . Vorstman, J. (2011). Practical guidelines for managing patients with 22q11.2 deletion syndrome. *Journal of Pediatrics, 159*(2), 332–339. doi:10.1016/j.jpeds.2011.02.039; Briggs, A. (2014). Primary care of a child with Rett syndrome. *Journal of the American Association of Nurse Practitioner, 26,* 471–480. doi:10.1002/2327-6924.12056; Burns, C. E. (2013). Genetic disorders. In C. E. Burns, A. M. Dun, M. A. Grady, N. B. Starr, & Blosser,C. G. (Eds.), *Pediatric primary care* (5th ed., pp. 1032–1054). Philadelphia, PA: Saunders; Chiu, S. (2011). *Basics to the approach of developmental delay.* Retrieved from http://learn.pediatrics.ubc.ca/body-systems/nervous-syste/basics-to-the-approach-of-developmental-delay; Hauk, P., J., Johnston, R. B., & Liu, A. H. (2011). Immunodeficiency. In W. W. Hay, M. J. Levin, J. M. Sondeheimer, & R. R. Deterding (Eds.), *Current diagnosis & treatment* (20th ed., pp. 920–942). New York, NY: McGraw-Hill; McDonald-McGinn, D. M., Fahiminiya, S., Revil, T., Nowakowska, B. A., Suhi, J., Bailey, A., . . . Jerome-Majewska, L. A. (2013). Hemizygous mutations in SNAP29 unmask autosomal recessive conditions and contribute to atypical findings in patients with 22q11.2DS. *Journal of Medical Genetics, 50*(2), 80–90. doi:10.1136/jmedgenet-2012-101320; Moeschler, J. B., Shevell, M., & Committee on Genetics. (2006). Clinical genetic evaluation of the child with mental retardation or developmental delays. *Pediatrics, 117*(6), 2304–2316; Moeschler, J. B., Shevell, M., & Committee on Genetics. (2014). Comprehensive evaluation of the child with intellectual disability or global developmental delays. *Pediatrics, 134,* e903–e918. doi:10.1542/peds.2014-1839; Tsai, A. C., Manchester, D. K., & Elias, E. R. (2011). Genetics & dysmorphology. In W. W. Hay, M. J. Levin, J. M. Sondeheimer, & R. R. Deterding (Eds.), *Current diagnosis & treatment* (20th ed., pp. 1020–1053). New York, NY: McGraw-Hill; U.S. Department of Health & Human Services, National Institute of Health. (n.d.). *How do health care providers diagnose down syndrome?* Retrieved from https://www.nichd.nih.gov/health/topics/down/conditioninfo/Pages/diagnosed.aspx

Turner, or Klinefelter, or a family reproductive history suggestive of specific chromosomal abnormalities. Satya-Murti, Cohen, and Michelson (2013) note that children with intellectual disabilities and dysmorphic feature may benefit from the results of CMA testing; CMA testing can provide a firm diagnosis in about 7% of the cases. Furthermore, CMA testing may provide the evidence needed to initiate or stop therapies as well as assist the family in planning for the child's future developmental and educational needs. In some cases, a decision may be made to limit care to palliative based on a diagnosis with poor prognosis (Cameron et al., 2013; Michelson et al., 2011; Satya-Murti, Cohen, & Michelson, 2013). In addition, the need for laboratory and imaging studies may be eliminated based on results from the CMA. Results may also provide guidance for families who need to determine whether there is a risk with future pregnancies. The AAP (2016) and the AAN (2011) note that there is no guideline that is comprehensive for all cases of GDD.

■ TREATMENT

Autism Spectrum Disorder

As with most other developmental disorders, multimodal treatment needs to be considered and must encompass physical, emotional, social, and psychological behavioral problems that may occur in relation to the diagnosis as well as family care. Early diagnosis and interventions are critical and should be introduced as early as possible. With the potential for comorbid conditions, early interventions are imperative in assisting the child to attain developmental progress and well-being (Warren et al., 2011; Zwaigenbaum et al., 2015). In some cases, and related to the experience and educational preparation of the P-PCP, referral to a specialist may be the first step. The P-PCP in a primary care role may be part of a multidisciplinary care team and in the role of ongoing monitoring and health maintenance. Interventions may include family training and support, psychopharmacological symptom support, a structured classroom setting for the older child, as well as interventions directed toward social, speech, and language skill development. In addition, the P-PCP needs to carefully monitor for associated gastrointestinal and feeding challenges as well as toileting and sleep difficulties.

Interventions may include nonpharmacological therapies and psychotropic medications and a family-based framework with focus on anticipatory guidance for effective parenting. Treatment goals should be broad-ranging and address not only immediate needs but also future planning. Long-term outcomes may target behavioral interventions that address reducing odd and/or disruptive behaviors, improving the child's abilities to integrate into schools, developing meaningful peer relationships, and increasing the likelihood of maintaining independent living as adults. Academic and language remediation may need to be considered.

Currently there are no specific medications available that have been proven to be efficient in the treatment of the core symptoms of ASD. Some medications have been shown to be promising in reducing hyperactivity, OCD behavior, irritability, aggression, and self-injurious behavior. Antipsychotics have been shown to reduce aggressive and self-injurious behaviors. Both risperidone and aripiprazole have received U.S. Food and Drug Administration (FDA) approval for the treatment of irritability in children who have been diagnosed with ASD (McPheeters et al., 2011; Napolitano & Brown, 2013; Volkmar et al., 2014). Atypical antipsychotics are known to have a lower risk of causing extrapyramidal adverse effects (risperidone, olanzapine, clozapine, ziprasidone, and quetiapine [Seroquel]). Adverse effects of antipsychotics may include dyskinesia, increased appetite, and weight gain. In 2006, the FDA approved the use of risperidone for treating irritability in children between the ages of 5 and 16 (Centers for Disease Control and Prevention [CDC], 2015). It is currently the only FDA-approved drug for treatment of ASD symptoms.

Selective serotonin reuptake inhibitors (SSRIs) have been used off-label in children with ASD. The term "off-label" refers to the use of pharmaceutical drugs not specified in the FDA's approved packaging label or insert. Off-label use may include unapproved indications, age groups, dosages, or route of administration. The use of SSRIs in the treatment of repetitive thoughts and behaviors associated with ASD has been suggested because of the similarity of those symptoms to obsessions and compulsions, which are noted to respond to SSRIs (Kaplan & McCracken, 2012). Though studies suggest improvement in symptoms such as anxiety, aggression, and repetitive behaviors, analysis found no evidence that SSRIs are effective in treating autism (McPheeters et al., 2011; Kaplan & McCracken, 2012). A major concern with using SSRIs is the potential for activation, which includes irritability, angry outbursts, excitability, manic symptoms, hyperactivity, agitation, nervousness, sleep disturbance, lability, and hostility.

In a systematic review of medical treatment for children with ASD, McPheeters et al. (2011) found that there was insufficient evidence to support the use of SSRIs or stimulants as treatments for ASD. They concluded that strength of evidence for the beneficial effect to citalopram or escitalopram in reducing repetitive behavior was insufficient. Furthermore, they noted that an increase in challenging behavior and loss of appetite occurred with the use of stimulants, also noting an insufficient strength of evidence in reducing hyperactivity.

Contemporary and alternative medicine has included use of a gluten-free, casein-free, and sugar free diets. Though commonly considered by families, most alternative treatments have limited empirical bases for use as treatment of children with ASD (Volkmar et al., 2014). An important role of the nurse practitioner in providing holistic care to the child includes educating family members on the potential benefits and risks associated with alternative and complementary treatments. Randomized controlled trials regarding the use of gluten-free and casein-free diets have not supported their benefit (Volkmar et al., 2014). Treatments with intravenous secretin and oral vitamin B6 have not been found to show any benefit (Volkmar et al., 2014).

Global Developmental Delay

While there is no cure for GDD, education, early intervention, and referral can help the child and family work toward optimal functioning. Treatment for GDD is based on careful diagnosis of the underlying cause, comorbid conditions, and is individualized based on the degree to which the child demonstrates characteristics of the disorder as well as the risks associated with the syndrome. Just as with

ASD, multimodal treatment needs to be considered and must encompass physical, emotional, social, and psychological behavioral problems that may occur in relation to the diagnosis as well as family care (Briggs, 2014). The P-PCP may also be in the role of a primary care provider as well as part of a multidisciplinary care team. The P-PCP can provide oversight for ongoing monitoring and health maintenance. Interventions may include family training and support, psychopharmacological symptom support, a structured classroom setting for the older child, as well as interventions directed toward social, speech, and language skill development. Genetic counseling may provide guidance and family planning options available for parents or relatives at risk for transmitting an inherited disorder, as well as to determine the probability of transmitting the disorder. Referral to community resources and support groups may be of value in helping parents adjust and cope with the diagnosis or disability.

■ SUMMARY

Early recognition of developmental disorders and intervention are key to helping the child and family lead a more productive life. Knowledge of individual variations in growth and in achieving developmental milestones enables the nurse practitioner to detect manifestations of delays and key red flags. Key to diagnosis is attention to parental concerns, as well as periodic developmental surveillance. According to the *DSM-5* both ASD and GDD are categorized as neurodevelopmental disorders. ASD is characterized by social deficits and repetitive behaviors. These characteristics lead to marked impairment in social functioning and difficulty in developing meaningful relationships. The diagnosis of GGD is reserved for children younger than age 5 when the clinical severity cannot be reliably assessed. The key to diagnosing this category is the child's failure to accomplish developmental milestones on two or more areas. Delays can occur in multiple areas such as fine and gross motor skills, social development, language development, reasoning, and adaptive skills. Both ASD and GDD may require a range of interventions based on severity. Treatment needs may encompass the physical, emotional, social, and psychological needs of the child, as well as care of the family. Health promotion should be the foundation of health supervision with children and families. The goal of healthcare supervision focuses on promotion of healthy outcomes and efforts to improve the child's ability to accomplish age-appropriate milestones, develop a positive self-esteem, and increase his or her ability to cope.

■ REFERENCES

Agency for Healthcare Research and Quality (U.S. Department of Health & Human Services. (2016). *Screening for autism spectrum disorder in young children: A systematic evidence review for the U.S. preventive series task force* (AHRQ Publication, 13-05185-EF-1, pp. 1–220).

American Academy of Neurology. (2011). *AAN summary of evidence-based report for clinicians: Genetic and metabolic testing in children with global developmental delay.* Retrieved from https://www.aan.com/Guidelines/Home/GetGuidelineContent/489

American Academy of Neurology. (n.d.). *AAN guideline summary for clinicians: Evaluation of the child with global developmental delay.* Retrieved from http://tools.aan.com/professionals/practice/guidelines/guideline_summaries/Global_Devlopmental_Delay_Clinicians.pdf

American Academy of Pediatrics. (2016). *Children are diagnosed with autism at younger ages since push for universal screening*. Retrieved from https://www.aap.org/en-us/about-the-aap/aap-press-room/pages/Children-are-Diagnosed-with-Autism-at-Younger-Ages-Since-Push-for-Universal-Screening.aspx

American Psychiatric Association. (2013a). *Diagnostic and statistical manual of mental disorders* (5th ed.). Washington, DC: Author.

American Psychiatric Association. (2013b). *Highlights of changes from DSM-IV to DSM-5*. Washington, DC: Author.

Bassett, A. A., McDonald-McGinn, D. M., Devriendt, K., Digilio, M. C., Goldenberg, P., Habel, A., . . . Vorstman, J. (2011). Practical guidelines for managing patients with 22q11.2 deletion syndrome. *Journal of Pediatrics*, 159(2), 332–339. doi:10.1016/j.jpeds.2011.02.039

Briggs, A. (2014). Primary care of a child with Rett syndrome. *Journal of the American Association of Nurse Practitioner*, 26, 471–480. doi:10.1002/2327-6924.12056

Burns, C. E. (2013). Genetic disorders. In C. E. Burns, A. M. Dun, M. A. Grady, N. B. Starr, & Blosser,C. G. (Eds.), *Pediatric primary care* (5th ed., pp. 1032–1054). Philadelphia, PA: Saunders.

Cameron, F., Xu, J., Jung, J., & Prasad, C. (2013). Array CGH analysis and developmental delay: A diagnostic tool for neurologists. *The Canadian Journal of Neurological Sciences*, 40(6), 777–782. doi:10.1017/S0317167100015882

Cangialose, A., & Allen, P. J. (2014). Screening for autism spectrum disorders in infants before 18 months of age. *Pediatric Nursing*, 40(1), 33–37.

Centers for Disease Control and Prevention. (2014). Screening for developmental delays among young children—National survey of children's health, United States, 2007. *Morbidity and Mortality Weekly Report*, 63(02), 27–35.

Centers for Disease Control and Prevention. (2015). *Autism spectrum disorder: Treatment*. Atlanta, GA: U.S. Department of Health & Human Services. Retrieved from https://www.cdc.gov/ncbddd/autism/treatment.html

Chiu, S. (2011). *Basics to the approach of developmental delay*. Retrieved from http://learn.pediatrics.ubc.ca/body-systems/nervous-syste/basics-to-the-approach-of-developmental-delay/

Crais, E. R., McComish, C. S., Humphreys, B. P., Watson, L. R., Baranek, G. T., Reznick, J., . . . Earls, M. (2014). Pediatric healthcare professionals' views on autism spectrum disorder screening at 12–18 months. *Journal of Autism and Developmental Disorders*, 44, 2311–2328. doi:10.1007/s10803-014-2101-2

Dreyer, B. (2016). *AAP statement on U.S. preventive services task force final recommendation statement on autism screening*. Retrieved from American Academy of Pediatrics: https://www.aap.org/en-us/about-the-aap/aap-press-room/Pages/AAP-Statement-on-US-Preventive-Services-Task-Force-Final-Recommendation-Statement-on-Autism-Screening.aspx

Hauk, P., J., Johnston, R. B., & Liu, A. H. (2011). Immunodeficiency. In W. W. Hay, M. J. Levin, J. M. Sondeheimer, & R. R. Deterding (Eds.), *Current diagnosis & treatment* (20th ed., pp. 920–942). New York, NY: McGraw-Hill.

Howe, Y. J., Palumbo, M. L., & Neumeyer, A. (2016) Medical evaluation of patients with autism spectrum disorder. In C. J. McDougle (Ed), *Autism spectrum disorder* (pp. 67–84). New York, NY: Oxford University Press. doi:10.1093/med/9780199349722.003.0005

Kaplan, G., & McCracken, J. T. (2012). Psychopharmacology of autism spectrum disorders. *Pediatric Clinics of North America*, 59, 175–187. doi:10.1016/j.pcl.2011.10.005

Lewis, N. (2017). Our role in early identification. *The ASHA Leader*, 22, 6–7. doi:10.1044/leader.FMP.22012017.6

Lingen, M., Alblers, L., Borchers, M., Haass, S., Gartner, J., Schroder, S., . . . Zirn, B. (2015). Obtaining a genetic diagnosis in a child with disability: Impact on parental quality of life. *Clinical Genetics*, 89, 258–266. doi:10.1111/cge.12629

Lowry, L. (2012). Early signs of autism. *The Hanen Centre*. Retrieved from http://www.hanen.org/SiteAssets/Helpful-Info/Articles/early-signs-of-autism.aspx

Mackrides, P. S., & Ryherd, S. J. (2011). Screening for developmental delay. *American Family Physician*, 84(5), 544–549.

McDonald-McGinn, D. M., Fahiminiya, S., Revil, T., Nowakowska, B. A., Suhi, J., Bailey, A., . . . Jerome-Majewska, L. A. (2013). Hemizygous mutations in SNAP29 unmask autosomal recessive conditions and contribute to atypical findings in patients with 22q11.2DS. *Journal of Medical Genetics*, 50(2), 80–90. doi:10.1136/jmedgenet-2012-101320

McPheeters, M. L., Warren, Z., Sathe, N., Bruzek, J. L., Krishnaswami, S., Jerome, R. N., & VanderWeele, J. V. (2011). A systematic review of medical treatments for children with autism spectrum disorders. *Pediatrics*, 127(5), e1312–e1321. doi:10.1542/peds.2011-0427

McPheeters, M. L., Weitlauf, A., Vehorn, A., Taylor, C., Sathe, N. A., Krishnaswami, S., . . . Warren, Z. E. (2016). *Screening for autism spectrum disorder in young children: A systematic evidence review for the U.S. Preventive Services Task Force.* Agency for Healthcare Research and Quality (13-05185-EF-1). Retrieved from https://www.ncbi.nlm.nih.gov/pubmed/26985520

Michelson, D. J., Shevell, M. I., Sherr, E. H., Moeschler, J. B., Gropman, A. L., & Ashwal, S. (2011). Evidence report: genetic and metabolic testing on children with global developmental delay. *American Academy of Neurology, 77,* 1629–1635. doi:10.1212/WNL.0b013e3182345896

Moeschler, J. B., Shevell, M., & Committee on Genetics. (2006). Clinical genetic evaluation of the child with mental retardation or developmental delays. *Pediatrics, 117*(6), 2304–2316. doi:10.1542/peds.2006-1006

Moeschler, J. B., Shevell, M., & Committee on Genetics. (2014). Comprehensive evaluation of the child with intellectual disability or global developmental delays. *Pediatrics, 134,* e903–e918. doi:10.1542/peds.2014-1839

Napolitano, D. A., & Brown, H. E. (2013). Autism and pervasive developmental disorders. In B. A. M. Melynk (Ed), *A practical guide to child and adolescent mental health screening, early intervention, and health promotion* (2nd ed., pp. 222–234). New York, NY: National Association of Pediatric Nurse Practitioners.

National Institute of Neurological Disorders and Stroke. (2015). *Autism spectrum disorder fact sheet* (NIH Publication No. 15-1877). Bethesda, MD: Author.

Plum, A. M., & Wetherby, A. M. (2013). Vocalization development in toddlers with autism spectrum disorder. *Journal of Speech, Language, and Hearing Research, 56,* 721–734. doi:10.1044/1092-4388(2012/11-0104)

Satya-Murti, S., Cohen, B. H., & Michelson, D. (2013). Chromosomal microarray analysis for intellectual disabilities. *American Academy of Neurology,* 1–11. Retrieved from https://www.aan.com/uploadedFiles/Website_Library_Assets/Documents/3.Practice_Management/1.Reimbursement/1.Billing_and_Coding/5.Coverage_Policies/13%20ChromoMicroIntelDisabil.pdf

Schaefer, G. B., & Mendelsohn, N. J. (2013). Clinical genetics evaluation in identifying the etiology of autism spectrum disorders: 2013 guideline revisions. *Genetics in Medicine, 15*(5), 399–407. doi:10.1038/gim.2013.32

Shevell, M., Ashwal, S., Donley, D., Flint, J., Gingolg, M., Hirtz, D., . . . Sheth, R. D. (2003). Practice parameter: Evaluation of the child with global developmental delay Report of the Quality Standards Subcommittee of the American Academy of Neurology and the Practice Committee of the Child Neurology Society. *Neurology, 60*(3), 367–380. doi:10.1212/01.WNL.0000031431.81555.16

Soares, N. S., & Patel, D. R. (2012). Office screening and early identification of children with autism. *Pediatric Clinics of North America, 59,* 89–102. doi:10.1016j.pcl.2-10/10/011

Srour, M., Mazer, M., & Shevell, M. L. (2006). Analysis of clinical features predicting etiologic yield in the assessment of global developmental delay. *Pediatrics, 118*(1), 139–145. doi:10.1542/peds.2005-2702

Tsai, A. C., Manchester, D. K., & Elias, E. R. (2011). Genetics & dysmorphology. In W. W. Hay, M. J. Levin, J. M. Sondeheimer, & R. R. Deterding (Eds.), *Current diagnosis & treatment* (20th ed., pp. 1020–1053). New York, NY: McGraw-Hill.

U.S. Department of Health & Human Services, National Institute of Health. (n.d.). *How do health care providers diagnose down syndrome?* Retrieved from https://www.nichd.nih.gov/health/topics/down/conditioninfo/Pages/diagnosed.aspx

Volkmar, F., Siegel, M., Woodbury-Smith, M., King, B., McCracken, J., State, M., & the American Academy of Child and Adolescent Psychiatry Committee on Quality Issues. (2014). Practice parameter for the assessment and treatment of children and adolescents with autism spectrum disorder. *Journal of the American Academy of Child & Adolescent Psychiatry, 53*(2), 237–257. doi:10.1016/j.jaac.2013.10.013

Warren, Z., McPheeters, M. L., Sathe, N., Foss-Feig, J. H., Glasser, A., & Veenstra-VanderWeele, J. (2011). A systematic review of early intensive intervention for autism spectrum disorders. *Pediatrics, 127*(5), e1303–e1311. doi:10.1542/peds.2011-0426

Wetherby, A., Woods, J., Allen, L., Cleary, J., Dickinson, H., & Lord, C. (2004/2012). Early indicators of autism spectrum disorders in the second year of life. *Journal of Autism and Developmental Disorders, 34,* 473–493. doi:10.1007/s10803-004-2544-y

Zero to Three. (2016). *DC:0-5 Diagnostic classification of mental health and developmental disorders of infancy and early childhood.* Washington, DC: Author.

Zwaigenbaum, L., Baurran, M. L., Choueiri, R., Fenn, D., Kasar, C., Pierce, K., . . . Wetherby, A. (2015). Early identification and interventions for autism spectrum disorder: Executive summary. *Pediatrics, 136*(Suppl 1), S1–S9. doi:10.1542/peds.2014-33667B

CHAPTER 15

Challenging Behaviors: Sleep Disorders in Children With Autism Spectrum Disorder and Attention Deficit Hyperactivity Disorder

SHAYLEIGH K. DICKSON

The diagnosis of autism spectrum disorder (ASD) previously precluded a diagnosis of attention deficit hyperactivity disorder (ADHD); however, the *Diagnostic and Statistical Manual of Mental Disorders, Fifth Edition (DSM-5)* recognizes that both conditions may occur together. While the overall prevalence of ADHD in the school-age population is approximately 5%, a recent analysis found that 21.3% of children with ASD also have a diagnosis of ADHD (Levy et al., 2010). Children with comorbid ASD and ADHD have more severe impairments in their social skills, adaptive and cognitive functioning, and are less responsive to standard treatment plans (Leitner, 2014). Challenging behaviors, which may include tantrums and aggression, can limit a child's participation in educational and recreational programs as well as negatively impact his or her functioning in school, home, and the community. Thus, behavioral concerns are a common presenting problem to the pediatric primary care provider (P-PCP) for children with ASD and ADHD. Careful history, clinical interview, and physical exam can identify areas where the P-PCP may *intercept* these problematic behaviors.

CASE PRESENTATION

This is a presentation of an unfolding case study of a 7-year-old male, previously diagnosed with ASD and ADHD, and now presents with recent onset of challenging behaviors including aggression and sleep problems.

Chief Complaint
Mother reports that her child has "aggressive behaviors for the past 2 months several times each week."

■ HISTORY OF PRESENT ILLNESS

The child's mother reports that she has been getting calls from his school several times per week for the past 2 months about her son hitting, pushing, and kicking other students and the teacher's aide. He also has tantrums that involve crying, screaming, and kicking his legs. The tantrums occur primarily during transitions between activities. At home, he is aggressive with his younger sister and his babysitter who cares for him after school. He throws tantrums during homework time and at bedtime. It typically takes 1 to 2 hours for him to fall asleep at night.

The mother reports no history of aggressive behaviors at home or school prior to this onset about 2 months ago. His previous teachers expressed concerns about hyperactive and inattentive behaviors during classroom activities. He did very well academically in his self-contained kindergarten program (nine students, one teacher, and two shared teacher's aides) and was moved to an inclusion setting for 1st grade. He is now in a class with 20 students, one teacher, and one shared teacher's aide. He has an individualized education plan (IEP) and receives speech therapy (ST) and occupational therapy (OT) one time each week in a small group (three students, one therapist). No concerns were reported by his speech and occupational therapists.

■ PAST MEDICAL HISTORY

He was born full term via uncomplicated vaginal delivery. He has no history of hospitalizations or surgeries. Routine labs, vision, and hearing examinations have been within normal limits. He was diagnosed with ASD at 2½ years old and ADHD at 6 years old by a developmental pediatrician who he follows up with every 6 months.

■ SCREENING TOOLS

The BEARS Sleep Screening Tool (Owens & Dalzell, 2005) was completed in the office with his mother, as follows:

Bedtime problems include difficulty falling asleep (1–2 hours) and bedtime resistance (tantrums) every day of the week. No excessive daytime sleepiness. Occasional nighttime awakenings occur one to two times per week. Bedtime and wake-up time are consistent on school days and weekends. He sleeps on average 8 hours per night. Loud snoring and occasional coughing at night are heard.

■ REVIEW OF SYSTEMS

Ear, nose, and throat (ENT): Positive history of snoring for about 6 months
Diet: Very selective about food choices; dislikes crunchy foods
Neurological: Sensory-avoidant (covers ears) to noises such as the blender, vacuum cleaner, doorbell, and large crowds
All other systems were reviewed and were noncontributory.

■ PHYSICAL EXAMINATION

Tonsils were plus (+) 3 without exudate or injection. Physical exam was otherwise noncontributory.

■ DISCUSSION OF THE BEHAVIORAL PROBLEM

Developmentally normative physical aggression typically appears around the ages of 2 to 3 years and declines shortly thereafter (Austerman, 2017). Aggressive behaviors occur in approximately 3% to 7% of children and adolescents (Zahrt & Melzer-Lange, 2011). The prevalence of aggressive behaviors in children diagnosed with ASD is significantly higher, with rates reported in the range of 53% to 68% in population-based studies (Kanne & Mazurek, 2011; Mazurek, Kanne, & Wodka, 2013). Aggressive behaviors in children with ASD and ADHD are more likely to be impulsive in nature as opposed to the premeditated aggressive behaviors that may be present in children with conduct disorder or other psychiatric diagnoses. In general, the causes of pathologic aggression, both impulsive and premeditated, are multifactorial. In children with ASD, it has been found that the presence of self-injurious behaviors, sleep problems, and sensory problems is strongly correlated with aggressive behaviors (Mazurek et al., 2013). Therefore, *intercepting* sleep and sensory problems may improve aggression.

Sleep Disturbances

Sleep disturbances, which may include difficulties with falling asleep or maintaining sleep, premature awakening, restlessness, and sleep-disordered breathing, result in sleep that is insufficient or of poor quality. Children with poor sleep habits have increased risk for problematic behavior (irritability, aggression) and performance (attention, cognition) during the daytime. Additionally, a child's poor sleeping habits can directly impact the quality and duration of parents' sleep and thereby negatively affect parental fatigue, mood, and functioning. Sleep disturbances occur in about one quarter to one third of typically developing children, but are significantly more common both in children with ASD and in children with ADHD (Konafal, Lecendreux, & Cortese, 2010; Malow et al., 2012). As such, routine screening for sleep disturbances is recommended for children diagnosed with ASD and/or ADHD. Given the link between poor sleep and problematic behavior, when the presenting complaint is a behavioral concern, careful assessment of sleep is important.

Screening for Sleep Disturbances

Screening for sleep disturbances can be easily completed in the pediatric office by either parent interview or questionnaire. Two commonly used tools are the BEARS Sleep Screening Tool and the Children's Sleep Habits Questionnaire (CSHQ; Owens & Dalzell, 2005; Owens, Spirito, & McGuinn, 2000). The BEARS Sleep Screening Tool, utilized in the case presented here, was developed for use in the primary care setting to assess five sleep domains (Owens & Dalzell, 2005). The sleep domains are bedtime problems (difficulty going to bed and falling asleep), excessive daytime sleepiness, awakening during the night, regularity of the sleep wake cycle (i.e., bedtime, wake time, and duration of sleep), and snoring. Each domain has a "yes" or "no" screening question that the parent is asked, and if a "yes" response is elicited, the parent is asked to describe the problem in further detail. The CSHQ is a 45-item questionnaire that identifies sleep problems in eight subscales: bedtime resistance, sleep onset delay, sleep duration, sleep anxiety, night wakings, parasomnias, sleep-disordered breathing, and daytime sleepiness (Owens et al., 2000).

Following identification of a sleep disturbance by screening, a review of systems can identify possible medical contributors to poor sleep habits and quality. Medical comorbidities underlying sleep disturbances may include sleep-disordered breathing, seizures, gastrointestinal distress, pain, and restless legs syndrome (RLS). Snoring is the most common symptom of sleep-disordered breathing, but other signs may include gasping or coughing. Physical examination can also reveal if the child has enlarged tonsils or adenoids. Children with ASD have an increased risk for seizure disorders, so evaluating for the presence of seizures, especially those that may occur at night, is important. This evaluation may include asking the parent about unusual movements that occur during the night, especially if the movements appear to occur in a similar way every time. Presence of these symptoms should prompt further evaluation by polysomnography (sleep study) with EEG.

Studies have also found associations between both RLS and periodic limb movements in sleep (PLMS) and ADHD in children (Konafal et al., 2010). The provider can ask the parent if he or she notices any leg or limb movements and the child may be able to describe unpleasant feelings in their legs. If RLS or PLMS are suspected, the provider may consider testing for serum ferritin as low levels have been associated with RLS and PLMS (Konafal et al., 2010). Careful attention to medication that the child is taking is also important, especially in children with ASD and ADHD because several medications often used to treat behavioral symptoms (i.e., stimulants, antipsychotics) have potential side effects that may cause or exacerbate sleep disturbances.

■ TREATMENT MANAGEMENT PLAN

While the presenting concern from his mother is aggressive behaviors, there are two factors that may be contributing to the emergence of these aggressive behaviors: sleep disturbances and behavioral rigidity (e.g., resistance to change, difficulty with transition). The P-PCP may concurrently *intercept* these two factors with the goal of reducing the resultant aggressive behaviors.

Sleep Disturbance

With respect to his sleeping, he presents with bedtime resistance, problematic sleep onset, and snoring/coughing during sleep. First, there is a medical comorbidity that requires further workup. A sleep study is recommended to rule out sleep-disordered breathing, and referral to an ENT specialist for evaluation of hypertrophied tonsils and snoring may also be considered. For the bedtime resistance and problematic sleep onset, behavioral strategies should be implemented first. Table 15.1 describes behavioral strategies for the management of sleep

TABLE 15.1

BEHAVIORAL STRATEGIES FOR COMMON SLEEP DISTURBANCES

Sleep Disturbance	Behavioral Strategies

Bedtime resistance	• Create a bedtime environment that promotes sleep
	  ▪ Turn off electronics at least 1 hour before bedtime
	  ▪ Keep the room cool, dark or dimly lit, and quiet
	  ▪ The bed should be used only for sleep (i.e., no playing with toys or watching TV in bed)
	• Establish a bedtime routine
	  ▪ Routine should take less than 1 hour, be enjoyable for the child, and gradually move toward the bed
	    – *Example:* Bath, brush teeth, read a story, lights out
	  ▪ A visual schedule may be utilized to remind child of bedtime routine

Delayed sleep onset	• Adjust bedtime: Temporarily move bedtime closer to the child's actual sleep onset. Every 3–4 days, move the bedtime earlier by 15 minutes until the child is falling asleep at the target bedtime.
	• Extinction: Place the child in bed and leave the room. The goal of this strategy is to eliminate the bedtime tantrums by ignoring the behavior. There are a few types:
	  ▪ Unmodified
	    – Monitor child to ensure safety, but do not return to room or "check in"
	  ▪ Gradual
	    – "Check in" on the child at defined intervals (e.g., every 5 minutes)
	    – "Check-in" times should become increasingly less frequent over time
	• A very anxious child may need the gradual extinction to begin with the parent sitting next to the bed, then close to the door before beginning the "check-ins" previously noted.
	• Bedtime "pass": Provide child with a "pass" that may be used for one time out of the room, such as for a small drink or hug from parent. If the child does not use the "pass" (i.e., they stay in their room), they can exchange the "pass" for a small prize in the morning.

Nighttime awakenings	• Scheduled awakenings: If the child consistently wakes up in the middle of the night, schedule an awakening about 30 minutes prior to the spontaneous awakening and calmly soothe the child back to sleep. • Eliminate sleep-onset associations: If child is awakening to drink milk, gradually reduce the amount of milk provided, then replace with a small amount of water, followed by no drink. If child is awakening to come into parent's room, consistently return the child to their own bed every time.
Premature awakening	• Adjust bedtime: If a child is also going to bed very early, try pushing back bedtime by 30–60 minutes to promote sleeping in later • Reduce light or noise that may awaken child in the morning: Blackout curtains or a "white noise" machine may be helpful.

Source: Adapted from Morgenthaler, T. I., Owens, J., Alessi, C., Boehlecke, B., Brown, T. M., Coleman, J., . . . Swick, T. J. (2006). Practice parameters for behavioral treatment of bedtime problems and night wakings in infants and young children. *Sleep, 29*, 1277–1281. Retrieved from https://aasm.org/resources/practiceparameters/pp_nightwakingschildren.pdf

disturbances. If behavioral strategies fail after consistent implementation, a trial of medication may be considered. Melatonin, antihistamines (diphenhydramine and hydroxyzine), and alpha-2 agonists (clonidine and guanfacine) are commonly prescribed, but it is important to note that there are presently no Food and Drug Administration–approved medications for sleep in children (Felt & Chervin, 2014). The effectiveness of these medications on sleep is variable in children and should be monitored closely when initiated.

Temper Tantrums

The child in this case study, like many children with ASD, has tantrums that are triggered by transitions and nonpreferred activities. He has also recently changed his classroom placement from a small structured setting to a larger less restrictive classroom environment. While it is the goal for all students to be educated in the least restrictive environment and placement in an inclusion setting is particularly beneficial for children with ASD to develop social skills, this type of change represents a significant change in routine and can trigger behavioral problems.

In the school setting, his parents may request a Functional Behavior Assessment (FBA). This type of assessment is typically completed by a school psychologist or behavior specialist and includes both interviews with parents and teachers as well as observations of the child's behavior in various school settings (e.g., classroom, playground). The goal is to identify the causes of problematic behavior (i.e., aggression) and create a behavioral intervention plan.

At home, he may benefit from implementing an after-school routine such that transitions (e.g., homework to play or dinner to bedtime) are clear and expected. Use of a visual schedule (Figure 15.1) is particularly helpful for children with ASD. Timers that clearly identify a start and end to an activity, such as homework, may also be utilized. Finally, ensuring that all caregivers, in this instance parents and babysitter, are following the same routines, enforcing the same rules, and utilizing the same discipline strategies is important.

Applied Behavior Analysis

He is currently receiving ST and OT in school; however, he may benefit from evaluation for private therapies. Applied behavior analysis (ABA), ST, and OT are three types of therapies that are commonly used to treat children with ASD and/or ADHD. ABA is the most scientifically validated treatment specific to ASD. The goal of ABA is to increase behaviors that are useful for learning (e.g.,

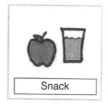
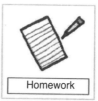
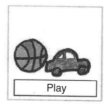

Snack   Homework   Play

FIGURE 15.1 Example of a visual schedule.

listening, transitioning) and decrease maladaptive behaviors (e.g., tantrums and aggression). Many teachers utilize ABA strategies in their classroom when teaching children with ASD. Parents can also seek private ABA therapy through their child's insurance provider. OT should be considered for children with deficits in fine motor skills, coordination, daily living skills, and sensory processing. Occupational therapists can work with children to improve attentional skills, decrease impulsivity, and reduce sensory-seeking or sensory-avoidant behaviors. Speech therapists can work to improve a child's language skills and thereby improve behaviors that may stem from a child not understanding or not being understood. Children who have deficits in their receptive language skills may have difficulty understanding and following directions and may appear disobedient or defiant. Children who have deficits in their expressive language skills may become frustrated when they cannot express themselves. The P-PCP should consider referring a child for ABA, ST, or OT evaluations when there are presenting behavioral concerns.

■ SUMMARY

Follow-Up Care

Follow-up in one month is recommended. At this visit, the provider should follow up on the effectiveness of the behavioral strategies recommended for both sleep and transitions, the results of a sleep study, and progress in school. Improvement in behavior can take time and parents should be encouraged to be patient and persistent when implementing behavioral strategies. It is likely that problematic behaviors will remain; however, in-office follow-up allows the family and provider to identify areas that have improved as well as areas that may require additional interventions or modified strategies.

■ REFERENCES

Austerman, J. (2017). Violence and aggressive behavior. *Pediatrics in Review, 38*, 69–80. doi:10.1542/pir.2016-0062

Felt, B. T., & Chervin, R. D. (2014). Medications for sleep disturbances in children. *Neurology Clinical Practice, 4*, 82–87. doi:10.1212/01.CPJ.0000442521.30233.ef

Kanne, S. M., & Mazurek, M. O. (2011). Aggression in children and adolescents with ASD: Prevalence and risk factors. *Journal of Autism and Developmental Disorders, 41*, 926–937. doi:10.1007/s10803-010-1118-4

Konafal, E., Lecendreux, M., & Cortese, S. (2010). Sleep and ADHD. *Sleep Medicine, 11*, 652–658. doi:10.1016/j.sleep.2010.02.012

Leitner, Y. (2014). The co-occurrence of autism and attention deficit hyperactivity disorder in children—What do you know? *Frontiers in Human Neuroscience, 8*, 1–8. doi:10.3389/fnhum.2014.00268

Levy, S. E., Giarelli, E., Lee, L., Schieve, L. A., Kirby, R. S., Cunniff, C., . . . Rice, C. E. (2010). Autism spectrum disorder and co-occurring developmental, psychiatric, and medical conditions among children in multiple populations of the United States. *Journal of Developmental & Behavioral Pediatrics, 31*, 267–275. doi:10.1097/DBP.0b013e3181d5d03b

Malow, B. A., Bryars, K., Johnson, K., Weiss, S., Bernal, P., Goldman, S. E., . . . Glaze, D. G. (2012). A practice pathway for the identification, evaluation, and management of insomnia in children and adolescents with autism spectrum disorders. *Pediatrics, 130*, S106–S123. doi:10.1542/peds.2012-0900I

Mazurek, M. O., Kanne, S. M., & Wodka, E. L. (2013). Physical aggression in children and adolescents with autism spectrum disorders. *Research in Autism Spectrum Disorders, 7,* 455–465. doi:10.1016/j.rasd.2012.11.004

Morgenthaler, T. I., Owens, J., Alessi, C., Boehlecke, B., Brown, T. M., Coleman, J., . . . Swick, T. J. (2006). Practice parameters for behavioral treatment of bedtime problems and night wakings in infants and young children. *Sleep, 29,* 1277–1281. Retrieved from https://aasm.org/resources/practiceparameters/pp_nightwakingschildren.pdf

Owens, J. A., & Dalzell, V. (2005). Use of the "BEARS" sleep screening tool in a pediatric residents' continuity clinic: A pilot study. *Sleep Medicine, 6,* 63-69. doi:10.1016/j.sleep.2004.07.015

Owens, J. A., Spirito, A., & McGuinn, M. (2000). The children's sleep habits questionnaire (CSHQ): Psychometric properties of a survey instrument for school-age children. *Sleep, 23,* 1043–1051. Retrieved from https://www.ncbi.nlm.nih.gov/pubmed/11145319 doi:10.1093/sleep/23.8.1d

Zahrt, D. M., & Melzer-Lange, M. (2011). Aggressive behavior in children and adolescents. *Pediatrics in Review, 32,* 325–322. doi:10.1542/pir.32-8-325

Toddler Impulsive Behaviors: A Case Study

ALEXANDRA BARBER, AMELIA BURKE, MAURA COBURN, JENNIFER KIEHL, AND ALEXANDRA LAURENZANO

CASE PRESENTATION

A mother presents to the primary care clinic with twin 28-month-old toddlers who she describes as "very active all day long." She described their behaviors as very impulsive, with little attention to her instructions, although she knows that they understand her. Time-out is ineffective, hitting them is also ineffective, putting them into their beds does not work—they just jump out. Two babysitters have quit.

Chief Complaint
"My toddlers are out of control."

■ HISTORY OF PRESENT ILLNESS (HPI)

These are 28-month-old twins, one male, one female, who present to the pediatric clinic for an initial primary care visit. The twins were born via normal spontaneous vaginal delivery at 37 weeks, without complication, went home with their mother from well-baby nursery at 2 days of life. They were "pretty easy babies," but after they started walking at 12 months old, they have been very active and their behavior has only "gotten worse" over the past few months. They never listen to directions and are always screaming and making a scene whenever she takes them out in public (i.e., grocery store, play in the park). Mom is never able to leave them alone with a babysitter because they scream and cry for more than an hour after she leaves, throw toys around the house, and hit their babysitter, which has caused two sitters to quit. Mom has tried time-outs, putting them to bed, and has hit them twice, which she says seems to only make their behavior worse. She has had to take them each to the emergency department (ED) twice for stitches and broken bones from jumping off furniture and jungle gym at the park. The twins some-times fight and push each other, but they usually feed off each other's impulsive behavior. Their mother has put them in a day-care program 3 days a week, but she has been called to speak about the twins' behavior twice and she is worried they may be asked to leave.

Past Medical History

The mother denies asthma, heart disease, seizures, other chronic medical condi-tions, and any recent acute illnesses.

ED Visits

Twin A: Stitches under chin 1 month ago
Twin B: Stitches on forehead and broken wrist (right) 6 months ago; casted and healed

■ SCREENING TOOLS

Toddler Care Questionnaire (TCQ)

The TCQ may benefit this mother and her twins. The TCQ is used to measure maternal confidence for mothers who have a toddler between 12 and 36 months of age (Gross & Rocissano, 1988). This screening tool consists of 37 questions the mother must answer. The answers are then rated from A to E, simultaneously with the numbers 1 to 5. The range of scores can be 37 to 185. Higher scores indicate higher maternal confidence. Examples of questions include knowing which toys are age appropriate for your child and knowing which situations are likely to upset your child (Gross & Rocissano, 1988).

Brigance Toddler Screen

The Brigance Toddler Screen is administered to toddlers who are between 12 and 33 months of age (Brigance & Glascoe, 2002). This screening tool consists of 10 questions that screen for social–emotional skills. Higher scores indicate higher social–emotional development. This screening tool can be completed in under 1 minute.

Modified Checklist for Autism in Toddlers, Revised (M-CHAT-R)

The American Academy of Pediatrics (AAP, 2017) recommends that all toddlers be screened for autism spectrum disorders (ASDs). Pediatric primary care providers (P-PCPs) should screen all toddlers using the M-CHAT-R at well-child visits (e.g., 16 months, 21 months, or 24 months) and/or if there is a concern from a parent or caregiver. P-PCPs must recognize the early signs of ASDs and inform parents of the latest research evidence that support better outcomes for toddlers whose conditions are diagnosed early and who participate in appropriate intervention programs. The M-CHAT-R (AAP, 2017) is a free tool that can be used by P-PCPs to support or oppose a diagnosis of autism.

Ages and Stages Questionnaire: Social–Emotional (ASQ-SE-2)

The ASQ-SE-2 (2017) is a very reliable screening tool that is used to evaluate social and emotional development in toddlers. The parents complete a questionnaire that focuses on the toddler's social and emotional behaviors. The results are evaluated by the P-PCP and a decision on steps to improve the social–emotional development of the toddler are made with the parent, who can then feel more in control of the toddler's behavior.

Lead-Exposure Risk Assessment Questionnaire for Children

All states require infants and toddlers to have a blood lead-level test performed, usually at age 1 and typically again at age 2. The lead exposure risk assessment questionnaire for children (New York State Department of Health, 2009) should also be documented at each well-infant/toddler visit until age 3, and then annually until the child's sixth birthday. If the caregiver answers "yes" to any questions in the risk assessment, the child should receive a blood lead-level test (Centers for Disease Control and Prevention (CDC), 2017). Toddlers and all children with elevated lead levels are at high risk for neurological changes in the brain and spinal cord, which can lead to adverse neurodevelopmental outcomes. Children with elevated lead levels also show changes in their behaviors. In this case, the toddlers did not have elevated blood lead levels.

Additional screening tools that may be used to assess toddlers' social–emotional development and other growth and development parameters are discussed in Chapter 20.

■ REVIEW OF SYSTEMS

> **Constitutional**: Increased activity level, fussiness, crying and tantrums in recent months; picky eaters
> **Head:** Denies trauma, lumps, abrasions, hair loss, headache
> **Gastrointestinal:** Denies vomiting, abdominal pain, change in appetite, diarrhea, or constipation
> **Musculoskeletal:** Denies limited range of motion, joint pain, swelling, or tenderness
> **Neurological:** Denies change in neuro status, numbness, tingling, or seizures
> **Skin:** Denies rashes, lesions, or abrasions

■ PHYSICAL EXAMINATION WITH BEHAVIORAL HEALTH FOCUS

> **General:** Alert, active, well-nourished children crying and screaming at times during the examination
> **Head:** Normocephalic, atraumatic

Abdominal: Abdomen is protuberant, soft, and nondistended. Bowel sounds audible and active in all four quadrants. No hepatomegaly or splenomegaly. No guarding or rebound tenderness.

Musculoskeletal: Upper and lower extremities with full active and passive ROM. Gait straight and erect. No limp; no toe walking.

Skin: Healing 2-cm scar underneath chin; no erythema or drainage noted.

Neurological: No tics or tremors. CN II-VII intact. Ignores two thirds of directions and questions asked by P-PCP. Opening drawers and attempting to jump off of examination table.

DIFFERENTIAL DIAGNOSES: BEHAVIORAL HEALTH

It is often difficult to establish behavioral diagnoses for the toddler population. The most important factor to consider is whether the behaviors are within normal limits for age, temperament, and general health when formulating a list of differential diagnoses.

Toddler Impulsive Behaviors

Toddlers are naturally impulsive. The determination of what is normal and abnormal impulsive behavior is not easy to make. The parents need to objectively observe the toddler, which may be difficult, as they are so immersed and stressed in the home environment that an objective reference frame is not possible. With the availability of advanced technology, parents can record their toddlers' activity and send the video to the P-PCP or bring a few brief videos to the pediatric office for the P-PCP to review with the parents. Sometimes the determination of what is the norm for a particular "impulsive" behavior is easy to decide for the P-PCP. For example, a toddler may be told that the stove is hot and experiences the heat by being near the stove and feeling the heat emitting from it. The same toddler may be running around with the parent thinking the toddler's impulsive behavior is out of control, but when the toddler comes near the hot stove, the toddler immediately stops and either says "hot" or in essence acknowledges that it is hot nonverbally by running away from the stove.

In this case study, toddler impulsive behaviors must be on top of the differential list. Other behavioral diagnoses to consider include separation anxiety, social aggression, attention deficit hyperactivity disorder (ADHD), lead exposure, and ASD.

Separation Anxiety

Separation anxiety is a normal developmental phenomenon that should be considered when examining the history of the twins' behavior (Daria-Wiener, 2004). The behavior described by the mother in this case is not unusual for toddlers. Toddlers act aggressively and even intentionally injure themselves in the absence of their primary caregiver (Goldman-Fraser, Fernandez, & Marfo, 2005). It is important to recognize that separation anxiety is differentiated from separation anxiety disorder by the history of toddler reactions that interfere with daily activities and developmental tasks. In addition, separation anxiety disorder typically manifests when the child is older, usually between 5 and 16 years old, when separation anxiety is no longer a normal developmental behavior (Burns et al., 2013).

Social Aggression

Social aggression is a pattern of social behavior with the intent to harm others (Leff et al., 2009). Social aggression is unusual in the toddler population. The behaviors displayed by the toddlers in the case study are not done with intent to harm, as the toddlers are just too young. Their overt behaviors are more consistent with the very active toddler who needs a more consistent level of parenting. Social aggression behaviors may appear in the preschool-age child whose parents are unable to change "aggressive" toddler behaviors or who lack parenting skills. In this case, the mother is actively seeking help for her toddlers' behaviors and would benefit from parent education and parenting anticipatory guidance counseling on ways to manage toddler behaviors during this office visit, with follow-up phone calls and at each subsequent visit (Hallas, Koslap-Petraco, & Fletcher, 2017).

Attention Deficit Hyperactivity Disorder

ADHD is the most commonly diagnosed behavioral disorder in childhood. According to the mom's description of the toddlers' behaviors, it is possible that they are exhibiting the core symptoms of inattention, hyperactivity, and impulsivity. However, it is difficult to diagnose a child with ADHD before the age of 4. Though many children who present with symptoms can grow out of them, research has shown that 3-year-olds who present with typical symptoms are more likely to meet the diagnostic criteria for ADHD by the time they are 13 years old (CHADD, 2017). The average age of diagnosis is typically later in childhood, usually 7 years old; however, children with severe symptoms may be diagnosed at an earlier age (AAP, 2017). There are no screening tools for a toddler with ADHD, as this is not a diagnosis of the toddler years. The Intercepting Behavioral Health (IBH; Hallas, 2018) conceptual model can be applied to these twins by providing guidance and parenting instructions about the toddlers' behaviors, which may be beneficial to both the mother and the toddlers, as coping skills are learned. See Chapter 18 for a detailed discussion of ADHD from age 4 years and older.

Lead Exposure

Lead exposure is a serious environmental health problem. Any amount of lead in a child's blood can have permanent toxic effects on multiple organ systems. However, a blood lead level must be 5 mcg/dL or greater for a diagnosis of lead poisoning. Toddlers may be prenatally exposed to lead and may also be exposed to lead in their homes, if the homes are older and the walls were covered with lead-based paint or the homes were built with lead pipes. There are other sources of lead that toddlers may be exposed to, which includes but is not limited to soil, air, children's jewelry or toys, imported candy, and imported cans of food (New York State Department of Health, n.d.). Parents or guardians should also always be given the basic personal-risk questionnaire as discussed previously, and should receive anticipatory guidance on prevention of lead exposure as part of their routine care.

Toddlers who have elevated lead levels and neurodevelopmental complications may display behavioral problems. In this case, the lead risk assessment was negative, and the toddlers' blood levels were normal, so lead exposure was not considered in the diagnosis.

Autism Spectrum Disorder

ASD is characterized, according to the *Diagnostic and Statistical Manual of Mental Disorders (fifth edition, DSM-5;* American Psychiatric Association [APA], 2013), as deficits in social communication and interaction across many contexts, as well as restrictive, repetitive patterns of behaviors, interests, and activities. Children from 16 months to 36 months should be screened for ASD using the M-CHAT-R. ASD can be reliably diagnosed at 2 years of age (CDC, 2016). Toddlers with ASD can present with severe behavior problems and excessive temper tantrums similar to the twins' behavior. However, the M-CHAT-R for the toddlers was not suggestive of ASD at this time; thus, parenting skills must be considered as one of the causes of the toddlers' behavior presentation, which is more consistent with toddler temper tantrums. See Chapters 14 and 15 for detailed discussions of ASD.

Temper Tantrums

Temper tantrums are ways that toddlers express their wishes and needs in ways that confuse parents and all who interact with the toddler. Toddlers have varying degrees of language reception and expression; thus, they cannot explain their wishes and needs, and often, have a temper tantrum until the confused parent figures out what the toddler wants. Temper tantrums look and sound rather violent, with head banging, thrashing around on the floor, and screaming and crying behaviors that persist. Toddlers often keep the parent in sight even during a temper tantrum. If a toddler is in a safe home environment, the parent should leave the visual sight of the toddler, while maintaining his or her view of the toddler. By staying out of the toddler's view, the toddler will typically self-regulate and stop the tantrum, as the toddler cognitively understands that the parent is not paying attention. As P-PCPs, most of us know that toddlers are seeking attention, and we have personally witnessed tantrums in our offices. Providing this information to parents may be helpful. In addition, using motivational interviewing to speak with parents about temper tantrums is also an effective strategy, as the parents begin to problem-solve how they can best manage the temper tantrums at home.

Daniels, Mandleco, and Luthy (2012) state that, since tantrums are hard to stop once started, theyrecommend that parents identify triggers that lead to tantrums and to avoid the triggers as often as possible. Creating a routine is one helpful method for preventing triggers. If the tantrum has started, Daniels et al. (2012) recommend that parents remain calm, try to distract the child, and ignore the tantrum if possible. Daniels et al. (2012) state that "many tantrums happen when children are asked to do something they do not want to do" (p. 572). With this knowledge, they recommend that parents do not give into the tantrum because it causes negative reinforcement and the child will continue to throw tantrums in an attempt to get their way. As toddlers continue to grow and develop, they learn how to better express themselves and understand their environment, which leads to fewer tantrums (Daniels et al., 2012).

■ TREATMENT PLAN

Parents of toddlers face many challenges on a daily basis. The toddler years are characterized by increased activity, play, and receptive and expressive language development. The toddler also begins to realize that he or she is a separate individual from his or her parents and caregivers (Hagan, Shaw, & Duncan, 2008). This drives toddlers to express likes and dislikes and their wants and needs, and to assert themselves and act independently. Although this is an age of learning and independence, they struggle to understand logic and the concepts of waiting and self-control (Hagan et al., 2008). The toddler's struggle with understanding self-control can be difficult to deal with as a parent, but there are a variety of ways parents and caregivers can interact with their toddlers that will foster appropriate behavior and enhance their self-confidence and aspiration to learn and explore.

To help the mother in this case feel less stressed and enjoy her very active twins, the P-PCP can help the mother consider ways to prioritize spending individual time with the twins, playing, hugging, and reading to them, to enjoy them and to help them begin to learn self-regulation and control. The mother also needs to listen to the toddlers, notice their body language, their expressions, their pleasures and frustrations, and, most importantly, praise the toddlers for good behavior and accomplishments. Toddlers need opportunities to assert themselves and to investigate the environment with the least amount of restrictions (Hagan et al., 2008). Toddlers enjoy making decisions. However, parents must understand that the choices must be acceptable to the parent and offered only when the toddler can have the choice (Hagan et al., 2008). Limiting choices to two equally acceptable options is best. For example, allow the toddler to choose between cleaning up his arts and crafts or cleaning up his blocks. In this case, offering the twins opportunities to assert themselves and act independently will help increase their self-confidence. Furthermore, in this case, the twins have not reached an age where they have developed the skills necessary to interact with other children (Hagan et al., 2008). Expectations must be realistic for how the twins will play with each other and share toys.

As previously mentioned, 2-year-olds are rapidly developing their use of language and enjoy communicating. Toddlers are able to follow simple one- or two-step commands such as "pick up the book and bring it to me," but many struggle with responding quickly (Hagan et al., 2008). Be sure to speak slowly and give the toddler the opportunity to respond and offer praise for his or her effort. Many times, challenging behavior by a toddler means that the toddler is not able to express personal feelings in an acceptable way (Hagan et al., 2008). Toddlers are beginning to experience feelings such as pride, shame, joy, and anger. It is important to encourage your toddler's self-expression and help the toddler describe these feelings (Hagan et al., 2008).

■ SUMMARY

As the toddler continues to grow and develop, self-control improves and the number and frequency of tantrums decrease. Parents play a critical role in helping their toddler "use their words" to express themselves. Parents also play a critical role in controlling the "out-of-control" toddler's behaviors. If a toddler's behavior does not improve with the suggestions for controlling impulsive behaviors and/or temper tantrums, the parent should be advised to return to the primary care office for further evaluation. The toddler may need a referral for a behavioral or neurodevelopmental evaluation. P-PCPs may refer a toddler for early intervention services, including behavior modification strategies. Parents can also be referred for parenting classes to assure that the toddler has every opportunity to grow and develop throughout the toddler years without adverse behavioral health outcomes. Parents who present with concerns about their toddler's behaviors should also be advised that respite for themselves is an important part of caring for themselves as well as their child. Respite can be as simple as having a relative, grandparent, aunt, uncle, or friend spend 3 hours with the toddler to permit the parents to go out to dinner, a movie, or any activity that they enjoy. Parents who spend some quality time together, while their toddler is safe at home, often feel refreshed when returning to the care of their toddler. This case study is an example of normal toddler behaviors that can be controlled with parental education and patience, thus intercepting potential adverse behavioral outcomes for the toddler.

■ REFERENCES

American Academy of Pediatrics. (2017). *Star center: Screening, technical assistance, and resource center*. Retrieved from https://www.aap.org/en-us/advocacy-and-policy/aap-health-initiatives/Screening/Pages/Screening-Tools.aspx

American Psychiatric Association. (2013). *Diagnostic and statistical manual of mental disorders* (5th ed.). Arlington, VA: American Psychiatric Publishing.

Brigance, A., & Glascoe, F. P. (2002). *Brigance infant toddler screen*. North Billencia, MA: Curriculum Associates, Inc.

Brookes Publishing Co. (2017). *Ages and stages questionnaire: Social-emotional (ASQ-SE-2)*. Retrieved from http://www.brookespublishing.com/resource-center/screening-and-assessment/asq/asq-se-2/

Burns, C. B., Dunn, A. M., Brady, M. A., Starr, N. B., Blosser, C. G., & Garzon, D. L. (2013). *Pediatric primary care* (5th ed.). St. Louis, MO: Elsevier.

Centers for Disease Control and Prevention. (2017). *What do parents need to know to protect their children?* Retrieved from https://www.cdc.gov/nceh/lead/acclpp/blood_lead_levels.htm

Centers for Disease Control and Prevention. (2016). *Autism spectrum disorder*. Retrieved from https://www.cdc.gov/ncbddd/autism/index.html

Children and Adults with Attention-Deficit/Hyperactivity Disorder (CHADD). (2017). Preschoolers and ADHD. Retrieved from http://www.chadd.org/understanding-adhd/for-parents-caregivers/preschoolers-and-adhd.aspx

Daniels, E., Mandelco, B., & Luthy, K. E. (2012). Assessment, management and prevention of childhood temper tantrums. *Journal of the American Academy of Nurse Practitioners*. doi:10.1111/j.1745-7599.2012.00755.x

Daria-Wiener, I. (2004). As they grow; 1 year: Why toddlers cling. *Parents*, 79, 201–202.

Goldman-Fraser, J., Fernandez, M. T., & Marfo, K. (2005). Separation and continuity in the lives of infants and toddlers: Introduction to the issue. *Zero to Three*, 25, 4–7.

Gross, D., & Rocissano, L. (1988). Maternal confidence in toddlerhood: A measurement for clinical practice and research. *Research in Nursing and Health*, 18, 489–499. doi:10.1002/nur.4770180605

Chapter 16 TODDLER IMPULSIVE BEHAVIORS: A CASE STUDY ■ 197

Hagan, J. F., Shaw, J. S., & Duncan, P. M. (2008). *Bright futures: guidelines for health supervision of infants, children, and adolescents* (3rd ed.). Elk Grove Village, IL: American Academy of Pediatrics.

Hallas, D. (2018). *Pediatric behavioral health: Intercepting abnormal behaviors...A textbook for primary care providers.* New York, NY: Springer.

Hallas, D., Koslap-Petraco, M., & Fletcher, J. (2017). Social emotional development of toddlers: Randomized control trial of an office-based intervention. *Journal of Pediatric Nursing, 33,* 33–40. doi:10.1016/j.pedn.2016.11.004

Leff, S. S., Tulleners, C., & Posner, J. C. (2009). Aggression, violence, and delinquency. In *Developmental-behavioral pediatrics* (pp. 389–396). Philadelphia, PA: Saunders.

New York State Department of Health. (2009). *Lead exposure risk assessment questionnaire for children.* Retrieved from https://www.health.ny.gov/environmental/lead/exposure/childhood/risk_assessment.htm

New York State Department of Health. (n.d.). *Sources of lead.* Retrieved from https://www.health.ny.gov/environmental/lead/sources.htm

Preschooler Population

CHAPTER 17

Intercepting Behavioral Health Problems in Preschool-Age Children

JANE A. FOX AND TRACI R. BRAMLETT

The preschool child is generally 3 to 5 years of age. At 3 years old, the child is becoming a real person. Children in this age range are described by their parents, preschool teachers, and healthcare providers as "awesome." This is an interesting and exciting time. During the preschool period, the child is able to perform self-care and fine motor tasks. An important step in the socialization process is the beginning of a conscience that slowly starts to emerge during this period. This allows children to have some control over their emotions. As preschool children begin to broaden their interactions beyond their family members, friendships and peers become more important (Marotz, 2014). These children are becoming more independent and are able to show affection.

The preschool years are an important time to prepare children to be successful in school. It is critical to identify and address the problem of social behavior readiness long before a child enters school. Parents need to be partners with other professionals in helping their children to succeed. They need to learn about their child's growth and development and to be aware of unusual behavior changes and/or regressions to work with pediatric primary care providers (P-PCPs) to *intercept* potential behavioral problems. P-PCPs must be diligent in assessing children in order to identify risk factors for behavioral challenges and/or school performance difficulties and educating parents. Children who are identified as "not ready" socially and/or behaviorally for school have a negative long-term impact on communities, families, schools, and themselves.

This chapter addresses the assessment, screening, diagnosis, and treatment of preschoolers with behavioral health problems. It also discusses assessing for school readiness and strategies to *intercept* potential and identified behavioral health problems in preschool-age children to help the child become ready to succeed in school.

■ DAY CARE VERSUS PRESCHOOL-AGE PROGRAM

A preschool is a licensed educational establishment or learning space offering early childhood education to children, usually between the ages of 3 and 5 years, prior to the commencement of compulsory education at primary school or kindergarten. Many preschools will start accepting children at around age 2½ years, but often require the child be toilet-trained. They are often not open full days or during vacations or in the summer. Day care centers can be a more convenient choice for working parents because they usually provide full-time care, even during school breaks.

■ BEHAVIORAL HEALTH ASSESSMENT OF THE PRESCHOOL-AGE CHILD

There are certain milestones and behaviors a child should exhibit to determine readiness for preschool. For example: Is the child fairly independent? Can he or she work on projects on his or her own (solo play)? Is the child able to participate in group activities? Children younger than 3 years may not be developmentally ready to play with others. Does the child have a regular schedule—breakfast, play, rest? Is physical stamina a concern? Does the child nap after lunch while in preschool? Is the child toilet-trained and able to use the toilet by him or herself? Can the child independently wash his or her hands? Can the child feed himself or herself? Is he or she able to calmly separate from his or her parent or caregiver?

Many counties and states have adopted a kindergarten entry assessment that will determine school readiness. Children may be evaluated for literacy skills, emerging math skills, technical adequacy, and social skills; for example, does the child know his or her name, address, and telephone number, ABCs, colors, how to count to 10 or 20, and show affection.

■ SCREENING TOOLS FOR BEHAVIORAL HEALTH PROBLEMS

P-PCPs strive to identify preschool children with behavioral health problems early in an effort to initiate early intervention strategies. Rodrigues, Binnoon-Erez, Plamondon, and Jenkins (2017) report that early identification of behavioral risk factors is crucial in the prevention and intervention of later psychopathology. Many informal checklists are currently used in practice, resulting in the overlooking of many children who are otherwise eligible for early intervention. The American Academy of Pediatrics (AAP) has issued a policy statement calling for detailed developmental surveillance of children (American Academy of Pediatrics, Council on Children With Disabilities, Section on Developmental Behavioral Pediatrics, & Bright Futures Steering Committee Medical Home Initiatives for Children With Special Needs Project Advisory Committee, 2006). Table 17.1 presents several reliable and valid surveillance tools which can be used in identifying preschool children with behavioral problems.

Early Childhood Behavior Screen (ECBS)–Challenging Behavior Scale (CBS)

The ECBS is used to quickly and efficiently identify young children who may be at risk for behavior disorders. This instrument is first-line screening for externalizing

TABLE 17.1

BEHAVIORAL SCREENING INSTRUMENTS FOR PRESCHOOL CHILDREN

Instrument	Target Age Group	Description
Early Childhood Behavior Screen–Challenging Behavior Scale	Toddlers and preschoolers	10-item questionnaire
Home Situations Questionnaire Website: blog.hawaii.edu/dop/files/2011/08/home-situations-questionnaire.doc	Children ages 4–11	16-item questionnaire parents rate
Child Behavior Checklist	Children ages 1.5–5	Parents rate child's behavior problems
Caregiver–Teacher Report Form	Children ages 1.5–5	Teachers rate child's behavior problems
Behavior Assessment Scale for Children-3 Emotional & Screening System	Children ages 2.5–18	Assesses behavioral and emotional strengths and weaknesses
Stressful Life Events Questionnaire	Children and adolescents	Screening questionnaire completed by parent
Pediatric Symptoms Checklist	Children ages 4–5	35-question screening questionnaire completed by parent

behavior problems in very young children. The instrument is short, simple to administer, easy to score, and may be used across settings (Glascoe & Robertshaw, 2007). The ECBS is a 20-item parent report measure that assesses behavior disorders in children living in poverty and included in that measure is a 10-item CBS.

The Child Behavior Checklist (CBCL) for Ages 1½ to 5 Years

This instrument measures two dimensions of child behavior problems: externalizing and internalizing behaviors. Examples of externalizing behaviors are aggression, noncompliance, and inattention. Internalizing behaviors are noted as anxiety, depression, and withdrawal. The CBCL contains a scale that parents use to rate the behavior problems of the child (Harris, Fox, & Holtz, 2016).

The Behavior Assessment Scale for Children-2 and Emotional Screening System (BASC-3 BESS)

The BASC-3 BESS evaluates behavioral and emotional strengths and weaknesses of preschool children. This tool is completed by the parent and identifies a child's risk of behavioral problems (Coke & Moore, 2016).

The Stressful Life Events Questionnaire

This tool is completed by the parent and asks if 13 stressful life events have occurred in the past 12 months, such as birth, death, illness/accident, employment, financial status change, family move, and trouble with law (Harris, Fox, & Holtz, 2016).

The Pediatric Symptoms Checklist

This tool is a psychosocial screen designed to initiate the recognition of cognitive, emotional, and behavioral problems in children. The parent-completed version consists of 35 questions with an assigned cut-off score. A positive score suggests further evaluation by a healthcare provider or behavioral health specialist (American Academy of Pediatrics, Council on Children With Disabilities, Section on Developmental Behavioral Pediatrics, & Bright Futures Steering Committee Medical Home Initiatives for Children With Special Needs Project Advisory Committee, 2006).

The Home Situations Questionnaire (HSQ)

This tool is a 16-item questionnaire that takes 5 minutes to complete. A list is provided of common circumstances at home in which behavior problems are likely to arise. Parents are asked to rate the severity of behavior problems for each situation (Harris, Fox, & Holtz, 2016).

■ FAMILY ASSESSMENT

Assessment of the family and a careful social history are critical to identifying potential mental health and behavioral problems in the preschooler. A genogram, including three generations, is very helpful in mapping family structure, health history, relationships, and identifying family health patterns. Specifically, significant to note are chronic, mental, or behavioral conditions in the family. An ecomap may also be useful in assessing resources and strengths of family relationships with significant others, organizations, and institutions. An assessment tool such as the Family Stressor Strength Inventory (Mischke & Hanson, 1991) helps identify specific stressors and strengths of the family, what resources are currently being utilized, and what other resources may be appropriate in the future. A second assessment tool, Home Situations Questionnaire, focuses on the family and where the parent rates home situations (see Table 17.1). For example, who lives in the home and what is his/her relationship to the child? How many siblings does the child have and what is the relationship (e.g. older, younger, full or half-sibling)? Are there adopted or foster children in the home currently or in the past? Discuss the home and living conditions in the social history. What is the socioeconomic status of the family? Are the parents employed? Does the child feel safe in the home? How are disagreements resolved? Are there guns in the home? A third assessment tool is Stressful Life Events Questionnaire (Coke & Moore, 2016) in which the parent identifies stressful life events within the family over the last year (see Table 17.1). Has any family member been incarcerated or had frequent interactions with law enforcement? Have there been changes in family dynamics? Has there been divorce, separation, violence in the family and or home? What is the education and employment status of the parents? Has the family ever been evicted from a home or apartment? Have they ever been homeless? Do they have reliable transportation? Is there any family history of substance abuse, mental illness, or violence? Describe parenting style. Do the family members feel stress? If so, why? Does the child live in poverty? What is the language spoken in the home? If the family is under extreme stress, lives in poverty, or the child is a witness to violence, referrals to social service and support groups should be made immediately. If there is a family history of substance abuse and/or mental illness, appropriate referrals and close follow-up of the family and child are imperative.

A careful history of the child should be obtained, including growth and development, nutrition, history of elevated lead level (if at risk), anemia, temperament (see Chapter 12), sibling rivalry, extreme anxiety, sleep problems, nightmares/night terrors (5–7 years old), bedwetting, bowel habits, temper tantrums, holding one's breath, aggression, cruelty to animals, impulse control, fears (imaginary figures, the dark, noises, sleeping alone, thunder, and others), separation anxiety, and physical problems or chronic disease. Chronic stress, poverty, and/or other traumatic events such as divorce, abuse, and separation can have a negative impact on development.

Low parent education has been associated with deficits in the development of self-control and self-regulation in the child. Poverty is associated with an increased incidence of parent psychopathology, specifically depression. Also, poverty impacts parenting by causing more stress, exposure to violence, and social isolation. Appropriate referrals that strengthen parenting and improve the child's school readiness, such as social services, programs that deliver home visits, center group meetings, parent group training, behavioral care services, church-based programs, domestic violence support, other community programs as needed, such as Alcholics Ananomous (AA) or AL Anon, and national and state programs, are required. The earlier the strategies are implemented, the greater the potential to intercept behavioral problems in the preschool-age child and enable the family to become a stronger family unit.

■ DETERMINING SCHOOL READINESS: WHY IS IT IMPORTANT?

School readiness is a multidimensional concept (Ackerman & Barnett, 2005). Research has shown that children who enter school with a basic knowledge of math and reading are more likely than their peers to experience later academic success (Duncan, Dowsett, & Claessens, 2007), attain higher levels of education, and secure employment (Rouse, Brooks-Gunn, & McLanahan, 2005). Absence of these and other skills may contribute to even greater disparities in the future. For example, one study found that gaps in math, reading, and vocabulary skills evident at elementary school entry explained at least half of the racial gap in high school achievement scores. School readiness is essential for promoting future academic success. Success in school relates to better emotional and physical well-being, better employment opportunities, and an improved quality of life.

The National Educational Goals Panel (1999) noted school readiness encompasses five dimensions: (a) physical well-being and motor development; (b) social and emotional development; (c) approaches to learning; (d) language development (including early literacy); and (e) cognition and general knowledge. The school readiness indicator reported here includes four skills related to early literacy and cognitive development: a child's ability to recognize letters, count to 20 or higher, write his or her first name, and read words in a book. While cognitive development and early literacy are important for children's school readiness and early success in school, other areas of development, like health, social development, and engagement, may be of equal or greater importance. However, although experts agree that social–emotional skills are critically important for school readiness, to date there are no nationally representative data in this area. Compared with Caucasian or African American children, Hispanic children are less likely to be able to recognize the letters of the alphabet, count to 20 or higher, or write their names before they start kindergarten. African American children are similar to Caucasian Head Start children on these measures, but are more likely than Caucasian children to be reading words in books (Child Trends Databank, 2015).

Age does not necessarily determine readiness for preschool, which has more to do with where the child is developmentally—specifically social, emotional, physical, and cognitive development level. A child's ability to control his or her emotions, interact with others, and help him or herself is an indicator of social and emotional development. A preschooler can follow simple rules during games, may approach other children and begin to play with them, and enjoy playing make-believe games.

■ IMPORTANCE OF PLAY

Play is important to children and it should be fun. It is how a child learns and explores feelings. It also provides an opportunity for them to escape reality, set new rules, and expand their world without the consequences of taking risks.

In 2012, Milteer, Ginsburg, the Council on Communications and Media Communications on Psychosocial Aspects of Child and Family Health, and Mulligan restated that parents should make child-directed nonstructured free play a priority over adult-driven play. Free play is especially important for children living in poverty (Milteer et al., 2012). Gray (2011) found that the decline in play time was accompanied by a decline in children's mental health. Veiga, Neto, and Rieffe (2016) studied the relationship between having opportunities for free play and social development in preschoolers. They found that less time for free play is related to more disruptive behaviors in this age group. Therefore, free play might help to prevent the development of disruptive behaviors. Free play is essential for positive social development. In free play, children have the freedom to guide their play by their own interests and needs and to act out aggressive tensions. Overall, free play is associated with better outcomes. In today's world, families are overscheduled and children often go from one activity to another. To *intercept* the problem of overscheduled parents, the parents need to provide more opportunities for nonstructured child-directed free play without electronic devices. Simple, inexpensive toys such as blocks, balls, jump ropes, and buckets are more effective in allowing children to be imaginative and creative than more expensive toys. Remind parents playtime is a way to engage fully with their children.

Advise parents to participate in physical activities with their children that are free or low cost. Connect parents to community resources that can offer opportunities or assistance (Milteer et al., 2012).

A preschool child plays next to another child rather than with the other child. This is parallel play and is the final stage before the child connects with another. To reach the next level of play, known as cooperative or associative play, a child needs to understand the concept of taking turns. Learning to play is learning how to relate to others. Parallel play lays the groundwork for cooperative play. Appropriate toys for this stage are sticker books and stacking and sorting blocks. In cooperative or associative play, the child plays with others but the play is not goal directed. The children understand taking turns and can handle small toys. Legos and erector sets are good choices to promote this play.

■ PREPARING PRESCHOOLERS FOR KINDERGARTEN

It is essential for the well-being of the preschool-age child that parents identify quality child care services within their own community. The American Academy of Pediatrics (AAP, 2016) "supports state and federal funding for quality pre-school, child care, and child development programs (e.g., Head Start) that pro-mote developmentally appropriate activities in a stimulating, nurturing, and safe environment" (p. 5). If a child has been identified "at risk," early educational preparation programs, such as Head Start, are beneficial. These programs help to close the education gap, help children to be better prepared for kindergarten, and avoid expensive remediation. One such program is More at Four. This nationally acclaimed community-based, high-quality prekindergarten initiative is for at-risk 4-year-olds. Eligibility includes both family income and educational need. Other programs are Head Start, Smart Start, and state- and federal-funded programs. Children who begin school with certain basic skills are more likely to succeed. Parents should read to their child beginning in infancy. Reading helps the child acquire basic skills such as recognizing and recalling letters, numbers, and colors. Parents should expose their child to various experiences such as playing with other children of both sexes, trips to the park and school playground, library, and other community programs. Allowing the child to "just play" or have free play opportu-nities helps the child prepare for entrance into school.

■ COMMON BEHAVIORAL PROBLEMS IN PRESCHOOL-AGE CHILDREN

Nocturnal Enuresis

Bedwetting, also known as nocturnal enuresis, is urinary incontinence in a child 5 years of age or older. Eighty percent of these children have primary enuresis, hav-ing never reached satisfactory dryness. Fifteen percent of 5-year-olds have mono-symptomatic nocturnal enuresis, meaning they do not have lower urinary track symptoms and no history of bladder dysfunction. There is a higher incidence if one or both parents had nocturnal enuresis. There is a high rate of spontaneous resolution, with the prevalence decreasing from 16% at 5 years, to 5% at 10 years, and 1% to 2% at age 15 years or older.

Treatment should begin with education, reassurance, and then motivational therapy. A sticker or star can be placed by the child on a calendar as a reward (motivator) for dry nights, with a greater reward for remaining dry for seven or more nights. Education to the parents and child should explain that enuresis is no one's fault. It is not the child or caregiver's fault. The child should never be punished or mocked for bedwetting. The impact of bedwetting can be reduced by using bed protection and washable/disposable products; using room deodorizers; thoroughly washing the child before dressing; and using emollients to prevent chafing. Keeping a calendar of wet and dry nights helps to determine the effect of interventions. It is important the child attempts to void regularly during the day and just before going to bed (a total of four to seven times); if the child wakes at night, the caregivers should take him/her to the toilet. High-sugar and caffeine-based drinks should be avoided in children with enuresis, particularly in the evening hours. Daily fluid intake should be concentrated in the morning and early afternoon; fluid intake should decrease during the evening. Some authors recommend that their enuretic patients drink 40% of their total daily fluid in the morning (7 a.m. to 12 p.m.), 40% in the afternoon (12 p.m. to 5 p.m.), and only 20% after 5 p.m. (Jalkut, Lerman, & Churchill, 2001).

Ample consumption of fluid in the morning and afternoon reduces the need for significant intake later in the day. Isolated nighttime fluid restriction, without compensatory increase in daytime fluid consumption, may prevent the child from meeting his or her daily fluid requirement and is usually unsuccessful (Jalkut, Lerman, & Churchill, 2001).

An enuresis alarm is the most effective long-term treatment. It is effective in 50% to 75% of the cases, with few adverse effects. However, an alarm requires a long-term commitment (usually 3 to 4 months). An enuresis alarm is an appropriate initial active therapy for highly motivated children and families when the child has frequent enuresis (more than twice per week) and short-term improvement is not a priority (Tu & Baskin, 2017).

Desmopressin (a synthetic vasopressin analog) is a first-line treatment for enuresis in children older than 5 years whose bedwetting has not responded to advice about fluid intake, toileting, or an appropriate reward system. It is an alternative to enuresis alarms for children and families who seek rapid or short-term improvement of enuresis; have failed, refused, or are unlikely to adhere to enuresis alarm treatment; and for whom an enuresis alarm is unsuitable. This treatment is the best choice for parents who are having emotional difficulty coping with the burden of bedwetting and/or parents expressing anger, negativity, or blame toward the child. This medication may be costly, but it is useful for sleepovers and overnight camp. A "trial run" of desmopressin is suggested if the child plans to use it for overnight camp. The trial should take place at least 6 weeks before camp in order to adequately titrate the dose and make sure it will be effective (O'Flynn, 2011). The dose and timing of administration depend upon the formulation. Regular tablets (the only formulation available in the United States) are given 1 hour before bedtime. The initial dose is 0.2 mg (one tablet); if needed after 10 to 14 days, the dose may be increased by 0.2 mg to a maximum dose of 0.4 mg. Oral melt tablets are given 30 to 60 minutes before bedtime. The initial dose is 120 mcg; if needed after 10 to 14 days, the dose may be increased by 120 mcg to a maximum dose of

240 mcg. The relapse rate is 60% to 70% after the medication is discontinued. It is important to evaluate bowel habits and treat any episodes of constipation.

Encopresis

Encopresis is fecal incontinence after toilet training has been completed. This generally occurs in a child 4 years of age or older (usually presents in children younger than age 7 years) and is the passage of stool in clothing and or in inappropriate places. Over 90% of encopresis is due to chronic functional constipation. *Intercept*: Children who suffer from constipation must be treated and closely followed. Encopresis is extremely upsetting to the parents and often to the child.

A careful history and physical exam are required to rule out organic or systemic causes of the constipation and incontinence. The history should explore if any stressful events precipitated the beginning of fecal soiling, such as toilet training, separation (beginning school), or other emotional events that may have interfered with the child's toilet habits. For example, any change in family (divorce, illness, death), school (new teacher or classroom), or peer relationships (bullying), places (school, bathroom), or the toilet itself may be stressors.

The abdominal exam may indicate an abdominal mass (stool) and the digital exam may show dilated rectum packed with stool. An abdominal radiograph may be indicated if the child is uncomfortable with the abdominal or digital exam or the history is vague. *Intercept*: Parents need to understand the child is not able to control the stool leaking and should not be ridiculed or blamed. This problem is not so unusual and can be successfully treated. Initially, the stool needs to be cleaned out with medication and the cycle of leaking stool needs to be broken. Treatment requires commitment from both the parents and the child. Regular bowel habits need to be established. The goal is to keep the rectum as near to empty as possible so the rectum can return to its normal size. The goal is to have the child pass stool before he or she feels the sensation of needing to stool. Constipation and encopresis are often long-term issues and may return after improvement with treatment. Children often require a laxative such as polyethylene glycol and/or high fiber supplements for an extended period of time. Children and parents who understand the signs of stool backup and *intercept* the problem by implementing a rescue plan as soon as the problem emerges, empower the child and parent in anticipating and treating recurrences.

Nightmares and Night Terrors

Night terrors (also called "sleep terrors") typically occur when a child is between 4 and 12 years of age. The events occur during the first third of nocturnal sleep. The child awakens abruptly from sleep with a loud scream, is agitated, and has a flushed face, sweating, and tachycardia. The child may jump out of bed as if running away from an unseen threat and is usually unresponsive to parental efforts at calming. The child usually does not remember the episode later.

Confusional arousals are episodes in which children behave in a confused way because they are in between sleeping and waking up. They sit up in bed, moan, or cry. The child is not able to be calmed. These episodes usually last 10 to

30 minutes. Both night terrors and confusional arousals happen in the first part of the night, are not dangerous, and the child does not remember them the next day. They are also more likely to happen in children who have a fever or are not getting enough sleep. Nightmares are very scary, sad, or upsetting dreams that wake a child up. After a nightmare, children often have trouble going back to bed. They usually happen in the second half of the night.

PARENTAL STRATEGIES TO INTERCEPT NIGHT TERRORS

If a child has a night terror or confusional arousal, the caregiver (*intercept*) should stay with the child until the episode stops but not try to wake the child. Once the episode stops, the child will go back to sleep.

If a child has a nightmare, parents should remind the child that it was only a dream and not real. Suggest they help the child think of a new, happy ending to the dream or draw a picture or write about the dream, which often makes it less scary. These strategies, consistently applied, may intercept the occurrence of future nightmares.

Breath Holding

About 5% of all children have breath-holding spells. They are common between 6 months and 6 years of age. There is a family history in 20% to 35% of cases. The most common type of breath-holding spell is cyanotic or type 1 and is precipitated by anger, pain, or frustration (Salerno, 2017). These occur most often in toddlers, last less than a minute, and recovery is spontaneous. These spells are self-limited and harmless and need to be differentiated from seizures. Carefully explain (*intercept*) and demystify breath-holding spells to parents and that the child is unable to control them (Zuckerman, 2013b). Iron supplementation is effective in the management of breath-holding spells. Non-anemic and iron-replete children with breath-holding spells also respond well to iron supplementation.

Anxiety

Fear and anxiety are a normal part of childhood development. The P-PCP may *intercept* to assist the parent in recognizing if the fear and anxiety are normal in development or excessive, therefore interfering with functioning. Anxiety disorders are commonly identified health problems in children. They are often underdiagnosed or even misdiagnosed (Brown & Melnyk, 2013a). Depression, oppositional defiant disorder, and learning disorders are comorbidities associated with anxiety. Parents may report that the child is a "worrier." The parent may also describe the preschooler as having episodes of sudden fear that intensifies in a short amount of time. Physical symptoms include agitation, fidgeting, headache, abdominal pain, sleep difficulties, fatigue, muscle tension, and dizziness. Behavioral symptoms often include crying, nail-biting, poor concentration, anger, and social skills deficits. Cognitive symptoms reported by parents are negative thinking, worrying about things before they happen, and constant worries and concerns (Swenson et al., 2016; AAP, 2015a). Careful screening and assessment is a high priority with the goal of determining the diagnoses and severity. When developing a treatment plan, the P-PCP should educate the parents and child about common signs and symptoms and environmental health strategies such as optimal sleep habits, decreasing stressors, and maintaining routines. Other treatment options are cognitive behavior therapy (CBT), psychopharmacological intervention, combined CBT and psychopharmacological interventions, family interventions such as parent anxiety management, and behavior intervention.

Depression

A common feature of depression is the presence of sad, empty, or irritable mood, which is associated with somatic and cognitive changes that interfere with functioning. Detection is low at less than 20% of cases, with less than 25% of affected children receiving treatment. An estimated 5% (males and females equally) of children are affected. Depression may also be misdiagnosed as attention deficit hyperactivity disorder (ADHD) in young children due to their inattention, impulsivity, and hyperactivity (Brown & Melnyk, 2013b). Common symptoms preschoolers may present with are sadness, irritability, impulsivity, crying spells, loss of interest in activities, sleep problems, frequent complaints that no one likes him or her, stomachaches or headaches, and acting-out behaviors (Swenson et al., 2016). The P-PCP should always assess for suicide ideations in the preschooler as well as *intercept* by working with the parent to identify safety precautions and mobilize social supports. As with anxiety, educating on the depressive condition and supporting the family is crucial. The P-PCP should work with the parents to involve school and after-care personnel in the treatment plan. In addition, careful and regular follow-up with the family is crucial. Medications should be reserved for moderate to severe depression not responding to psychotherapy and/or cognitive behavioral skills–building programs.

Anger and Aggression

Anger is a normal emotion in preschoolers. Common situations associated with a preschooler becoming angry are not getting what they want, others not understanding them, having hurt feelings, or feeling left out. Parents are encouraged to acknowledge angry feelings and take notice of the changes in the body when anger is evident. The child's heart will beat faster and their faces will become hot and sweaty. Finding it hard to breathe may also be exhibited as they try to release energy through immediate action. The AAP (2015b, 2015c) recommends working with parents to encourage children to put feelings into words; to let children know it takes more courage to walk away from a fight; to know that it is not good to hit someone, break things, or say things that hurt; to encourage children to think about the problem and of ways to fix it; to explain themselves to others when they are not understood; and to stop, think, listen, avoid, and move on before acting with violence.

The AAP (2015b) describes an aggressive child as one who hits, bites, bullies, demands, and/or destroys. Preschoolers most likely will exhibit signs of aggression during times of threat, anger, rage, and/or frustration. An important task in early childhood is mastering the skills needed to manage aggression effectively. By kindergarten, a child whose aggressive behavior is a threat to others or to him or herself should receive professional help (AAP, 2015b). Displays of aggressive behavior that are concerning in the preschooler are hitting, throwing objects, threatening peers, or having tantrums, which means they may have feelings of frustration, anger, or humiliation. These kinds of worrisome behaviors may have serious implications for later functioning. Their presence should involve an evaluation by a behavioral care specialist.

■ SUMMARY

A preschool child is generally 3 to 5 years of age. An important step in the socialization process is the beginning of a conscience that slowly starts to emerge during this period. A conscience allows children to have some control over their emotions, become independent, and show affection. The preschool age is an important time to prepare children to be successful in school. It is critical to identify and address the problem of social behavior readiness long before a child enters school. Parents need to be partners with other professionals in helping their children to succeed. Performing preschool-age behavioral health assessments and family assessments is an important role of P-PCPs. Assessing for school readiness is another important task performed by P-PCPs and the local school districts that provide education for children in day-care or preschool environments. Common behavioral problems identified in the preschool years include nocturnal enuresis, encopresis, nightmares and night terrors, breath holding, first evidence of anxiety or depression, anger, and aggressive behaviors. P-PCPs play a critical role in early identification of these behaviors to recommend evidence-based interventions to *intercept* them as early as possible to prevent adverse outcomes and potential long-term problems.

■ REFERENCES

Ackerman, D. J., & Barnett, W. S. (2005). *Prepared for kindergarten: What does "readiness" mean?* New Brunswick, NJ: National Institute for Early Education Research.

American Academy of Pediatrics. (2015a). *How to ease your child's separation anxiety.* Retrieved from https://www.healthychildren.org/English/ages-stages/toddler/Pages/Soothing-Your-Childs-Separation-Anxiety.aspx

American Academy of Pediatrics. (2015b). *Aggressive behavior.* Retrieved from https://www.healthychildren.org/English/family-life/family-dynamics/communication-discipline/Pages/Aggressive-Behavior.aspx

American Academy of Pediatrics. (2015c). *Everybody gets mad: Helping your child cope with conflict.* Retrieved from https://www.healthychildren.org/English/healthy-living/emotional-wellness/Pages/Everybody-Gets-Mad-Helping-Your-Child-with-Conflict.aspx

American Academy of Pediatrics. (2016). *Policy statement: American Academy of Pediatrics highlights impact of children's earliest experiences on school readiness.* Retrieved from https://www.aap.org/en-us/about-the-aap/aap-press-room/Pages/American-Academy-of-Pediatrics-Highlights-Impact-of-Children's-Earliest-Experiences-on-School-Readiness.aspx

American Academy of Pediatrics, Council on Children With Disabilities, Section on Developmental Behavioral Pediatrics, & Bright Futures Steering Committee Medical Home Initiatives for Children With Special Needs Project Advisory Committee. (2006). Identifying infants and young children with developmental disorders in the medical home: An algorithm for developmental surveillance and screening. *Pediatrics, 118,* 405–420. doi:10.1542/peds.2006-1231

Brown, H., & Melnyk, B. M. (2013a). Depressive disorders. In B. M. Melnyk & P. Jensen (Eds.), *A practical guide to child and adolescent mental health screening, early intervention, and health promotion* (pp. 99–105). New York, NY: National Association of Pediatric Nurse Practitioners.

Brown, H., & Melnyk, B. M. (2013b). Anxiety disorders. In B. M. Melnyk & P. Jensen (Eds.), *A practical guide to child and adolescent mental health screening, early intervention, and health promotion* (pp. 61–63, 67, 81–82, 89). New York, NY: National Association of Pediatric Nurse Practitioners.

Coke, S. P., & Moore, L. C. (2016). Factors influencing female caregivers' appraisals of their preschoolers' behaviors. *Journal of Pediatric Health Care, 31*, 46–56. doi:10.1016/j.pedhc.2016.01.006

Duncan, G. J., Dowsett, C. J., & Claessens, A. (2007). School readiness and later achievement. *Developmental Psychology, 43*(6), 1428–1446. doi:10.1037/0012-1649.43.6.1428

Glascoe, F. P., & Robertshaw, N. S. (2007). New AAP policy on detecting and addressing developmental and behavioral problems. *Journal of Pediatric Health Care, 21*, 4107–4412. doi:10.1016/j.pedhc.2007.08.008

Gray, P. (2011). The decline of play and the rise of psychopathology in children and adolescents. *American Journal of Play, 3*, 443–463.

Harris, S. E., Fox, R. A., & Holtz, C. A. (2016). Screening for significant behavior problems in diverse young children living in poverty. *Journal of Child and Family Studies, 25*, 1076–1085. doi:10.1007/s10826-015-0300-x

Jalkut, M., Lerman, S., & Churchill, B. (2001). Enuresis. *Pediatric Clinics of North America, 48*, 1461–1488. doi:10.1016/S0031-3955(05)70386-2

Marotz, L. R. (2014). *Health, safety, and nutrition for the young child* (9th ed.). Boston, MA: Cengage Learning.

Milteer, R. M., Ginsburg, K. R., Council on Communications and Media Communications on Psychosocial Aspects of Child and Family Health, & Mulligan, D. A. (2012). Clinical report: The importance of play in promoting healthy child development and maintaining strong parent–child bonds. *Pediatrics, 129*, e204–e213. Retrieved from http://pediatrics.aappublications.org/content/129/1/e204

National Education Goals Panel. (1999). *National education goals report: Building a nation of learners.* Washington, DC: Retrieved from http://govinfo.library.unt.edu/negp/reports/99rpt.pdf

O'Flynn, N. (2011). Nocturnal enuresis in children and young people: NICE clinical guideline. *The British Journal of General Practice, 61*(586), 360–362. Retrieved from http://doi.org/10.3399/bjgp11X572562

Rodrigues, M., Binnoon-Erez, N., Plamondon, A., & Jenkins, J. M. (2017). Behavioral risk assessment from newborn to preschool: The value of older siblings. *Pediatrics, 140*(2). doi:10.1542/peds.2016-4279

Rouse, C., Brooks-Gunn, J., & McLanahan, S. (2005). School readiness: Closing racial and ethnic gaps; Introducing the issue. *Future of Children, 15*(1). Retrieved from http://www.princeton.edu/futureofchildren/publications/docs/15_01_FullJournal.pdf

Salerno, J. (2017). Causes of syncope in children and adolescents. In T. W. Post (Ed.), *UptoDate.* Retrieved from http://www.uptodate.com

Sood, M. (2017). Chronic functional constipation and fecal incontinence in infants and children: Treatment. In T. W. Post (Ed.), *UptoDate.* Retrieved from http://www.uptodate.com

Swenson, S., Ho, G. W., Budhathoki, C., Belcher, H. M., Tucker, S., Miller, K., & Gross, D. (2016). Parents' use of praise and criticism in a sample of young children seeking mental health services. *Journal of Pediatric Health Care, 30*, 49–56. doi:10.1016/j.pedhc.2015.09.010

Tu, N., & Baskin, L. S. (2017). Nocturnal enuresis in children: Management. In T. W. Post (Ed.), *UptoDate.* Retrieved from http://www.uptodate.com

Veiga, G., Neto, C., & Rieffe, C. (2016). Preschoolers' free play—Connections with emotional and social functioning. *The International Journal of Education, 8*, 48–62.

Wright, L. M., & Leahey, M.L. (2012). *Nurses and families: A guide to family assessment and intervention.* Philadelphia: F.A. Davis.

Zuckerman, B. (2011a). Breath holding. In M. Augustyn, B. Zuckerman, & Caronna, E. (Eds.), *The Zuckerman Parker handbook of developmental and behavioral pediatrics for primary care* (pp 158–159). Philadelphia, PA: Lippincott.

Zuckerman, B. (2011b). Nightmares and night terrors. In M. Augustyn, B. Zuckerman, & Caronna, E. (Eds.), *The Zuckerman Parker handbook of developmental and behavioral pediatrics for primary care* (pp. 280–281). Philadelphia, PA: Lippincott.

CHAPTER 18

Attention Deficit Hyperactivity Disorder and Coexisting Disorders

SUSAN R. OPAS

Attention deficit hyperactivity disorder (ADHD) is a neurodevelopmental disorder that can be diagnosed as early as toddlerhood (American Psychiatric Association [APA], 2013; Banaschewski et al., 2017). The American Academy of Pediatrics (AAP) revised guidelines for diagnosis and treatment of ADHD in children between 4 and 6 years old, since the management of children in this age range is considerably different than children older than 6 years (AAP, 2011a). However, ADHD is most often identified and diagnosed as children enter and proceed through their primary school years. As early as kindergarten, children are expected to follow classroom and play-yard rules as they further socialize and build cognitive learning skills outside their homes and familiar settings. Once enrolled in schools, teachers and parents may begin to identify children's learning and/or social and behavioral differences that are incongruent with those expected by developmental age and stage, or academic skills corresponding to their chronological age and expected school grade learning level. The incidence is believed to be 5% of children, boys being identified in a ratio of 2:1 to girls (Albert, Rui, & Ashman, 2017; Faraone et al., 2003).

■ ADHD: A HISTORICAL PERSPECTIVE

The Story of Fidgety Philip, a German children's poem, is of the oldest identified descriptions of ADHD (Hoffman, 1848; http://germanstories.vcu.edu/struwwel/philipp-e.html).

From first recognition of childhood ADHD, the disorder's name and characterizations have gone through a wide range of terms, some rather punitive such as "Defect of Moral Control" (Still, 1902), to the *Diagnostic and Statistical Manual of Mental Disorders* (third edition; *DSM-III*), which suggested that all with ADHD also had learning disabilities (APA, 1980). The *DSM-IV* more precisely explained ADHD subtypes (APA, 1994). These subtypes were again more clearly described in the most recent, fifth edition, of the *DSM* (*DSM-5*; APA, 2013).

This chapter provides an overview of the assessment, diagnosis, and treatment of children and adolescents with a diagnosis of ADHD. In addition, common coexisting or comorbidities that are seen in children and adolescents with a diagnosis of ADHD are presented.

■ UNDERSTANDING ADHD

There are three subtypes of ADHD (APA, 2013). Within the three subtypes, the child with ADHD exhibits a persistent pattern of inattention and/or hyperactivity-impulsivity that interferes with daily development or functioning. Additionally, at least six behaviors have been noted before the age of 12, most persisting at least 6 months to a point inconsistent with the child's developmental level, and causing negative impact on social and academic activities within at least two settings. Five identified behaviors form the basis when assessing an adolescent age 17 or older (APA, 2013).

The common subtypes of ADHD include the following: (a) a predominance of inattentive behaviors; (b) a combination of hyperactive and impulsive behaviors; and (c) a combination of inattentive and hyperactive/impulsive behaviors.

ADHD: Inattentive Behaviors

The child or adolescent with ADHD and inattentive behaviors often fails to give close attention to details; has difficulty sustaining attention in tasks or play; does not seem to listen when spoken to directly; does not follow through on instructions and fails to complete the associated task; has difficulty organizing tasks and activities; avoids, dislikes, is reluctant to engage in tasks requiring sustained mental efforts; loses items needed for tasks or activities; is easily distracted by extraneous stimuli; and is forgetful in daily activities (APA, 2013).

ADHD: Hyperactive/Impulsive Behaviors

The child or adolescent with ADHD and hyperactive-impulsive or ADHD combined presentation often fidgets, squirms, taps hands and feet; leaves seat when expected to remain seated; runs about, climbs in inappropriate settings; cannot play or engage in leisure activities quietly; on the go "as if driven by a motor"; talks excessively; blurts out answers before the question is completed; has difficulty waiting turn; and interrupts/intrudes on others (APA, 2013).

■ EXECUTIVE BRAIN FUNCTION AND ADHD

Theoretically, experts in ADHD research have shifted the focus of ADHD from uncontrolled physical hyperactivity to identifying the role of the brain in managing cognitive functions of self-regulation. Thomas Brown identified six related cognitive behaviors (activation, focus, effort, emotion, memory, and action) necessary for positive executive function (Brown, 2005) in his executive function diagram of cognitive functions, with examples, that work toward smooth and steady task initiation through completion. Neurologically and biochemically, the primary behaviors of ADHD arise from a deficiency of dopamine (DA) and norepinephrine (NE) transport within the synaptic vesicles of the arousal networks (Stahl, 2008). This deficiency leads to inefficient information processing within the prefrontal cortical areas. Cortical-striatal-thalamic-cortical (CSTC) loops link thought and action to other parts of the brain when the neurotransmitter charges are constant. Stahl (2008) identifies the cortical areas and their regulatory function of ADHD behaviors as follows: (a) dorsal anterior cingulate cortex (ACC) → selective attention; (b) dorsolateral prefrontal cortex (DLPFC) → sustained attention responsible for problem solving; (c) prefrontal motor cortex (PMC) → motor hyperactivity; and (d) orbital frontal cortex (OFC) → impulsivity.

■ ESTABLISHING THE DIAGNOSIS OF ADHD

ADHD diagnosis is both subjective and objective. Since by diagnostic criteria, ADHD behaviors must be noted in at least two of the child's attended settings, those most frequented are the best information source of a child's performance. Use of standardized, validated reporting screening tools addressing key target ADHD behaviors set by the versions of the *DSM* began in the 1969s (Table 18.1). Each set of authored questionnaires includes forms for the parent, teacher, and, occasionally, child to complete. All screening tools have been validated for reliability, although the person responsible for completing the form is doing so subjectively, based on recent interactions with the child or adolescent.

Once completed, the screening tools or forms are scored to determine the direction of the ADHD evaluation process. A diagnosis is not established if criteria are not sufficiently noted in one of the two reported settings. If a child does not meet criteria in one of the settings, the diagnosis is delayed. The child's home and school are the most frequently selected settings. Additional documentation of criteria or concerns of potential coexisting problems can be gathered by reviewing copies of the child's previous and current report cards (including teacher comments), classroom observations, standardized district or state academic and achievement testing results, school district or private psychoeducational testing reports (including individual education programs [IEPs]), and clinic-based psychological or neurodevelopmental testing. Rarely is there need for laboratory tests, unless the pediatric primary care provider (P-PCP) suspects an exposure to a neurotoxin, such as living in lead-based painted housing.

Initial evaluation begins with a general health assessment by the child's P-PCP or a school district's physician, nurse practitioner, or other healthcare provider. Definitive diagnosis depends on state licensure or institutional algorithms. P-PCPs may collaborate with developmental pediatricians, child psychiatrists, neurologists, or clinical psychologists. The AAP published practice guidelines for the evaluation and diagnosis of ADHD in 2000, treatment in 2001, and updated the guidelines in 2011 (AAP, 2000, 2001, 2011a). Simultaneously the "Work Group on Quality Issues" of the American Academy of Child and Adolescent Psychiatry developed and published similar practice parameters for assessment and treatment of childhood and adolescent attention deficit (Greenhill et al., 2002; Plizska, 2007).

TABLE 18.1

SELECTED SCREENING AND DIAGNOSTIC ASSESSMENTS FOR ATTENTION DEFICIT HYPERACTIVITY DISORDER AND COEXISTING DISORDERS

General Pediatric Assessments	
Adolescent Mental Health Questionnaire	Reynolds (1998)
ASQ-3: Ages and Stages Questionnaire	Squires, Bricker, and Twonbly (2009)
CBCL: Child Behavior Checklist	Achenbach and Rescorla (2001)
CGAS: Children's Global Assessment Scale	Shaffer et al. (1983)
C-3GI: Conners 3 Global Index	Gallant (2008)
Peds-QL: Paediatric Quality of Life Inventory	Varni et al. (2001)
PSC-17: Pediatric Symptom Checklist-17 item	Murphy et al. (2016)
PSC-35: Pediatric Symptom Checklist-35 item	Jellinek et al (1999)
SDQ: Strengths and Differences Questionnaire	Goodman et al. (2009)
Attention Deficit Hyperactivity Disorder	
ACTeRS: ADD-H Comprehensive Teachers Rating Scale	Carini and Parks (1993)
ADHD Rating Scale-IV	DuPaul et al. (1998)
Conners CPT-3: Child, Parent, Teacher (ADHD) Rating Scales	Conners (n.d.; 1998)
SKAMP: Swanson, Kotkin, Agler, M-Flynn, & Pelham Scale	Murray (2009)
SNAP-IV: Swanson, Nolan & Pelham Rating Scale	Bussey et al (2008)
SWAN: Strengths & Weaknesses of ADHD-Sx & Normal Behavior	Swanson et al. (2012)
VADRS: Vanderbilt Diagnostic Rating Scales	Wolraich et al. (2003)
Executive Function	
BRIEF: 2 Behavior Rating Inventor of Executive Function	Gioia et al. (2017)
Learning Disabilities	
Jordan Left–Right Reversals	Jordan (2011)
KTEA-3: Kaufman Tests of Educational Achievement-3rd ed.	Kaufman and Kaufman (2014)
TVPS-4: Test of Visual–Perceptual Skills-Rev.	Martin (2017)
VMI-6: Beery Test of Visual–Motor Integration	Beery, Buktenica, and Beery (2010)

(continued)

TABLE 18.1 *(CONTINUED)*

SELECTED SCREENING AND DIAGNOSTIC ASSESSMENTS FOR ATTENTION DEFICIT HYPERACTIVITY DISORDER AND COEXISTING DISORDERS

WIAT-3: Wechsler Individual Achievement Test-3rd ed.	Wechsler (2009)
WISC-V: Wechsler Intelligence Scales for Children-5th ed.	Wechsler (2014)
WJ-3: Woodcock-Johnson Tests of Cognitive Abilities-4th ed.	Woodcock, Schrank, McGrew, and Mathes (2007)
WRAT-4: Wide Range Achievement Test-4th ed.	Wilkenson and Robertson (2017)
Anxiety	
BYI-2: Beck Youth Inventory-2nd ed.	Beck, Beck, Jolly, and Steer (2005)
SCARED: Screen for Childhood Anxiety Related Disorders	Birmaher et al. (1997)
Obsessive-Compulsive Disorder	
Y-BOCS-2: Yale-Brown Obsessive Compulsive Scale	Storch et al. (2010)
Depression	
BDI-PC: Beck Depression Inventory for Primary Care	Beck et al. (1997)
CDI-2: Children's Depression Inventory	Kovacs (2010)
Kutcher Adolescent Depression Scale 6 Item	LeBlanc, Almudevar, Brooks, and Kutcher (2002)
PHQ-9/A: Patient Health Questionnaire-Adolescent	Johnson, Harris, Spitzer, and Williams (2002)
Oppositional Defiant Disorder	
DBRS: Disruptive Behavior Rating Scale	Silva et al. (2005)
Conduct Disorder	
CDS: Conduct Disorder Scale	Gilliam (2002)
Bipolar Disorder	
BSDS: Bipolar Spectrum Diagnostic Scale	Nasser Gaemi et al. (2005)
Autism Spectrum Disorder	
ADOS-2: Autism Diagnostic Observation Schedule-2nd ed.	Lord et al. (2012)
CARS-2: Childhood Autism Rating Scales	Schopler, VanBourgondien, Wellman, and Love (2010)

(continued)

TABLE 18.1 *(CONTINUED)*

SELECTED SCREENING AND DIAGNOSTIC ASSESSMENTS FOR ATTENTION DEFICIT HYPERACTIVITY DISORDER AND COEXISTING DISORDERS	
M.CHAT-R/F: Modified Checklist for Autism in Toddlers-R/F	Robins, Fein, and Barton (2009)
SCQ: Social Communication Quotient	Rutter, Bailey, and Lord (2003)
Sleep Disorders	
CSHQ: Children's Sleep Habits Questionnaire	Owens, Spirito, and McGuinn (2000)

Editions, dates, and authors reflect most current resource information and can be found in the Reference list.

■ TREATMENT FOR ADHD

In 2011, the Subcommittee on Attention Deficit/Hyperactivity Disorder of the AAP published a new comprehensive Clinical Practice Guidelines for ADHD (AAP, 2011a), which include the current algorithm and process of evaluation, diagnosis, treatment, and monitoring for children and adolescents (AAP, 2011b).

Clinical research on the pharmacologic treatment for children of all ages with ADHD has been conducted for decades (Conners, 2002; Efron et al., 1997, Greenhill et al., 2006; Kavale, 1982; Scheffler et al., 2009, Swanson et al., 1993; Zuvekas & Vitiello, 2012). The most well-known clinical investigation is the multimodal, multisite MTA study by Jensen et al. (2001). The researchers investigated the differences among four treatment strategies to determine the most effective treatments for children and adolescents with a diagnosis of ADHD. The treatment groups consisted of the following treatment and control groups: (a) medication only; (b) behavioral therapy only; (c) a combination of medication and therapy; and (d) community standard of care (control group). Results of this study revealed that subjects receiving combination medication and therapy had slightly better control of ADHD symptoms than those in the medication-alone group. However, in a 3-month follow-up, results were equal for these two groups. Greenhill et al. (2006) selectively studied the effects of stimulant medication in a preschool population, from which a cohort continued to be followed into their adolescence (Riddle et al., 2013). Using alternatives to medication is often at the forefront of parents' treatment questions (see Silverman & Hinshaw, 2008 for a 10-year update of evidence-based nonpharmacological therapies). Mohammadi et al. (2016) studied 47 children diagnosed with ADHD who were receiving methylphenidate. The mothers of 22 children were enrolled in a parent behavioral management training (PBMT) program. Between groups, children of mothers participating in the PBMT program had a significant reduction in ADHD behaviors.

Neurofeedback is another consistently discussed non-medication alternative therapy for children with ADHD. Gelade et al. (2016) investigators reported the use of methylphenidate to be superior in improving neurocognitive functioning over theta/beta neurofeedback training. Encouraging behavioral support and therapy along with ADHD medication has been found to play an important role in developing executive function strategies, for example, organization and time management (Mattingly & Anderson, 2016).

■ MEDICATION FOR MANAGEMENT OF ADHD

The initial practice of treating ADHD with the stimulant Benzedrine was reported in 1937 (Bradley, 1937). Methylphenidate research began in 1954 and was used for treating hyperkinesis of childhood in 1957. Neurochemically, stimulants boost firing of dopamine and norepinephrine signals across pre- and post-synaptic neurons to enhance ineffectively processed ADHD cognitive thoughts and actions. The methylphenidate class of stimulant is of the most highly researched and supported for use in childhood (Conners, 2002; Jensen et al., 2001; Riddle et al., 2013; Swanson et al., 1993). The C-II stimulant class is the gold standard, with atomoxetine and the alpha-2-adrenergic as second-line treatment (Greenhill, Pliszka, Dulcan, & the Work Group on Quality Issues, 2002; see Chapter 3 for further discussion on stimulant and psychotropic medications). Stimulants are available as full or partial immediate onset and short, intermediate, or long-acting duration. When selecting and prescribing a medication, it is important to inform families that finding the right medication, dose strength, and duration is a balancing process of seeing the child experience positive outcomes without experiencing negative side effects. Additionally, undiagnosed coexisting cognitive or behavioral problems, or medications used to treat known behavioral issues, may further complicate the effects of the ADHD stimulants (March et al., 2000).

■ COEXISTING DIAGNOSES OF ADHD

Children with a diagnosis of ADHD may have one or more coexisting or comorbid disorders that further complicate these children's diagnosis, treatment, and management. Banaschewski et al. (2017) reported the results of a meta-analysis on the diagnosis and treatment of individuals with a diagnosis of ADHD. The authors reported up to 75% of children diagnosed with ADHD had at least one coexisting disorder and 60% were diagnosed to have two or more coexisting disorders. Concurrently, researching the National Ambulatory Medical Care Survey, Albert et al. reported 29% of child and adolescent visits identified a coexisting mental health disorder (2017). Most of the coexisting disorders were most likely present prior to the child's initial diagnosis of ADHD. However, underlying characteristics of the coexisting disorders may have been overshadowed by ADHD behaviors. Thus, symptoms of coexisting disorders may not have been noticed until medications that targeted ADHD behaviors effectively improved ADHD symptoms, leading to the recognition of behaviors consistent with coexisting disorder(s) (Biederman, Newcorn, & Sprich, 1991). Occasionally, the medication prescribed for a child's

ADHD can heighten the behaviors of a coexisting diagnosis, causing the need to address those newly exhibited behaviors. Table 18.2 lists the more commonly co-occurring diagnoses and their best reported incidence of co-occurrence. It is important to follow the AAP's ADHD process-of-care algorithm to identify and coordinate care for the child or adolescent with ADHD and coexisting disorders as a child/youth with special healthcare needs (CYSHCN; AAP, 2011b).

TABLE 18.2

ATTENTION DEFICIT HYPERACTIVE DISORDER: PERCENTAGE OF COEXISTENCE REPORTED BY DISORDER

Disorder	Percentage
Executive Function Impairment	50
Learning Disabilities	10–20 to 40–60
Anxiety	34
Generalized Anxiety Disorder	34–50
Tic/Tourette's	5–10
Obsessive-Compulsive Disorder	25–50
Depression	13–27 to 60
Persistent Depressive Disorder–Dysthymia	0.5
Autism Spectrum Disorder	30–50
Disruptive Mood Dysregulation Disorder	2–5
Intermittent Explosive Disorder	2.7
Oppositional Defiance Disorder	40–60
Conduct Disorder	11
Bipolar Disorder	≤1
Sleep Disorders	25–50

American Psychiatric Association. (2013). *Diagnostic and statistical manual of mental health disorders* [DSM-5]. (5th ed.). Arlington, VA: Author. Retrieved from https://doi.org/10.1176/appi.books.9780890425596; Brown, T. E. (2005). *Attention deficit disorder: The unfocused mind in children and adults*. New Haven, CT: Yale University Press; Brunsvold, G. L., Oepen, G., Federman, E. J., & Akins, R. (2008) Comorbid depression and ADHD in children and adolescents. Psychiatric Times, 1-8; Leitner, Y. (2014). The co-occurrence of autism and attention deficit hyperactivity disorder in children—What do we know? *Frontiers in Human Neuroscience, 8*, 1–8. doi:10.3389/fnhum.2014.00268; Lougy, R. A., & Rosenthal, D. K. (2016) Co-existing conditions commonly found with ADHD. *2016 Annual CHADD international conference* (11-11-16). Costa Mesa, CA; Sciberras, E., Lycett, K., Effron, D., Mensah, F., Gerner, B., & Hiscock, H. (2014). Anxiety in children with attention deficit/hyperactivity disorder. *Pediatrics, 133*, 801–808. doi:10.1542/peds.2013-3686; Wang, Y. F., Huang, F., Sun, L., Qian, Y., Liu, L., Ma, Q.-G., . . . Qian, Q.-J. (2016). Cognitive function of children and adolescents with attention deficit hyperactivity disorder and learning difficulties: A developmental perspective. *Chinese Medical Journal, 129*, 1922–1928. doi:10.4103/0366-6999.187861; *DSM-5* states not to be diagnosed with ADHD.

Specific Learning Disabilities (SLDs)

Most often, the child's teacher is the first person to notice the child's classroom behaviors that are consistent with a possible diagnosis of ADHD and coexisting learning difficulties. Unless the child is hyperactive or impulsive, it may be difficult to determine if the child is having problems in processing and learning information presented, or is unable to attend and maintain focus on content presented. An experienced teacher who identifies persistent ADHD behaviors may suggest to parents that the child be evaluated by the P-PCP. While the P-PCP or specialist will determine if the child has ADHD, the child's public education setting is responsible for identifying areas of learning difficulty, specific learning disabilities, followed by an educational learning plan.

DIAGNOSIS OF SLD COEXISTING WITH ADHD

An SLD presents as persistent difficulty in learning or using academic skills, for at least 6 months, despite the child receiving targeted interventions in one or more of the following areas of difficulty: slow and/or inaccurate word reading; understanding what one has read; spelling; written expression; mastering number sense, facts, and calculations; and mathematical reasoning (APA, 2013). Approximately 20% to 60% of children with ADHD also have coexisting learning disorders (Huang et al., 2016). In a large cohort study, children with ADHD were found to have higher learning risks in reading, spelling, and math (Czamara et al., 2013). In addition, the academic skill deficits were both significantly and quantifiably below the child's expected chronological age. Difficulty learning causes significant interference with academic and occupational performance, as well as in activities of daily living. Learning disabilities are often present in the early school years, but may not fully manifest until specific academic demands exceed a child's cognitive capacity. Learning disability diagnoses are confirmed by standardized achievement and comprehensive clinical assessments such as the Woodcock-Johnson-3, an assessment comparing a child's achievement in several learning areas with the child's chronological age. (See Table 18.1 for a list of other commonly used academic assessments.)

TREATMENT OF SLD COEXISTING WITH ADHD

When ADHD and SLD are coexisting, appropriate use of stimulants to treat the ADHD behaviors often has a positive influence on achievement (Scheffler et al., 2009). However, remediation of learning disabilities is provided by educators, in and outside educational settings. P-PCPs working with families of children with coexisting ADHD and SLD must understand federal laws as they relate to children's ADHD and learning disabilities. The Individuals with Disabilities Education Act (IDEA; Federal Law 101-476 1990) established the basis for planning a child's learning through appropriate learning settings and learning accommodations and modifications. Parents may be aware that their child is not meeting grade-level benchmarks, regardless of ADHD treatment, but may not know the process for requesting academic services. Support begins at school with a Student Study/Success Team (SST) meeting where learning difficulties and gaps are identified. From this meeting, an informal plan to include supportive accommodations is written for school and home implementation. However, at this time, formalized assessments for an SLD might not be offered and learning problems can persist, regardless of ADHD treatment efficacy. Left unidentified, learning gaps can widen. Thus the next step for the family is a written request for a formal school district educational assessment. This request can be a tedious and intimidating process for parents due to the burdens of time and costs placed on the child's school and district. Often parents must be assertive to keep the process timely. If a child is identified with either an SLD or history of falling behind in learning by at least approximately 2 academic years, the child will qualify for an IEP. In an initial meeting, a formalized plan will address specific learning needs, goals, and appropriate modifications and accommodations to meet learning goals within the least restrictive environment. Section 504 of the Rehabilitation Act (1973) is a less structured but important supportive document of specifically identified learning accommodations when IEP qualifications are not met. The P-PCP can use knowledge about a child's identified learning disability to offer the family suggestions for learning accommodations as well as to better evaluate the effectiveness of prescribed ADHD medications.

Oppositional Defiant Disorder (ODD)

Children with ODD are noted to be in an angry, irritable mood; argumentative and defiant; and have a vindictive personality persisting for 6 months or more, directed toward at least one individual—not a sibling. It is not uncommon for this disorder to be identified only at home or with family. When pervasive beyond the home, symptoms and severity may significantly affect a child's academic and social functioning. ODD often begins in preschool as temper outbursts and becomes a healthcare issue when the child is repeatedly dismissed from child care or learning centers. Forty percent of children with ADHD will also express ODD behaviors (Lougy & Rosenthal, 2016).

DIAGNOSIS OF ODD COEXISTING WITH ADHD

The eight key oppositional characteristics are found within three categories. Category one is an angry, irritable mood with frequent loss of temper; "touchy" mood, easily annoyed; angry and resentful. This child may not see self as oppositional due to an underlying mood disorder such as anxiety or depression. The second category is argumentative and defiant. The child argues with persons of authority—known peers placed in positions of decision making, adults including parents and teachers—shows active defiance or refusal to comply with an authoritative figure; deliberately annoys others; places blame on others for personal mistakes or misbehaviors. The third category is vindictiveness and spite directed toward at least two persons. This behavior is further specified in frequency and intensity and exhibited outside the child's expected developmental age and stage. Children younger than age 5 will express characteristics daily. Children 5 years or older will express characteristics at least weekly. Persistence and severity expand when coexisting with ADHD when the ADHD symptoms are not adequately supported by medication and therapeutic behavioral interventions. Left untreated, opposition can lead to conduct disorder (CD; APA, 2013).

TREATMENT FOR ODD COEXISTING WITH ADHD

Medication intervention will require a combination of ADHD medication and those for modulating mood. Choosing medications can be challenging due to the overlap of ADHD impulsivity and mood dysregulation. Since opposition may be an expression of unidentified underlying anxiety and/or depression, a first-line medication added to stimulant medication might be a selective serotonin reuptake inhibitor (SSRI; see Chapter 3). Unfortunately, SSRIs can take up to 4 weeks to relieve the underlying anxiety or depression and presenting ODD behaviors. If the ODD behaviors are more impulsive, they may be more quickly reduced with the addition of an alpha-2-adrenergic agonist such as guanfacine or clonidine. The alpha-2-adrenergic action of clonidine can cause more sedation and hypotension than guanfacine. Both bond to alpha-2 receptors in the prefrontal cortex mediating ADHD behaviors also (Stahl, 2008). Oppositional behaviors that do not respond to this medication class may require stronger psychotropic medications such as nortriptyline, a tricyclic antidepressant, or an atypical antipsychotic such as risperidone and aripiprazole. In addition to monitoring the child's ADHD and ODD behaviors, a baseline ECG is suggested before using nortriptyline due to arrhythmia risk, which occurs more often when given in large doses. The atypical antipsychotics can cause unsatiated appetite and rapid weight gain. This side effect adds the need for metabolic risk monitoring of hemoglobin A1c and lipid profiles, and encouragement for healthy diet and exercise habits. Individual and group behavioral therapy will be important for the child to understand and learn age-appropriate social and interaction skills.

Conduct Disorder (CD)

CD is seen as repetitive and persistent patterns of behavior where a child violates major age-related societal norms and rules that impact the basic rights of others. The *DSM-5* places 15 clearly identified behaviors into four categories: aggression toward people and/or animals; destruction of property; deceitfulness and/or theft; and serious violation of rules. Although the *DSM-5* reports the occurrence of CD as 2% to 4%, the incidence of coexisting CD with ADHD has been reported as 11% (Lougy & Rosenthal, 2016).

DIAGNOSIS OF CD COEXISTING WITH ADHD

The child with CD will have exhibited at least one of the following behaviors within the past 6 months, and three of the 15 within the past 12 months. Toward others, the child frequently bullies, threatens, intimidates; initiates fights; has used a harmful weapon; is physically cruel; has confronted and stolen (robbed); or forced another into sexual acts. Property destruction is deliberate, including fire setting with intent to damage. Deceit and theft include breaking and entering homes and cars, stealing after entry, and lying to gain favor or avoid obligations. Designating CD in relation to rule violations is more age-dependent and before the teen years involves staying out overnight despite lack of parental consent; running away from home overnight twice or for an extended time period; and frequent truancy from school. Characteristically, the child with a coexisting CD is more often a young boy, physically aggressive toward others, exhibiting disturbed peer relationships. This child often has been previously diagnosed with ODD. The prognosis is poor with high risk of CD persisting into adulthood (Table 18.1 provides examples of ODD and CD screening tools).

TREATMENT FOR CD COEXISTING WITH ADHD

The child with coexisting ADHD and CD behaviors may have already been taking medications to manage ODD. If the SSRI, alpha-2-adrenergic, tricyclic, and atypical antipsychotic medications have not remediated negative CD behaviors, the choice of medications may be either mood stabilizers and/or anticonvulsants. Among these are lithium, valproic acid, carbamazepine, oxcarbazepine, and lamotrigine (see Chapter 3). Each of these carries a significant side-effect profile with potential long-term problems. Thus, in addition to laboratory monitoring for unwanted metabolic and end-organ effects, there are serum therapeutic ranges to guide peak behavioral response.

Generalized Anxiety Disorder

Childhood anxiety presents as persistent worry in multiple domains of performance. There is excessive worry or apprehension experienced more days than not, over 6 or more months, about a wide range of events or activities. The child cannot control the worry which intrudes on attention to daily tasks at hand. There are notable clinical signs of distress or inability to attend to academic and social functions. Anxiety coexisting with ADHD has been reported as 34% (Lougy & Rosenthal, 2016). March et al. (2000) studied the coexisting prevalence of anxiety and ADHD as both a predictor and outcome variable within the MTA study, establishing the foundation for diagnosing this coexisting condition and the need for further investigations. A study by Sciberras et al. (2014) reported that children with ADHD and two or more coexisting anxieties demonstrated poorer quality of life, daily functioning, and negative behaviors.

DIAGNOSIS OF GENERALIZED ANXIETY DISORDER COEXISTING WITH ADHD

A single behavior is all that is needed to diagnose childhood anxiety. Notable physiological expressions include: restlessness, irritability, muscle tension, feeling keyed up or on edge, difficulty concentrating or mind going blank, and becoming easily fatigued but finding it difficult to fall asleep or stay asleep (APA, 2013). The frequency, intensity, and duration of the behaviors seen are out of proportion to the actual importance of the child's intended performance or likelihood of it being unsuccessful. In the general population, girls are more affected with generalized anxiety disorders than boys (55%–60% females to 40%–45% males; APA, 2013).

There are a number of validated childhood anxiety screening tools (Table 18.1). The Childhood Behavioral Checklist (CBCL; Achenbach & Rescorla, 2001) is a parent-response checklist covering a broad base of childhood behaviors. A more specific anxiety screening tool is the parent and child (self-report) checklist, SCARED: Screen for Childhood Anxiety-Related Emotional Disorders (Birmaher et al., 1997). This 41-item child (items 1–20) and parent (items 21–41) checklist quantifies item scoring as 0–never or hardly; 1–somewhat or sometimes true; or 2–very or often true, over the past 3 months. A total of more than 25 indicates probable anxiety and need for further investigation. Additionally, questions are grouped to more specifically identify the relationship of anxiety to separation, social, school, or somatic.

TREATMENT OF GENERALIZED ANXIETY COEXISTING WITH ADHD

Adding SSRIs and psychotherapeutic intervention like cognitive behavioral therapy (CBT) to the management of children with ADHD may significantly lower the risk of the anxiety becoming more pervasive and pronounced (Walkup et al., 2008). Anxiety might lead to somatic, physiological distress such as irritable bowel disorder or recurrent headaches. Psychological compensatory behaviors may be adopted such as overly conforming, seeking perfection, or expressing unsureness through an overzealous need for approval and reassurance. Left untreated, frequency increases with thoughts of recurring precipitants, and duration becomes longer. CBT might take several months to reach desired effects. Eldar et al. (2012) researched a computer-based self-therapy to help children identify and reduce anxious behaviors. By shifting attention from threatening images, anxiety symptoms decreased while subjects practiced sustaining attention.

Persistent Depressive Disorder–Dysthymia

A diagnosis of persistent depressive disorder–dysthymia is not currently included in the literature as coexisting with ADHD (APA, 2013); however, this diagnosis should be considered when a child with or without a diagnosis of ADHD is not meeting criteria for diagnosis of another depressive diagnosis. Dysthymia is noted in children age 2 or older, expressing a depressed mood most of the day more days than not, for a period longer than a year (APA, 2013). Note that irritability may be the mode of expressing the depression.

DIAGNOSIS OF PERSISTENT DEPRESSIVE DISORDER–DYSTHYMIA COEXISTING WITH ADHD

A child or adolescent must present with at least two of the following behaviors: poor or absent appetite; insomnia or hypersomnia; low energy and fatigue; low self-esteem; poor concentration or decision making; and feelings of hopelessness. By history, major depressive disorder (MDD) behaviors may have been expressed previously or coexisting for more than 2 years. However, a manic or hypomanic episode or cyclothymia has never been noted. Onset may be insidious, thus not fully recognized, and may be persistent in 0.5% of diagnoses (APA, 2013).

TREATMENT OF PERSISTENT DEPRESSIVE DISORDER–DYSTHYMIA COEXISTING WITH ADHD

As with all mood disorders, a first line of treatment may include behavioral therapy. However, as this diagnosis is persistent by nature, early start of an SSRI could benefit potential long-term behavior (Emslie et al., 2004).

Disruptive Mood Dysregulation Disorder (DMDD)

DMDD presents as severe and recurring verbal and/or behavioral temper outbursts inconsistent with developmental level and grossly out of proportion in intensity and duration relative to the situation or provocation. Outbursts occur at least thrice weekly; manifest in at least two settings and are generally more severe in one setting; and have been present for at least 12 months, without a calm period of greater than 3 months. Mood between outbursts is perceived by others to be persistently irritable or angry most of the day, nearly every day. When coexisting with ADHD, DMDD's childhood prevalence is 2% to 5% (Lougy & Rosenthal, 2016).

DIAGNOSIS OF DMDD COEXISTING WITH ADHD

A DMDD is defined by onset, not earlier than age 6 and not later than age 18 (APA, 2013). Boys are more frequently identified than girls, during school-age years more than adolescence. By history and observations, onset is most prevalent within ages 6 to 10 years. When diagnostic criteria is not met, behaviors might better be explained by autism and the spectrum disorders, posttraumatic stress, separation anxiety, and persistent depressive disorder or dysthymia. DMDD can coexist with ADHD, MDD (major depressive disorder), CD, and substance use disorder, but cannot coexist with ODD, intermittent explosive disorder, or bipolar disorder diagnoses (APA, 2013). Thus, when considering a diagnosis of DMDD, it is relevant to carefully select which disorder will best meet treatment objectives. It is important to note that bipolar disorder, which can be overdiagnosed, has less than 1% prevalence before adolescence and is episodic in its presentation.

TREATMENT OF DMDD COEXISTING WITH ADHD

Medication intervention in coordination with ADHD medications easily includes atypical antipsychotics, for example, risperidone and aripiprazole (see Chapter 3). Because the child's underlying mood is perceived by others to be persistently irritable or angry, taking ADHD medication holidays may cause a neurochemical imbalance when stimulants are not present. School- and/or community-based child and family behavioral support should be considered. The goal is to develop consistent limits that include appropriate rewards and consequences. Contacting the child's school district regarding eligibility for an IEP based on emotional disability and the daily support of a one-on-one aide, in addition to local regional center eligibility for applied behavioral analysis (ABA) services in the home, is not the responsibility of the P-PCP, but is certainly a direction to suggest the family to explore.

Intermittent Explosive Disorder

Typically, intermittent explosive disorder presents as recurrent verbal or physical outbursts resulting from failure to control aggressive impulses. The magnitude of the outburst is grossly out of proportion to the provocation or any precipitating psychosocial stressors. Outbursts are not premeditated and do not occur for the purpose of receiving tangible objects. Most often, children are 6 years or older by chronological or developmental age. Occurrence is two to three times weekly over a 3-month period resulting in no property damage or injury to people or animals, or three recurrences within 12 months involving property damage or destruction and/or injury to persons or animals. When the occurrences are less frequent, but more injurious or destructive, the disorder can lead to marked personal distress and impaired interpersonal or occupational functioning, and potentially end in legal or financial consequences (APA, 2013).

DIAGNOSIS OF INTERMITTENT EXPLOSIVE DISORDER COEXISTING WITH ADHD

Explosive outbursts have a rapid onset, typically without warning and last less than 30 minutes. They are initiated by a minor provocation from a closely associated person. When first incidence is in later childhood or early adolescence, outbursts often persist. Prevalence is 2.7%. The diagnosis can be made along with ADHD, autism, ODD, or CD (APA, 2013).

TREATMENT OF INTERMITTENT EXPLOSIVE DISORDER COEXISTING WITH ADHD

Similar to other diagnoses bearing oppositional mood and behaviors, it may be necessary to cautiously add atypical antipsychotics to ADHD medications. Treatment-resistant behaviors may require use of anticonvulsants.

Additional Disorders Coexisting With ADHD

Anxiety, obsessive-compulsive disorder (OCD), tic disorders and Tourette's syndrome, MDDs, and autistic spectrum disorders (ASD) may also coexist in a child or adolescent with a diagnosis of ADHD. Refer to Chapter 14 for autism and global developmental delays; Chapter 15 for case studies for challenging behaviors in children with ADHD and ASD; and Chapter 25 for specific detail of selected neurological disorders (see Table 18.1 for examples of screening tools for these disorders, and Table 18.2 for their frequency when coexisting with ADHD).

■ SUMMARY

The AAP's clinical practice guidelines provide for ADHD diagnosis as early as 4 years old (AAP, 2011a). It has been reported that between 29% and 70% of children and adolescents diagnosed with ADHD will have at least one coexisting behavioral diagnosis to complicate the ADHD diagnosis and treatment, as well as that of the coexisting condition (Albert et al., 2017; Banaschewski et al., 2017). It is imperative that P-PCPs carefully identify behaviors suggestive of ADHD and coexisting disorders in an effort to assist parents with first-line behavioral and learning strategies at home and at day care or school settings (AAP, 2011b). Early behavioral intervention may assist young children to learn self-management of actions before they might escalate to levels disrupting the child's learning, peer interactions, and family life. When behavioral strategies are not effective or learning is compromised, stimulant medication becomes the gold standard of ADHD therapy, with the adjunct of behavioral therapy and/or disorder-targeted medications to mediate hyperactivity, mood, or negative outcomes. The child or adolescent with coexisting ADHD requires a team approach led by the P-PCP to include other medical and behavioral consultants, members from the child's school to identify and diagnose coexisting disorders, and to establish an evidence-based, family-centered treatment plan.

■ REFERENCES

Achenbach, T. M., & Rescorla, L. A. (2001). *Manual for ASEBA school age forms and profiles*. Burlington, VT: University of Vermont Research Center for Children, Youth and Families.

Albert, M., Rui, P., & Ashman, J. J. (2017). Physician office visits for attention-deficit/hyperactivity disorder in children and adolescents aged 4-17 years: United States 2012–2013. *NCHS Data Brief, 269*, 1–7.

American Academy of Pediatrics. (2000). Clinical practice guidelines: Diagnosis and evaluation of the child with attention-deficit/hyperactivity disorder. *Pediatrics, 106*, 1158–1170. doi:10.1542/peds.105.5.1158

American Academy of Pediatrics. (2001). Clinical practice guidelines: Treatment of the school-aged child with attention-deficit/hyperactivity disorder. *Pediatrics, 108*, 1033–1044. doi:10.1542/peds.108.4.1033

American Academy of Pediatrics. (2011a). ADHD: Clinical practice guideline for the diagnosis, evaluation, and treatment of attention–deficit/hyperactivity disorder in children and adolescents. *Pediatrics, 128*, 1007–1022. doi:10.1542/peds.2011-2654

American Academy of Pediatrics. (2011b). Supplemental Information: Implementing the Key Action Statements: An algorithm and explanation for process of care for the evaluation, diagnosis, treatment and monitoring of ADHD in children and adolescents. *Pediatrics, 128*(Suppl. 5), S11–S121. Elk Grove Village, IL: American Academy of Pediatrics.

American Psychiatric Association. (1980). *Diagnostic and statistical manual of mental health disorders* (3rd ed.). Washington, DC: Author.

American Psychiatric Association. (1994). *Diagnostic and statistical manual of mental health disorders* (4th ed.). Washington, DC: Author.

American Psychiatric Association. (2013). *Diagnostic and statistical manual of mental health disorders* (5th ed.). Retrieved from doi:10.1176/appi.books.9780890425596

Banaschewski, T., Becker, K., Dopfner, M., Holtmann, M., Rosler, M., & Romanos, M. (2017). Attentiondeficit/hyperactivity disorder: A current overview. *Deutsches Arztablatt International, 114*, 149–159. doi:10.3238/arztebl.2017.0149

Beck, A. T., Steer, R. A., Ball, R., Ciervo, C. A., & Kabat, M. (1997). Use of the Beck anxiety and Beck depression inventories in primary care with medical outpatients. *Assessment, 4*, 211–219. doi:10.1177/107319119700400301

Beck, J. S., Beck, A. T., Jolly, J. B., & Steer, R. A. (2005). *Beck youth inventory for children and adolescents* (2nd ed.). San Antonio, TX: Psychological Corporation.

Beery, K. E., Buktenica, N. A., & Beery, N. A. (2010). *Developmental test of visual-motor integration* (6th ed.). Bloomington, MN: Pearson Education.

Biederman, J., Newcorn, J., & Sprich, S. (1991). Comorbidity of attention deficit hyperactivity disorder with conduct, depression, anxiety and other disorders. *American Journal of Psychiatry, 148*, 564–577. doi:10.1176/ajp.148.5.564

Birmaher, B., Khetarpal, S., Brent, D., Cully, M., Balach, L., Kaufman, J., & McKenzie Neer, S. (1997). Screen for child anxiety related emotional disorders (SCARED): Scale construction and psychometric characteristics. *Journal of the American Academy of Child and Adolescent Psychiatry, 36*, 369–385. doi:10.1097/00004583-199704000-00018

Bradley, C. (1937). The behavior of children receiving benzedrine. *American Journal of Psychiatry, 94*, 577–585. doi:10.1176/ajp.94.3.577

Brown, T. E. (2005). *Attention deficit disorder: The unfocused mind in children and adults*. New Haven, CT: Yale University Press.

Brunsvold, G. L., Oepen, G., Federman, E. J., & Akins, R. (2008) Comorbid depression and ADHD in children and adolescents. Psychiatric Times, 1-8.

Bussey, R., Fernandez, M., Harwood, M., Wei Hou, Garvan, C. W., Eyberg, S. M., & Swanson, J. M. (2008). Parent and teacher SNAP-IV ratings of attention deficit hyperactivity disorder symptoms and psychometric properties and normative ratings from a school district sample. *Assessment, 15*, 317–328. doi:10.1177/1073191107313888

Carini, R. J., & Parks, T. W. (1993). ADD-H comprehensive teacher's rating scale. *Journal of Psychoeducational Assessment, 11*, 95–97. doi:10.1177/073428299301100114

Conners, C. K. (n.d). CPT 3, Conners Continuous Performance Test (3rd ed.). Retrieved from https://web.teaediciones.com/CPT-3--Conners-Continuous-Performance-Test-3rd-Edition.aspx

Conners, C. K. (2002). Forty years of methylphenidate treatment in attention-deficit/hyperactivity disorder. *Journal of Attention Disorders, 6*(S1):S17–S30. doi:10.1177/070674370200601S04

Conners, C. K., Sitarenios, G., Parker, J. D., & Epstein, J. (1998). The revised Conners' parent rating scales (CPRS-R): Factor, structure, reliability and critical validity. *Journal of Abnormal Child Psychiatry*, 26, 257–268. doi:10.1023/A:1022602400621

Czamara, D., Tiesler, C. M. T., Kohlbock, G., Berdel, O., Hoffmann, B., Bauer, C. P., . . . Heinrich, J. (2013). Children with attention deficit hyperactivity disorder symptoms have a higher risk for reading, spelling, and math difficulty in the GINIplus and LISAplus cohort studies. *PLOS ONE*, 8, 1–7. doi:10.1371/journal.pone.0063859

DuPaul, G. G., Power, T. J., Anastopoulos, A. D., & Reid, R. (1998). *ADHD rating scale-IV: Checklists, norms and clinical interpretations.* New York, NY: Guilford Press.

Efron, D., Jarman, F., & Barker, M. (1997). Side effects of methylphenidate and dexedrine in children with attention deficit hyperactive disorder: A double-blind crossover trial. *Pediatrics*, 100, 662–666. doi:10.1542/peds.100.4.662

Eldar, S., Apter, A., Lotan, D., Perez-Edgar, K., Naim, R., Fox, N. A., Pine, D. S., & Bar-Haim, Y. (2012). Computer-based treatment eases anxiety symptoms in children. *American Journal of Psychiatry*, 169, 213–230. doi:10.1176/appi.ajp.2011.11060886

Emslie, G. J., Hughes, C. W., Crismon, M. L., Lopez, M., Pliszka, S., Toprac, M. G., & Boemer, C. (2004). A feasibility study of the childhood depression medication algorithm: The Texas children's medication algorithm project (CMAP). *Journal of the American Academy of Child and Adolescent Psychiatry*, 43, 519–527. doi:10.1097/00004583-200405000-00005

Faraone, S., Sergeant, J., Gillberg, C., & Biederman, J. (2003). Worldwide prevalence of ADHD: Is it an American condition? *World Psychiatry*, 2, 104–113. doi:10-1176/ajp.2007.164.6.942

Gallant, S. (2008). Conners 3: Psychometric properties and practical applications. National Association of School Psychologists, February, New Orleans, LA.

Gelade, K., Bink, M., Janssen, T. W. P., Van Mourik, R., Maras, A., & Oosterlaan, J. (2016). An RCT into the effects of neurofeedback on neurocognitive function compared to stimulant and physical activity in children with ADHD. *European Child and Adolescent Psychiatry*, 26, 457–468. doi:10.1007/s00787-016-0902-x

Gilliam, J. E. (2002). *Conduct disorder scale.* Austin, TX: PRO-Education.

Gioia, G. A., Isquith, P. K., Guy, S. C., & Kenworthy, L. (2017). Behavior rating inventory of executive function, Second Edition Gerard A. Gioia, Peter K. Isquith, Steven C. Guy, and Lauren Kenworthy. *Journal of Pediatric Neuropsychology*, 3, 227–231. doi:10.1007/s40817-017-0044-1

Goodman, A., & Goodman, R. (2009). Strengths and differences as a dimensional measure of child mental health. *Journal of the American Academy of Child and Adolescent Psychiatry*, 48(4), 400–403. doi:10.1097/CHI.0b013e3181985068

Greenhill, L., Kollins, S., Abikoff, H., McCracken, J., Riddle, M., & Swanson, J. (2006). Efficacy and safety of immediate-release methylphenidate treatment for preschoolers with ADHD. *Journal of the American Academy of Child and Adolescent Psychiatry*, 45, 1284–1293. doi:10.1097/01.chi.0000235077.32661.61

Greenhill, L. I., Pliszka, S., Dulcan, M. K., & the Work Group on Quality Issues. (2002). Practice parameter for the use of stimulant medications in the treatment of children, adolescents and adults. *Journal of the American Academy of Child and Adolescent Psychiatry*, 41, (S2), 26S–49S. doi:10.1097/00004583-200202001-00003

Hoffman, H. (1848). *The Story of Fidgety Philip*. Der Struwwelpeter. Philadelphia: J.C. Winston & Co.

Jellinek, M. S., Murphy, J. M., Little, M., Pagano, M. E., Comer, D. M., & Kelleher, K. J. (1999). Use of the pediatric symptom checklist to screen for psychosocial problems in pediatrics. *Archives of Pediatric and Adolescent Medicine*, 153, 254–260. doi:10.1001/archpedi-153.3.254

Jensen, P. S., Hinshaw, S. P., Swanson, J. M, Greenhill, L. L., Conners, C. K., Arnold, L. E., . . . Wigal, T. (2001). Findings from the NIMH multimodal treatment study of ADHD (MTA): Implications and applications for primary care providers. *Journal of Developmental and Behavioral Pediatrics*, 22, 60–73. doi:10.1097/00004703-200102000-00008

Johnson, J. G., Harris, E. S., Pitzer, R. L., & Williams, J. B. (2002). The patient health questionnaire for adolescents: Validation of an instrument for the assessment of mental disorders among adolescent primary care patients. *Journal of Adolescent Health*, 30, 196–204. doi:10.1016/S1054-139X(01)00333-0

Jordan, B. T. (2011). *Jordan left-right reversal test – 3.* Novato, CA: Academic Therapy Publications.

Kaufman, A. S., & Kaufman, N. L. (2014). *Kaufman test of educational achievement* (3rd ed.). Retrieved from https://www.pearsonclinical.com/education/products/100000777/kaufman-test-of-educational-achievement-third-edition-ktea-3.html

Kavale, K. (1982). The efficacy of stimulant drug treatment for hyperactivity: A meta-analysis. *Journal of Learning Disabilities*, 15, 280–289. doi:10.1177/002221948201500508

Kovacs, M. (2010). *CDI-2: Children's Depression Inventory* (2nd ed.). Bloomington, MN: Pearson Clinical.

LeBlanc, J. C., Almudevar, A., Brooks, S. J., & Kutcher, S. (2002). Screening for adolescent depression: Comparison of the Kutcher adolescent depression screen with the beck depression inventory. *Journal of Child and Adolescent Psychopharmacology, 12*, 113–126. doi:10.1089/104454602760219153

Lord, C., Rutter, M., Di Lavore, P. C., Risi, S., Gotham, K., & Bishop, S. L. (2012). Inform diagnosis, treatment planning, and educational placement with an observational assessment of autistic spectrum disorder. *Autism diagnostic evaluation schedule (ADOS™-2)*. Retrieved from Multi-Health Systems, Inc.; https://www.mhs.com/MHS-Assessment?prodname=ados2

Lougy, R. A., & Rosenthal, D. K. (2016) Co-existing conditions commonly found with ADHD. *2016 Annual CHADD international conference* (11-11-16). Costa Mesa, CA.

March, J. S., Swanson, J. M., Arnold, L. E., Hoza, B., Conners, C. K., Hinshaw, S. P., . . . Pelham, W. C. (2000). Anxiety as a predictor and outcome variable in the multimodal treatment study of children with ADHD (MTA). *Journal of Abnormal Child Psychology, 28*, 527–541. doi:10.1023/A:1005179014321

Martin, N. A. (2017). *TPVS-4: Test of visual-perceptual skills* (4th ed.). Novato, CA: Academic Therapy Publications.

Mattingly, G. W., & Anderson, R. H. (2016). Optimizing outcomes in ADHD Treatment: From clinical targets to novel delivery systems. *CNS Spectrums, 21*, 48–58. doi:10.1017/S1092852916000808

Mohammadi, M. R, Soleimani, A., Ahmadi, N., & Davoodi, E. (2016). A comparison of effectiveness of parent behavior management training and methylphenidate on reduction of symptoms of attention deficit hyperactivity disorder. *ACTA Medica Iranica, 54*, 503–509.

Murray, D. W., Bussing, R., Fernandez, M., Hou, W., Garvan, C. W., Swanson, J. M., & Eyberg, S. M. (2009). Psychometric properties of teacher SKAMP ratings from a community sample. *Assessment, 16*, 193–208. doi:10.1177/1073191108326924

Murphy, J. M., Bergmann, P., Chiang, C., Sturner, R., Howard, B., Abel, M. R., . . . Jellinek, M. (2016). The PSC-17: Subscale scores, reliability and factor structure in a new national sample. *Pediatrics, 138*, 1–8. doi:10.1542/peds.2016-0038

Nasser Ghaemi, S., Miller, C. J., Berv, D. A., Klugman, J., Rosenquist, K. J., & Pies, R. W. (2005). Sensitivity and specificity of a new bipolar spectrum disorder scale. *Journal of Affective Disorders, 84*, 273–277. doi:10.1016/s0165-0327(03)00196-4

Owens, J. A., Spirito, A., & McGuinn, M. (2000). The child sleep habits questionnaire (CSHQ): Psychometric properties of a survey instrument for school-aged children. *Sleep, 23*, 1–9. doi:10.1093/sleep/23.8.1d

Plizska, S., & the Work Group on Quality Issues. (2007). Practice parameters for the assessment and treatment of children and adolescents with attention-deficit/hyperactivity disorder. *Journal of the Academy of Child and Adolescent Psychiatry, 46*, 894–921. doi:10.1097/chi.0b013e318054e724

Reynolds, W. M. (1998). *Adolescent mental health questionnaire*. Lutz, FL: PAR.

Riddle, M. A., Yershova, K., Lazzaretto, D., Paykina, N., Yenokyan, G., Greenhill, L., . . . Posner, K. (2013). Preschool ADHD treatment study (PATS) 6-year follow-up. *Journal of the American Academy of Child and Adolescent Psychiatry, 52*, 264–278. doi:10.1016/j.jaac.2012.12.007

Robins, D., Fein, D., & Barton, M. (2009). *Modified checklist for autism in toddlers–Revised/follow-up* (M-CHAT-R/F). Retrieved from www.mchat.com

Rutter, M., Bailey, A., & Lord, C. (2003). *The social communications questionnaire*. Los Angeles, CA: Western Psychological Systems.

Scheffler, R. M., Brown, T. T., Fulton, B. D., Hinshaw, S. P., Levine, P., & Stone, S. (2009). Positive association between attention deficit/hyperactivity disorder medication use and academic achievement during elementary school. *Pediatrics, 123*, 1273–1279. doi:10.1542/peds.2008-1597

Schopler, E., Van Bourgondien, M. E., Wellman, J., & Love, S. R. (2010). *Childhood autism rating scales* (2nd ed.). Los Angeles, CA: Western Psychological Services.

Sciberras, E., Lycett, K., Effron, D., Mensah, F., Gerner, B., & Hiscock, H. (2014) Anxiety in children with attention deficit/hyperactivity disorder. *Pediatrics, 133*, 801–808. doi:10.1542/peds.2013-3686

Shaffer, D., Gould, M. S., Brasic, J., Ambrosini, P., Fisher, P., Bird, H., & Aluwahlia, S. (1983). The children's global assessment scale (CGAS). *Archives of General Psychiatry, 40*, 128–1231. doi:10.1001/archpsyc.1983.01790100074010

Shrank, F. A., Mather, N., & McGrew, K. S. (2016) *Woodcock-Johnson tests of cognitive abilities* (4th ed.). Rolling Hills, IL: Riverside Publishing.

Silva, R. R., Alport, M., Pouget, E., Silva, V., Trosper, R., Reyes, K. & Dummit, S. (2005). A rating scale for disruptive behavior disorders, based on the DSM-IV item pool. *Psychiatric Quarterly, 76*, 327–339. doi:10.1007/s11126-005-4966

Silverman, W. K., & Hinshaw, S. P. (2008). The second special issue on evidence-based psychosocial treatments for children and adolescents: A ten-year update. *Journal of Clinical Child and Adolescent Psychology, 37*, 2–7. doi:10.1080/15374410701817725

Squires, J., Bricker, D. D., & Twombly, E. (2009). *Ages & stages questionnaires: A parent-completed child monitoring system.* Baltimore, MD: Paul H. Brooks.

Stahl, S. M. (2008). *Essential psychopharmacology: Neuroscientific basis and practical approaches* (3rd ed.). New York, NY: Cambridge University Press.

Still, G. F. (1902). Some abnormal psychical conditions in children. *Lancet, 1*, 1008–1012.

Storch, E. A., Larson, M. J., Goodman, W. K., Ras, S. A., Price, L. H., & Murphy, T. H. (2010). Development and psychometric evaluation of the Yale-Brown obsessive-compulsive scale–2nd ed. *Psychological Assessment, 22*, 223–232. doi:10.1037/a0018492

Swanson, J. M., McBurnett, K., Wigal, T., Pfiffner, L. J., Lerner, M. A., Williams, L., . . . Fisher, T. D. (1993). Effects of stimulant medication on children with attention-deficit disorder—A review of reviews. *Exceptional Children, 60*, 154–162. doi:10.1177/001440299306000209

Swanson, J. M., Schuck, S., Mann Porter, M., Carlson, C., Hartman, C. A., Sergeant, J. A., . . . Wigal, T. (2012). Categorical and dimensional definitions and evaluation of symptoms of ADHD: History of the SNAP and SWAN rating scales. *International Journal of Educational Psychology Assessment, 10*, 51–70.

Varni, J. M., Seid, M., & Kurtin, P. S. (2001). Ped QL 4.0: Reliability and validity of the Pediatric Quality of Life Inventory version 4.0 generic core scales in healthy and patient populations. *Medical Care, 39*, 800–812. doi:10.1097/00005650-2001080000-00006

Walkup, J. T., Albano, A. M., Piacentini, J., Birmaher, B., Compton, S. N., Sherrill, J. T., . . . Kendall, P. C. (2008). Cognitive-behavioral therapy, sertraline or a combination in childhood anxiety. *New England Journal of Medicine, 359*, 2753–2766. doi:10.1056/NEJMoa0804633

Wang, Y. F., Huang, F., Sun, L., Qian, Y., Liu, L., Ma, Q.-G., . . . Qian, Q.-J. (2016). Cognitive function of children and adolescents with attention deficit hyperactivity disorder and learning difficulties: A developmental perspective. *Chinese Medical Journal, 129*, 1922–1928. doi:10.4103/0366-6999.187861

Wechsler, D. (2009). *Wechsler individual achievement test* (3rd ed.). Bloomington, MN: Pearson Clinical.

Wechsler, D. (2014). *Wechsler intelligence scales for children* (5th ed.). Bloomington, MN: Pearson Clinical.

Wilkenson, G. S., & Robertson, G. J. (2017) *Wide range achievement test* (4th ed.). Bloomington, MN: Pearson Clinical.

Wolraich, M. L., Lambert, W., Doffling, M. A., Bickman, L., Simmons, T, & Worley, K. (2003). Psychometric properties of the Vanderbilt ADHD diagnostic parent rating scale in a referred population. *Journal of Pediatric Psychiatry, 28*, 559–568. doi:10.1093/jpepsy/jsg046

Woodcock, R. W., Schrank, F. A., Mather, N., & McGrew, K.S. (2007). *Woodcock-Johnson III Tests of Achievement, Form C/Brief Battery.* Rolling Meadows, IL: Riverside.

Zuvekas, S. H., & Vitiello, B. (2012). Stimulant medication use in children: A 12-year perspective. *American Journal of Psychiatry, 169*, 160–166. doi:10.1176/appi.ajp.2011.11030387

CHAPTER 19

Onychophagia: A Case Study of Body-Focused Repetitive Behavior

ELIZABETH MANDEL, YINI KONG, AND ISABEL GONZALEZ

CASE PRESENTATION

A 7-year-old male presents to the pediatric primary care office with his mother for his annual well-child visit. The mother is concerned with his constant nail biting. She reports that "most of his nails are gone" and she is worried about a possible infection.

Chief Complaint: 7-year-old male with constant nail biting. Mother reports, "Most of his nails are gone!"

■ HISTORY OF PRESENT ILLNESS

The mother describes her son as "an anxious child." He is an active participant in sports, has many friends, has a stable family life, and is currently on summer vacation. The mother reports that they have a planned vacation, and the child is not able to sleep through the night because he is so worried about flying. His nail biting seems to increase during times of stress.

■ RELEVANT HISTORY

Social History

The child is on summer vacation from school and his mother reports that he had a good academic year. The child reports feeling safe at home and school. He also reports that sometimes his stomach feels funny before soccer games or even before vacations. He is active, participating in swimming lessons, soccer, and piano lessons. The child reports that he enjoys all these activities and that his favorite thing to do in the summer is play with his siblings and friends.

Sleep Patterns

The child reports sleeping about 8 to 9 hours a night which the mother confirms but also reports that he occasionally wakes up from a "scary dream" and has a difficult time returning to sleep. The mother further reports that the majority of nights he sleeps without disturbance.

■ SCREENING TOOLS

The Screen for Child Anxiety Related Disorders (SCARED) was used to assess this child for anxiety (Birmaher, 1999). The purpose of the tool is to screen children for anxiety disorders including generalized anxiety disorders, panic/somatic, school phobia, and separation anxiety. SCARED contains a 41-item parent questionnaire as well as a child questionnaire. The child's screen was negative for anxiety disorder (www.midss.org/content/screen-child-anxiety-related-disorders-scared).

■ REVIEW OF SYSTEMS

General: The child says he feels well. The mother denies concerns aside from nail biting.
Head: Denies headache, pain, or trauma. Denies any history of sinus infection.
Respiratory: Denies increased dyspnea shortness of breath (SOB) or wheezing.
Cardiovascular: Denies syncope, palpitation. Denies cardiac history of murmurs. Denies chest pain or other referred pain. Is able to keep up with his peers.
Abdomen: Denies nausea, vomiting, diarrhea, and constipation or abdominal pain.
Skin: Denies rashes, lesions, or bruising. Mother reports nails are very short from constant biting.

■ PHYSICAL EXAMINATION

Skin

Nails measure approximately 1 cm from the cuticle to the upper portion of the nail. No bleeding or exudate.

■ DIFFERENTIAL DIAGNOSES

The differential diagnosis to consider for this case presentation include the following: onychophagia, nail lichen planus, nail psoriasis, onychotillomania, nail-patella syndrome, chronic paronychia.

Additional differential diagnoses to consider are generalized anxiety disorder and obsessive-compulsive disorder (OCD), both of which are discussed in Chapter 25; thus, only nail biting is discussed in this case.

■ DISCUSSION OF ONYCHOPHAGIA

Description

Onychophagia, more commonly known as nail biting, is a chronic behavior usually beginning in childhood or early adulthood. It is characterized by the act of placing the nail into the mouth thus creating contact between the fingernail and one or more teeth (Siddiqui, Qureshi, Marei, & Mahfouz, 2017). In the clinical setting, onychophagia may be the chief complaint; however, it is more commonly noted as an incidental finding. If there is mild nail biting, it may not be bothersome to the individual; yet if it is severe the behavior may lead to several negative sequelae (Halteh, Scher, & Lipner, 2017). Along with hair-pulling and skin picking, nail biting is classified as a body-focused repetitive behavior (BFRB), which children often find satisfying (Singal & Daulatabad, 2017).

Incidence

Nail biting is rarely seen in children younger than 3 years old. The incidence of nail biting peaks in childhood and adolescence, followed by a decrease through adulthood (Tanaka, Vitral, Tanaka, Guerrero, & Camargo, 2008). Pacan, Grzesiak, Reich, Kantorska-Janiec, and Szepietowski (2014) studied onychophagia and reported that the majority (86.2%) of participants with onychophagia had an onset before the age of 13, and only 13.8% had a later onset. A review of the literature on the incidence of nail biting reveals that 23% of preschoolers bite their nails, 20% to 33% of children ages 7 to 10 engage in the activity, which increases to 45% during adolescence followed by a steadily decline with age, approaching 10% in adulthood (Foster, 1998; Ghanizadeh & Shekoohi, 2011; Massler & Malone, 1950; Wechsler, 1931). More recently, Pacan et al. (2014) found a 47.2% lifetime prevalence of onychophagia among their study participants. However, one must realize that the prevalence may be under-recognized due to a wide variety in clinical course as well as feelings of shame and embarrassment that prevent seeking care (Pacan et al., 2014; Siddiqui et al., 2017).

Etiology

A long-standing belief concerning nail biting is that it occurs while a person is stressed or anxious in the attempt to relieve tension. It has also been theorized to be an impulse control disorder, hence the reason that onychophagia is grouped under the BFRB subgroup of obsessive-compulsive-related disorders (Siddiqui et al., 2017; Singal & Daulatabad, 2017). Yet the association of onychophagia with anxiety and OCD is controversial. Some studies highlight a higher lifetime prevalence of these disorders among nail biters as compared to non–nail biters, while other research shows no difference in the prevalence of these conditions (Halteh et al., 2017).

Selles et al. (2015) state that internalizing behaviors, including anxiety and poor adaptive skills, are higher in those youth who bite their nails. Kessler et al. (2005) found the lifetime prevalence of anxiety disorders was 24.2% and Bienvenu et al. (2000) found a higher prevalence of nail biting among subjects with OCD in comparison with control subjects.

Yet Williams, Rose, and Chisholm (2006) found that college students often bite their nails while bored or frustrated. Children tend to bite their nails more often when alone or watching television as compared to nail biting while engaging in other activities (Woods & Miltenberger, 1996). Similarly, Pacan et al. (2014) also found that for the majority of subjects (92.2%), nail biting is an automatic behavior that they perform during other activities, such as reading or watching TV. Pacan et al. (2014) also found that for others nail biting is an intentional activity. These individuals usually give up other kind of activities in order to bite their nails. These may include those who have the desire for perfect nails, and yet for others it may serve as a form of self-stimulation while they are bored or inactive. Interestingly, the precipitating factors for onychophagia differ in the male and female populations. Pacan et al. (2014) studied 339 medical students, both males and females, to determine the prevalence, the clinical picture of nail biting, and the comorbidities. Onychophagia was present in 46.9% of the study participants. Of these individuals, 92.2% reported nail biting as an automatic behavior. Among female subjects, intentional nail biting occurred only occasionally. In contrast, for more than half of males, nail biting was an intentional activity while they were not engaging in other forms of activity. More than 40% of females stated that they had always bitten their nails automatically without thinking about it, compared to less than 10% of males (Pacan et al., 2014).

Ghanizadeh (2008) found that comorbid psychiatric conditions were present in more than two thirds of youth who nail bite. The highest incident rates were for attention deficit hyperactivity disorder (ADHD), oppositional defiant disorder, and separation anxiety disorder. In addition, in 65% of youth who bite their nails, at least one other stereotypical behavior was present, including lip biting and head banging (Ghanizadeh, 2008). Despite the common belief that anxiety disorders or OCD contribute to nail biting, Ghanizadeh (2008) found that only 11% of youth who bite their nails were diagnosed with OCD, and separation anxiety disorder was the only anxiety disorder identified. Interestingly for roughly half the children who NB, either the mother or father were suffering from at least one psychiatric disorder, most commonly major depressive disorder (Ghanizadeh, 2008). Even though Pacan et al. (2014) found that tension before nail biting was reported by 65.7% of nail biters and feelings of pleasure after nail biting in 42% among their participants with lifetime onychophagia, the prevalence of anxiety disorders and OCD was nearly identical between those participants who did bite their nails and the control group who did not bite their nails. Therefore, Pacan et al. (2014) concluded that there was no correlation between nail biting and other anxiety disorders or OCD, but rather multiple factors were involved (Pacan et al., 2014).

There may even be a genetic component related to nail biting. The prevalence rates for children whose parents NB is almost three times greater than for children whose parents did not bite their nails (Bakwin, 1971). Although modeling could be an influence, many parents no longer engage in nail biting, which suggests that genetics may play a role (Ellington, 2017). This is supported by a survey of 743 parents of primary school students assessing rates of nail biting in their children and themselves, showing that 36.8% of nail biters had at least one family member with the habit (Ghanizadeh & Shekoohi, 2011). Additionally, twin studies show a higher concordance rate in the monozygotic group as compared to the dizygotic group (Bakwin, 1971; Ooki, 2005).

■ CLINICAL MANIFESTATIONS

The act of NB typically involves all the fingernails equally, with the toenails rarely being involved (Halteh et al., 2017). Interestingly, the biter typically bites the nail off and throws it out instead of swallowing it (Singal & Daulatabad, 2017). In mild and moderate cases, patients present with significantly short, ragged, uneven nails (Singal & Daulatabad, 2017). Hangnails, damaged nail folds which may be in various stages of healing, and splinter hemorrhages are also commonly seen. Additionally, the cuticles may be absent or ragged (Halteh et al., 2017; Singal & Daulatabad, 2017). In severe situations, the complete nail may be absent (Singal & Daulatabad, 2017). Frequent nail biters are prone to secondary skin infection of the nail folds known as paronychia, or dental and orthodontic complications, which are discussed in the "Complications" section in this chapter. It is also important to note that there are often periods of remission and exacerbation, which may mirror times of stress (Singal & Daulatabad, 2017).

■ DIAGNOSIS

The diagnosis of onychophagia is typically straightforward, especially when the patient offers it as a chief complaint, bites the nails in the exam room, or is honest when questioned regarding exam findings. However, due to shame and stigmatism, many may not admit to biting their nails.

Onychophagia is classified in the *Diagnostic and Statistical Manual of Mental Disorders* (fifth edition; *DSM-5*) under the subcategory of "Other Specified Obsessive-Compulsive and Related Disorders," specifically as a BFRB, which also includes lip biting and cheek chewing. To meet the criteria for this diagnosis, the patient must also repeatedly attempt to suppress or halt the activity, and it must have negative effects on their social and occupational life (American Psychiatric Association [APA], 2013).

Nail biopsy is rarely performed in the diagnosis of onychophagia. However, it can be offered if the patient is a poor historian or the provider is considering other diagnoses that would affect management. Usual biopsy findings are consistent with trauma. The biopsy specimen may show hyperkeratotic scale and focal hyperkeratosis. The epidermis shows hypergranulosis and a mild papillomatous configuration. There may be serum extravasation with entrapped red blood cells (Halteh et al., 2017).

■ COMPLICATIONS

Left unrecognized or untreated, nail biting can lead to serious complications, ranging from local trauma to dental abnormalities and systemic infections (Halteh et al., 2017; see Table 19.1).

■ TREATMENT PLAN

Selecting the appropriate treatment approach is challenging for parents and providers. Most children with mild nail-biting behavior may grow out of it with the

TABLE 19.1

POSSIBLE COMPLICATIONS OF NAIL BITING

Condition	Clinical Manifestations
Trauma (to nail bed, or nail matrix)	
Increased rate of nail growth	Longer nail plates
Nail bed shortening	Shorter nail plates due to loss of nail bed
Intraosseous epidermoid cyst	Pain/redness and swelling of distal digit
Longitudinal melanonychia	Faint bands on multiple fingernails
Infection	
Acute paronychia	Pain/redness, warmth, ± pus
Acute osteomyelitis	Pain/redness, warmth, fever
Herpetic whitlow	Clear vesicles on the distal digit, preceded by pain
Subungual warts	Verrucous papules in subungual area
Effect on Oral Bacterial Carriage	
Increased carriage of Enterobacteriaceae and Escherichia coli	Increased risk of dissemination
Increased carriage of methicillin resistant Staphylococcus epidermidis (MRSE) in healthcare workers	Health hazard for high-risk patients in hospitals
Dental/Orthodontic Complications	
Gingival infections (swelling, abscess)	Redness, bleeding/pus, foreign body (nail plate)
Apical root resorption	Changes of jaw shown on x-ray
Malocclusion, crowding of incisors	Overbite/underbite
Pain Disorder	
Temporomandibular joint disorder (TMJ)	Jaw pain, clicking/locking of jaw joints
Mimic of Infection	
Croup-like presentation	Barking cough for 7 or more days

Source: Adapted from Halteh, P., Scher, R. K., & Lipner, S. R. (2016). Onychophagia: A nail-biting conundrum for physicians. *Journal of Dermatological Treatment, 28*(2), 166–172. doi:10.1080/0954 6634.2016.1200711

wait and watch approach. However, in severe cases, persistent nail biting can lead to serious consequences, and require nonpharmacological or pharmacological interventions (Ellington, 2017). Beginning with the least intensive and noninvasive interventions is encouraged. Punishment is one of the most used nonpharmaco-logical methods in treating nail biting (Halteh et al., 2017). However, studies have shown that punishment is not effective and may result in poor self-esteem or an increase in nail-biting habit (Ellington, 2017).

The effectiveness of habit reversal (HR) and object manipulation (OM) for treating nail biting have been studied in several randomized control trials. Ninety-one children and adolescents with nail-biting behaviors were included in a randomized controlled trial that aimed to compare the effectiveness of OM training and HR training in Shiraz, Iran (Ghanizadeh, Bazrafshan, Firoozabadi, & Dehbozorgi, 2013). Children in both intervention groups received training on being aware of the nail-biting behavior and its warning signs, and picking someone as his or her social support throughout the study. Thirty participants in the HR group learned to hold an object, such as a pencil or a toy, with their hands immediately after recognizing the nail biting behavior or its warning signs. Children in the OM group were instructed to play with a toy instead of biting nails after the occurrence of nail biting or the warning signs. The outcome was measured by the length of their nails over a 3-month period. The study received positive responses from both intervention groups compared to the comparison group in increasing nail length in the long term. Additionally, the children in the HR group had longer nails than those in the OM group, that is, HR training is more effective than OM training. Another smaller study included 30 children with identified onychophagia and assigned them into either a placebo group who only discussed their nail-biting problems or the experimental group who received HR training, similar to the Ghanizadeh, Derakhshan, and Berk (2013) study. The results showed that after 5 months of therapy, HR demonstrated efficacy in treating onychophagia.

Bitter-tasting lacquer is described as "aversive therapy used to deter from nail biting due to bad taste of the substance" and commonly used by dermatologists (Halteh et al., 2017). One study put over-the-counter denatonium benzoate and sucrose octaacetate onto patients' fingers to discourage the behavior. The author concluded that the bitter-tasting lacquer method improved onychophagia. Using a nonremovable reminder, such as a wristband, to hinder nail biting is another non-pharmacological approach that has been found to be effective. However, neither the bitter-tasting lacquer technique nor the nonremovable reminder method were tested in a pediatric population.

There are no U.S. Food and Drug Administration (FDA)-approved medications for children with onychophagia. Since onychophagia is categorized as "Other Specified Obsessive-Compulsive and Related Disorders" in the *DSM-5*, the medications that have been used to treat OCD may be applicable to treat onychophagia (Ellington, 2017). Based on this theory, selective serotonin reuptake inhibitors (SSRI), tricyclic antidepressants (TCA), N-acetyl cysteine (NAC), dopamine agonists, and lithium have been studied to treat nail biting.

■ SUMMARY

The diagnosis for the child in this case presentation was onychophagia without other comorbidities, such as anxiety disorder or OCD. Thus, it was decided to use a family-centered treatment model with the pediatric primary care provider

(P-PCP) empowering the mother and child to be the decision makers and select the best treatment for the child. The parent and child determined that HR training was the option of choice. Since the child was 7 years old, he selected a favorite handheld toy (a miniature red car) to keep in his pocket and planned to hold the toy each time he realized that he was biting his nails. The mother also agreed to keep a visible record in the child's bedroom on a white board, awarding stars each time he reported holding his car instead of biting his nails. Behavior modification is most effective when the child and parent both feel they are in control of the situation and work collaboratively together and with their P-PCP to seek the healthcare outcome they desire.

■ REFERENCES

American Psychiatric Association. (2013). *Diagnostic and statistical manual of mental disorders* (5th ed.). Washington, DC: Author. doi:10.1176/appi.books.9780890425596

Bakwin, H. (1971). Nail-biting in twins. *Developmental Medicine and Child Neurology, 13*, 304–307.

Bienvenu, O. J., Samuels, J. F., Riddle, M. A., Hoehn-Saric, R., Liang, K. Y., Cullen, B. A. M., . . . Nestadt, G. (2000). The relationship of obsessive-compulsive disorder to possible spectrum disorders: Results from a family study. *Biological Psychiatry, 48*(4), 287–293. doi:10.1016/S0006-3223(00)00831-3

Birmaher, B. (1999). *Measurement instrument data bases for the social sciences.* doi:10.13072/midss.289

Ellington, E. (2017). Chronic nail biting in youth. *Journal Of Psychosocial Nursing & Mental Health Services, 55*(2), 23–27. doi:10.3928/02793695-20170210-03

Foster, L. G. (1998). Nervous habits and stereotyped behaviors in preschool children. *Journal of the American Academy of Child & Adolescent Psychiatry, 37*(7), 711–717. doi:10.1097/00004583-199807000-00010

Ghanizadeh, A. (2008). Association of nail biting and psychiatric disorders in children and their parents in a psychiatrically referred sample of children. *Child and Adolescent Psychiatry and Mental Health, 2*, 13. doi:10.1186/1753-2000-2-13

Ghanizadeh, A., Bazrafshan, A., Firoozabadi, A., & Dehbozorgi, G. (2013). Habit reversal versus object manipulation training for treating nail biting: A randomized controlled clinical trial. *Iranian Journal of Psychiatry, 8*(2), 61–67.

Ghanizadeh, A., Derakhshan, N., & Berk, M. (2013). N-acetylcysteine versus placebo for treating nail biting, a double blind randomized placebo controlled clinical trial. *Anti-Inflammatory and Anti-Allergy Agents In Medicinal Chemistry, 12*(3), 223–228. doi:10.2174/1871523013112030003.

Ghanizadeh, A., & Shekoohi, H. (2011). Prevalence of nail biting and its association with mental health in a community sample of children. *BMC Res Notes, 4*, 116. doi:10.1186/1756-0500-4-116

Halteh, P., Scher, R. K., & Lipner, S. R. (2017). Onychophagia: A nail-biting conundrum for physicians. *Journal of Dermatological Treatment, 28*(2), 166–172. doi:10.1080/09546634.2016.1200711

Kessler, R. C., Berglund, P., Demler, O., Jin, R., Merikangas, K.R., & Walters, E. E. (2005). Lifetime prevalence and age-of-onset distributions of DSM-IV disorders in the National Comorbidity Survey Replication. *Archives of General Psychiatry, 62*(6), 593–602. doi:10.1001/archpsyc.62.6.593

Massler, M., & Malone, A. J. (1950). Nailbiting—A review. *American Journal of Orthodontics, 36*(5), 351–367. doi:10.1016/0002-9416(50)90075-3

Ooki, S. (2005). Genetic and environmental influences on finger-sucking and nail-biting in Japanese twin children. *Twin Research and Human Genetics, 8*, 320–327. doi:10.1375/twin.8.4.320

Pacan, P., Grzesiak, M., Reich, A., Kantorska-Janiec, M., & Szepietowski, J. C. (2014). Onychophagia and onychotillomania: Prevalence, clinical picture and comorbidities. *Acta Derm-Venereol, 94*, 67–71. doi:10.2340/00015555-1616

Selles, R. R., Nelson, R., Zepeda, R., Dane, B. F., Wu, M. S., Novoa, J. C., . . . Storch, E. A. (2015). Body focused repetitive behaviors among Salvadorian youth: Incidence and clinical correlates. *Journal of Obsessive-Compulsive and Related Disorders, 5*, 49–54. doi:10.1016/j.jocrd.2015.01.008

Siddiqui, J. A., Qureshi, S. F., Marei, W. M., & Mahfouz, T. A. (2017). Onychophagia (nail biting): A body focused repetitive behavior due to psychiatric co-morbidity. *Journal of Mood Disorders, 7*(1), 47–49. doi:10.5455/jmood.20170204031431

Singal, A., & Daulatabad, D. (2017). Nail tic disorders: Manifestations, pathogenesis and management. *Indian Journal of Dermatology, Venereology & Leprology, 83*(1), 19–26. doi:10.4103/0378-6323.184202

Tanaka, O. M., Vitral, R. W., Tanaka, G. Y., Guerrero, A. P., & Camargo, E. S. (2008). Nailbiting, or onychophagia: A special habit. *American Journal of Orthodontics and Dentofacial Orthopedics, 134,* 305–308. doi:10.1016/j. ajodo.2006.06.023

Wechsler, D. (1931). The incidence and significance of fingernail biting in children. *Psychoanalytic Review, 18,* 201–209.

Williams, T. I., Rose, R., & Chisholm, S. (2006). What is the function of nail biting: An analog assessment study. *Behaviour Research and Therapy, 45,* 989–995. doi:10.1016/j.brat.2006.07.013

Woods, D. W., & Miltenberger, R. G. (1996). Are persons with nervous habits nervous? A preliminary examination of habit function in a non-referred population. *Journal of Applied Behavior Analysis, 29,* 259–261. doi:10.1901/jaba.1996.29-259

School-Age Population

CHAPTER 20

Behavioral Health Assessment: School-Age Children

KATIE PINK TOLLEY

School-age children with behavioral and mental health disorders struggle every day in relationships with adults and/or peers at home, school, and during formal and informal activities. Data from the 2011 to 2012 National Survey of Children's Health revealed that one out of seven children in the United States between the ages of 2 and 8 years old have a diagnosed mental, behavioral, or developmental disorder (MBDD; Centers for Disease Control and Prevention, National Center on Birth Defects and Developmental Disabilities, 2017). Pediatric primary care providers (P-PCPs) need to identify signs struggling children display, ant then assess and *intercept* the behaviors that adversely affect normal developmental patterns in social, emotional, and behavioral health. This chapter provides the best available evidence for the assessment, diagnosis, and treatment for school-age children with behavioral health problems and disorders.

■ IDENTIFICATION OF BEHAVIORAL HEALTH PROBLEMS

During a well-child or episodic primary healthcare visit, the parents or child may describe behaviors that provide the first level of evidence for an undiagnosed behavioral or emotional health problem (Table 20.1). Based on the precipitating factors, the child may experience the problem in one or more settings, such as home but not school; school but not home; or during or after school activities such as school gym classes, after-school organized sports, or other activities. Once a problem is identified, the P-PCP must begin the process of assessment, including the use of appropriate screenings to identify and intercept the problem. The P-PCP must also determine a diagnosis and treatment plan with the goal of restoring and normalizing behavioral health problems in school-age children.

■ BEHAVIORAL HEALTH ASSESSMENT

One goal in the assessment process for school-age children is to capture an understanding of the child's present and past world to determine underlying

<table>
<tr><td colspan="2">

TABLE 20.1

</td></tr>
<tr><td>

BEHAVIORS THAT ARE A "CRY FOR HELP"

</td></tr>
<tr><td>

The kindergartener that knows the right answer, but won't raise his hand.
The seventh grader that goes to the nurse for a "Band-Aid" a little too often.
The student with a headache before math class EVERY day.
The kid that just keeps making jokes and disturbing class.
The second grader that STOPPED and put her pencil down on the second problem.
The eighth grader avoiding class because there're just TOO many people.
The sixth grader with more than occasional stomachache.
The class clown that's avoiding what he doesn't know.
The third grader that's pretty damn smart, but says, "I can't do that!" when faced with a more mentally challenging task.
The first grader that runs in school even after being told to STOP, not because he's defiant or has ADHD, but because there is thunder and lightning outside!
The nineth grader who can't pay attention in class because she can't fall asleep at night worrying about her grades.
The first grader that resists help and completely melts down.
The eighth grader that thinks life is going to end when she gets a C.
The kid that asks to go to the bathroom, but talks to every adult and child along the way to avoid the unknown and awkward feeling of going back to class and NOT fitting in.
Kids don't have panic attacks...

</td></tr>
</table>

ADHD, attention deficit hyperactivity disorder.

components of the behavioral health problem. The assessment process begins with the parent(s). This meeting provides an opportunity for the P-PCP to obtain pertinent details about the current behavioral/mental health issues and relevant past medical and behavioral health history, including birth, developmental, educational, environmental, and social histories. The next step is to interview the child in a comfortable, nonthreatening setting. Based on the age of the child, and the parental concerns, the parent(s) may or may not be present. During the child's interview, all questions should be directed to the child, not the parents. The P-PCP must make it clear to the child that this interview is taking place in a "safe space" and that the goal is to listen to the child to help the child feel better about himself or herself at home, school, or just anywhere and everywhere.

A successful child behavioral health interview is predicated on the belief that the child who feels safe and trusts the examiner will begin to establish a relationship with the examiner in which the child feels comfortable as a participant in changing adverse behaviors. Successful strategies include permitting the child to play, draw, color, fidget, spin in a chair (safely), and speak freely at his or her own pace. Silence during conversation and play allows the child an opportunity to think about the questions raised and then respond. No two children are alike during a behavioral health assessment. Some children take longer than others to become comfortable with the P-PCP and to speak freely about their behaviors and concerns, as school-age children may be afraid of being punished for their behaviors. They need assurance that the goal is to help them, not punish them. The P-PCP should watch body language, reflect on the child's thought process, and observe everything the child does throughout the interview. The old adage "Actions speak

TABLE 20.2

ASSESSMENT GOALS

1. Create a professional working relationship with the parent(s) and the child.
2. Develop an understanding of the parent(s) and child's perspective of the behavioral health problem(s).
3. Collect all relevant data from the parent(s), child, and teacher(s).
4. Formulate differential diagnoses and the definitive diagnosis.
5. Formulate a treatment plan.
6. Decrease anxiety and increase hope that the behavioral health problem will respond to treatment.
7. Evaluate the treatment plan and make decisions for changes based on the evaluation.

louder than words" directly applies to understanding the child's behavioral issues. In addition, while listening to the child, the P-PCP should begin the process of comparing and contrasting the perspectives of the parents and the child on the presenting behavioral health problem.

Assessment Goals

There are seven major goals for completing a comprehensive behavioral health assessment for a school-age child, which are listed in Table 20.2. To achieve these goals, P-PCPs conduct an organized interview, do an assessment, and develop a comprehensive differential diagnostic list considering the physiological basis for physical, psychosocial, emotional, and behavioral health problems.

■ COMPONENTS OF BEHAVIORAL HEALTH INTERVIEW

The purpose of the behavioral health interview is to obtain a comprehensive behavioral health history. An approach for successful interviews with the child begins with getting to know the child. Toys in the room help the child relax and assume play behaviors. Play therapy is a successful way to conduct the interview for a school-age child. Observe the ways the child interacts with the toys and which specific toys interest the child. Allow the child's interaction with toys to guide the initial interview. Box 20.1 provides an example of the values of play therapy.

Begin with questions that offer the child an opportunity to talk about things that the child enjoys. Avoid asking questions about the problem and personal feelings until the child displays signs of comfort with the interview process. During the interview, the P-PCP should phrase questions to determine the disposition of the troubling actions and behaviors: Are the behaviors natural and involuntary or thoughtful and voluntary?

One of the easiest ways to learn more about a child is to ask the well-known "Who, What, When, Where, Why and How" questions. Table 20.3 provides an example of specific questions to ask the parent(s) and child.

Document the parent(s)' and child's "own words." Avoid making assumptions, interrupting the conversation or story, or making comments as the parent(s) or

BOX 20.1

EXAMPLES OF THE VALUE OF PLAY THERAPY
Several children were in a primary care waiting area and were playing with a dollhouse and miniature doll figures. One of the older children lined up several doll figures in rows, with one of the dolls behind a table. Suddenly, the older child yelled, "Order in the court! Order in the court!" The children immediately stopped their play activity and focused on the older child and the small figurine behind the table. The P-PCP quickly realized the stress these children had experienced when they accompanied their parent(s) to family court.

child tell their story. To clarify any part of the story that may have been unclear, consider saying, "I am not clear about what you just said, can you please tell me once more what happened?" At the end of the conversation, verify what has been said by summarizing the story and asking if what has been summarized is correct. Always ask if there is anything else the parent(s) or child would like to share prior to ending the interview.

■ DEVELOPMENTAL HISTORY FROM CONCEPTION TO SCHOOL AGE

Collecting or reviewing a detailed prenatal, birth, and developmental history guides the inquiry process for a possible relationship between physical and behavioral health problems. For example, a child who experienced an intrauterine exposure to drugs or alcohol may first exhibit signs of this exposure at school age when

TABLE 20.3

INTERVIEW QUESTIONS FOR THE PARENT AND CHILD

1. What?
   - What is the specific action/situation?
   - What precipitates it?
   - What are the physical symptoms associated with it?
2. Who?
   - Who is with the child?
   - Who has been with the child in this environment before?
3. Where?
   - Home/school/public places/car/public transportation/closed spaces?
4. When?
   - Time of day/transitions/nighttime/bedtime/separation from a loved one?
5. How?
   - Describe how the situation unfolds.
   - Who acts?
   - Who "re-acts"?
   - How long has this been happening?
6. Why?
   - Why does the parent and/or child think this is happening?

diagnosed with a learning disability. Details for obtaining prenatal, birth, and early developmental and social histories can be found in Chapter 6.

Social and Environmental History

Past and present bonding patterns of the child and other family members, including parents, siblings, grandparents, and other caregivers, should be obtained. Questions that will gather data about the social and environmental history that may provide clues to the current behavioral health problems include the following: Are the parents married, separated, divorced, living together, present in the child's life? Has there been a change in the physical and mental health history of the parents, grandparents, aunts, uncles, cousins, and siblings since the initial comprehensive history? Who are the primary caregivers of the child now and in the past? Who does the child live with, and who else lives in the house with the child? Does the child interact well with family members, adults, children, and strangers? Does the child engage in social situations? Does the child have friends? Does the child make friends easily? Does the child react the same in crowds and when alone? How does the child handle difficult situations, scary situations, emergency situations, and punishment/consequences? Is there any history of abuse (physical, emotional, sexual)?

Educational History

When discussing school, always pay attention to the child's nonverbal as well as verbal communication. Nonverbal and verbal communication will assist in discovering different special needs issues. Collect basic information about the child's education, such as school, grade, type of school (public vs. private, small vs. large, special needs, etc.). Ask the child if he or she enjoys school, what about school does he or she like and dislike. Give the child permission to "not" like some things. Ask about school performance, participation in class, work habits, homework habits, strengths, and challenges.

Gathering information about the education of the school-age child is an important aspect of the behavioral health assessment.

Food Intolerances and Links to Behavioral Health

There is a growing body of evidence that food intolerance and overuse of some medications can lead to inflammation in the gastrointestinal (GI) tract that is a precursor to multiple mental health diseases (Edwards, 2005). Are there foods the child does not tolerate? Does the child complain of stomach pain or headaches? Are there foods the child will not eat? Are there foods the child only eats? Does the child have food texture issues? All of these little details help determine any history of food intolerances and eating patterns that can lead to mental health challenges if not appropriately treated.

Sleep Problems

In my years of practice, sleep became a main topic of concern with many parents, especially parents of early school-age children. A child that doesn't get enough sleep will be at risk for behavior problems, decreased immune function, increased irritability, inability to play independently, inability to learn from the environment, and possible interference with proper growth and development. Lack of sleep can also increase a child's risk for physical disease. It can also affect emotional well-being, performance, productivity, and cognitive ability (Simola, Liukkonen, Pitkäranta, Pirinen, & Aronen, 2014).

There are medical reasons that a child may not sleep well. Children diagnosed with attention deficit hyperactivity disorder (ADHD) often have trouble falling asleep; they have trouble turning their brain off. The neurochemical imbalance that can be a problem in ADHD can also be a problem with sleep. When it comes to sleep and ADHD, each affects the other: ADHD can interfere with sleep patterns (Tolley, 2012). Another common cause of sleep problems in children is allergies. Children with allergies have trouble sleeping because of nagging symptoms like cough and runny nose, along with chronic airway obstruction that can accompany chronic allergies. Treating the cause of the problem is more beneficial than treating the symptoms, and that requires further testing and investigation.

There are multiple treatment options to help children resume a normal sleep schedule. Children do best when they are on a proper sleep schedule. Children that do not get adequate amounts of sleep often have trouble falling and staying asleep. There is a time each evening (and during the day for younger children) in the natural circadian rhythm when signs of fatigue are obvious. These signs include decreased social interaction, rubbing of the eyes, and slowing of cognitive functions and motor skills. When signs of fatigue are present, it is the ideal time for a child to go to sleep for the night. Bedtimes vary for different age groups, but young children may need to go to bed as early as 7:30 p.m., but teenagers much later. When a child misses their "window of opportunity" to go to sleep at the body's natural time, he or she will get a surge of energy trying to keep himself or herself awake; this can last a couple hours, delaying bedtime and decreasing the total amount of sleep the child requires to perform at his or her best throughout the day.

One of the natural treatment options for sleep can be melatonin. In my experience, melatonin can be useful starting at the lowest possible dose when used on a consistent basis. Melatonin is naturally made by the body, and helping the body stimulate this natural phenomenon is the philosophy behind melatonin treatment. Additional pharmaceutical treatment options are discussed in Chapter 3.

The most important thing to remember when it comes to sleep is to keep your child safe. If you are dealing with a child that wakes at night or sleepwalks, consider locks on doors that are high enough so the child cannot reach them. Night terrors are another common childhood occurrence. They are normal, but the parents are going to be more terrified than the child. The best advice is to comfort the child during the episode.

■ PERFORMING THE ASSESSMENT

It is critical to evaluate the child for possible physical disorders prior to diagnosing and treating the child for a behavioral/mental health disorder. The medical history and physical examination with appropriate testing may be a long process and requires patience from the parents and the child. Once physical diagnoses are ruled out, the process for screening and assessing for behavioral/mental health disorders can start. An example of this is as simple as untreated chronic allergies that may look like ADHD. A child with chronic allergies will have trouble sleeping, trouble concentrating, and this can look like ADHD. Once a child's allergies are adequately treated, he or she is better able to sleep, concentrate, eat, and focus.

The objective part of the behavioral health assessment for the school-age child is the sum total of clinical observations and impressions during the interview and the reports by parents, teachers, and others who interact with the child. Assessment of the child's appearance, actions, thought patterns, and speech patterns all play a significant part in determining the differential diagnoses (Tolley, 2012).

1. Appearance and behavior: Is the child clean, nourished, rested, cared for? Does the child exhibit normal childhood behaviors?
2. Affect and mood: Does the child interact easily? Is the child happy, sad, angry, or frustrated? Does the child smile?
3. Speech and thought pattern (process and content): Is the child's speech pattern rapid, slow, pressured, or mumbled? Is there a flow to his/her thought pattern or are his/her thoughts scattered? Are there situations that the child is blocking/repressing? Are there patterns representative of delusions, hallucinations, compulsions, or obsessions? Has the child shown or stated any suicidal ideations, spoken about suicide? If so, *ask* if they have a plan. Have there been past suicide attempts?
4. Does the child report any unusual thoughts, sightings, perceptions, or hallucinations (auditory, visual, tactile)? Does the child misinterpret actual experiences; is there a depersonalization/detachment in the child's interactions?
5. Cognitively, is the child alert and oriented, able to focus, and concentrate? Assess memory and calculations.
6. Does the child have age-appropriate insight and judgment? Does the child have an understanding of current situation and illness?

■ MOST COMMON BEHAVIORAL HEALTH DIAGNOSES

Approximately 5% to 15% of children will have a psychological disorder or disturbance severe enough to require treatment or that is impairing to their function (Melnyk & Moldenhauer, 2006). The most common behavioral/mental health diagnoses in childhood are ADHD, learning disabilities, autism, oppositional defiant disorder, conduct disorder, anxiety, and Tourette's syndrome (Melnyk & Moldenhauer, 2006). When these disorders continue into adulthood, the adult may be even more dysfunctional and the disorders may interfere with daily life performance and activities. In adults, these childhood disorders manifest as ADHD, anxiety, depression, substance abuse, bipolar disorer, obsessive-compulsive disorder, and schizophrenia (Melnyk & Moldenhauer, 2006).

■ DIAGNOSTIC SCREENING TOOLS

There are a variety of diagnostic screening tools available for use with school-age children. While using any of these tools, the P-PCP should make an effort to engage the child in the activity. One of the most widely used diagnostic tools in pediatric mental health is the Pediatric Symptoms Checklist (PSC) from Bright Futures (American Academy of Pediatrics [AAP], 2017). The PSC is a one-page checklist for providers to utilize that lists a wide range of children's emotional and behavioral concerns by parents. The checklist is completed by the parent prior to the visit or while he or she is waiting to see the provider. It helps guide the conversation; it is not meant to be a primary tool in diagnosis.

The ultimate authority on diagnoses of mental health disorders is the *Diagnostic and Statistical Manual of Mental Disorders, Fifth Edition (DSM-5)*. *DSM-5* provides guidelines for each of the separate disorders that are of concern in childhood. *DSM-5* does not offer treatment guidelines or recommendations, but is the first step in accurate diagnosis and appropriate care.

It is important to keep in mind that parents play an integral role in the diagnostic process, as many of the known symptom criteria require observation by them or individuals who interact regularly with the child. The PSC (AAP, 2017) can be completed by the parent prior to the visit and evaluated by the P-PCP before conducting the in-person health history (see Table 20.4). Please refer to Figure 20.1 for details to obtain a comprehensive behavioral health history for the child.

TABLE 20.4

PEDIATRIC SYMPTOM CHECKLIST				
Please mark under the heading that best fits you:				
		Never	Sometimes	Often
1. Complain of aches or pains	1.	_____	_____	_____
2. Spend more time alone	2.	_____	_____	_____
3. Tire easily, little energy	3.	_____	_____	_____
4. Fidget, unable to sit still	4.	_____	_____	_____
5. Have trouble with teacher	5.	_____	_____	_____
6. Less interested in school	6.	_____	_____	_____
7. Act as if driven by motor	7.	_____	_____	_____
8. Daydream too much	8.	_____	_____	_____
9. Distract easily	9.	_____	_____	_____
10. Am afraid of new situations	10.	_____	_____	_____

(continued)

TABLE 20.4 (*CONTINUED*)

PEDIATRIC SYMPTOM CHECKLIST

11. Feel hopeless	11.	_____	_____	_____
12. Am irritable, angry	12.	_____	_____	_____
13. Feel hopeless	13.	_____	_____	_____
14. Have trouble concentrating	14.	_____	_____	_____
15. Less interested in friends	15.	_____	_____	_____
16. Fight with other children	16.	_____	_____	_____
17. Absent from school	17.	_____	_____	_____
18. School grades dropping	18.	_____	_____	_____
19. Down on yourself	19.	_____	_____	_____
20. Visit doctor with doctor finding nothing wrong	20.	_____	_____	_____
21. Have trouble sleeping	21.	_____	_____	_____
22. Worry a lot	22.	_____	_____	_____
23. Want to be with parent more than before	23.	_____	_____	_____
24. Feel that you are bad	24.	_____	_____	_____
25. Take unnecessary risks	25.	_____	_____	_____
26. Get hurt frequently	26.	_____	_____	_____
27. Seem to be having less fun	27.	_____	_____	_____
28. Act younger than children your age	28.	_____	_____	_____
29. Do not listen to rules	29.	_____	_____	_____
30. Do not listen to rules	30.	_____	_____	_____
31. Do not understand other people's feelings	31.	_____	_____	_____
32. Tease others	32.	_____	_____	_____
33. Blame others for your troubles	33.	_____	_____	_____
34. Take things that do not belong to you	34.	_____	_____	_____
35. Refuse to share	35.	_____	_____	_____

Source: Pediatric Symptom Checklist. Retrieved from https://www.brightfutures.org/mentalhealth/pdf/professionals/ped_sympton_chklst.pdf. ©1988, M. S. Jellinek and J. M. Murphy, Massachusetts General Hospital.

Patient Name: _____   Date of Evaluation: _____

DOB: ____   Time In: ____ Time Out: ____

Accompanied by: _____   Informed Consent: Y/N

Chief Complaint: _____   Diagnostic Tools used

Vital Signs:

HT_____ WT_____ HR _____ RR_____ BP_____

History of Present Illness: Behavioral Health Problem

Medical History:

Provider: _____

Allergies: _____

Current Medications: _____

Family History: (mental health)

Mother: _____

Father: _____

Siblings: _____

Extended Family: _____

Review of Systems: (WNL unless documented)

Fever, headache, sore throat, rhinorrhea, cough, shortness or breath, chest pain, abdominal pain, nausea/vomiting/diarrhea, dizziness, or rash

Behavioral Health patterns of social emotional growth and development:

Mental Health History:

Diagnosis: _____

Past Medications: _____

   Any Side Effects: _____

History of tics? _____

History of suicide attempts/threats? _____

Birth and Developmental History

Vaginal or cesarean section: _____

Premature/Complications: (required oxygen, intubation, special feedings, etc.) _____

FIGURE 20.1 Mental health assessment for the school-age child.

Temperament as an infant/toddler: _____

Milestones: (sitting at 6 mo, walking ~ 1 yr, potty training ~ 2-3 yrs, bed wetting?) _____

Social History:

Living situation and home atmosphere: Past? Present? Recent changes/loss? Who works in the family? Guns in the house (locked)? _____

Parents married, divorced, never married? _____

Any step-parents or step siblings? Relationship with step? _____

School: Grade: Performance: (Special needs, GT, LD, behavior issues, retentions) _____

Homework habits: _____

Favorite/least favorite subject: _____

Extracurricular activities /Hobbies/Sports: _____

Sleep hygiene: How many hours daily? Trouble falling asleep? Where does child sleep? (own bed, sofa, shares room) _____

Eating Habits: caffeine intake? TID meals? Fruit/veg? Protein? Processed Foods? Food Dye? Milk? Dairy Products? Bread/pasta products?
Abuse or Trauma (physical/sexual/emotional): _____

Religion: _____

Legal Issues: (child or family, custody, legal guardianship, etc.) _____

Misc: _____

Mental Status Exam:

Alert/Oriented: Person/Place/Time/Situation

Affect: Labile/Flat/Blunted/Sad/Silly/Euthymic/WNL

Mood: Irritable/Angry/Sad/Happy/Elevated/Euphoric

Psychomotor Activity: Hyperactive/Agitated/Calm/

Psychomotor Slowing/Other_____

Thought Flow: Logical/Sequential/Goal-Directed/ Tangential

Circumstantial/Loose Associations

Hallucinations: Auditory/Visual/None

Other Sensory/Perceptual Disturbances: Racing Thoughts

Flight of ideas/Intrusive Thoughts/Grandiosity

Attention/Concentration: Good/Fair/Poor

Insight: Good/Fair/Poor

IQ: Above avg/Average/Below avg/Deficit

Speech: Rapid/Abnormal Prosody/WNL

Dimin Prosody/Increased Latency

Thought Content: SI/HI Yes or No

Memory: WNL/STM/LTM/Slightly

Impoverished/Grossly Impaired

Immediate Recall_____

_____ # recalled after 5 minutes

FIGURE 20.1 *(continued)*

Paranoia/Suspicions/Delusional Content   Self-Attitude: Poor/Low/Inflated/WNL

Other Thought Activity: Recurrent Intrusive Thoughts

            Obsessions/Compulsions/ Phobias/Excessive Fears
Diagnosis:

Treatment Recommendations/Plan:

Discussed with parent/guardian and patient: Y/N Agrees: Y/ N

Reviewed risk/benefits and side effects of medication: Y/N

Follow-up:

Clinician signature _____   Date _____

FIGURE 20.1 *(continued)*

BP, blood pressure; DOB, date of birth; GT, gifted/talented; HR, heart rate; HT, height; LD, learning disability; RR, respiratory rate; TID, three times a day; WNL, within normal limits; WT, weight.

Diagnosis can take weeks to months. It is not beneficial to the child or family to rush to a diagnosis or treatment plan prematurely. It can actually be harmful to the child emotionally and physically to administer therapies that are misguided. Always do a thorough assessment—physical, mental, and maybe even genetic— prior to forming a treatment plan.

▪ TREATMENT

Treatment includes creating a plan with the family, with ongoing interaction and consultation to determine the appropriate treatment path, and then, if needed, provide any necessary referral (i.e., underlying physical health issues, further mental health treatment).

The first line of mental health treatment should *always* be behavior modification with help and guidance from a capable mental health therapist. The plan will need to be continually modified in the beginning. It will be important for the therapist to help the parents/caregiver troubleshoot the behavioral interventions and provide support. Making changes may be difficult in the beginning; consistent effort is crucial for positive results.

▪ EFFECTIVE PARENTING

Establishing the Daily Routine

Establishing daily routines is an unbelievably important part of parenting a child with behavioral health problems. Planning a schedule helps a child learn what to anticipate day after day. Using lists or pictures can be helpful to remind the child of his or her responsibilities and keeps the child on task. Remind the child about one task at a time. Once a task is completed, then present the next task rather than giving multiple tasks at one time.

Make sure the rules are clear and followed consistently. If parents have rules that are only enforced some of the time, the child will not know when he or she does or does not have to follow the rules. This lack of consistent enforcement of the established rules leads to frustration for the child and the parent, and results will be inconsistent or nonexistent.

Assign the child a role in the house. Examples of roles include helping to care for pets, taking out the trash, making the beds, or other chores the child can most likely do well around the house. Chores help the child feel important, learn responsibility, and build self-esteem and self-confidence (Figure 20.2).

Praise and Positive Reinforcement

Praise and positive reinforcement is a must reward for all children, especially children with ADHD. Recognize and praise good behavior and accomplishments. Completing homework assignments or even small household chores can be challenging for some children.

Screen Time

There is a significant amount of research supporting limiting "screen time" for all children, including school-age children (American Academy of Pediatrics [AAP], 2009, 2017; Tolley, 2012). This recommendation covers anything with electronic screens, such as television, video games, computers, smartphones, and/or tablets. For school-age children, screen time should be limited to just 2 to 3 hours per day. All screen time activities should be stopped at least 1 hour before bedtime. This routine is easier to enforce during the school year because the child may have limited free time after school. It is more challenging during the summer. Be advised that more liberal screen exposure can affect dopamine levels in the brain and will affect the child's behavior (Weinstein, 2010). Initiate a weaning period prior to the start of school for a smoother transition into the school year (Tolley, 2012).

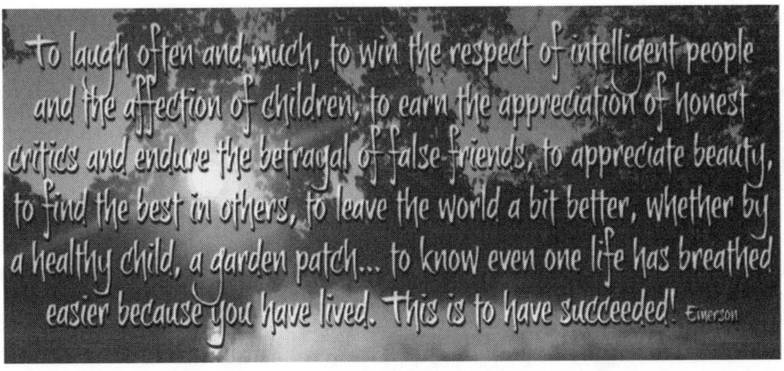

FIGURE 20.2 *To Laugh Often and Much.* A poem by Ralph Waldo Emerson.

Bedtime Routines

Have a good bedtime routine with an acceptable bedtime. Kids in preschool and early elementary grades should be in bed by 7:30 p.m. to 8:30 p.m.; upper elementary, by 8:30 p.m. to 9:00 p.m.; middle school, by 9:00 p.m. to 9:30 p.m.; and high school, by 9:00 p.m. to 10:00 p.m. A tired child has trouble focusing, paying attention, and retaining information (Tolley, 2012).

Nutrition

Eating three healthy meals and snacks are important for good cognitive function. Adding essential fatty acids (EFAs) to a child's diet helps promote brain growth and development. The most important of these fatty acids are the omega-3 fatty acids (DiPasquale, 2009). Omega-3 fatty acids are alpha-linolenic acids. There are other essential fatty acids as well, and the body needs all of them, but the one most often deficient in the standard American diet is omega-3. Some examples of EFAs are salmon, tuna, olive oil, coconut oil, flax seeds, chia seeds, farm fresh eggs, and walnuts (Axe, 2017).

Artificial Food Dyes in the Diet

Artificial food dyes (AFDs) should be eliminated from the child's diet. AFDs have been shown to increase hyperactivity in the majority of children. A study conducted in Great Britain revealed that approximately 74% of children demonstrated hyperactive behavior correlated with ingestion of AFDs and sodium benzoate. AFDs have been outlawed in Canada, Britain, Germany, and a few other countries (Arnold, Lofthouse, & Hurt, 2012; McCann et al., 2007; Tolley, 2012).

Exercise

Exercise, exercise, exercise! Physical activity helps to regulate neurotransmitters. Telling kids to run a few laps around the house really does help get the wiggles out. Encourage the child to pursue what they do well. Whether one's forte is math, sports, or building things, encourage it (Tolley, 2012).

■ NUTRITION AND THE GUT–BRAIN CONNECTION

There is a growing body of scientific evidence that nutrition plays a substantial role in brain development, brain health, and mental health. The balance of normal flora (bacterial, viral, and fungal) within the GI tract is crucial to the maintenance of the process of homeostasis in the body's digestion, absorption, and metabolic processes, including weight management, bowel habits, and nutrient delivery. Nutritional deficiencies and intolerances have been linked to an imbalance in gut and brain chemistry (Campbell, 2014). Thus, the gut–brain axis is being rigorously investigated as an approach to assess and treat behavioral and mental health problems (Figure 20.3).

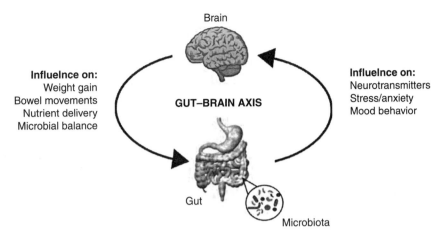

FIGURE 20.3 Gut–brain axis.

The connection between the central nervous system and the GI tract is recip-rocal. The brain relies on a healthy GI tract for partial regulation of neurotrans-mitters. Neurotransmitters, such as serotonin and melatonin, are present in the lining of the gut (Thor, Krolczyk, Gil, Zurowski, & Nowak, 2007). When there is a GI imbalance, symptoms of neurologic and metabolic deregulation occur. This deregulation may present as anxiety symptoms, sleep disorders, mood imbal-ances, hormone imbalances, attention disorders, difficulty with social communi-cations, thyroid problems, digestive problems, and behavior problems (Cryan & O'Mahony, 2011).

There is evidence that these problems result from a breakdown in intestinal permeability. This breakdown affects not only the GI system but also the immune and neurological systems, altering neurotransmitter balance, hormone regulation, and metabolic function (Fasano, 2012). The breakdown in intestinal permeability can occur from multiple assaults on the GI tract, including but not limited to food intolerance, some strains of bacteria, and antibiotic exposure.

Role of Vitamin D

Low levels of vitamin D have been shown to adversely affect overall physical and behavioral/mental health. Vitamin D is a hormone that affects neurocognitive func-tions such as sleep, mood imbalance, and anxiety. Adequate intake of vitamin D is now believed to be essential for mental health stability (Penckofer, Kouba, Byrn, & Ferrans, 2010). Further discussion on vitamin D is included in Chapter 35.

Food Intolerances

Food intolerances and overindulgence are two of the biggest causes of intesti-nal hyperpermeability. Gliadin (gluten) binds to CXCR3 and leads to MyD88-dependent zonulin release and increased intestinal permeability (Lammers et al., 2008). CXCR3 is a chemokine receptor that is highly expressed on effector T cells and plays an important role in T cell trafficking and function (Groom & Luster, 2012). The *MYD88* gene is essential for making a protein involved in signaling within immune cells (U.S. Department of Health & Human Services, National Institute of Health, 2017).

The consumption of gluten is problematic for individuals who are gluten sensitive. Individuals who are gluten sensitive may experience complaints if too much gluten is consumed. Studies examining dietary analysis of gluten consumption by children revealed that the majority of children have diets high in gluten (see Figure 20.4; Tolley, 2016a, 2016d). Researchers conclude that gliadin/gluten activates zonulin signaling, irrespective of the genetic expression of autoimmunity, leading to increased intestinal permeability to macromolecules (gluten, dairy, soy, sugar, and other foreign substances; Drago, 2006). Zonulin is used as a biomarker of impaired gut barrier function for several autoimmune, neurodegenerative, and humoral diseases (Fasano, 2011). Intestinal hyperpermeability is the just the beginning of the immune breakdown responsible for the disruption of the gut–brain axis (Arrieta, Bistritz, & Meddings, 2006; Tolley, 2016a, 2016b, 2016c, 2016d).

▪ GENE MUTATIONS THAT AFFECT ABSORPTION AND METABOLISM

There has been a longstanding belief that genetics influence behavioral/mental health. However, until the recent discovery of the methylenetetrahydrofolate reductase (MTHFR) gene mutation, this belief was not substantiated. The MTHFR mutation occurs on the short arm of chromosome 1, in position 677 or 1298. Gene 677 mutates when thymine replaces cytosine, and gene 1298 mutates when cytosine replaces adenine. One or both of these genetic mutations create problems for cellular metabolism, including elimination of toxins from the body, creation of neurotransmitters, production and proper function of blood cells and immune cells, and/or hormone production. The inhibition of methylation, a necessary cellular function, is one of the main problems associated with these gene mutations (Leclerc, Sibani, & Roze, 2000–2013).

The report of how many people in the United States have this mutation varies. However, it is estimated that between 30% and 70% of our population has this mutation in a heterogeneous or homogenous form (Lynch, 2014). If behavioral and mental health problems are to be effectively treated, the significant impact of this mutation must be identified and treated accordingly.

▪ SUMMARY

It is critically important to consider the nutritional and metabolic impact on behavioral and mental health to reduce the statistical incidence of children with behavioral health problems and to design strategies to intercept the onset of problems. Current treatment interventions are not effectively enabling many children to find and maintain normal daily functioning. The number of children placed on drug therapy for management of mental health behaviors has significantly increased over the past several years. P-PCPs need to view behavioral and mental health

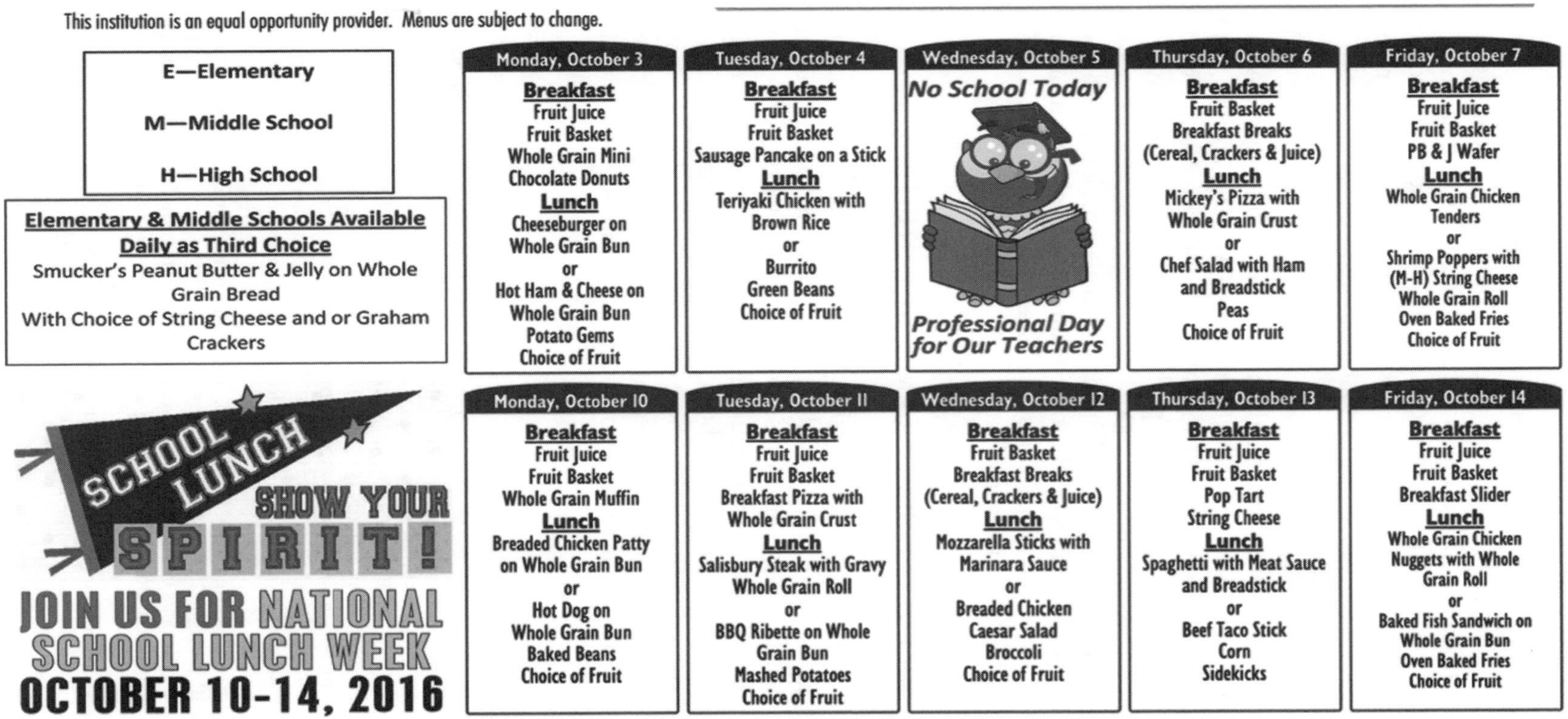

FIGURE 20.4 School breakfast and lunch menu.

Source: From Tolley, K. (2016c). *Wellness is nutrition.* [PowerPoint slides].

with the same lens that physical health and well-being are viewed if the outcomes for children with behavioral health problems are to improve.

The nutrition and gene mutation information must be considered in the diagnostic process to establish a full picture of the underlying cause of a child's presenting problems. P-PCPs must also consider the cause of neurotransmitter imbalance: Is the cause genetic? Is the cause from nutritional deficiencies caused by malabsorption? Is the cause from food intolerances and the inability to detox these foods from the gut and brain?

If P-PCPs do not diagnose and treat children with behavioral and mental health problems effectively, these children grow into adults who have difficulty functioning in society. Children with diagnoses of ADHD, anxiety, depression, conduct disorder, and/or oppositional defiant disorder become adults with anxiety, depression, bipolar disorder, addiction problems, and a variety of physical health problems (Melnyk & Moldenhauer, 2006).

Children with mental health challenges also have problems with social relationships. Children with unresolved social relationship problems as a child most often continue to have similar problems as adults, which often affects their ability to maintain adult relationships and jobs.

■ LOOKING AHEAD: THE SIGNIFICANCE OF NUTRITION

I, Katie Tolley, truly believe the missing link in child and adolescent mental health is nutrition. I think it is crucial for all P-PCPs to incorporate nutrition and digestive challenges as part of a standard medical workup. We must start learning more about and considering the gut–brain connection in the diagnostic process when evaluating and treating both physical and mental health problems. If we target nutrition for children in the early years of their life, we may be saving them from medical issues and interventions in the future. I think we need to focus on the cause of mental health disorders to be better able to avoid disorders.

■ REFERENCES

American Academy of Pediatrics. (2009). *More screen time and less activity can mean more distress*. Retrieved from https://www.aap.org/en-us/about-the-aap/aap-press-room/Pages/More-Screen-Time-and-Less-Activity-Can-mean-More-Distress.aspx

American Academy of Pediatrics. (2017). *Bright futures: Guidelines for health supervision of infants, children, and adolescents, pocket guide* (4rd ed.). Retrieved from http://www.acmh-mi.org/get-information/childrens-mental-health-101/common-diagnosis/, https://www.brightfutures.org/

Arnold, L. E., Lofthouse, N., & Hurt, E. (2012). Artificial food colors and attention deficit/hyperactivity disorder symptoms: Conclusions to dye for. *Neurotherapeutics, 9*, 599–609. doi:10.1007/s13311-012-0133-x

Arrieta, M. C., Bistritz, L., & Meddings, J. B. (2006). Alterations in intestinal permeability. *Gut, 55*(10), 1512–1520. doi:10.1136/gut.2005.085373

Axe, J. (2017). *15 omega-3 foods your body needs now*. Retrieved from https://draxe.com/omega-3-foods/

Campbell, A. W. (2014). Autoimmunity and the gut. *Autoimmune Disease, 2014*, 1–12. doi:10.1155/2014/152428

Centers for Disease Control and Prevention, National Center on Birth Defects and Developmental Disabilities. (2017). *Children's mental health: Data & statistics*. Retrieved from https://www.cdc.gov/childrensmentalhealth/data.html

Cryan, J. F., & O'Mahony, S. M. (2011). The microbiome-gut-brain axis: From bowel to behavior. *Neurogastroenterology & Motility, 23,* 187–192. doi:10.1111/j.1365-2982.2010.01664.x

Di Pasquale, M. G. (2009). The essentials of fatty acids. *Journal of Dietary Supplements, 6,* 143–161. doi:10.1080/193902861841

Drago, S. (2006). Gliadin, zonulin and gut permeability: Effects on celiac and non-celiac intestinal mucosa and intestinal cell lines. *Scandinavian Journal of Gastroenterology, 41,* 408–419. doi:10.1080/00365520500235334

Edwards, T. (2005). Inflammation, pain, and chronic disease: An integrative approach to treatment and prevention. *Alternative Therapies in Health and Medicine, 11,* 20–27. Retrieved from https://www.ncbi.nlm.nih.gov/pubmed/16320856

Fasano, A. (2011). Zonulin and its regulation of intestinal barrier function: The biological door to inflammation, autoimmunity, and cancer. *Physiological Review, 91,* 151–175. doi:10.1152/physrev.00003.2008

Fasano, A. (2012). Leaky gut and autoimmune disease. *Clinical Review of Allergy and Immunology, 42,* 71–78. doi:10.1007/s12016-011-8291-x

Groom, J. R., & Luster, A. D. (2012). CXCR3 in T cell function. *Experimental Cell Research, 317,* 620–631. Retrieved from https://www.ncbi.nlm.nih.gov/pmc/articles/PMC3065205/ doi:10.1016/j.yexcr.2010.12.017

Lammers, K. M., Lu, R., Brownley, J., Lu, B., Gerard, C., Thomas, K., . . . Fasano, A. (2008). Gliadin induces an increase in intestinal permeability and zonulin release by binding to the chemokine receptor CXCR3. *Gastroenterology, 135,* 194–204.e3. doi:10.1053/j.gastro.2008.03.023

Leclerc, D., Sibani, S., & Roze, R. (2000–2013). *Molecular biology of methylenetetrahydrofolate reductase (MTHFR) and overview of mutations/polymorphisms.* Retrieved from https://www.ncbi.nlm.nih.gov/books/NBK6561/

Lynch, B. (2014). *Mthfr.net: Your expert resource on MTHFR gene mutation.* Retrieved from www.mthfr.net

McCann, D., Barrett, A., Cooper, A., Crumpler, D., Dalen, L., Grimshaw, K., . . . Stevenson, J. (2007). Food additives and hyperactive behaviour in 3-year-old and 8/9-year-old children in the community: A randomised, double-blinded, placebo-controlled trial. *Lancet, 370,* 95981560–95981567. doi:10.1016/S0140-6736(07)61306-3

Melnyk, B., & Moldenhauer, Z. (2006). *The KySS (keep your children/yourself safe & secure) guide to child and adolescent mental health screening, early intervention and health promotion.* Cherry Hill, NJ: National Association of Pediatric Nurse Practitioners (NAPNAP).

Penckofer, S., Kouba, J., Byrn, M., & Ferrans, C. E. (2010). Vitamin D and depression: Where is all the sunshine? *Issues in Mental Health Nursing, 31,* 385–393. doi:10.3109/01612840903437657

Simola, P., Liukkonen, K., Pitkäranta, A., Pirinen, T., & Aronen, E. T. (2014). Psychosocial and somatic outcomes of sleep problems in children: A 4-year follow-up study. *Child Care Health Dev, 40,* 60–67. doi:10.1111/j.1365-2214.2012.01412.x

Thor, P. J., Krolczyk, G., Gil, K., Zurowski, D., & Nowak, L. (2007). Melatonin and serotonin effects on gastrointestinal motility. *Journal of Physiology and Pharmacology, 58*(Suppl 6), 97–103. Retrieved from https://www.ncbi.nlm.nih.gov/pubmed/18212403

Tolley, K. (2012). *Effective Parenting… Important for all kids, but especially important for ADHD kids.* Retrieved from https://katiepinktolley.com/2012/08/09/effective-parenting-especially-important-for-raising-kids-with-adhd/

Tolley, K. (2016a). *Digestive health lesson #1: Leaky gut.* Retrieved from https://katiepinktolley.com/2016/05/22/digestive-health-lesson-1-leaky-gut/

Tolley, K. (2016b). *Digestive health lesson #2: It all starts with inflammation.* Retrieved from https://katiepinktolley.com/2016/06/23/digestive-health-lesson-2-it-all-starts-with-inflammation/

Tolley, K. (2016c). *Wellness is nutrition.* [Powerpoint slides].

Tolley, K. (2016d). *You're wrong, that's not it at all…* Retrieved from https://katiepinktolley.com/2016/02/13/youre-wrong-thats-not-it-at-all-2/

Touchette, E., Cote, S. M., Petit, D., Liu, X., Boivin, M., Falissa, B., . . . Montplaisir, J. Y. (2009). Short nighttime sleep-duration and hyperactivity trajectories in early childhood. *Pediatrics, 124,* 5. doi:10.1542/peds.2008-2005

U.S. Department of Health & Human Services, National Institute of Health. (2017). *Your guide to understanding genetic conditions.* Retrieved from file:///Users/donnahallas/Downloads/MYD88_gene.pdf

Weinstein, A. M. (2010). Computer and video game addiction—A comparison between game users and non-game users. *American Journal of Drug and Alcohol Abuse, 36,* 268–276. doi:10.3109/00952990.2010.491879

CHAPTER 21

Bullying and Other Behavioral Problems at School

SALLY S. COHEN AND JAMES J. WEIDEL

Schools are intended to enrich students' cognitive, emotional, and social development. But for some children and youth, schools pose behavioral challenges. Behavioral problems in school can signal emotional issues that adversely affect children or youth and persist through adulthood. Such problems are often the result of complex interactions among genetic, individual, home, school, and community factors.

In addition to posing behavioral challenges, schools can be pivotal as settings where children's behavioral and other psychosocial issues are detected and treated. Many schools provide mental health services, which is important for youth, especially adolescents, who lack access to mental healthcare in their communities. Moreover, teachers observe students in various contexts, ranging from structured classrooms to more informal settings such as cafeterias, hallways, and playgrounds, where students interact with peers.

The purpose of the chapter is to provide an overview of behavioral issues in school settings. Major topics covered are explanations of why school settings can pose challenges for behavior; etiology, manifestations, and consequences of behavioral challenges in school settings; and bullying among children and youth as an example of a challenging behavior at school. The chapter concludes with a summary of recommendations for pediatric primary care providers (P-PCPs) who, with the correct knowledge about bullying behaviors, can *intercept* the problems while working with children who are affected by behavioral challenges at school.

■ DETECTION AND INTERVENTION

Children spend at least 32 hours a week in school, not including time spent on the school bus, doing homework online through school information technology platforms, participating in sports or other extracurricular activities, or attending before- and after-school programs. Teachers, administrators, and other personnel at the nation's approximately 98,000 public schools and 34,000 private schools

(U.S. Department of Education, Institute for Education Statistics, National Center for Education Statistics, 2015a) play a vital role in the health and development of children and youth.

Education is primarily the responsibility of state governments and local educational agencies (LEAs), which are public boards of education, schools, or other public authorities legally designated by a state to direct or administer public primary or secondary schools (Legal Information Institute, n.d.). Although there is no federal law requiring children to attend school, essentially every state has a compulsory education law that stipulates, with some exceptions, the ages that children must attend school. State compulsory education laws, combined with certain federal policies, ensure that every child in the United States has the right to an equal education opportunity, making education one of the few entitlements for all children (American Civil Liberties Union [ACLU], n.d.; U.S. Department of Education, Office for Civil Rights, 2010; U.S. Department of Education and U.S. Department of Justice, 2014). No comparable entitlement exists for access to child healthcare, health insurance coverage, or other children's services.

Schools nationwide enroll children of diverse ethnicities, socioeconomic status, sexual orientation, gender preference, and with varying health and immigration status. For example, many schools, especially public schools, enroll students whose primary language is not English. For academic year 2014–2015, over four million children (approximately 9.3%) enrolled in public schools had difficulty communicating in English (U.S. Department of Education, Institute for Education Science, National Center for Education Statistics, 2017a). Difficulties communicating with teachers and peers can negatively affect children's behavior, development, and learning.

In caring for children who present with behavioral problems in schools, P-PCPs need to partner with parents, teachers, and other school personnel. They also need to know how to access national, state, and local policies and resources regarding behavioral issues in school settings. Knowledge of the most recent evidence and best practices for managing behavioral challenges in schools is also important. The sections that follow offer resources and guidance in these areas.

Protective Factors

The Centers for Disease Control and Prevention (CDC) experts in school and adolescent health have addressed the importance of "protective factors" in preventing "adverse health and educational outcomes" (CDC, 2016a). Protective factors are "individual or environmental characteristics, conditions, or behaviors that reduce the effects of stressful life events." Such factors also have the potential to reduce or eliminate risks or hazards, and promote social and emotional competence so that children and youth can "thrive in all aspects of life, now and in the future" (CDC, 2016a). P-PCPs can explore youth's and parents' perceptions of how well their schools promote development of protective factors. If deficits are noted or suspected, then P-PCPs might guide parents and youth in how to discuss the importance of protective factors with teachers and other school personnel, beginning the process of *intercepting* potential adverse behavioral outcomes.

Recognizing the importance of physical and emotional health on students' ability to learn, several government and nonprofit organizations have formed innovative partnerships to enhance students' health outcomes (National Association of Chronic Disease Directors [NACDD], 2017; CDC, n.d.). One such partnership is between the CDC and the Association for Supervision and Curriculum Development (ASCD), which culminated in the *Whole School, Whole Child, Whole Community* model, an integration of health and education perspectives to ensure that children are ready to learn (CDC, n.d.; Lewallen, Hunt, Potts-Datema, Zaza, & Giles, 2015). Two of the 10 components of the model are of particular relevance to behavioral and mental health: (a) counseling, psychological, and social services and (b) a school's social and emotional climate (CDC, n.d.; Demissie & Brenner, 2017).

School Nurses

School nurses are often the main liaisons among parents, students, P-PCPs, school administrators, teachers, and other education professionals. Their offices offer safe havens for students dealing with emotional or behavior challenges. School nurses may be the first to identify signs and symptoms as a cause or consequence of behavioral challenges (National Association of School Nurses [NASN], 2017a).

Each state has policies regarding educational requirements for school nurses and the maximum allowed ratio of students to school nurses. Nonetheless, many schools or school districts lack adequate numbers of school nurses to meet students' physical and behavioral health needs. Approximately 25% of all U.S. schools do not employ a school nurse at all (NASN, 2017a). When a school has a nurse, P-PCPs should consider that person a major ally in working with parents, educators, and school personnel to prevent behavioral risks and guide parents to appropriate interventions if needed: the first step in intercepting potential behavioral problems.

■ ETIOLOGY, MANIFESTATIONS, AND CONSEQUENCES OF BEHAVIORAL CHALLENGES AT SCHOOL

Early childhood, between birth and 5 years of age (Carson et al., 2016), is increasingly recognized as a critical stage for shaping development across the life course (Duncan, Kalil, & Ziol-Guest, 2013). The sooner in life that behavioral problems are identified and addressed, the greater the likelihood they do not impede education attainment, work productivity, or lead to criminality in adulthood. Behaviors at school deemed problematic are those that hinder students' ability to learn or distract teachers' efforts to develop the entire class's academic progress (Thompson, 2011). Common problematic behaviors such as harassment, fighting, disrespect, defiance, and physical and verbal aggression (Conley, Marchant, & Caldarella, 2014) may manifest under many conditions and in various locations throughout a school (Thompson, 2011).

Risk Factors, Characteristics, and Types of Behavioral Challenges

DISRUPTIVE BEHAVIORS

Disruptive behaviors (e.g., defiance of authority, lying, cheating) have the potential to cause serious harm to students' emotional and social well-being, to disrupt the classroom environment, and to limit students' ability to achieve their full academic potential (Barth, Dunlap, Lochman, & Wells, 2004). A complex interplay of demographic, family, psychosocial, and biological risk factors are implicated in the etiology of problematic and disruptive behaviors. Among them are intellectual disability (Soedjatmiko, Kadim, Madiyono, & Said, 2016), aggression and violence in childhood (Muratori et al., 2015), anxiety disorders, poor problem-solving skills (Smith et al., 2014), and parental smoking (Keyes Legrand, Iacono, & McGue, 2008). Children who exhibit disruptive and problematic behavior are at greater risk for subsequent psychopathology, substance use (Miettunen et al., 2014), and criminal behaviors (Dodge et al., 2014) during adolescence and adulthood. Although complex in origin and presentation, disruptive and problematic behaviors fall along a continuum between low and high severity marked by aggression (Andrade, Sorge, Na, & Wharton-Shukster, 2015).

Aggression

Aggression refers to any form of behavior with the goal of harming or injuring another living being that is motivated to avoid such treatment. Aggressive actions or behaviors can be verbal or physical and include physical assault, homicide, destruction of property, and violence against humans and animals (Tahirovic, 2015). In children, aggressive behaviors typically deviate from normal developmental aggression for specific ages with respect to frequency, intensity, and duration of aggressive behavior, the extent of which also disrupts various aspects of a child's development like speech development, communication with peers, and academic success (Shechtman & Tutian, 2016).

Aggression among children often occurs in schools. Given universal access to schools for all children in the United States, schools are an important location for the identification and treatment of aggressive behaviors (Wilson & Lipsey, 2007). But identifying and addressing aggressive behavior in children can be difficult, especially because of the varying forms of aggression. Examples of aggressive behavior in schools include cyber-aggression (Shapka & Maghsoudi, 2017) and bullying (Ledwell & King, 2015).

CAUSES OF AGGRESSION

Causes of aggressive behavior vary. Temperaments and environmental factors can influence the development of aggression (Farnicka & Grzegorzewska, 2016). Aggressive behavior may be acquired through learning by observing and imitating (Hasan, Bègue, Scharkow, & Bushman, 2013), which makes parents and their discipline styles important to note (Gershoff, 2013). Aggression generally begins with the emotion of anger, which once evoked is expressed as overt or covert aggression (verbal or physical). When anger is suppressed, feelings of resentment, suspicion, and alienation develop (Rubio-Garay, Carrasco, & Amor, 2016).

HOSTILITY

Hostility is often a combination of internal impulses and external stimuli or triggers (Walters & Espelage, 2018). In children, both anger and hostility are important antecedents to aggression (Rubio-Garay et al., 2016).

CHARACTERIZATIONS OF AGGRESSIVE BEHAVIORS

Characterizations and definitions of aggressive behaviors in schools typically depend on teachers' observations of students who display such behaviors and parental reports. Adults have their own varying emotional states, resulting in different perceptions of observed behaviors. Likewise, children who are targets of aggression view such actions differently depending on the child's perceived threat and own emotional reactions (Crotty, Doody, & Lyons, 2014).

Use of aggressive behavior itself is an instrument to achieve a particular goal such as better status among school peers. Associated with later social dominance, delinquency, and disruptive behaviors, proactive aggression is a learned phenomenon reinforced by the positive outcomes (Fite, Rubens, Preddy, Raine, & Pardini, 2014). Proactive aggression occurs in early childhood, a time when aggression is often proactive with a goal of gaining desired objects such as toys (Sroufe, Coffino, & Carlson, 2010), although hostile and proactive aggressions exist concomitantly, which explains why children express the variety of aggressive behaviors in isolation or in combination (Angus, Schutter, Terburg, van Honk, & Harmon-Jones, 2016).

In contrast to hostile or proactive aggression, reactive or "hot-blooded" aggression is impulsive and is typically motivated by an angry emotional response to some external stimulus event or a perceived offense (Card & Little, 2006). Reactive aggression results from external provocation without thought to personal gain. The external stimulus may not in reality pose a real danger, but rather results from a child's perception of a situation or event. Development of reactive aggression is connected with parenting styles, exposure to violence, and social and economic factors in the family (Ledwell & King, 2015). Children expressing reactive aggression often have underdeveloped skills for emotional and behavior control (Rosell & Siever, 2015). In schools, reactively aggressive children and adolescents tend to misjudge others' intentions as provoking and hostile, increasing their risk for overreactive, aggressive responses (Jung, Krahe, & Busching, 2017).

Aggressive behaviors are also characterized in terms of their expressed forms. Physical aggression includes harmful behaviors directed toward another person, such as punching, kicking, or shoving (Fite et al., 2014). Physical aggression is perhaps the most pronounced of all the subtypes because it is the most socially costly of aggressive behaviors (Broidy et al., 2003; Juvonen & Graham, 2014). Direct physical aggression or open aggression, which is most often employed by young males (Ledwell & King, 2015), typically takes the form of pushing, hitting, kicking, or the use of weapons (Rajan, Namdar, & Ruggles, 2015). Adolescent and adulthood physical aggression trace back to behaviors identified in early childhood (Racz, O'Brennan, Bradshaw, & Leaf, 2016).

VERBAL AGGRESSION

Verbal aggression is conditional on personal subjectivity, cultural beliefs, and intrinsic predisposition (Aloia & Solomon, 2016). Direct verbal aggression uses words and insults to threaten to injure the victim rather than physically harming them (Card, Stuckey, Sawalani, & Little, 2008; Tackett, Kushner, Herzhoff, Smack, & Reardon, 2014). Unlike a more persistent type of abuse, verbal abuse, verbal aggression is a single incident of verbal or nonverbal (but not physical) aggressive threatening behavior. A nonconfrontational form of aggression, hidden aggression, takes place in secret like stealing, running away from school or home, or setting something on fire (Catanzaro, 2011). Shy children and children with weak family emotional support are more prone to such acts than their peers (Thomas, Bierman, & Powers, 2011).

RELATIONAL AGGRESSION

Relational aggression involves using the relationship as the means of harm, such as social exclusion, spreading rumors and malicious gossip, giving the silent treatment, or threatening to withdraw friendship (Mathieson, Klimes-Dougan, & Crick, 2014). Relational aggression encompasses manipulation, rejection, shunning, ostracism, slander, and social exclusion. Examples include sending the target cruel notes, telling lies, spreading destructive rumors, peer exclusion, and shunning (Clinton et al., 2014). In early childhood, relational aggression is carried out in a direct fashion when the identity of the perpetrator is known. For example, a child may tell a peer "you're not my friend anymore" or spread rumors about a peer within close proximity. Because relational aggression is evoked with a desired goal of disrupting human relationships (circulating malicious rumors, for instance), relational aggression is considered a subtype of proactive aggression (Kawabata, Tseng, & Crick, 2014). Relational aggression occurs most frequently in girls (Loflin & Barry, 2016; Pitula, Murray-Close, Banny, & Crick, 2015). Victims of relational aggression are not able to meet basic needs for friendship, they feel unhappy and desperate, and they often react impulsively (Swearer, Espelage, Vaillancourt, & Hymel, 2010).

■ BULLYING

In the past 15 years, public recognition of the devastating effects of bullying and the need for effective ways of preventing it have soared. Public service announcements, books, movies, rigorous scientific studies, and education laws on bullying enacted in all 50 states demonstrate the growing concern about peer bullying (National Academies of Science, Engineering, and Medicine, 2016; The Bully Project, 2014). Bullying prevention policies are usually the responsibility of state and local education authorities; they also are a growing part of public health and juvenile justice policies (Gladden, Vivolo-Kantor, Hamburger, & Lumpkin, 2014; Masiello & Schroeder, 2014; National Academies of Science, Engineering, and Medicine, 2016; Vessey, DeFazio & Strout, 2013).

The CDC developed an evidence-based uniform definition of bullying as

> any unwanted aggressive behavior(s) by another youth or group of youths who are not siblings or current dating partners that involves an observed or perceived power imbalance and is repeated multiple times or is highly likely to be repeated. Bullying may inflict harm or distress on the targeted

youth including physical, psychological, social, or educational harm. (Gladden et al., 2014, p. 7)

National surveys provide data on prevalence and types of bullying. For 2015, among students between 12 and 18 years of age, the highest rates of bullying were for students in sixth and seventh grade (31% and 25%, respectively). The lowest rates were reported by students in 11th and 12th grades (16% and 15%, respectively; U.S. Department of Education, Institute for Education Science, National Center for Education Statistics, 2017b).

In the 2014–2015 academic year, approximately 20% of all students between 12 and 18 years reported being bullied at school. This is a decrease from the high figure of 32% reported in 2007 (U.S. Department of Education, Institute of Education Statistics, National Center for Education Statistics, 2017a). One of the factors most likely to "limit schools' efforts to reduce or prevent crime" was lack of effective alternative placements or programs for "disruptive students" (30%; Diliberti, Jackson, & Kemp, 2017, p. 4). Indeed, students who bully or display other forms of aggression or disruptive behavior should be assessed for underlying etiologies and referred to appropriate social and mental health services.

Scholars, educators, clinicians, and policy makers have increasingly viewed bullying as a group phenomenon involving the child or youth who is bullied, the one who bullies, and those who observe or witness the bullying behavior (National Academy of Science, Engineering, and Medicine, 2016; Salmivali, 2010). This framework is useful for education and healthcare professionals because it acknowledges how bullying can have negative impacts on children and youth bullied, as well as those who bullied and observed bullying. This view further supports the importance of addressing the emotional and other health needs of all children involved in bullying (Salmivali, 2010).

Cyberbullying, Suicide, and Related Issues

There is consensus among bullying scholars that cyberbullying has similar dynamics as bullying on playgrounds and other settings but is different because it can be anonymous and has the potential to be rapidly and widely disseminated. Despite widespread concern about the dangers of cyberbullying, an evidence-based definition has yet to be determined (National Institute of Justice, 2016). P-PCPs can provide anticipatory guidance and recognize possible signs of bullying, including cyberbullying. (e.g., avoiding school, academic struggles, increased anxiety, reporting health problems, and detachment from friends; Moreno & Vaillancourt, 2017). Because children might not know that P-PCPs care about bullying, clinicians need to include it as part of anticipatory guidance and well-child visits (Moreno & Vaillancourt, 2017; Vessey, DeFazio, & Strout, 2017).

The relationship between suicide and bullying is another emerging area of inquiry. Although many children and youth who committed suicide had histories of being bullied or bullying, there is insufficient evidence to establish a consistent causal relationship. Moreover, confounding factors, such as depression and social isolation, need to be considered. Further research is needed to establish the pathways between bullying and suicide (National Academies of Science, Engineering, & Medicine, 2016).

■ THE ROLE OF P-PCPs

The chapter has addressed behavioral problems in a school setting. Major points are that such issues require engagement of diverse stakeholders including students, parents, educators, health and social service personnel, and sometimes juvenile justice experts. Behavioral problems of one child can affect other children and require assessment of etiology, manifestations, and consequences as they pertain to a child's family and home, school, community, and lifelong trajectory.

To effectively work with students who exhibit behavioral challenges in school settings, P-PCPs need to communicate with many individuals including parents, teachers, school health and psychosocial personnel (such as social workers, psychologists, nurses, and guidance counselors). P-PCPs also need to know their state policies on bullying prevention and reporting, school health, school nursing, and juvenile justice as it pertains to students whose disruptive behavior results in suspension, expulsion, or placement in a juvenile justice facility. Familiarity with federal policies, such as the Individual Disabilities Education Act (Pub.L. 101-476) and the Family Educational Rights and Privacy Act (Pub.L. 93-380), which protect privacy of students' educational records, is also important.

■ SUMMARY

P-PCPs can encounter difficulties with assessment, intervention, and appropriate referral for children who exhibit aggressive behaviors. Initially, P-PCPs may have difficulty differentiating between "normal" aggression as part of growing up and "abnormal" aggressive behavior that leads to pathology. Later challenges arise when P-PCPs must define or characterize the exact problematic nature of a child's behavior (Crotty, Dood, & Lyns, 2013). The ability of P-PCPs, including school nurses, to recognize, understand, assess, and document various types of aggressive behaviors remains essential for directing prevention intervention and management of aggressive behavior in school settings (Oliver, Wehby, & Reschly, 2011) to intercept problem behaviors.

In discussing behavioral problems with teachers and parents, it's important for P-PCPs to remember that descriptions of aggressive behaviors vary in severity, frequency, and seriousness of the acts themselves. Urge teachers and parents to observe and report the exact behaviors, their duration, possible catalysts, and impacts of the behaviors on the student, peers, and classroom learning. Observers of behaviors should describe behaviors along a continuum from moderately challenging to aggressive in nature. Observers should also remark on the possible perceived social outcomes or impacts of the respective behaviors (Thomas, Connor & Scott, 2015).

Bullying is one form of aggression that frequently occurs in schools. Knowledge of risk factors, manifestations, and possible consequences of bullying is important. Children may not think that P-PCPs are interested in bullying experiences. Hence, it is important for P-PCPs to convey to educators and family members that bullying and other aggressions require a team approach that includes healthcare professionals.

■ REFERENCES

Aloia, L. S., & Solomon, D. H. (2016). Emotions associated with verbal aggression expression and suppression. *Western Journal of Communication, 80*(1), 3–20. doi:10.1080/10570314.2014.943428

American Civil Liberties Union. (n.d.). *Your right to equality in education.* Retrieved from https://www.aclu.org/other/your-right-equality-education

Andrade, B. F., Sorge, G. B., Na, J. J., & Wharton-Shukster, E. (2015). Clinical profiles of children with disruptive behaviors based on the severity of their conduct problems, callous–unemotional traits and emotional difficulties. *Child Psychiatry & Human Development, 46*(4), 567–576. doi:10.1007/s10578-014-0497-8

Angus, D. J., Schutter, D. J. L. G., Terburg, D., van Honk, J., & Harmon-Jones, E. (2016). A review of social neuroscience research on anger and aggression. In E. Harmon-Jones & M. Inzlicht (Eds.) (pp. 223–246). New York, NY: Routledge.

Barth, J. M., Dunlap, S. T., Dane, H., Lochman, J. E., & Wells, K. C. (2004). Classroom environment influences on aggression, peer relations, and academic focus. *Journal of School Psychology, 42*(2), 115–133.

Broidy, L. M., Nagin, D. S., Tremblay, R. E., Bates, J. E., Brame, B., Dodge, K. A., . . . & Lynam, D. R. (2003). Developmental trajectories of childhood disruptive behaviors and adolescent delinquency: A six-site, cross-national study. *Developmental Psychology, 39*(2), 222–245. doi:10.1037/0012-1649.39.2.222

Card, N. A., & Little, T. D. (2006). Proactive and reactive aggression in childhood and adolescence: A meta-analysis of differential relations with psychosocial adjustment. *International Journal of Behavioral Development, 30*(5), 466–480.

Card, N. A., Stucky, B. D., Sawalani, G. M., & Little, T. D. (2008). Direct and indirect aggression during childhood and adolescence: A meta-analytic review of gender differences, intercorrelations, and relations to maladjustment. *Child Development, 79*(5), 1185–1229. doi:10.1111/j.1467-8624.2008.01184.x

Carson, V., Hunter, S., Kuzik, N., Wiebe, S. A., Spence, J. C., Friedman, A., . . . Hinkley, T. (2016). Systematic review of physical activity and cognitive development in early childhood. *Journal of Science and Medicine in Sport, 19*(7), 573–578. doi:10.1016/j.jsams.2015.07.011

Catanzaro, M. F. (2011). Indirect aggression, bullying and female teen victimization: A literature review. *Pastoral Care in Education, 29*(2), 83–101. doi:10.1080/02643944.2011.573495

Crotty, G., Doody, O., & Lyons, R. (2014). Identifying the prevalence of aggressive behaviour reported by Registered Intellectual Disability Nurses in residential intellectual disability services: an Irish perspective. *Advances in Mental Health and Intellectual Disabilities, 8*(3), 174–187.

Centers for Disease Control and Prevention. (n.d.). *The whole school, whole child, whole community model.* Retrieved from https://www.cdc.gov/healthyyouth/wscc/pdf/wscc_fact_sheet_508c.pdf?s_cid=tw-zaza-1081

Centers for Disease Control and Prevention. (2016a). *Adolescent health: Protective factors.* Retrieved from https://www.cdc.gov/healthyyouth/protective/index.htm

Centers for Disease Control and Prevention. (2016b). *Understanding bullying (fact sheet).* Retrieved from https://www.cdc.gov/violenceprevention/pdf/Bullying_Factsheet.pdf

Clinton, A., Crothers, L. M., Kolbert, J. B., Hughes, T. L., Schreiber, J. B., Schmitt, A. J., . . . Field, J. E. (2014). A cross-cultural investigation of relational and social aggression in female college students from Puerto Rico and the United States. *Journal of Aggression, Maltreatment & Trauma, 23*(2), 99–115. doi:10.1080/10926771.2014.872745

Conley, L., Marchant, M., & Caldarella, P. (2014). A comparison of teacher perceptions and research-based categories of student behavior difficulties. *Education, 134*(4), 439–451.

Crotty, G., Doody, O., & Lyons, R. (2014). Aggressive behaviour and its prevalence within five typologies. *Journal of Intellectual Disabilities, 18*(1), 76–89. doi:10.1177/1744629513511356

Demissie, A., & Brenner, N. (2017). Mental health and social services in schools: Variations by school characteristics—United States, 2014. *Mental Health and Prevention, 5*, 5–11. doi:10.1016/j.mhp.2016.11.002

Diliberti, M., Jackson, M., & Kemp, J. (2017). Crime, violence, discipline, and safety in U.S. public schools: Findings from the school survey on crime and safety: 2015–16 (NCES 2017-122). Retrieved from https://nces.ed.gov/pubs2017/2017122.pdf

Dodge, K. A., Bierman, K. L., Coie, J. D., Greenberg, M. T., Lochman, J. E., McMahon, R. J., . . . Conduct Problems Prevention Research Group. (2014). Impact of early intervention on psychopathology, crime, and well-being at age 25. *American Journal of Psychiatry, 172*(1), 59–70. doi:10.1176/appi.ajp.2014.13060786

Duncan, G. J., Kalil, A., & Ziol-Guest, K. M. (2013). Early childhood poverty and adult achievement, employment and health. *Family Matters*, *93*, 27–35.

Farnicka, M., & Grzegorzewska, I. (2016). Intrapersonal correlates of aggression in adolescents: Determinants of undertaking the role of the perpetrator and the victim. *Current Issues in Personality Psychology*, *3*, 25–35. doi:10.5114/cipp.2015.49940

Fite, P. J., Rubens, S. L., Preddy, T. M., Raine, A., & Pardini, D. A. (2014). Reactive/proactive aggression and the development of internalizing problems in males: The moderating effect of parent and peer relationships. *Aggressive Behavior*, *40*(1), 69–78. doi:10.1002/ab.21498

Gershoff, E. T. (2013). Spanking and child development: We know enough now to stop hitting our children. *Child Development Perspectives*, *7*(3), 133–137. doi:10.1111/cdep.12038

Gladden, R. M., Vivolo-Kantor, A. M., Hamburger, M. E., & Lumpkin, C. D. (2014). *Bullying surveillance among youths: Uniform definitions for public health and recommended data elements, Version 1.0*. Retrieved from https://www.cdc.gov/violenceprevention/pdf/bullying-definitions-final-a.pdf

Hasan, Y., Bègue, L., Scharkow, M., & Bushman, B. J. (2013). The more you play, the more aggressive you become: A long-term experimental study of cumulative violent video game effects on hostile expectations and aggressive behavior. *Journal of Experimental Social Psychology*, *49*(2), 224–227. doi:10.1016/j.jesp.2012.10.016

Jung, J., Krahé, B., & Busching, R. (2017). Differential risk profiles for reactive and proactive aggression. *Social Psychology*, *48*(2), 71–84. doi:10.1027/1864-9335/a000298

Juvonen, J., & Graham, S. (2014). Bullying in schools: The power of bullies and the plight of victims. *Annual Review of Psychology*, *65*, 159–185. doi:10.1146/annurev-psych-010213-115030

Kawabata, Y., Tseng, W. L., & Crick, N. R. (2014). Mechanisms and processes of relational and physical victimization, depressive symptoms, and children's relational-interdependent self-construals: Implications for peer relationships and psychopathology. *Development and Psychopathology*, *26*(3), 619–634. doi:10.1017/S0954579414000273

Keyes, M., Legrand, L. N., Iacono, W. G., & McGue, M. (2008). Parental smoking and adolescent problem behavior: An adoption study of general and specific effects. *American Journal of Psychiatry*, *165*(10), 1338–1344. doi:10.1176/appi.ajp.2008.08010125

Ledwell, M., & King, V. (2015). Bullying and internalizing problems: Gender differences and the buffering role of parental communication. *Journal of Family Issues*, *36*(5), 543–566. doi:10.1177/0192513X13491410

Legal Information Institute. (n.d.). *Local educational agency*. CFR Title 34, Subtitle B, Chapter III, Part 303, Subpart A, Section 303.23. Retrieved from https://www.law.cornell.edu/cfr/text/34/303.23

Lewallen, T. C., Hunt, H., Potts-Datema, W., Zaza, S., & Giles, W. (2015). The whole school, whole community, whole child model: A new approach for improving educational attainment and healthy development for students. *Journal of School Health*, *85*, 729–739. doi:10.1111/josh.12310

Loflin, D. C., & Barry, C. T. (2016). "You can't sit with us": Gender and the differential roles of social intelligence and peer status in adolescent relational aggression. *Personality and Individual Differences*, *91*, 22–26. doi:10.1016/j.paid.2015.11.048

Masiello, M. G., & Schroeder, D. (Eds.). (2014). *A public health approach to bullying prevention*. Washington, DC: American Public Health Association. doi:10.2105/9780875530413

Mathieson, L. C., Klimes-Dougan, B., & Crick, N. R. (2014). Dwelling on it may make it worse: The links between relational victimization, relational aggression, rumination, and depressive symptoms in adolescents. *Development and Psychopathology*, *26*(3), 735–747. doi:10.1017/S0954579414000352

Miettunen, J., Murray, G. K., Jones, P. B., Mäki, P., Ebeling, H., Taanila, A., . . . & Veijola, J. (2014). Longitudinal associations between childhood and adulthood externalizing and internalizing psychopathology and adolescent substance use. *Psychological Medicine*, *44*(8), 1727–1738. doi:10.1017/S0033291713002328

Moreno, M., & Vaillancourt T. (2017). The role of health care providers in cyberbullying. *The Canadian Journal of Psychiatry*, *62*(6), 364–367. doi:10.1177/0706743716684792

Muratori, P., Bertacchi, I., Guili, C., Lombardi, L., Bonetti, S., Nocentini, A., . . . Lochman, J. E. (2015). First adaptation of Coping Power program as a classroom-based prevention intervention on aggressive behaviors among elementary school children. *Prevention Science*, *16*(3), 432–439.

National Academies of Science, Engineering, and Medicine. (2016). *Preventing bullying through science, policy, and practice*. Retrieved from https://www.nap.edu/catalog/23482/preventing-bullying-through-science-policy-and-practice

National Association of Chronic Disease Directors. (2017). *Local health departments and school partnerships: Working together to build healthier schools.* Retrieved from http://c.ymcdn.com/sites/www.chronicdisease.org/resource/resmgr/school_health/NACDD_Health_Department_and_pdf

National Association of School Nurses. (2017a). Behavioral health of students, the school nurse's role in (Position Statement). Retrieved from https://www.nasn.org/advocacy/professional-practice-documents/position-statements/ps-behavioral-health

National Association of School Nurses. (2017b). *School nurses in the U.S.* Retrieved from https://higherlogicdownload.s3.amazonaws.com/NASN/3870c72d-fff9-4ed7-833f-215de278d256/UploadedImages/PDFs/Advocacy/2017_School_Nurses_in_the_Nation_Infographic_.pdf

National Institute of Justice. (2016). *Understanding cyberbullying: Developing an evidence-based definition.* Retrieved from http://nij.gov/topics/crime/pages/understanding-cyberbullying.aspx

Oliver, R. M., Wehby, J. H., & Reschly, D. J. (2011). Teacher classroom management practices: Effects on disruptive or aggressive student behavior. Society for Research on Educational Effectiveness. *Campbell Systematic Reviews.* doi:10.4073/csr.2011.4

Pitula, C. E., Murray-Close, D. Banny, A. M. & Crick, N. R. (2015). Prospective associations between peer aggression and victimization: The moderating roles of physiological stress reactivity and gender. *Social Development,* 24(3), 621–639.

Racz, S. J., O'Brennan, L. M., Bradshaw, C. P., & Leaf, P. J. (2016). The influence of family and teacher factors on early disruptive school behaviors: A latent profile transition analysis. *Journal of Emotional and Behavioral Disorders,* 24(2), 67–81. doi:10.1177/1063426615599541

Rajan, S., Namdar, R., & Ruggles, K. V. (2015). Aggressive and violent behaviors in the school environment among a nationally representative sample of adolescent youth. *Journal of School Health,* 85(7), 446–457. doi:10.1111/josh.12272

Rosell, D. R., & Siever, L. J. (2015). The neurobiology of aggression and violence. *CNS Spectrums,* 20(3), 254–279. doi:10.1017/S109285291500019X

Rubio-Garay, F., Carrasco, M. A., & Amor, P. J. (2016). Aggression, anger and hostility: Evaluation of moral disengagement as a mediational process. *Scandinavian Journal of Psychology,* 57(2), 129–135. doi:10.1111/sjop.12270

Salmivali, C. (2010). Bullying and the peer group: A review. *Aggression and Violent Behavior,* 15, 112–120. doi:10.1016/j.avb.2009.08.007

Shapka, J. D., & Maghsoudi, R. (2017). Examining the validity and reliability of the cyber-aggression and cyber-victimization scale. *Computers in Human Behavior,* 69, 10–17. doi:10.1016/j.chb.2016.12.015

Shechtman, Z., & Tutian, R. (2016). Teachers treat aggressive children: An outcome study. *Teaching and Teacher Education,* 58, 28–34. doi:10.1016/j.tate.2016.04.005

Smith, S. W., Daunic, A. P., Barber, B. R., Aydin, B., Van Loan, C. L., & Taylor, G. G. (2014). Preventing risk for significant behavior problems through a cognitive-behavioral intervention: Effects of the Tools for Getting Along curriculum at one-year follow-up. *The Journal of Primary Prevention,* 35(5), 371–387. doi:10.1007/s10935-014-0357-0

Soedjatmiko, S., Kadim, M., Madiyono, B., & Said, M. (2016). Behavior and emotional problems in children with mental retardation. *Paediatrica Indonesiana,* 44(3), 90–94. doi:10.14238/pi44.3.2004.90-4

Sroufe, L. A., Coffino, B., & Carlson, E. A. (2010). Conceptualizing the role of early experience: Lessons from the Minnesota longitudinal study. *Developmental Review,* 30(1), 36–51. doi:10.1016/j.dr.2009.12.002

Swearer, S. M., Espelage, D. L., Vaillancourt, T., & Hymel S. (2010). What can be done about school bullying? Linking research to educational practice. *Educational Researcher,* 39(1), 38–47.

Tackett, J. L., Kushner, S. C., Herzhoff, K., Smack, A. J., & Reardon, K. W. (2014). Viewing relational aggression through multiple lenses: Temperament, personality, and personality pathology. *Development and Psychopathology,* 26(3), 863–877. doi:10.1017/S0954579414000443

Tahirovic, S. (2015). Teachers' perception of aggressive behaviour in children: Case of Bosnia and Herzegovina. *Epiphany,* 8(1), 149–165. doi:10.21533/epiphany.v8i1.132

The Bully Project. (2014). *The bully project.* Retrieved from http://www.thebullyproject.com/

Thomas, D. E., Bierman, K. L., & Powers, C. J. (2011). The influence of classroom aggression and classroom climate on aggressive–disruptive behavior. *Child Development,* 82 (3), 751–757. doi:10.1111/j.1467-8624.2011.01586.x

Thomas, H. J., Connor, J. P., & Scott, J. G. (2015). Integrating traditional bullying and cyberbullying: Challenges of definition and measurement in adolescents–A review. *Educational Psychology Review,* 27(1), 135–152. doi:10.1007/s10648-014-9261-7

Thompson, A. M. (2011). A systematic review of evidence-based interventions for students with challenging behaviors in school settings. *Journal of Evidence-Based Social Work*, 8(3), 304–322. doi: 10.1080/15433714.2010.531220

U.S. Department of Education and U.S. Department of Justice. (2014). *Dear colleague letter: School enrollment procedures*. Retrieved from https://www2.ed.gov/about/offices/list/ocr/letters/colleague-201405.pdf

U.S. Department of Education, Institute for Education Science, National Center for Education Statistics. (2015a). *Number of educational institutions, by level and control of institution: Selected years, 1980–81 through 2013–14 (Table 105.50)*. Retrieved from https://nces.ed.gov/programs/digest/d15/tables/dt15_105.50.asp

U.S. Department of Education, Institute for Education Science, National Center for Education Statistics. (2015b). *Percentage of students ages 12–18 who reported being bullied at school during the school year, by type of bullying and selected student and school characteristics: Selected years, 2005 through 2013 (Table 230.45)*. Retrieved from https://nces.ed.gov/programs/digest/d14/tables/dt14_230.45.asp

U.S. Department of Education, Institute for Education Science, National Center for Education Statistics. (2017a). *English language learners in public schools*. Retrieved from https://nces.ed.gov/programs/coe/pdf/coe_cgf.pdf

U.S. Department of Education, Institute for Education Science, National Center for Education Statistics. (2017b). Student reports of bullying: Results from the 2015 school crime supplement to the national crime victimization survey (Web tables) (NCES 2017-015). Retrieved from https://nces.ed.gov/pubs2017/2017015.pdf

U.S. Department of Education, Office for Civil Rights. (2010). *Free appropriate public education for students with disabilities: Requirements under section 504 of the Rehabilitation Act of 1973*. Retrieved from https://www2.ed.gov/about/offices/list/ocr/docs/edlite-FAPE504.html

Vessey, J. A., DeFazio, R. L., & Strout, T. D. (2013). Youth bullying: A review of the science and a call to action. *Nursing Outlook*, 61, 337–345. doi:10.1016/j.outlook.2013.04.011

Walters, G. D., & Espelage, D. L. (2018). From victim to victimizer: Hostility, anger, and depression as mediators of the bullying victimization–bullying perpetration association. *Journal of School Psychology*, 68, 73–83.

Wilson, S. J., & Lipsey, M. W. (2007). School-based interventions for aggressive and disruptive behavior: Update of a meta-analysis. *American Journal of Preventive Medicine*, 33(2), S130–S143. doi:10.1016/j.amepre.2007.04.011

CHAPTER 22

Social Media and Behavioral Health: Normal and Abnormal Behaviors

MARY M. ROCK

The use of social media is as much a part of child and adolescent lifestyles today as paper, pencils, and books were used decades ago. Anticipatory guidance regarding the appropriate and beneficial use of social media to nurture developing minds, and the protection of children while using social media, is a critical focus of the advanced practitioner. Seventy-five percent of teenagers own cell phones, the most widely used social means for texting, messaging, and social media (Hinduja & Patchin, 2007), and that number is undoubtedly on the rise today with school-age children.

The definition of social media is "any website that allows social interaction, including Facebook, MySpace, Twitter, Snapchat, gaming sites, and video sites such as YouTube and blogs" (O'Keefe & Clarke-Pearson, 2011). Media no longer is a term exclusive to television and music videos—the past generation's influence on developing children. Practitioners are asked repeatedly by families for advice and guidelines regarding use of these social media sites and monitoring for potential problems (O'Keeffe & Clarke-Pearson, 2011).

Girls Matter!, research conducted by the Substance Abuse and Mental Health Service Administration (SAMHSA), found that girls ages 14 to 17 send and receive 100 texts daily, with information that is persistent, visible, searchable, and spreadable (https://www.samhsa.gov/women-children-families/trainings/girls-matter). Social media use may lead to an emotional roller coaster of connection as well as exclusion from peers. Practitioner education to families regarding the opportunities for social media use for mental and physical activity, writing, journaling, connecting, and relaxation is a way to promote positive mental health. There are multiple educational and self-esteem-building sites for children and adolescents, as well as online resources for parents. Examples include conversation tips and resources regarding social media, bullying, and underage drinking that can be used as reinforcement of anticipatory guidance on well-child visits. The nurse practitioner (NP) is in a unique position to help families explore these sites and also monitor for problems such as bullying, depression, sexting, and inappropriate or fraudulent sites (O'Keeffe & Clarke-Pearson, 2011).

■ LITERATURE REVIEW

We are just now beginning to see the results of research studies demonstrating negative and positive effects of social media use (Rosen, 2011). Positive effects include learning "virtual empathy" for others, the practice of socialization for introverted individuals, and the availability of innovative tools for educational learning and advancing technical skills (Lenhart, 2015). Safety reasons for cell phone use include the allowance of cell phones for family contact when away from home and even in the school setting, with an increase in allowed school use after the recurrent incidences of school shootings.

The potential harmful effects of social media plague parents and clinicians alike. Daily overuse of social media makes children prone to psychological disorders such as anxiety, depression, and sleep disorders. Health issues such as poor diet and exercise habits and obesity can occur with the habitual overuse of social media. Research shows teens that obsessively overuse social media, including gaming and Facebook, tend to develop narcissistic tendencies, aggression, mania, and antisocial tendencies. Last, the dangers of sexting are all too real, with worst-case scenarios of children becoming victims of child pornography, assaults, and abduction (Kaiser Family Foundation, 2010).

The American Academy of Child and Adolescent Psychiatry (AACAP) reports that 60% of 13- to 17-year-olds spend more than 2 hours per day on social networking sites. Although connection to friends, developing new contacts, sharing self-expression, and developing an individual identity are benefits of social networking, it also exposes children and adolescents to the risks of cyberbullying, vulnerability to predators, sharing information that cannot be retrieved or rescinded, and reduced time for physical activities (AACAP, 2011). Recent studies document increased media use, with the average child between 8 and 18 years old spending 7.5 hours daily using media. Children take in and imitate media behavior, including violence (Kaiser Family Foundation, 2010). Excessive media use also results in increased alcohol and tobacco use (Gidwani, Sobol, DeJong, Perrin, & Gortmaker, 2002).

Vulnerable children are learning to use social media sites, and today, toddlers can be seen using and accessing their own tablets in restaurants, shopping centers and preschools. The ability to click access sites is appealing to children's impulsive curiosity and needs for immediate gratification (AACAP, 2015). NP guidance regarding safe restricted use for developmental ages and stages is imperative.

The Pew Research Center 2015 study researched social media use by a national representative sample of thousands of teens. The study reveals that 88% of teens have access to a mobile phone, with the highest use by African Americans at 71%. Up to 20% of teens go online constantly, with Facebook remaining the most used site. There is a distinct pattern of increased use in households with a family income of less than $50,000 annually. Girls dominate social media, with 84% of boys choosing video games instead. The typical teen has at least 145 Facebook friends. Facebook remains the favorite social media site, but in higher income families, Instagram is also used for sharing photos, as well as Twitter and Snapchat (Lenhart, 2015).

■ DANGERS OF SOCIAL MEDIA USE BY CHILDREN AND ADOLESCENTS

Genetic makeup is known to be an important component of the development of positive mental health in children; however, environmental exposure, social circumstances, and behavioral patterns account for 70% of mental health determinants. Prevention of mental health issues includes anticipatory guidance related to wise social media use. Clinic-based interventions focus on positive use of social media, mitigating risks, and the prevention of rampant bullying to build healthier communities as a whole. Addressing social media use with families in clinical practice through counseling, education, and intervention is a vital. Social media use can also be a springboard to address socioeconomic, cultural, and political issues in families, just as radio and television were in the past.

Promotion of accessing health information is part of health information technology building regarding subjects such as sexually transmitted diseases, depression, suicide prevention, and addiction, which are all readily available on social media, as well as resource information and hotlines. Applications better known as "apps" are available for such things as healthcare adherence, sleep and rest, better disease understanding, and communicating with health practitioners (Lenhart, Purcell, Smith, & Zickur, 2010). The NP can promote health information technology and web sharing of laboratory and healthcare data. Optimal up-to-date practitioners today are building websites with information for their individual practices.

■ RISKS OF SOCIAL MEDIA USE

Most pediatric primary care providers (P-PCPs) recall the mantras of their parents:, "Don't talk to strangers," "Don't open the door if you are home alone," but social media has left the door wide open to every opportunistic adventure, some of which can be deadly. Parents can monitor children who come to play, meet families at school events, but they are unable to meet or screen social media friends and strangers their child may wander upon. For children and preteens in particular, social media access can be no different than a walk alone in the woods, or wandering the city alone at night. Dangers include accessing inappropriate sites, exposure to hate violence and pornography, and loss of private information including demographic and identifying information (AACAP, 2015). Teaching a child to *never* meet someone they have met online is imperative. Anticipatory guidance to parents and children that everything seen or read online is not true is also important. Children are very aware of school guidelines for Internet use and homes should follow similar guidelines.

Decreased personal social skills, physical activity, and lack of exercise are known risk factors of overuse of social media. Children have limited capacity for self-regulation and are susceptible to peer pressure on media sites. Sexting and sexual experimentation online is a very real problem. Teens rank media as the second leading source of information regarding sexual activity after sex education in the school. Increased exposure to sexually explicit social media increases the risk of pregnancy twofold (Escobar-Chaves, Tortolero, Markham, Low, & Eitel, 2005). Cybersex is defined as a virtual sexual encounter via social media and contributes to the growing threat of sex crimes against children (Wolak, Mitchell, & Finkelhor, 2003).

■ SOCIAL MEDIA OVERUSE

A problem of social media overuse is Internet addiction and sleep deprivation. Overuse of social media takes away from adequate quantity and quality of sleep, with adolescents often sleeping with phones turned on and texting throughout the night-time. Poor sleep leads to impaired regulation of metabolism and immune function, and leads to school and behavior problems (Zimmerman, 2008). Texting while driving can be deadly. "No texting while driving" education and contracts have helped to decrease accidents due to texting, along with devices in newer cars and smartphone apps which include automobile phone shut off devices.

■ KNOWLEDGE AND TECHNICAL SKILL GAP

A knowledge and technical skill gap between parents and children, and even providers, can create a disconnect between the child's social media world and adults (Jenkins, Clinton, Purushotma, Robinson, & Weigel, 2006). Some parents may need guidance regarding social media monitoring. One directive for guidance is the Children's Online Privacy Protection Act (COPPA), which prohibits by law the collection of information on children younger than 13 years and regulates the prohibition of social profiles by children younger than 13. The American Academy of Pediatrics strongly encourages use of that guideline (O'Keeffe & Clarke- Pearson, 2011).

Risks to social media use do occur, and worst-case scenarios are often seen and advertised by the media itself. Cyberbullying, the deliberate use of social media to communicate hostile information about another person, is quite common and can lead to profound psychosocial problems including depression, isolation, and suicide (Hinduja & Patchin, 2010). Over half of today's adolescents have been cyberbullied, and 25% of them repeatedly. Nine out of 10 adolescents never report this to anyone, and multiple studies have found a relationship between cyberbullying and suicidality (Kim & Leventhal, 2008).

■ SEXTING

Sexting is defined as the "sending and receiving of sexually explicit messages or images via phone, computer or digital device." Surveys have found that 20% of teens have sent or received nude pictures, an act that has led to school suspensions, dismissals, and felony charges (Berkshire District Attorney, 2010).

■ FACEBOOK DEPRESSION

Facebook depression is a new term identified in research for preadolescents who surf Facebook and blogs for help, and find blogs that may promote substance abuse, unsafe sexual practices, or aggressive and dangerous behaviors (Davida & Starr, 2009). These children may be the risk takers, socially awkward, or "lost souls" that try to find a place to identify and often wander into the wrong people or places on social media. They may find themselves in a dark hole that leads them further and further away from family and personal contact, and into the hands of dangerous strangers.

Last, pop-up ads target viewers based on their roving social media activity and can be powerful influences on children and adolescents. Educating families on these tactics and manipulation of young minds is important. The digital footprint of online exploring can cause future reputation issues and put children at risk for fraudulent activity. Today schools and future employers may follow their nonerasable social media footprint. Social media has even been used to make arrests for underage or illegal activities.

■ SUMMARY OF GUIDANCE FOR P-PCPs

The role of the P-PCPs in shaping the health of children and adolescents regarding social media is to educate families on the healthy use of social media to promote and expand development while avoiding the dangers. New opportunities for children and adolescent engagement in charity, political, and philanthropic community events exist, and social media provides rich opportunities for children, adolescents, and families to look outside themselves. Sharing creative ideas with others in interest groups exposes children to diverse backgrounds and cultures they may have not been able to connect with in the past.

Developmental guidance, especially for young children who are particularly vulnerable due to difficulty discriminating between reality and fiction, is needed (American Academy of Pediatrics [AAP], 2001). Adolescence and preadolescent social media overuse and cyberbullying are risk factors for depression and suicide. The AACAP also recommends that children and adolescents restrict public access of their sites, omit full identifying data, and only post what they would want seen by *anyone*. Parents need to keep open communication regarding appropriate use, not just police their posts. Guidelines on rules that are clearly defined and limits on time and type of use are a frequent topic at provider well-child check-ups.

Helping parents to understand child and adolescent issues on and off social media can seem like a complex task to practitioners. Serious issues include bullying, depression, risk taking, social anxiety, substance abuse, and suicide. Practitioners can help parents to understand how to use social media as a bridge to a more solid family connection. Talking to children about today's social pressures in a nonjudgmental way, developing a family online-use plan, regular family meetings to discuss online topics, and emphasizing healthy behaviors and respect for others is healthy promotion of social media. Use of the American Academy of Pediatrics online resources and development of a practitioner website connecting these resources are optimal ways of providing expansive information for families (O'Keeffe & Clarke-Pearson, 2011). The advanced practitioner that learns, uses, and demonstrates social media use for families is the bridge to positive physical and mental health for today's developing families.

■ **REFERENCES**

American Academy of Child and Adolescent Psychiatry. (2011). *Children and social networking.* Facts for Families No. 100. Retrieved from http://www.aacap.org

American Academy of Child and Adolescent Psychiatry. (2015). *Internet use in children.* Facts for Families No. 59. Retrieved from http://www.aacap.org

American Academy of Pediatrics. (2001). Children, adolescents, and television. *Pediatrics, 107*(2), 423–425. doi:10.1542/peds.107.2.423

Berkshire District Attorney. (2010). *Sexting.* Pittsfield, MA. Retrieved from https://www.mass.gov/?pageid=berterminal&L=3&L1=crime+awareness+%26+prevention+L2=parents+%26+Youth&sid=Dber

Davida, J. S., & Starr, L. E. (2009). Romantic and sexual activities, parent–adolescent stress, and depressive symptoms in early adolescent girls. *Journal of Adolescence, 32*(4), 909–924. doi:10.1016/j.adolescence.2008.10.004

Escobar-Chaves, S., Tortolero, S., Markham, C., Low, B., & Eitel, P. (2005). Impact of the media on media on adolescent sexual attitudes and behaviors. *Supplement to Pediatrics, 116*(1), 297–331.

Gidwani, P., Sobol, A., DeJong, W., Perrin, J., & Gortmaker, S. (2002). Television viewing and initiation of smoking among youth. *Pediatrics, 110*(3), 505–508. doi:10.1542/peds.110.3.505

Hinduja, S., & Patchin, J. (2007). Offline consequences of online victimization: School violence and delinquency. *Journal of School Violence, 6*(3), 89–112. doi:10.1300/J202v06n03_06

Hinduja, S., & Patchin, J. (2010). Bullying, cyberbullying, and suicide. *Archives of Suicide Research, 14*(3), 206–221. doi:10.1080/13811118.2010.494133

Jenkins, H., Clinton, K., Purushotma, R., Robinson, A., & Weigel, M. (2006). *Empowering parents and protecting children in an evolving media landscape.* Retrieved from MacArthur Foundation; http://digitallearning.macfound.org/atf/cf/{7E45C7E0-4B89-AC9C-E807E4E}/JENKINS_WHITE_PAPER.PDF

Kaiser Family Foundation. (2010). *Generation M2: Media in the lives of 8- to 18-year-olds.* A Kaiser Family Foundation Study. Retrieved from http://kaiserfamilily foundation.files.wordpress.com/2013/01/8010.pdf

Kim, Y., & Leventhal, B. (2008). Bullying and suicide: A review. *International Journal of Adolescent Mental Health, 20*, 133–154. doi:10.1515/IJAMH.2008.20.2.133

Lenhart, A. (2015). *Teens, social media & technology overview 2015.* Retrieved from Pew Research Center; http://www.pewinternet.org/2015/04/09/teens-social-media-technology-2015/

Lenhart, A., Purcell, K., Smith, A., & Zickur, K. (2010). *Social media and young adults.* Retrieved from Pew Research Center; http://pewinternet.org/Reports/2010/Social_Media_and_Young_Adults.aspx

O'Keeffe, G. S., & Clarke- Pearson, K. (2011). Clinical report—The impact of social media on children, adolescents and families. *Pediatrics,* 800–804. doi:10.1542/peds.2011-0054

Rosen, L. (2011). *Social networking's good and bad impact on kids.* Retrieved from http://www.apa.org

Wolak, J., Mitchell, K., & Finkelhor, D. (2003). *Internet sex crimes agianst minors: The response of law enforcement.* University of New Hampshire: National Center for Missing and Exploited Children. Alexandria, VA: National Center for Missing & Exploited Children

Zimmerman, F. (2008). *Children's media use and sleep problems: Issues and unanswered questions.* Retrieved from Kaiser Family Foundation; http://www.kff.org

SECTION VI

Adolescent Population

CHAPTER 23

Identifying and Intercepting Behavioral Health Problems in Adolescents

JEANETTE F. GREEN

Adolescence is a critical transition period within the life course during which adolescents experience rapid and substantial changes in physical, sociocultural, psychological, emotional, behavioral, and cognitive growth and development. Typically, this period is considered the transition from childhood toward adulthood (Dunn & Fisher, 2004; Lassi, Salam, Das, Wazny, & Bhutta, 2015; Rew, 2005; Sawyer et al., 2012). The World Health Organization (WHO) considers adolescence to encompass ages 10 to 19 years. However, other authors suggest more distinct phases within adolescence consisting of early adolescence (10–13 years), middle adolescence (14–17 years), and late adolescence (18–21 years; Rew, 2005) or emerging adulthood (18–29 years), a widely known concept in developmental psychology (Arnett, Žukauskienė, & Sugimura, 2014). While aforementioned age ranges may be distinct, the timing and tempo of adolescent development varies among individuals (Golub et al., 2008; Graber, Nichols, & Brooks-Gunn, 2010; Malina, Rogol, Cumming, Coelho e Silva, & Figueiredo, 2015). Variance among adolescents' development is particularly salient for provision of healthcare by pediatric primary care providers (P-PCPs). The long-term effects of physical and behavioral health or disorders and risks for behavioral health disorders during adolescence and emerging adulthood (EA) impact health in later adult life (Viner et al., 2015). Assessment of the adolescent requires knowledge about typical developmental stages among adolescents and immediate recognition of atypical development to *intercept* atypical behaviors to improve healthcare outcomes. This chapter provides an analysis of adolescent brain growth and development, typical physical development, and the interrelationship of brain growth and physical development to social, emotional, and behavioral development during the entire adolescent and emerging adult age span, with a focus on evidence-based behavioral interventions to immediately *intercept* atypical behaviors.

■ ADOLESCENT BRAIN DEVELOPMENT

Adolescence is a period of rapid brain growth and development across body systems, second only to fetal and infant development. This period results in rapid somatic growth, brain development, sexual maturation, and attainment of reproductive capacity. Advanced understanding of brain parenchyma maturation throughout the life course has been facilitated by technological advancements in diagnostic testing such as functional MRI, structural MRI, and diffusion tensor imaging. Typical adolescent brain structural changes include cortical thinning and white matter maturation in adjacent neural tracks (Tamnes et al., 2010). Cortical areas involved with complex thinking and fine motor skills are fully developed while areas controlled by the frontal lobe involved with abstract thinking, emotion, and judgment continue to develop into adulthood (Toledo et al., 2012). During this time frame, significant neural synaptic pruning and substantial neural circuitry reorganization occurs (Konrad, Firk, & Uhlhaas, 2013). To that end, the adolescent brain experiences substantial growth and development, especially the prefrontal cortex that is responsible for executive functions of abstract thinking, reasoning, judgment, decision making, emotions, and personality.

■ ONSET OF PUBERTY

The physiologic underpinning of adolescent biologic development is the onset of puberty. Puberty, a phase in the continuum of normative gonadal development, is the activation of the hypothalamus–pituitary–gonadal (HPG) system that began in utero. The trigger of HPG system activation is unknown to date, but has been found to initiate complex processes that result in gene expression and changes in neurotransmitter and hormonal activity such as increased release of gonadotropin-releasing hormone (GnRH) resulting in physical changes (Holder & Blaustein, 2014). Physical changes follow a typical, sequential pattern with thelarche (e.g., breast tissue development), adrenarche (e.g., pubic hair development), and menarche (e.g., first menstruation). The timing and onset of neuroendocrine changes are influenced by both modifiable (e.g., nutrition, sleep, physical activity, stress) and nonmodifiable factors (e.g., sex, genetics, race/ethnicity) accounting for variation amongst adolescent development. HPG activation has been found to be interconnected with other physiological changes associated with adolescent growth and maturation (Andersen, 2016).

Cognitive Control and Brain Development

Refinement of cognitive control over behavior and emotional reactions is a primary task among adolescents. Contemporary models of emotional changes during adolescence consider a gradually emerging modulatory control neural system (Guyer, Silk, & Nelson, 2016). Emotionality peaks in early adolescence followed by adolescents' emerging ability to exert greater self-control over behaviors and emotions (Guyer et al., 2016) due to increasing inhibitory control over striatal and limbic regions (Casey et al., 2016; Shulman et al., 2016). Substantial neural remodeling occurs predominantly in brain areas involved in emotion and learning, such as the prefrontal cortex, hippocampus, amygdala, and nucleus accumbens (Guyer et al., 2016). The dopaminergic system and cognitive control processes differ in their developmental timing, thus leading to heightened responses to socio-emotional cues while cognitive controls (e.g., executive function and emotional regulation) lag behind. Additionally, salient memories are made during adolescence, in part due to the interrelationships between the anterior cingulate cortex and other brain regions.

As adolescence is a critical period for brain development, the adolescent brain is uniquely vulnerable to socio-environmental factors (Brenhouse et al., 2008). Socio-environmental factors include peer relationships (Kilford et al., 2016), rewarding stimuli (e.g., substance or alcohol use or abuse), or sexual activity (Steinberg, 2008). The dose–response of these factors may lead to a depressive phenotype, addiction, early pregnancy, or even premature death (Beltz, Corley, Bricker, Wadsworth, & Berenbaum, 2014). Thus, it is critically important for P-PCPs to consider factors that may be influential to behavioral health, such as pubertal timing, genetics, quality of family and peer relationships, stress processes, social determinants of health, and other health concerns to provide comprehensive healthcare for each adolescent and to intercept behavioral problems with evidence-based interventions.

Disruptions in typical developmental processes may negatively influence adolescent brain development, manifesting as behavioral problems or psychopathology. Pubertal timing has been associated with a range of internalizing and externalizing behaviors and disorders such as depression, substance abuse, and eating disorders in adolescents among both males and females (Graber et al., 2010). Timing of pubertal development is important for psychological development in adolescence and beyond and serves as a source of psychological risk, as a contributor to normative change, and as a trigger for psychopathology in vulnerable youth (Ge & Natsuaki, 2009; Graber et al., 2010; Gunnar et al., 2009; Negriff & Susman, 2011; Trotman et al., 2013). Typical ages for pubertal changes differ for children based on the area of the world in which they live; presence of secondary sex characteristics in U.S. girls younger than age 6 (Black girls) or age 7 (White girls) or boys younger than age 9 are considered abnormal pubertal onset (Golub et al., 2008). Presence of secondary sexual characteristics at an earlier age than one's peer group leads to physical differences observable to their peers. Despite the normality of puberty and the development of sexual characteristics, the impact on *psychological health* among those who appear different than their peers should not be underestimated. Early pubertal timing among girls has been associated with higher internalizing disorders such as anxiety, depressive symptoms, and eating disorders (Pomerantz, Parent, Forehand, Breslend, & Winer, 2017), or externalizing disorders such as substance use and conduct disorders (Kaltiala-Heino et al., 2003). Evidence related to the tempo of progressing through pubertal Tanner stages and behavioral health is conflicting (Marceau, Ram, Houts, Grimm, & Susman, 2011); however, emerging evidence suggests a rapid tempo through Tanner stages may influence internalizing disorders.

In general, biological development and physical characteristics do not occur with perfect synchrony, with approximately half of girls exhibiting breast development prior to the onset of other morphological changes, for example, body composition, acceleration in skeletal growth, genital development, and the growth of body hair. Although some degree of asynchrony in morphological development is not uncommon, these variations have long been theorized to influence psychological well-being. Pubertal asynchrony may contribute to *depressive symptoms*, especially among girls (Thompson, Hammen, & Brennan, 2016).

With the emergence of advanced technology to study the adolescent brain, research related to factors influential to adolescent brain development and consequential onset of behavioral health issues continues to develop. An extensive review of this literature is beyond the scope of this text; thus, brief descriptions about such factors will sensitize P-PCPs to consider a comprehensive assessment of the adolescent. For example, pro-inflammatory responses may impact brain development and behavior, suggesting immune regulation during brain development may be an important consideration for care management (Bilbo & Schwarz, 2012).

Self-Identity Versus Identify Diffusion

The most significant psychosocial task of adolescence is construction of an identity through integration of physical, social, cognitive, behavioral, and psychological experiences acquired during earlier ages and developmental phases (Erickson, 1950, 1959; Wright, Betz, & Yearwood, 2012). Erickson's description of developmental tasks across the life span remain integral in healthcare provider assessment of the adolescent (Hagan, Shaw, & Duncan, 2017). The developmental task of adolescence is to establish identity or experience identity diffusion (Rew, 2005; Wright et al., 2012). Identity diffusion refers to an adolescent who has not realized his or her social identity and is not ready to accomplish this task. The development of self-identity is a dynamic, interactive process between one's self and the social world that is constructed over time through social interaction (Bowers, 1989; Rew, 2005). Self-identity is directly and indirectly interdependent on multiple factors such as genetics, physical appearance, experience, temperament, reciprocal relationships, and environments (Bronfenbrenner, 1979, 1994a, 1994b, 2005; Lau, Fox, & Cheung, 2006; Rew, 2005).

Cognitive, Moral, and Spiritual Development

Adolescence is also a period of cognitive, moral, and spiritual development, with distinct processes to achieve each developmental phase. Cognitively, concrete thinking in early adolescence transitions to more abstract thoughts throughout the developmental process. Information processing, critical thinking, and ascertaining consequences of actions evolve during adolescence. Adolescents begin to consider values and morals and become observant of contradictory behaviors, for example, parents drinking alcohol but telling the adolescent not to drink because it is bad for him or her. Faith development theorists describe adolescence as the period in which they operationalize faith or beliefs lived out through their personal experiences. Adolescents embark on their personal journey to form and operationalize a spirituality, and morality, that is their own and separate from their parents. Through this process, adolescents incorporate their past experiences when projecting their meaningful future pursuits. Spirituality among adolescents has been described in terms of wisdom, connectedness, joy, wonder, moral sensitivity, and compassion (Michaelson, Brooks, & Jirasek, 2016).

Risk behaviors consisting of actions that may jeopardize physical, cognitive, emotional, or behavioral health are often present during adolescence. While many adolescents engage in experimentation and risky behaviors, not all will encounter negative outcomes. Socio-ecological factors are influential in risk behaviors; for example, adolescents whose role models engage in risk behaviors, such as physical, emotional, or sexual abuse and illiteracy, whereas protective behaviors may include academic success, parental support, and/or, community engagement (Table 23.1).

■ DEVELOPMENTAL SCREENING AND ASSESSMENT

At least 20% of U.S. adolescents and emerging adults have experience with a behavioral health, mental health, or substance use disorder. These disorders among adolescents and emerging adults are associated with risks for eating disorders, mood disorders, suicide, injury, risky sexual or drug activity, early pregnancy, and inability to reach their academic or employment potential. Despite the implications of these disorders among adolescents, only one third of adolescents with a diagnosable disorder receive the appropriate care (Richardson, McCarty, Radovic, & Ballonoff Suleiman, 2017). Therefore, screening for physical, emotional, social, behavioral, and psychological problems that represent normal behaviors and behaviors that provide the initial evidence of behavioral health problems are important considerations for P-PCPs. The intercepting behavioral health (IBH) hypothesizes that the earlier a behavioral health problem can be identified and intercepted, the more likely the adolescent will have improved healthcare outcomes.

TABLE 23.1

BEHAVIORAL HEALTH SCREENING TOOLS FOR ADOLESCENTS

Instrument	
Personal Health Questionnaire–2 (PHQ-2)	Two-item questionnaire for depression
Personal Health Questionnaire–9 (PHQ-9)	Nine-item questionnaire for depression. The PHQ-9 is used if the PHQ-2 is positive
CRAFFT	Specific questions screen for drug and alcohol use
Audit-C	Specific questions only for alcohol use
Generalized Anxiety Disorder–7 (GAD-7)	Seven-item screen for anxiety

Information and public access for each of these screening tools can be found on the SMASHA website (https://www.samhsa.gov).

■ HEALTHCARE DECISION MAKING BY ADOLESCENTS

While parents or caregivers may accompany adolescents to their healthcare visits, it is imperative that P-PCPs recognize the dynamics of the parent–adolescent and parent–emerging adult dyads. Many adolescents express the desire for a larger role in their healthcare decision making; however, data reveal that healthcare providers often direct communication to parents rather than the adolescent (Lipstein, Muething, Dodds, & Britto, 2013). Another concern is that parents may not initiate or follow up on health concerns expressed by an adolescent (Anthony, 2014; Klein, Wild, & Cave, 2005), which is reflective of differing priorities between parent and adolescent. While individual state laws vary in the area of adolescent rights, it is critically important that P-PCPs know individual state laws and adhere to confidentiality laws for adolescent healthcare. Some adolescents describe a desire to address healthcare concerns independently from their parents (Atkins, Bluebond-Langner, Read, Pittsley, & Hart, 2010; Ginsburg, Menapace, & Slap, 1997), preferring to make autonomous decisions about their own health (Lipstein et al., 2013). Therefore, P-PCPs should respect adolescent physical and behavioral healthcare needs and should interview adolescents independently from parents or caregivers. However, insufficient understanding of health problems and consequences may diminish the importance of seeking healthcare (Atkins et al., 2010; Beresford & Sloper, 2003). While health literacy has been identified among adults as a factor for poorer health outcomes and health service utilization (Berkman et al., 2011), health literacy has not been widely studied in children (Driessnack et al., 2014). Preliminary findings suggest adolescents may lack skills to arrange healthcare appointments (Klein et al, 2005) or articulate their health concerns to providers (Beresford & Sloper, 2003). Acknowledging these findings, P-PCPs should enact practice policies that assist adolescents in making appointments and use texting or other technology-driven methods, per the adolescent's personal preference, for reminders of scheduled appointments or follow-up care, thus *intercepting* missed appointments and delay in essential adolescent healthcare.

Additional factors influencing adolescent healthcare engagement include the use of technology within the healthcare office, with tablets and computers perceived to guard privacy more than a shared desktop computer, or paper and pencil survey to gather patient health information (Kadivar et al., 2014). Other factors that prevent adolescent engagement with the healthcare system include system barriers such as inaccessibility to transportation (Ambresin, Bennett, Patton, Sanci, & Sawyer, 2013; Ginsburg et al., 1997), lack of health insurance (Ginsburg et al., 1997), office hours during school hours (Anthony, 2014), and prolonged office wait times (Klein et al., 2005). Preserving confidentiality of the adolescent during healthcare visits is vitally important, yet the adolescent needs to be made aware that certain disclosures may be reportable such as when the adolescent presents a harm to self or others, child abuse, and in some states human trafficking.

Health-Seeking Behaviors of Adolescents

An adolescent's decision to seek professional healthcare services for health promotion, acute injury treatment, and/or chronic illness management is influenced by personal, social, community, cultural, economic, and political factors reflective of a socio-ecological model (Sawyer et al., 2012). Despite recommendations for annual health visits for adolescents, episodic care for acute illnesses and injuries is more prevalent among this population (Dempsey, 2010; Mulye et al., 2009). The decision to seek episodic healthcare is often related to quality of life issues such as unrelieved pain (Lipstein et al., 2013), especially pain with extended duration and intensity (Rathleff et al., 2013). Decisions against seeking healthcare include fear of health information being used against them or perceived inability for healthcare providers to understand adolescent experiences (Atkins et al., 2010; Draucker, 2005). Trust, confidentiality, and mutual respect are priorities for the adolescent when considering their relationship with a healthcare provider. Adolescents want to seek healthcare without feeling judged or treated unequally based on insurance status or race (Ginsburg et al., 1997).

Multiple factors have been found to influence healthcare-seeking behaviors of adolescents in general, including individual, social, school, and community factors. Individual factors, such as adolescent growth and development, health literacy, access to provider, ability to pay, confidentiality, and perceived respect and open communication by healthcare providers, have been described as significant factors for adolescents when seeking healthcare (Ambresin et al, 2013; Anthony, 2014; Atkins et al., 2010; Ginsburg et al., 1997). Adolescent peer groups may influence adolescent decision making based on health beliefs and stigma placed on a particular illness or injury (Anthony, 2014), although peer opinions may not be a factor for all adolescents (Klein et al., 2005).

■ SCREENING TOOLS

Behavioral health screening tools are widely available for P-PCPs for early detection of behavioral health problems, school and home experiences, environmental risks, known adolescent high-risk behaviors, or prior exposure to toxic stress or trauma (see Table 23.2; Hagan, Shaw, Duncan, 2017). Appropriate screening tools should be used at each primary care visit. These tools are designed to elicit adolescent participation in his/her personal healthcare needs and problems as perceived by the adolescent. Additional screenings and assessments using valid and reliable screening tools may be used to provide P-PCPs with additional information to intercept identified behavioral health problems prior to their escalation into a behavioral or mental health disorder or diagnosis. If a potential concern emerges during the screening process, psychometrically tested instruments may be utilized to further assess and monitor emotional and behavioral concerns such as depression or suicide risk.

A well-known screening tool is the called the HEEADSSS assessment (Smith & McGuinness, 2017) and refers to questions about **h**ome, **e**ducation/**e**mployment, **a**ctivities, **d**rugs, **s**exuality, **s**uicide/depression, and **s**afety (HEEADSSS) relevant to adolescents' feelings and perceptions of themselves and their environments (Bright Futures, 2017). Nurse practitioners should be alert for red flags in physical, emotional, social, and psychological and behavioral health to intercept as early as possible the problem, thus optimizing healthcare outcomes (Table 23.2).

The SSHADESS tool was introduced for adolescent screenings since the introduction of the Internet, social media, and new and ever-changing ways of

TABLE 23.2

HEEADSSS ASSESSMENT SAMPLE QUESTIONS

Domain	Sample Questions
Home	Who lives with you? Where do you live? What are relationships like where you live? Who can you talk to where you live about stressful things in your life? Have you ever lived away from home? (Why?)
Education and Employment	Tell me about school. How are your grades at school? What classes do you do well in? What are your challenges at school? Do you feel connected with people at your school? Have you missed any school this month/quarter/semester? If so, why? What are your future education/employment plans? Do you work? (If so, tell me how much do you work? How do you balance school and work responsibilities?)
Eating	What are typical meals for you during the week? On the weekend? Tell me about your exercise routine. How do you like your body? (What do you like about your body? What do you want to change about your body?) Have you had any recent changes in weight? Have you "dieted" during the past year? (If yes, how often? What was the diet? Have you ever taken diet pills, energy drinks? If yes, how often and how much?)
Activities	What do you do for fun? (With whom, when, where?) How do you spend time with friends? Family? How much time do you spend on the Internet or in front of a screen (TV, computer, video games, smartphone?) What types of things do you use the Internet for? What types of books do you read for fun? What music do you like to listen to? Do you regularly attend religious or spiritual activities? Have you sent messages or photographs through text or social media that you wished you hadn't sent? How do you feel after playing video games? How often do you view nude images or videos online? Tell me about your sleep.
Drugs	Do any of your friends or family smoke cigarettes? E-cigarettes? Smoke marijuana? Drink alcohol? Use drugs? How often? Do you smoke cigarettes? E-cigarettes? Smoke marijuana? Drink alcohol? Use drugs? How often? Have you ever used energy drinks, performance enhancing drugs or steroids, or medication prescribed to someone else? If so, what are those products and how often are they used? (Assess type, frequency, intensity, patterns of use, method of payment?)

(continued)

TABLE 23.2   (CONTINUED)

HEEADSSS ASSESSMENT SAMPLE QUESTIONS

Domain	Sample Questions
Sexuality	Have you ever been in a romantic relationship? Tell me about the people that you have dated. Tell me about your sexual life. What does the term "safe sex" mean to you? Have you ever been pressured into doing something sexual that you did not want to? Have you ever been touched in a way that made you uncomfortable?
Suicide and Depression	Do you feel stressed or more anxious than usual? Do you feel sad or down more than usual? Are you bored much of the time? Have you thought about hurting yourself or someone else? Tell me about a time that someone made you feel uncomfortable online. Tell me about a time that you felt sad while using social media (Facebook, Instagram, Snapchat, Twitter). Have you ever tried to hurt yourself to calm down or feel better? Have you ever thought about or tried to kill yourself?
Safety	Have you ever been seriously injured? Tell me about that experience. Do you use safety equipment for your sport? How often do you wear a seatbelt when you ride/drive a car? Where do you keep your phone when you drive? Tell me what it is like to be in a car with someone who was driving while drunk or high. Have you ever met or plan to meet someone that you met online? How safe is your neighborhood? Have you ever felt picked on or bullied? Have you ever gotten into a physical fight with someone?

HEEADSSS, home, education/employment, activities, drugs, sexuality, suicide/depression, and safety.

communication placed adolescents at new risks for behavioral health problems. The SSHADESS acronym stands for questions about **s**trength, **s**chool, **h**ome, **a**ctivities, **d**rugs/substance **a**buse, **e**motions/eating/depression, **s**exuality, and **s**afety. Sample questions are included in Table 23.3.

■ DIAGNOSIS OF SOCIAL, EMOTIONAL, AND BEHAVIORAL PROBLEMS

Behavioral health disorders among adolescents are an important public health issue due to prevalence, early onset, and impact on the child, family, and community (Centers for Disease Control and Prevention [CDC], 2013). In the United States, behavioral and mental health disorders result in substantial healthcare costs, use of services such as special education and juvenile justice, and decreased

TABLE 23.3

SSHADESS ASSESSMENT SAMPLE QUESTIONS

Domain	Sample Questions
S strength	What do you like doing? How would you describe yourself? Tell me what you're most proud of. How would your best friends describe you?
S school	What do you enjoy most/least about school? How many days have you missed or had to be excused early or arrived late to school? How are your grades? Any different from last year? Do you feel like you are doing your best at school? If not, why not? What's getting in the way? Do you feel safe on the way to school and in school? Do you participate in gym class? What would you like to do when you get older?
H home	Who do you live with? Any changes in your family? Could you talk to your family if you were stressed? Who would you go to first?
A activities	Are your friends treating you well? Do you have a best friend or adult you can trust outside your family? Are you still involved in the activities you were doing last year? What kinds of things do you do just for fun? Are you spending as much time with your friends as you used to?
D drugs/ substance abuse	Do any of your friends talk about smoking cigarettes, taking drugs, or drinking alcohol? Do you smoke cigarettes? Drink alcohol? Have you tried sniffing glue, smoking weed, or using pills or other drugs? When/if you smoke, drink, or get high, how does it make you feel, or what does it do for you?
E emotions/ eating/ depression	Have you been feeling stressed? Do people get on your nerves more than they used to? Are you feeling more bored than usual? Do you feel nervous a lot? Have you been having trouble sleeping lately? If yes, what kind of trouble? Would you describe yourself as a healthy eater? Have you been trying to gain or lose weight? Tell me why. Have you been feeling down, sad, or depressed? Have you thought of hurting yourself or someone else? Have you ever tried to hurt yourself? How?
S sexuality	Are you attracted to anyone? Tell me about that person. (Using gender-neutral language) Are you comfortable with your sexual feelings? Are you attracted to guys, girls, or both?

(continued)

TABLE 23.3 *(CONTINUED)*

SSHADESS ASSESSMENT SAMPLE QUESTIONS

Domain	Sample Questions
	What kinds of things have you done sexually? Kissing? Touching? Oral sex? Have you ever had sexual intercourse? Have you enjoyed it? What kind of steps do you take to protect yourself? Have you ever been worried that you could be pregnant? Have you ever been worried about or had a sexually transmitted infection?
S safety	Are there a lot of fights at your school? Do you feel safe at school? Is there bullying? Have you been bullied? Do you carry weapons? What kinds of things make you mad enough to fight? Has anyone ever touched you physically or sexually when you didn't want them to? Does your boyfriend/girlfriend get jealous? (Jealousy is an early sign of controlling, potentially abusive, relationships.) Do you ever get into fights with your boyfriend/girlfriend? Physical fights? Have you ever seen people in your family or home hurt each other? Say mean things? Throw things or hit each other?

productivity among adolescents and their families; therefore, early recognition and intercepting of the behavior with evidence-based interventions is essential to minimizing health burdens. Diagnosis of behavioral and mental health disorders by P-PCPs will be facilitated by analysis of the chief complaint(s), a thorough adolescent and family history, comprehensive adolescent interview, and physical examination.

Physical examination should include observations about the adolescent's general appearance, Tanner staging, growth charts (height, weight, body mass index), menstrual history, behavior, mood, affect, thinking, social interaction, language, and evidence of injury and substance or physical abuse. History should include growth and development, medication (prescription, over the counter, and any herbal supplements), nutritional intake, sleep patterns, physical and social activity, social media use, substance use, sexual experiences, risk behaviors, and duration and extent of problematic symptoms. Once information is synthesized and evaluated according to the typical developmental stage, the P-PCP formulates a differential diagnosis. Psychiatric diagnoses are organized on the *Diagnostic and Statistical Manual of Mental Disorders, Fifth Edition* (DSM-5; APA, 2013) or International Statistical Classification of Diseases and Related Health Problems (ICD) taxonomies. Diagnoses will guide management through evidence-informed patient-centered decision making for nonpharmacological therapies, psychotropic medication, a combination of approaches, or referral to psychiatric nurse practitioner. Factors that may influence referral include comorbid symptoms or presence of more than one psychiatric disorder, history of trauma, high-risk symptoms (i.e., hallucinations, suicidal or homicidal ideation), substance abuse or addiction, or persistent symptoms unresponsive to initial psychotropic medications.

■ INTERCEPTING ADOLESCENT BEHAVIORAL HEALTH PROBLEMS

Risk behaviors are often the hallmark of adolescent life. Adolescents often feel that "nothing will happen to them" and it is acceptable to "try things out." Risky behaviors often include attraction to tobacco products, street drugs, alcohol, speeding while driving, drag racing, and sexual activity with numerous partners placing them at risk for sexually transmitted infections and HIV, as well as placing females at risk for pregnancy.

The goal of behavioral healthcare is for early identification through screeing of adolescents who are participating in high-risk behaviors and implementation of evidence-based interventions that will intercept these behaviors, thus reducing the adolescents risk for behavioral problems that may lead to mental health disorders.

■ TREATMENT STRATEGIES

Treatment for behavioral and mental health disorders may include nonpharmacological therapies (Chapter 35) and psychotropic medications (Chapter 3). It is important to ascertain health goals, knowledge, and beliefs of the adolescent and family to facilitate treatment adherence. Internalization of public stigma may influence perception of diagnosis and treatment options (Kranke, Floersch, Kranke, & Munson, 2011), thus impacting adherence to treatment modality (Timlin, Hakko, Heino, & Kyngas, 2014). When considering psychotropic medications, it is important to consider both the patient and family in decision making based on comorbid conditions, risks and benefit profile of side effects, potential drug interactions with other over-the-counter and prescription medications, monitoring recommendations, and dosing strategies.

■ SUMMARY

Adolescence is a unique time for individuals to explore their personal feelings, beliefs, emotions, and social interactions, to cultivate new friendships, and to consider decisions regarding their career, personal healthcare, and health behaviors that confront them in their everyday lives. Adolescence is a period of rapid brain growth and development leading to the refinement of cognitive control over behaviors and emotional reactions, which is their primary task during the adolescent years. Disruptions in typical development processes may negatively influence adolescent brain development, manifesting as behavioral problems or psychopathology. P-PCPs play a critical role in identifying and intercepting adverse behaviors through screening adolescents at all healthcare visits and implementing evidence-based interventions and referral to treatment as needed.

■ REFERENCES

Ambresin, A. E., Bennett, K., Patton, G. C., Sanci, L. A., & Sawyer, S. M. (2013). Assessment of youth-friendly health care: A systematic review of indicators drawn from young people's perspectives. *Journal of Adolescent Health, 52,* 670–681. doi:10.1016/j.jadohealth.2012.12.014

American Psychological Association. (2013). *Diagnostic and statistical manual of mental disorders* (5th ed.). Arlington, VA: American Psychiatric Publishing. doi:10.1176/appi.books.9780890425596

Andersen, S. L. (2016). Commentary on the special issue on the adolescent brain: Adolescence, trajectories, and the importance of prevention. *Neuroscience and Biobehavioral Reviews, 70,* 329–333. doi:10.1016/j.neubiorev.2016.07.012

Anthony, I. (2014). Discreet and indiscreet barriers to adolescent health seeking efforts. *Clinical Pediatrics, 53,* 601–602. doi:10.1177/0009922813497426

Arnett, J. J., Žukauskienė, R., & Sugimura, K. (2014). The new life stage of emerging adulthood at ages 18–29 years: Implications for mental health. *The Lancet Psychiatry, 1*(7), 569–576. doi:10.1016/S2215-0366(14)00080-7

Atkins, R., Bluebond-Langner, M., Read, N., Pittsley, J., & Hart, D. (2010). Adolescents as health agents and consumers: Results of a pilot study of the health and health-related behaviors of adolescents living in a high-poverty urban neighborhood. *Journal of Pediatric Nursing, 25,* 382–392. doi:10.1016/j.pedn.2009.07.001

Beltz, A. M., Corley, R. P., Bricker, J. B., Wadsworth, S. J., & Berenbaum, S. A. (2014). Modeling pubertal timing and tempo and examining links to behavior problems. *Developmental Psychology, 50*(12), 2715–2726. doi:10.1037/a0038096

Beresford, B. A., & Sloper, P. (2003). Chronically ill adolescents' experiences of communicating with doctors: A qualitative study. *Journal of Adolescent Health, 33,* 172–179. doi:10/1016/S1054-139X(03) 00047-8

Berkman, N. D., Sheridan, S. L., Donahue, K. E., Halpern, D. J., & Crotty, K. (2011). Low literacy and health outcomes: An updated systematic review. *Annals of Internal Medicine, 155,* 97–107. doi:10.7326/0003-4819-155-2-201107190-00005

Bilbo, S. D., & Schwarz, J. M. (2012). The immune system and developmental programming of brain and behavior. *Frontiers in Neuroendocrinology, 33*(3), 267–286. doi:10.1016/j.yfme.2012.08.006

Bowers, B. (1989). The grounded theory method: From conceptualization to research process. In B. Sarter (Ed.), *Paths to knowledge: Innovative research methods in nursing.* Washington, DC: National League for Nursing.

Brenhouse, H. C., Sonntag, K. C., & Andersen, S. L. (2008). Transient D1 dopamine receptor expression on prefrontal cortex projection neurons: Relationship to enhanced motivational salience of drug cues in adolescence. *Journal of Neuroscience, 28,* 2375–2382. doi:10.1523/JNEUROSCI.5064-07.2008

Bronfenbrenner, U. (1979). *The ecology of human development.* Cambridge, MA: Harvard University Press.

Bronfenbrenner, U. (1994a). Ecological models of human development. *International Encyclopedia of Education, 3,* 1643–1647.

Bronfenbrenner, U. (1994b). Nature-nurture reconceptualized in developmental perspective: A bioecological model. *Psychological Review, 101,* 568–586. doi:10.1037/0033-295X.101.4.568

Bronfenbrenner, U. (2005). *Making human beings human: Bioecological perspectives on human development.* Thousand Oaks, CA: Sage.

Casey, B. J., Galvánb, A., & Somerville, L. H. (2016). Beyond simple models of adolescence to an integrated circuit-based account: A commentary. *Developmental Cognitive Neuroscience, 17,* 128–130. doi:10.1016/j.dcn.2015.12.006

Centers for Disease Control and Prevention. (2013). *Mental health surveillance among children—United States, 2005–2011.*

Dempsey, A. F., & Freed, G. L. (2010). Health care utilization by adolescents on Medicaid: Implications for delivering vaccines. *Pediatrics, 125,* 43–49. doi:10.1542/peds.2009-1044

Draucker, C. B. (2005). Processes of mental health service use by adolescents with depression. *Journal of Nursing Scholarship, 37,* 155–162. doi:10.1111/j.1547-5069.2005.00028.x

Driessnack, M., Chung, S., Perkhounkova, E., & Hein, M. (2014). Using the "newest vital sign" to assess health literacy in children. *Journal of Pediatric Health Care, 28,* 165–171. doi:10.1016/j.pedhc.2013.05.005

Dunn, A. M., & Fisher, J. W. (2004). Developmental management of adolescents. In C. E. Burns, A. M. Dunn, M. A. Brady, N. Barber Starr, & C. G. Blosser (Eds.), *Pediatric primary care: A handbook for nurse practitioners* (3rd ed.). St. Louis, MO: Elsevier.

Erickson, E. (1950). *Childhood and society*. New York, NY: Norton.

Erickson, E. (1959). *Identity and the life cycle: Selected papers, psychological issues* (Vol. 1). New York, NY: International Press.

Ge, X., & Natsuaki, M. N. (2009). In search of explanations for early pubertal timing effects on developmental psychopathology. *Current Directions in Psychological Science, 18*, 327–331. doi:10.1111/j.1467-8721.2009.01661.x

Ginsburg, K. R., Menapace, A. S., & Slap, G. B. (1997). Factors affecting the decision to seek health care: The voice of adolescents. *Pediatrics, 100*, 922–930. doi:10.1542/peds.100.6.922

Golub, M. S., Collman, G. W., Foster, P. M. D., Kimmel, C. A., Rajpert-De Meyts, E., Reiter, E. O., . . . Toppari, J. (2008). Public health implications of altered puberty timing. *Pediatrics, 121*(Suppl 218), S218–S230. doi:10.1542/peds.2007-1813G

Graber, J. A., Nichols, T. R., & Brooks-Gunn, J. (2010). Putting pubertal timing in developmental context: Implications for prevention. *Developmental Psychobiology, 52*(3), 254–262. doi:10.1002/dev.20438

Gunnar, M. R., Wewerka, S., Frenn, K., Long, J. D., & Griggs, C. (2009). Developmental changes in hypothalamus–pituitary–adrenal activity over the transition to adolescence: Normative changes and associations with puberty. *Developmental Psychopathology, 21*, 69–85. doi:10.1017/S0954579409000054

Guyer, A. E., Silk, J. S., & Nelson, E. E. (2016). The neurobiology of the emotional adolescent: From the inside out. *Neuroscience and Biobehavioral Reviews, 70*, 74–85. doi:10.1016/j.neubiorev.2016.07.037

Hagan, J. F., Shaw, J. S., & Duncan, P. M. (2017). *Bright Futures: Guidelines for health supervision of infants, children and adolescents* (4th ed.). Elk Grove, IL: American Academy of Pediatrics.

Holder, M. K., & Blaustein, J. D. (2014). Puberty and adolescence as a time of vulnerability to stressors that alter neurobehavioral processes. *Neuroendocrinology, 35*, 89–110. doi:10.1016/j.yfrne.2013.10.004

Kilford, E. J., Garrett, E., & Blakemore, S. J. (2016). The development of social cognition in adolescence: An integrated perspective. *Neuroscience Biobehavior Review, 70*, 106–120. doi:10.1016/j.neubiorev.2016.08.016

Kadivar, H., Thompson, L., Wegman, M., Chisholm, T., Khan, M., Eddleton, K., . . . Shenkman, E. (2014). Adolescent views on comprehensive health risk assessment and counseling: Assessing gender differences. *Journal of Adolescent Health, 55*, 24–32. doi:10.1016/j.jadohealth.2013.12.002

Kaltiala-Heino, R., Kosunen, E., & Rimpelä, M. (2003). Pubertal timing, sexual behaviour and self-reported depression in middle adolescence. *Journal of Adolescence, 26*(5), 531–545.

Klein, D., Wild, T. C., & Cave, A. (2005). Understanding why adolescents decide to visit family physicians. *Canadian Family Physician, 51*, 160–169.

Konrad, K., Firk, C., & Uhlhaas, P. J. (2013). Brain development during adolescence: Neuroscientific insights into this developmental period. *Dtsch Arztebl Int, 110*(25), 425–431. doi:10.3238/arztebl.2013.0425

Kranke, D. A., Floersch, J., Kranke, B. O., & Munson, M. R. (2011). A qualitative investigation of self-stigma among adolescents taking psychiatric medication. *Psychiatric Services, 62*(8), 893–899. doi:10.1176/ps.62.8.pss6208_0893

Lassi, Z. S., Salam, R. A., Das, J. K., Wazny, K., & Bhutta, Z. A. (2015). An unfinished agenda on adolescent health: Opportunities for interventions. *Seminars in Perinatology, 39*(5), 353–360. doi:10.1053/j.semperi.2015.06.005

Lipstein, E. A., Muething, K. A., Dodds, C. M., & Britto, M. T. (2013). "I'm the one taking it": Adolescent participation in chronic disease treatment decisions. *Journal of Adolescent Health, 2013*, 253–259. doi:10.1016/j.jadohealth.201302.004

Malina, R. M., Rogol, A. D., Cumming, S. P., Coelho e Silva, M. J., & Figueiredo, A. J. (2015). Biological maturation of youth athletes: Assessment and implications. *British Journal of Sports Medicine, 49*(13), 852–859. doi:10.1136/bjsports-2015-094623

Marceau, K., Ram, N., Houts, R. M., Grimm, K. J., & Susman, E. J. (2011). Individual differences in boys' and girls' timing and tempo of puberty: Modeling development with nonlinear growth models. *Developmental Psychology, 47*(5), 1389–1409. doi.org/10.1037/a0023838

Michaelson, V., Brooks, F., Jirásek, I., Inchley, J., Whitehead, R., King, N., . . . HBSC Child Spiritual Health Writing Group. (2016). Developmental patterns of adolescent spiritual health in six countries. *SSM-Population Health, 2*, 294–303. doi:10.1016/j.ssmph.2016.03.006

Mulye, T. P., Park, M. J., Nelson, C. D., Adams, S. H., Irwin, C. E., & Brindis, C. D. (2009). Trends in adolescent and young adult health in the United States. *Journal of Adolescent Health, 45*(1), 8–24. doi:10.1016/j.jadohealth.2009.03.013

Negriff, S., & Susman, E. J. (2011). Pubertal timing, depression, and externalizing problems: A framework, review, and examination of gender differences. *Journal of Research on Adolescence, 21*, 717–746. doi:10.111/j.1532-7795.2010.00708x

Pomerantz, H., Parent, J., Forehand, R., Breslend, N., & Winer, J. P. (2017). Pubertal timing and youth internalizing psychopathology: The role of relational aggression. *Journal of Child and Family Studies, 26*(2), 416–423. doi:10.1007/s10826-016-0598-z

Rathleff, M. S., Skuldbol, S. K., Rasch, M. N., Roos, E. M., Rasmussen, S., & Olesen, J. L. (2013). Care-seeking behaviour of adolescents with knee pain: A population-based study among 504 adolescents. *BMC Musculoskeletal Disorders, 14*, 1–8. doi:10.1186/1471-2474-14-225

Rew, L. (2005). *Adolescent health: A multidisciplinary approach to theory, research, and intervention.* Thousand Oaks, CA: Sage.

Richardson, L. P., McCarty, C. A., Radovic, A., & Ballonoff Suleiman, A. (2017). Research in the integration of behavioral health for adolescents and young adults in primary care settings: A systematic review. *Journal of Adolescent Health, 60*(3), 261–269. doi:10.1016/j.jadohealth.2016.11.013

Sawyer, S. M., Afifi, R. A., Bearinger, L. H., Blakemore, S. J., Dick, B., Ezeh, A. C., & Patton, G. C. (2012). Adolescence: A foundation for future health. *Lancet, 379*, 1630–1640. doi:10.1016/S0140-6736(12)60072-5

Shulman, E. P., Harden, K. P., Chein, J. M., & Steinberg, L. (2016). The development of impulse control and sensation-seeking in adolescence: Independent or interdependent processes? *Journal of Research on Adolescence, 26*, 37–44. doi:10.1111/jora.12181

Smith G., & McGuinness T. (2017). Adolescent psychosocial assessment: The HEEADSSS. *Journal of Psychosocial Nursing and Mental Health Services, 55*(5) 24–27. doi:10.3928/02793695-20170420-03

Steinberg, L. (2008). A social neuroscience perspective on adolescent risk-taking. *Developmental Review, 28*(1), 78–106. doi:10.1016/j.dr.2007.08.002

Tamnes, C., Ostby, Y., Fjell, A., Weslye, T., Due-Tonnessen, P., & Walhovd, K. (2010). Brain maturation in adolescence and young adulthood: Regional age-related changes in cortical thickness and white matter volume and microstructure. *Cerebral Cortex, 20*, 534–548. doi:10.1093/cercor/bhp118

Thompson, S. M., Hammen, C., & Brennan, P. (2016). The impact of asynchronous pubertal development on depressive symptoms in adolescence and emerging adulthood among females. *Journal of Youth and Adolescence, 45*, 494–504. doi:10.1007/s10964-015-0402-1

Timlin, U., Hakko, H., Heino, R., & Kyngas, H. (2014). A systematic narrative review of the literature: Adherence to pharmacological and nonpharmacological treatments among adolescents with mental disorders. *Journal of Clinical Nursing, 23*(23–24), 3321–3334. doi:10.1111/jocn.12589

Toledo, E., Lebel, A., Becerra, L., Minster, A., Linnman, C., Maleki, N., & Borsook, D. (2012). The young brain and concussion: Imaging as a biomarker for diagnosis and prognosis. *Neuroscience and Biobehavioral Reviews, 36*, 1510–1531. doi:10.1016/j.neubiorev.2012.03.007

Trotman, H. D., Holtzman, C. W., Ryan, A. T., Shapiro, D. I., MacDonald, A. N., Goulding, S. M., . . . Walker, E. F. (2013). The development of psychotic disorders in adolescence: A potential role for hormones. *Hormones and Behavior, 64*(2), 411–419. doi:10.1016/j.yhbeh.2013.02.018

Viner, R. M., Ross, D., Hardy, R., Kuh, D., Power, C., Johnson, A., . . . Batty, G. D. (2015). Life course epidemiology: Recognizing the importance of adolescence. *Journal of Epidemiology & Community Health, 69*(8), 719–720. doi:10.1136/jech-2014-205300

Wright, S., Betz, C. L., & Yearwood, E. L. (2012). Child, adolescent, and family development. In E. L. Yearwood, G. S. Pearson, & J. A. Newland (Eds.), *Child and adolescent behavioral health: A resource for advanced practice psychiatric and primary care practitioners in nursing.* West Sussex, UK: Wiley-Blackwell. doi:10.1002/9781118704660.ch1

CHAPTER 24

Eating Disorders in Children and Adolescents

JULIE SCHREINER

Eating disorders are the most common psychiatric illnesses among adolescent women and the most lethal of all psychiatric conditions within every age group, including children and the elderly (Martin & Golden, 2014). The incidence and prevalence of anorexia nervosa (AN), bulimia nervosa (BN), and other eating disorders in children and adolescents continue to increase, calling for an emergent need for pediatric primary care providers (P-PCPs) to be familiar with early detection and evidence-based management of these disorders. As focus has turned to the dramatic increase in childhood obesity, so too has come a greater emphasis on dieting and weight loss among children and adolescents. This focus has shifted the epidemiology of eating disorders among children and adolescents, with a greater prevalence of males and minority populations in the United States than ever before suffering from eating disorders (Raevuoni, Keski-Rahkonen, & Hoek, 2014). P-PCPs play an important role in combating the statistics that have led these disorders to continue to have the highest mortality rate of any psychiatric illness.

An estimated 0.5% of adolescent girls in the United States have AN, approximately 1% to 2% of girls meet criteria for BN, and between 5% to 10% of all cases of eating disorders occur in males (Campbell & Peebles, 2014). An even larger percentage of children and adolescents fall in the subclinical categories of eating disorders but face many similar challenges of those that meet criteria for these life-altering diseases. Unfortunately, treatment for eating disorders is extremely limited and often excluded from insurance coverage, leaving patients with even more risk to medical complications, chronic illness, and ultimately death. This deficit in treatment is further limited by the lack of funding for more research on these deadly diseases. As previously mentioned, eating disorders are the most common and most deadly psychological disorders, yet the funding for research is the most limited (Thomas, 2017).

This chapter describes eating disorders in children and adolescents, appropriate screening to assess for eating disorders in this population, the medical and psychological evaluation, the medical complications, and current treatment recommendations. P-PCPs must know how to assess and diagnose children and adolescents who present with a possible diagnosis of an eating disorder, to intercept patients from the potential long-term damage of these deadly diagnoses, and to establish a referral to a psychiatric provider as soon as identified. P-PCPs continue to provide primary care to individuals with a diagnosis of eating disorders; however, treatment of eating disorders must be managed by a psychiatric provider.

■ TYPES OF EATING DISORDERS

The *Diagnostic and Statistical Manual of Mental Disorders, Fifth Edition* (*DSM-5*; American Psychiatric Association [APA], 2013) defines five types of eating disorders that exist among children and adolescents. The *DSM-5* criteria for AN include the following: restriction of energy intake leading to low body weight; fear of gaining weight or behavior that interferes with weight gain; and self-evaluation influenced by weight and body shape. There are two subtypes of AN: restricting type and binge-eating/purging type. In the *DSM-5*, amenorrhea is no longer required to meet diagnostic criteria; that ommission provides more opportunities for children and adolescents to be diagnosed and treated for eating disorders.

The *DSM-5* (APA, 2013) criteria for BN include the following: recurrent binge eating in which a binge is defined as consuming a very large amount of food in a specific period of time, such as within 2 hours, and a sense of loss of control over eating during that episode; recurrent compensatory behavior, such as vomiting, fasting, exercise, laxative use, diuretic use, diet pill use; and self-evaluation influenced by weight and body shape. The binge-eating and compensatory behaviors both occur, on average, at least once a week for 3 months.

Binge-eating disorder (BED), the newest eating disorder to be added to the *DSM-5* (APA, 2013), is characterized by recurrent binge-eating episodes accompanied by a sense of loss of control over eating during the episode. In BED, these episodes are associated with at least three of the following: eating more rapidly, eating until uncomfortably full, eating when not hungry, eating alone because of embarrassment about the amount of food consumed, and feelings of disgust, depression, or guilt. According to the *DSM-5*, binge-eating episodes need to occur, on average, at least once a week for 3 months, and must be associated with marked distress, to meet diagnostic severity levels. BED is distinguished from BN in part because the binge-eating episodes are not associated with inappropriate compensatory behaviors.

The *DSM-5* (APA, 2013) criteria for avoidant restrictive food intake disorder (ARFID) include food restriction or avoidance, without shape or weight concerns or intentional efforts to lose weight that results in significant weight loss and nutritional deficiencies, associated with disturbances in psychological development and functioning. Some patients present with highly selective eating, the fear of new things related to food types, or hypersensitivity to food texture, appearance, and taste. For some patients, fear of swallowing or choking contributes to food avoidance; a specific event can sometimes be identified as triggering that fear, such as a choking episode or a vomiting episode (Nicely, Lane-Loney, Masciulli, Hollenbeak, & Ornstein, 2014). About 20% of patients with AFRID have autism spectrum disorder (ASD), about one third of children with this disorder have a mood disorder, and three quarters have an anxiety disorder (Fisher et al., 2014).

In the *DSM-IV* (APA, 1994), an eating disorder not otherwise specified (EDNOS) was the broad diagnostic category that encompassed atypical and sub-threshold presentations of AN, BN, BED, and other atypical eating problems. In the *DSM-5* (APA, 2013), many of the patients who would previously have been diagnosed with EDNOS will now meet the revised criteria for AN, BN, BED, and ARFID. The remaining patients will be diagnosed under the general diagnosis of Other Specified Feeding or Eating Disorder (OSFED).

■ SCREENING FOR EATING DISORDERS IN CHILDREN AND ADOLESCENTS

Timely screenings and implementation of early interventions for eating disorders have the potential to prevent and *intercept* future development of clinically sig-nificant eating disorders and their complications. Reductions in complications and improved outcomes are reported with timely diagnosis, underscoring the impor-tance of timely routine screening, diagnosis, and referral of eating disorders by P-PCPs and those caring for children and adolescents. For P-PCPs, prevention of eating disorders truly rests on the recognition of early risk factors and intercepting the patterns of eating disorders by prompt and effective interventions for those with disordered eating before potential complications arise. Bright Futures (American Academy of Pediatrics [AAP], 2017) offers helpful screening questions for chil-dren and adolescents and provides a good basis for appropriate questions to ask the patient. The SCOFF (sick, control, one, fat, and food) questionnaire, although validated only in adults, provides a good working framework for screening in the primary care setting and offers a short and effective screening for disordered eat-ing (Campbell & Peebles, 2014). The underlying goal of any screening tool like the SCOFF questionnaire is the appropriate screening of disordered eating behaviors that serves as a launching pad for appropriate medical and psychological evaluation.

■ MEDICAL AND PSYCHOLOGICAL EVALUATION

As with any behavioral health and/or psychiatric condition, all medical conditions for the current and past presenting symptoms must be ruled out prior to deter-mining if the current symptoms are a true eating disorder. To begin the diagnostic process, a complete history and mental health assessment must be performed for the child or adolescent in which an eating disorder is suspected. The mental health assessment should include an evaluation of the patient's eating habits, including a 24-hour food recall, use of compensatory behaviors, and evaluation of any comor-bid factors that may exist and possibly underlie the patient's current eating habits. In addition to assessing the eating habits of the child or adolescent, current mental status should be evaluated by a psychiatric specialist and must include screening for suicidal thoughts or behaviors.

Suicide attempts and completed suicide are relatively common among patients with eating disorders, especially in those with binge/purge or purging behaviors. Death from suicide is 50 times more likely in patients with AN, 25% to 35% of patients with BN report a history of attempted suicide, and patients with BED have been found to be at greater risk of early death due to suicide (Fichter & Quadflieg, 2016; Zerwas et al., 2015).

When the P-PCP determines a possibility of an eating disorder in the child or adolescent, further workup and evaluation must be done including a thorough medical evaluation. In most patients with eating disorders, laboratory results will often be normal; however, normal laboratory results do not dismiss a serious illness. Initial laboratory assessment should include a complete blood count (CBC), a comprehensive metabolic panel, liver function tests (LFTs), and thyroid (TFP with TSH) tests. In adolescents presenting with amenorrhea, further studies including urine pregnancy, serum luteinizing and follicle-stimulating hormones, serum prolactin, and serum estradiol may be warranted. Bone densitometry is recommended for adolescents who have not had a menstrual cycle for more than 6 to 12 months (Sjögren, 2015). An ECG is recommended for any patient with cardiovascular signs and symptoms, for everyone whose laboratory results reveal electrolyte abnormalities, as well as for anyone who has severe weight loss or significant purging (Rosen, 2010).

■ MEDICAL COMPLICATIONS OF EATING DISORDERS

No organ system is spared when it comes to the complications of eating disorders. As early as 2003, the Society for Adolescent Medicine (2003) reported the following medical concerns secondary to eating disorders, which remain a major problem today:

> Irreversible medical complications are associated with eating disorders left untreated, including growth retardation if the disorder occurs before closure of the epiphyses, loss of dental enamel with chronic vomiting, structural brain changes noted on cerebral tomography, magnetic resonance imaging and single-photon computerized tomography studies, pubertal delay or arrest, and impaired acquisition of peak bone mass, predisposing adolescents and young adults to osteoporosis and increased fracture risk. (pp. 496–497)

Fortunately, most of the medical complications resolve once the patient is re-fed or has stopped purging. However, for children and adolescents, a major concern exists in the growth and development problems that may arise when an eating disorder presents at a young age. Growth retardation and pubertal delay can be seen in children and adolescents with eating disorders. These delays may contribute to endocrine abnormalities such as abnormal thyroid function, abnormal adrenal function, and low levels of sex steroids that are secondary to eating disorders. Low bone mass density is cause for concern due to the risk of fractures that may be potentially irreversible and cause for concern later in life. Patients with eating disorders have also been found to have volume deficits of both gray and white matter of the brain, leading to cognitive impairment and potentially irreversible changes of the brain. Cardiovascular complications of eating disorders include bradycardia, orthostatic hypotension, conduction abnormalities, and repolarization abnormalities, which can be life threatening. Gastrointestinal changes are a very common presentation in children and adolescents with eating disorders, and in particular, common problems seen are delayed gastric emptying, constipation, and bloating. Many patients with BN suffer from severe gastroesophageal reflux, upper intestinal bleeding, and potentially severe bleeding secondary to a tear of the esophagus called a Mallory–Weiss tear. Many children and adolescents with eating disorders also suffer from fluid and electrolyte disturbances, including severe dehydration and hypokalemia, which can lead to cardiac arrhythmias. Hypomagnesemia is also a severe risk for those in severely malnourished states. Hyponatremia can be seen in those who "water load" rather than eat or in order to manipulate their weight during weigh-ins for treatment. Skin changes in patients with eating disorders are also common and include lanugo, dry skin, and acrocyanosis (Golden & Ornstein, 2016).

The complications of these life-threatening diseases are real and must be intercepted through early treatment and management. The primary goal of treatment for the patient with an eating disorder is to be re-fed. Often these complications resolve, but for many with eating disorders referrals to specialists for further management must be done in a timely manner and a potential for hospitalization should always be considered in those with severe complications.

■ TREATMENT RECOMMENDATIONS

Medical complications of eating disorders must be managed at an appropriate level of care with a goal of providing the best supervision and medical management for each child, adolescent, and their families. If the child or adolescent is able to be managed on an outpatient basis, the treatment of children and adolescents with eating disorders is best provided by a multidisciplinary team consisting of P-PCPs, dieticians, psychotherapists, and a psychiatrist or psychiatric nurse practitioner (Golden & Ornstein, 2016). Goals for weight gain for individuals managed on the outpatient setting are to establish food intake that provides a 1- to 2-pound weight gain per week (Marzola et al., 2013). An appropriate target weight for children and adolescents with eating disorders is 90% of average weight expected for their age, height, and sex. Many eating disorder experts recommend the minimum objective weight be at the time of resumption of the menstrual cycle for females (Harrington, Jimerson, Haxton, & Jimerson, 2015). The use of hormone replacement therapy is not recommended for resumption of menses, as there is no evidence that this treatment modality is effective in increasing bone mass density and it also has the possibility of falsely causing menses, which can obstruct the goal weight of a patient who had previously had amenorrhea (Bergstrom et al., 2013).

Medication Considerations for Eating Disorders

Psychotropic medications are not considered first-line treatment in eating disorders and no medications have been approved by the U.S. Food and Drug Administration (FDA) for the treatment of children and adolescents with AN. Selective serotonin uptake inhibitors (SSRIs) are most often used in patients with AN but may not be effective in severely malnourished patients (Harrington et al., 2015). The use of atypical neuroleptic agents, especially olanzapine, has been shown to improve both weight gain and dysfunctional, obsessive thinking in patients with AN, but no drugs have received FDA approval for use in children and adolescents with eating disorders (Flament, Bissada, & Spettigue, 2012). In contrast to AN, several medications have been shown to be effective in the treatment of BN in adults. Although fluoxetine remains the only medication approved by the FDA for the treatment of BN, other SSRIs, seratonin and norepinephrine reuptake inhibitors (SNRIs), and tricyclic antidepressants have been shown to decease binge-eating and purging cycles in BN (Flament et al., 2012). Certainly, the use of medications for treatment of comorbid conditions of eating disorders is recommended and has been shown to improve overall functioning in children and adolescents with eating disorders (Harrington et al., 2015).

Cognitive Behavior Therapy Essential for Improvement in Eating Disorders

Along with medical and dietary management of eating disorders, psychotherapeutic services are at the core of eating disorder treatment and management. Individual cognitive behavior therapy (CBT) has shown to be moderately effective in treating eating disorders, especially when the patient is provided a specific form of CBT that focuses on modifying abnormal eating behaviors and distorted perceptions of weight (Campbell & Peebles, 2014). For children and adolescents, family-based therapy (FBT) has been shown to be a very effective evidence-based treatment (Harrington et al., 2015). In FBT, there are three phases with very distinct goals: Phase 1, the goal is weight restoration; Phase 2, the goal is returning control over eating back to the child or adolescent; and Phase 3, the goal is for child or adolescent development and treatment termination. A major role for the P-PCP in FBT is to be the point person for parents and therapists, to monitor medical stability, and to offer ongoing guidance to the patient and family (Katzman, Peebles, Sawyer, Lock, & Le Grange, 2013). P-PCPs collaborating with the child's or adolescent's therapeutic team and family provide the best support for the child and adolescent with a diagnosis of an eating disorder.

■ ROLE OF P-PCPs IN CARING FOR CHILDREN AND ADOLESCENTS WITH EATING DISORDERS

P-PCPs play an important role in the care of the child or adolescent with an eating disorder. Practice parameters include the following:

- P-PCPs must be knowledgeable about the risk factors and early signs and symptoms of disordered eating and eating disorders.
- Healthy eating behaviors and building self-esteem should be the primary focus when counseling families on preventing obesity, since children and adolescents may misunderstand the discussion, and that may lead to eating disorders.
- All children and adolescents should be screened for disordered eating behaviors. Evidence-based practice guidelines for the treatment and management of eating disorders should be implemented for all children and

adolescents who screen positive for an eating disorder, with an immediate referral to a psychiatric specialist for further evaluation.

■ P-PCPs should investigate local treatment resources for eating disorders to appropriately coordinate multidisciplinary interprofessional team members in the care of children and adolescents with an eating disorder.

■ P-PCPs play a vital role in the primary prevention and education about eating disorders for children, adolescents, their families, communities, and their fellow medical providers.

■ SUMMARY

Fortunately, the outcomes for children and adolescents with eating disorders are significantly better than those reported in adults. However, positive outcomes require early interception of potential problems through early recognition of symptoms, early treatment, and quality care management and follow-up. Shorter duration of symptoms and appropriate management of these symptoms lead to improved prognosis for children and adolescents with eating disorders (Campbell & Peebles, 2014). P-PCPs who provide the best available evidence-based and empathetic care to children and adolescents with diagnoses of eating disorder have the potential to decrease this growing number of children and adolescents suffering from these life-altering disorders and their adverse outcomes, including untimely death.

■ REFERENCES

American Academy of Pediatrics. (2017). *Bright Futures: Guidelines for health supervision of infants, children, and adolescents* (4th ed.). Elk Grove Village, IL: Author.

American Psychiatric Association. (1994). *Diagnostic and statistical manual of mental disorders* (4th ed). Washington, DC: Author.

American Psychiatric Association. (2013). *Diagnostic and statistical manual of mental disorders* (5th ed.). Washington, DC: Author. doi:10.1176/appi.books.9780890425596

Bergstrom, I., Crosby, M., Engstrom, A., Holcke, M., Fored, M., Kruse, P. J., & Sandberg, A. (2013). Women with anorexia nervosa should not be treated with estrogen or birth control pills in a bone-sparing effect. *Acta Obstetricia et Gynecologica Scandinavica, 92*, 8. doi:10.1111/aogs.12178

Campbell, K., & Peebles, R. (2014). Eating disorders in children and adolescents: State of the art review. *Pediatrics, 134*, 582–592. doi:10.1542/peds.2014-0194

Fichter, M. M., & Quadflieg, N. (2016). Mortality in eating disorders—Results of a large prospective clinical longitudinal study. *International Journal of Eating Disorders, 49*, 391–401. doi:10.1002/eat.22501

Fisher, M. M., Rosen, D. S., Ornstein, R. M., Mammel, K. A., Katzman, D. K., Rome, E. S., . . . Walsh, B. T. (2014). Characteristics of avoidant/restrictive food intake disorder in children and adolescents: A "new disorder" in DSM-5. *Journal of Adolescent Health, 55*, 49–52. doi:10.1016/j.jadohealth.2013.11.013

Flament, M. F., Bissada, H., & Spettigue, W. (2012). Evidence-based pharmacotherapy of eating disorders. *International Journal of Neuropsychopharmacology, 1592*, 189–207. doi:10.1017/s14611457110000381

Golden, N. H., & Ornstein, R. M. (2016). Eating problems in children and adolescents. In B. T. Walsh, E. Attia, D. R. Glasofer, & R. Sysko (Eds.), *Handbook of assessment and treatment of eating disorders* (pp. 45–61). Arlington, VA: American Psychiatric Association.

Harrington, B. C., Jimerson, M., Haxton, C. A., & Jimerson, D. C. (2015). Initial evaluation, diagnosis, and treatment of anorexia nervosa and bulimia nervosa. *American Family Physician, 91*, 46–52. Retrieved from https://www.ncbi.nlm.nih.gov/pubmed/25591200

Katzman, D. K., Peebles, R., Sawyer, S. M., Lock, J., & Le Grange, D. (2013). The role of the pediatrician in family-based treatment for adolescent eating disorders: Opportunities and challenges. *Journal of Adolescent Health, 53,* 433–440. doi:10.1016/j.jadohealth.2013.07.001

Martin, S. P., & Golden, N. H. (2014). Eating disorders in children, adolescents, and young adults. *Contemporary Pediatrics, 31,* 12–16.

Marzola, E., Nasser, J. A., Hashim, S. A., Shih, P. A., & Kaye, W. H. (2013). Nutritional rehabilitation in anorexia nervosa: Review of the literature and implications for treatment. *BMC Psychiatry, 13,* 290. doi:10.1186/1471-244X-13-290

Nicely, T. A., Lane-Loney, S., Masciulli, E., Hollenbeak, C. S., & Ornstein, R. M. (2014). Prevalence and characteristics of avoidant/restrictive food intake disorder in a cohort of young patients in day treatment for eating disorders. *Journal of Eating Disorders, 2,* 1. Retrieved from https://jeatdisord. biomedcentral.com/articles/10.1186/s40337-014-0021-3

Raevuoni, A., Keski-Rahkonen, A., & Hoek, H. (2014) A review of eating disorders in males. *Current Opinions on Psychiatry, 27–26,* 426–430. doi:10.1097/YCO.0000000000000113

Rosen, D. S. (2010). Identification and management of eating disorders in children and adolescents. *Pediatrics, 126*(6), 1240–1253.

Sjögren, M. (2015) The diagnostic work-up of eating disorders. *Journal of Psychology and Clinical Psychiatry, 4*(5), 00234. doi:10.15406/jpcpy.2015.04.00234

Society for Adolescent Medicine. (2003). Eating disorders in adolescents: Position paper. *Journal of Adolescent Health, 33,* 496–503. Retrieved from http://www.jahonline.org/article/S1054-139X%2803%2900326-4/fulltext

Thomas, M. (2017). *Eating disorder treatment: Even when it works, its hard to access and afford.* Retrieved from Public Health Post; https://www.publichealthpost.org/research/eating-disorder-treatment-hard-to-access-afford/

Zerwas, S., Larsen, J. T., Petersen, L., Thornton, L. M., Mortensen, P. B., & Bulik, C. M. (2015). The incidence of eating disorders in a Danish register study: Associations with suicide risk and mortality. *Journal of Psychiatric Research, 65,* 16–22. doi:10.1016/j.jpsychires.2015.03.003

CHAPTER 25

Neurological and Psychiatric Mental Health Disorder

INGRID G. COOK

Pediatric primary care providers (P-PCPs) are involved in the primary care of children and adolescents with developmental and behavioral issues. According to LaRosa (2017), the American Academy of Pediatrics (AAP) recommends screening for developmental and behavioral problems to promote early identification at well-child visits. The primary care medical home model (Windel, Anderko, & Konetzka, 2011) presents the P-PCP with the unique opportunity to identify mental health problems as early as possible through appropriate evidence-based screenings and observations made during well-child exams as well as sick visits. The purpose of ongoing developmental–behavioral screening in a primary care medical home is to identify problems early so interventions can be provided in a timely manner to *intercept* adverse behavioral health outcomes. These early interventions improve the long-term outcomes for children and adolescents.

When the P-PCP identifies a developmental or behavioral problem in a child or adolescent, the P-PCP can intercept and evaluate whether treatment can be provided in the primary care medical home setting. However, if the evaluation or treatment of the disorder is beyond the capabilities of the P-PCP, a referral can be initiated to specialty providers such as developmental–behavioral pediatrics, child and adolescent psychiatry, mental health specialists, early intervention programs, and special education programs within the school system. The P-PCP must be knowledgeable of the behavioral mental health resources available within their community and school systems for children and their families. P-PCPs can also play a key role in providing follow-up visits in collaboration with the specialists to help monitor the effectiveness of the treatments and plan of care.

Most of the disorders listed in this chapter are not typically managed within the primary care medical home setting. However, the P-PCP should be aware of the more common neurological and psychiatric disorders. The ability to recognize potential problems early in the child and adolescent can lead to earlier interventions and promote better outcomes. When diagnosing neurological and psychiatric disorders within the pediatric population, the *Diagnostic and Statistical Manual of Mental Disorders, Fifth Edition* (*DSM-5*; American Psychiatric Association [APA],

2013) is the most widely used evidence-based guide. The *DSM-5* contains detailed criteria and symptoms common to mental health disorders; however, the *DSM-5* does not contain any information concerning the treatment of the mental health disorders.

This chapter focuses on some of the more common neurological and psychiatric disorders that are encountered by children and adolescents in the primary care medical home setting and the ways in which the P-PCP can better identify a mental health disorder as early as possible through screening and intercept the problem with evidence-based interventions to promote better behavioral health outcomes. However, even with early intervention, some of the mental health disorders are chronic, long-term disorders requiring lifelong attention and treatment. Some of the topics covered in this chapter include bipolar I disorder, depressive disorder, conduct disorder (CD), obsessive-compulsive disorder (OCD), schizophrenia, and trauma- and stressor-related disorders.

■ BIPOLAR I DISORDER

Bipolar I disorder is defined as recurrent episodes of elevated mood including mania and hypomania that exceed the normal developmental stage for a child or adolescent. To meet the guidelines for bipolar I disorder, the symptoms must not be related to any other type of mental health or medical condition. Youth with bipolar I disorder often experience major depression episodes in addition to the mania. Symptoms often appear in early childhood; however, initiation of treatment does not typically occur for about 10 years on average after being identified. *DSM-5* (APA, 2013) criteria include persistently elevated or irritable mood with persistently increased energy for 1 week or longer and three or more of the following mania core symptoms of inflated self-esteem or grandiosity; decreased need for sleep (<4 hours); pressured speech; racing thoughts; distractibility or risk-taking behavior (Birmaher, 2017).

Research suggests bipolar I disorder has a genetic link with the estimated heritability of over 80%. This link means children whose parents have been diagnosed with bipolar I disorder have a 25-fold increase in rates of developing bipolar I disorder when compared to children whose parents do not have the disorder. In addition, studies have shown children from low-socioeconomic environments who have also been exposed to negative events and who exhibit high expressed emotion have a poor prognosis (Birmaher, 2016). Youth at risk for bipolar I disorder often present early with increased levels of mood lability and manic symptoms that are not categorized as severe enough for a diagnosis to be made clinically. Children with bipolar disorder often initially present with other symptoms that may include irritability, depression, anxiety, and sleep disturbances and that may mimic other psychiatric disorders. However, if these symptoms are present, along with one or more of the parents having bipolar I disorder, the child is at greater risk of developing the disorder (Birmaher, 2016). Knowledge of these statistics provides P-PCPs with opportunities to intercept potential problems by referring children of parents with a diagnosis of bipolar I disorder or other behavioral health problems to the school psychologist or to a qualified mental health specialist.

Nierengarten (2015) reports early onset of bipolar disorder in childhood has been shown to be associated with a "higher risk of suicide; severe mood lability and polarity; lower quality of life and greater functional impairment; higher rates of comorbidity; and a higher risk of substance use compared with adult-onset disease" (p. 1). Unfortunately, some children fall outside of the *DSM-5* (APA, 2013) criteria, which makes diagnosis in children even more problematic for the healthcare provider. Nierengarten (2015) notes that the lack of research concerning bipolar disorder in children and adolescents makes this disorder controversial because the presentation of childhood bipolar disorder can differ greatly from adult bipolar disorder presentation.

Assessment and Screening for Bipolar I Disorder

Initially, a physical assessment is performed along with laboratory tests that include a thyroid panel with free T4 to rule out a hypothyroidism or hyperthyroidism disorder; a complete blood count (CBC) to rule out fatigue due to anemia: a comprehensive metabolic profile (CMP) to alert the provider of any metabolic abnormalities from the liver or kidneys; and, lastly, urine drug analysis. Furthermore, a careful review of medications is also helpful to ensure the mania is not merely a side effect of medications, for example, steroids or asthma medications. Once the *DSM-5* (APA, 2013) criteria are met for one manic episode, the clinician must ensure that the occurrences of both the manic and major depressive episodes are not related to schizophrenia or some other type of psychotic disorder (Melnyk & Jenson, 2013).

Birmaher (2017) reported the use of clinician administered rating scales, for example, the Young Mania Rating Scale (YMRS; Youngstrom, 2005) and the KSADS Mania Rating Scale (KSADS-MRS; Youngstrom, 2005). These scales do not provide a diagnosis of bipolar disorder but identify symptoms that need further evaluation to rule out the disorder. Birmaher suggests using the *DSM-5* (APA, 2013) criteria as a guide to diagnosing bipolar mood episodes and disorders. In addition to the *DSM-5* (APA, 2013) criteria, the World Health Organization's *International Statistical Classification of Diseases and Related Health Problems*, 10th revision (ICD-10) uses similar criteria for the diagnosis of bipolar disorder.

Intercepting Problems for Children and Adolescents With Bipolar I Disorder

According to Axelson (2016), P-PCPs must be aware of symptoms that may suggest the likelihood of bipolar I disorder. Once the child has been screened and identified to have symptoms consistent with bipolar disorder, the P-PCP needs to initiate a referral to a child psychiatrist or other mental health specialist. The P-PCP is encouraged to remain involved with the management of this child because he or she can help educate children and families about the diagnosis, pharmacotherapy, and the importance of compliance with the prescribed plan of care. When mood stabilizers are used, the P-PCP can collaborate with the mental health specialist by monitoring side effects, including changes in height, weight, and waist circumference, and intercept weight gain with nutritional support during anticipatory guidance sessions and medication reviews.

Evidence-Based Management (EBM) and Treatment for Bipolar I Disorder

In addition to psychotherapy, a mental health specialist primarily manages children and adolescents with bipolar I disorder. Axelson (2016) describes initial pharmacotherapy for pediatric mania to be a "second-generation antipsychotic, such as aripiprazole, asenapine, olanzapine, quetiapine, risperidone, or ziprasidone" (p. 2), starting with one drug initially and monitoring for a response within 4 to 8 weeks (see Chapter 3 for more details on these drugs). It is not uncommon for pediatric mania to not respond to multiple second-generation antipsychotics. In addition, treatment-resistant patients are often treated with lithium. However, increased levels of lithium in the blood can have effects on kidneys, thyroid, and heart; the mental health provider should order baseline tests prior to starting lithium including "blood urea nitrogen, creatinine, electrolytes, thyrotropin (thyroid stimulating hormone), and an electrocardiogram" (Axelson, 2016, p. 3). If pediatric mania does not respond to second-generation antipsychotics and lithium, medication combinations are recommended and managed by the mental health specialist.

■ DEPRESSIVE DISORDERS

Major Depressive Disorder (MDD)

Bonin (2016) describes the *DSM-5* (APA, 2013) criteria necessary to meet the diagnosis for MDD, also known as unipolar major depression. The child or adolescent must present with five or more depressive symptoms during the same 2-week time frame with at least one of the symptoms including depressed mood (dysphoria) or loss of interest or pleasure (anhedonia). These symptoms include "change in appetite or weight; insomnia or hypersomnia; psychomotor agitation or retardation, fatigue or loss of energy; feelings of worthlessness or guilt; impaired thinking or concentration, indecisiveness; suicidal ideation or behavior" (Bonin, 2016, p. 6).

The depressive symptoms typically develop after a comorbid disorder. The comorbid disorders of anxiety and oppositional defiant disorder (ODD) are considered strong predictors of subsequent depression. Melnyk and Jenson (2013) report the mean age of onset for MDD is 14 years, with an estimated 40% to 70% of affected children and teens having other mental health comorbidities including anxiety, attention deficit hyperactivity disorder (ADHD), CD, and substance use. Comorbidities are associated with a longer "duration of illness, poorer response to treatment, and increased recurrence of depressive episodes" (Bonin, 2016, p. 4).

Assessment and Screening for MDD

When considering a diagnosis of MDD, the P-PCP should (a) obtain a comprehensive medical and psychiatric history; (b) perform a complete physical exam including mental status; and (c) obtain laboratory specimens that include thyroid stimulating hormones (TSH), CBC, chemistries, urinalysis, and urine toxicology to screen for substance abuse (Bonin, 2016). The initial evaluation involves ruling out any other psychiatric or medical conditions that may be causing the depressive symptoms. Other medical differential diagnoses for depressive mood include migraines, multiple sclerosis, brain neoplasm, epilepsy, head trauma, thyroid disorder, infectious mononucleosis, and drug or alcohol exposure.

Depression increases with age and affects approximately twice as many females as males. Diagnosis should also include data gathered using standardized screening tools and rating scales from the child or adolescent, with supplemental information provided by the parents and teachers. One of the most common screening tools used for depression is the self-report Patient Health Questionnaire-Nine Item (PHQ-9). In addition to the PHQ-9, Melnyk and Jenson (2013) recommend the Center for Epidemiological Studies Depression Scale (CES-DC) to be used as a screening tool for older children and teens. Both these tools are available for free and can assist the provider in establishing the diagnosis through a validated instrument. Another helpful tool in identifying symptoms common with depressive disorder is the mnemonic called "SIGE-CAPS" which stands for **S**-sleep disturbances, **I**-interest deficit, **G**-guilt, **E**-energy deficit, **C**-concentration deficit, **A**-appetite disorder, **P**-psychomotor retardation, and **S**-suicidality (Moses, 2017).

Intercepting Problems for Children and Adolescents With MDD

P-PCPs in primary care settings must be comfortable diagnosing depressive disorders by using standardized screening instruments, as identified above, combined with interview skills that question the child or adolescent about any suicidal, homicidal, or self-harming thoughts. In addition, P-PCPs should remain conscious of differential diagnoses and other psychiatric comorbidities. Initiating and managing antidepressant medications and referral of the child or adolescent for psychotherapy are also within the P-PCPs scope of practice (Tang & Pinsky, 2015). In addition, the P-PCP should also be sensitive to the child's age and cultural background because depression may often present with nonspecific symptoms and be misunderstood by the child and parents. Additionally, MDD episodes typically go an average of 7 to 9 months untreated. This lag in treatment often leads to problems with school functioning, activities of daily living, and relationships with family and friends.

EBM and Treatment for MDD

Identifying depression is the first step in developing a treatment plan of care. Depression can be a primary disorder or, less frequently, a secondary disorder due to another medical condition. Tang and Pinsky (2015) state one of the first steps in the treatment of MDD is to educate the child and family concerning the diagnosis and treatment options, including advice about nutrition, exercise, and sleep. In addition, the P-PCP must involve parents and children in the informed consent process and allow them to share in decision making to ensure the benefits of medication outweigh the risks to the child.

First-line treatment for mild to moderate depression is psychotherapy. Antidepressant medication is used in conjunction with psychotherapy to treat moderate to severe depression and mild to moderate depression that has not responded to psychotherapy after 6 to 8 weeks. The Food and Drug Administration

(FDA) has approved selective serotonin reuptake inhibitors (SSRIs) for the treatment of pediatric depression. Examples of FDA-approved SSRIs for the treatment of pediatric depression are fluoxetine (Prozac) in children 8 years and older, starting with an initial dosage of 5 mg daily in preadolescent and 10 mg daily in an adolescent, and escitalopram (Lexapro) in children 12 years and older, with an initial dosage of 10 mg daily. Once initiating SSRIs, common side effects to monitor include nausea, vomiting, diarrhea, constipation, headaches, sleep difficulties, and sexual adverse effects (Tang & Pinsky, 2015). Other SSRI options may often be used by providers but are considered off-label. Mitchell, Davies, Cassesse, and Curran (2014) point out that fluoxetine (Prozac), when compared to other SSRIs, has the best response rate due to the longer half-life that leads to fewer withdrawal symptoms. SSRIs with shorter half-lives require extreme caution in monitoring due to associated risk of *suicidality* when used in children and adolescents.

Response to antidepressant medication is defined as having "no symptoms for at least 2 weeks and remission for 2 to 8 weeks with no or few depressive symptoms" (Tang & Pinksly, 2015, p. 56). When initiating a trial of antidepressant medication, there is a potential to induce mania symptoms in susceptible children who have a positive family history of bipolar illness (Smiga & Elliott, 2011). However, evidence has shown there is no indication that a trial of antidepressants should be avoided even when there is a suspicion of bipolar disorder. If manic symptoms do occur within the first to fourth week of antidepressant treatment, discontinuing the medication is suggested, followed by clinical reassessment.

Serotonin syndrome is another concern when prescribing high doses of SSRIs. Serotonin syndrome leads to an increase of total brain serotonin concentrations and is considered a medical emergency requiring immediate medical attention. Symptoms of the potentially lethal syndrome include confusion, disorientation, agitation, excessive salivation, tremors, muscle twitching, and flu-like symptoms with fever (Smiga & Elliott, 2011).

Indications for prompt referral to a mental health specialist after pediatric depression has been treated by P-PCPs include suicidal or homicidal thoughts; any past history of suicidal attempts; psychotic symptoms; bipolar depression; any psychiatric comorbidity disorders; lack of response to initial SSRI; or discomfort managing child or adolescent depression. In conclusion, early treatment of depression can minimize morbidity, mortality, and lead to better outcomes in school functioning, activities of daily living, and relationships with families and peers.

■ CONDUCT DISORDER (CD)

CD is defined by the *DSM-5* (APA, 2013) as "repetitive and persistent pattern of behavior in which the basic rights of others or major age-appropriate societal norms or rules are violated" (Melnyk & Jensen, 2013, p. 309). The child must exhibit three of the following criteria within the past 12 months with one in the past 6 months: aggression toward people and animals; destruction to property; deceitfulness or theft; and serious violations of rules. Possessing two or more of the characteristic traits for longer than 12 months results in a poorer prognosis. Simply stated, CD is often a failure of parental authority and rejection of available motivations to be good.

Child onset CD must be present with at least one symptom characteristic of CD occurring prior to 10 years of age. Children who present with early onset of CD symptoms have a poorer prognosis than children who present with CD symptoms diagnosed as occurring after the age of 10. The median age of onset for adolescent type of CD is 11.6 years in those who present with no CD symptoms prior to 10 years. CD is more common in males and has been linked to comorbidities such as ADHD, depression, and bipolar disorder (p. 304). CD often follows the diagnosis of ODD. In addition to comorbidities, an estimated 25% of girls and 40% of boys diagnosed with CD will eventually develop adult antisocial personality disorder (Black, 2016).

Another form of adolescent CD, that is characteristically less severe, involves teenage peer pressure groups. According to Black (2016), adolescents within peer groups who have no prior history of earlier CD (except being associated with a peer group) manage to improve suddenly. This sudden improvement in their CD symptoms supports the data explaining why the majority of adolescents do not develop adult antisocial personality disorder even when CD is present at earlier ages (Black, 2016). Interestingly, neurodevelopmental research has shown individuals who are psychopathic require greater sensory input to produce normal brain functioning as compared to normal individuals, causing the psychopathic individuals to seek out potentially dangerous or risky situations. Black further explains that youth with CD typically have "low resting pulse rates, low skin conductance, and increased amplitude on event-related potentials" (Black, 2016, p. 4).

Assessment and Screening for CD

To meet criteria for a diagnosis of CD, two or more of the following characteristics must be present at least 12 months in more than one setting: (a) lack of remorse or guilt; (b) callous lack of empathy; (c) unconcerned about performance; and (d) shallow or deficient affect (Melnyk & Jenson, 2013). The P-PCP must assess the potential for violence in these children and adolescents. Other age-linked behaviors for the P-PCP to monitor for CD in school-age children includes bullying or threatening others, cruelty to animals, fire setting, and any type of property destruction. Adolescents who have a diagnosis of CD often present with a history of truancy, elopement, criminal behaviors such as household invasions, stealing cars and other personal property, and conning behaviors (Hill, 2016). Social and school contributing factors associated with CD often involve academic failure, community violence, bullying, peer rejection, and associating with other children who display violent behaviors. Family influences also play a role in CD and may consist of poor supervision, harsh discipline, parental disharmony, limited involvement in the child's life, providing negative attention for tantrums, being unresponsive to emotional needs of the child, and lacking confidence in parent–child bond (Hill, 2016).

Intercepting Problems for Children and Adolescents With CD

Melnyk and Jenson (2013) report early recognition of warning signs during history taking by the P-PCP can increase the likelihood of identifying the potential for violence in children as young as toddlers. Potential warning signs for violence may include excessive tantrums; withdrawal from social contacts; fascination with weapons; bullying behaviors as well as a history of being bullied; low interest in school; violent writing and drawings; disciplinary problems; intolerance to differences like race, religion, gender, sexual orientation, or physical appearance; and increased risk-taking behaviors. Furthermore, warning signs of potential violence can then lead to warning signs of imminent violence requiring the P-PCP to immediately contact police. Signs include reports of severe physical fighting; severe property destruction; rage for minor reasons; detailed plan to commit violent acts; possession of weapons; and self-injurious behaviors. Other warning signs for potential violence toward humans that require immediate action include fire setting and animal cruelty.

EBM and Treatment for CD

Melnyk and Jenson (2013) recommend the following resource from the AAP titled "Connected Kids" (https://www.aap.org/en-us/advocacy-and-policy/aap-health-initiatives/resilience/Pages/Prevention.aspx). This program addresses violence prevention related to anticipatory guidance with a systematic approach that includes four elements: a clinical guide that provides a program review; a color-coded counseling schedule for different age groups of children; educational brochures to support the topics of Connected Kids; and a PowerPoint presentation titled "Clinical Guide" for use prior to implanting Connected Kids within the P-PCP practice. In addition to the "Connected Kids" training, Melnyk and Jenson (2013) recommend P-PCPs utilize four prevention strategies detailed in the CDC's "Best Practices for Violence Prevention" plan (Centers for Disease Control and Prevention [CDC], 2017). The four strategies for reducing youth violence include (a) family-based strategies involving parenting skills training to enhance communication with their children and nonviolent conflict resolution; (b) a home visiting strategy to bring community resources to at-risk families; (c) social–cognitive strategies helping children develop skills needed to develop nonviolent techniques to deal with difficult situations; and (d) a mentoring strategy promoting positive adult role models lowering their risk for violent behaviors.

Black (2017) reports there is limited evidence of efficacy in reducing aggression in children and adolescent CDs with medications like lithium, risperidone, and divalproex. When treatment is indicated in children, early family therapy interventions involving parent training have shown to offer the best help in preventing adult antisocial personality disorder. Parent training can assist the parents in dealing with misbehaviors in children with CD. However, recommendations do include first treating any psychiatric comorbidities that may also be noted, such as ADHD, depression, anxiety, irritability associated with autism, and bipolar disorder.

▨ OBSESSIVE-COMPULSIVE DISORDER (OCD)

Rosenberg (2015) defines OCD as "a severe, prevalent and most often chronically debilitating disorder characterized by repetitive, ritualistic, and distressing thoughts, ideas, and behaviors over which a person typically has very little if any control" (p. 1). Obsessions are repetitive and persistent thoughts, images, or urges considered to not be pleasurable or voluntary leading to anxiety in the majority of individuals. Rosenberg explains individuals attempt to ignore the thoughts or urges by attempting to counteract the urges that lead to performing a compulsion. Compulsions are referred to as rituals that are repetitive behaviors or mental acts that are performed in response to the obsession. Examples of physical acts of compulsions in children include repetitive behaviors like washing hands repeatedly, going in and out of doorways a certain number of times, tapping or touching in a specific row, arranging objects, or rechecking homework repeatedly. Examples of mental acts of compulsion may include counting or repeating words silently with very rigid rules. Unfortunately, performing the compulsion may provide temporary relief from fear and worry but ultimately this repetitive behavior will not bring as much relief to the child as it did initially, thus leading to a vicious cycle of repeating the ritual (Rosenberg, 2015).

Research suggests approximately 50% of OCD cases occur during childhood with the mean age of onset for boys to be between age 9 and 11 years and the mean age for girls to be between 11 and 13 years. Interestingly, pediatric OCD is more common in males but seems to be equal between both sexes in adulthood. Childhood presentation of OCD has been found to continue into adulthood with symptoms frequently subsiding and flaring up over the life span. As a note, prior to the current edition of the *DSM-5* (APA, 2013), the *DSM-IV* categorized OCD under the anxiety disorder section. However, the *DSM-5* has placed OCD within its own chapter and no longer classifies OCD as an anxiety disorder.

Assessment and Screening for OCD

Diagnosis of pediatric OCD can be very difficult. Observing a compulsion in younger children is easier to identify than obsessions because younger children are unlikely to be able to verbalize and describe obsessive thoughts or their reasoning behind carrying out the compulsive act. Diagnosis is more difficult compared to adults. When children and adolescents present with symptoms of OCD, the P-PCP should obtain a comprehensive medical history and include a neurological examination to rule out any other medical condition. In addition, when screening for possible OCD, the P-PCP should assess for any repeated streptococcal infections, especially if they correspond with the onset of obsessive or compulsive behaviors. Research has reported a link between streptococcal infections and OCD in some children. This pediatric autoimmune neuropsychiatric syndrome is referred to as Pediatric Autoimmune Neuropsychiatric Disorders Associated with Streptococcal Infection (PANDAS) and is managed by treating the underlying psychiatric symptoms in addition to treatment for the streptococcal infection (Rosenberg, 2016).

The diagnosis of OCD is based on *DSM-5* (APA, 2013) criteria including the presence of obsessions, compulsions, or both. When conducting the psychiatric assessment for OCD, the parent and child should be asked about each of the following *DSM-5* OCD diagnostic criteria, including if the obsessions or compulsions "take more than 1 hour per day or cause clinically significant distress or impairment in social, occupational, or other important areas of functioning" (Rosenberg, 2015, p. 5). In addition, the obsessive or compulsive symptoms should not have been associated with any type of medical conditions or due to drug abuse or medications. Furthermore, the P-PCP needs to ensure the symptoms are not associated with any other mental health disorders like anxiety, body dysmorphic disorder, hoarding, trichotillomania, excoriation, stereotypic movement, eating disorders, paraphilic disorders, impulse-control or CD, depression, delusional psychotic disorders, and autism spectrum disorder.

Research shows more than half of children with OCD have been found to have at least one comorbid psychiatric disorder, such as mood disorder, anxiety disorder, disruptive behavior disorder, Tourette's syndrome, speech/developmental disorder, enuresis, pervasive developmental disorder, and eating disorder. Furthermore, separation anxiety disorder can be linked as a precursor to OCD in childhood (Rosenberg, 2015).

Intercepting Problems for Children and Adolescents With OCD

P-PCPs have the opportunity to assist children who may be experiencing OCD symptoms because OCD signs may be nonspecific functional impairments such as poor school performance, loss of interest in activities, and the appearance of unusual habits (Sarvet, 2013). Children may have fear of being ridiculed by family or friends if they verbalize their obsessions or display the compulsive acts, so they might hide the behavior from others. Since the compulsive act causes anxiety or worry, the child will avoid situations that trigger the rituals. Direct questioning of the parent and child is needed to assess the symptoms of OCD. Hilt and Nussbaum (2016) recommend the following screening questions for OCD: "Do you ever get unwanted thoughts, urges, or pictures stuck in your mind and repeating so that you cannot get rid o themf?" or "Is there anything you feel you have to check, clean, or organize over and over again in order to feel okay?" (p. 110). If yes, then the P-PCP can further investigate by asking, "Do these experiences or behaviors ever cause you significant trouble with your friends or family, at school, or in another setting?" (p. 111).

One common general mental health screening instrument used in the primary care setting is the Pediatric Symptom Checklist (PSC). Children who have been identified as having positive signs of distress and functional impairments by the PSC should receive further screening by the P-PCP and referral to a mental health specialist. Rosenberg (2015) recommends a more detailed rating scale called the Children's Yale-Brown-Obsessive-Compulsive Scale (CY-BOCS; www.cappcny.org/home/media/CYBOCS.pdf) to identify symptoms specific to OCD (www.stlocd.org/handouts/YBOC-Symptom-Checklist.pdf).

EBM and Treatment for OCD

Rosenberg (2016) recommends cognitive behavioral therapy (CBT) as first-line treatment for mild to moderate cases of pediatric OCD. CBT sessions may be weekly for up to 5 months to achieve results. SSRIs may also be used in cases where CBT is unavailable. However, severe cases of pediatric OCD are better treated with both CBT and SSRIs and require lifetime treatment due to high relapse rates after SSRI withdrawal. The prescribed SSRI can help decrease the OCD symptoms and any related anxiety enabling CBT to be beneficial for the child.

There are three demonstrated SSRIs used as monotherapy for the treatment of child and adolescent OCD: fluoxetine, fluvoxamine, and sertraline. SSRIs are the treatment of choice due to their demonstrated efficacy and well-tolerated side effects profile that has been shown to be safe for children and adolescents (Rosenberg, 2016). The most common side effects for SSRIs in children and adolescents include headaches, abdominal pain, nausea, diarrhea, sleep changes, and jitteriness or agitation, which are dose dependent and improve over time. Recommendations for SSRIs are to initiate the drug at the lowest dose for week one and increase gradually every 2 to 4 weeks until a therapeutic dose is reached. The therapeutic dose is then administered for a 12-week trial. When prescribing fluoxetine, the P-PCP should be aware the dosage ranges are higher when treating pediatric OCD (20 to 60 mg/day) as compared to treating pediatric major depression (10 to 20 mg/day; Rosenberg, 2016).

Improvements in OCD symptoms may take more than 8 weeks to be achieved. Children and adolescents being treated with SSRIs should be monitored weekly during the first month of initiating treatment, and then monthly visits are recommended. To intercept problems in children with OCD, close monitoring by the P-PCP and family should include listening and observing for any suicidal thoughts or symptoms of mania. Suicidal thoughts or behaviors are rare adverse events but must be monitored closely due to the FDA boxed warning concerning the relationship between SSRI use and suicidality in children. SSRI induced mania is another controversial issue that must be closely monitored when prescribing SSRI medications due to a higher risk of mania in children aged 10 to 14 when treated with antidepressants compared to adolescents and young adults. These adverse events are rare; however, sexual side effects such as decreased libido and erectile dysfunction are common, leading to discontinuation of SSRIs in adolescents.

■ SCHIZOPHRENIA SPECTRUM

Fischer and Buchanan (2017) define schizophrenia as a "psychiatric disorder involving chronic or recurrent psychosis" (p. 1). Schizophrenia is considered a syndrome that presents with more than one symptom including cognitive impairments as well as mood and anxiety symptoms. Abidi (2013) explains the two types of childhood onset schizophrenia as very-early-onset schizophrenia (VEOS), which is rare but can begin in childhood occurring prior to age 13. The mean age of onset for VEOS is 6.9 years and is more common in boys. The psychotic symptoms of VEOS appear primarily as auditory hallucinations. When schizophrenia begins after age 13 but prior to age 17, it is termed early onset schizophrenia (EOS). The author further explains a psychotic experience as a perception that occurs in the absence of a stimulus. Hallucinations are defined by "hearing, seeing, tasting, smelling, or feeling something without the occurrence of an actual stimulating event" (Abidi, 2013, p. 297). Schizophrenic symptoms termed EOS that begin in adolescence and young adulthood is clustered into four distinct symptom domains as follows: "psychotic or positive symptom domain includes hallucinations, delusions, disorganized thoughts, and behaviors"; second, "negative system domain is marked by apathy, anhedonia, reduced or absent affect"; third, "altered cognition domain is marked by new difficulties in working memory, attention, processing speed, and executive function"; and last, "mood domain includes altercations in emotion or affect regulation, often secondary to the psychotic symptoms themselves" (Fischer & Buchanan, 2017, p. 297).

Fischer and Buchanan (2017) explain delusions to be false beliefs typically present in approximately 80% of cases. Cognitive impairments usually precede the onset of positive symptoms. Mood and anxiety symptoms have been reported to occur at higher rates in schizophrenia. Other associated physical manifestations associated with schizophrenia include neurological (impairment of sensory integration, motor coordination, and sequencing) and metabolic disturbances (diabetes, hyperlipidemia, and hypertension) due to side effects of antipsychotic medications and catatonia.

Assessment and Screening for Schizophrenia

Diagnosing psychotic-type symptoms is very difficult in younger children and pre-schoolers because most exhibit illogical thinking with transient hallucinations but do not have a true psychotic disorder. In fact, when there is evidence of a problem, metabolic issues are the most likely cause before the age of 6 (Otto, 2017, p. 1). Assessment should include a detailed medical history and neurological assessment with the following labs for the screening of a child who presents with psychotic symptoms: CBC to identify any infection, particularly meningitis or encephalitis; liver function test (LFT) to identify any metabolic disorders; chemistry panels to rule out abnormalities in sodium, calcium, magnesium, and glucose; urine toxicology to identify any substance-induced psychosis; TSH and free T4 to identify hyperthyroidism; and last, erythrocyte sedimentation rate (ESR) to identify autoimmune disorders like lupus (Sikich, 2013). Obtaining the recommended labs is useful in ruling out any medical condition that might explain the psychotic behavior. However, there are "no laboratory or physical examination findings or other biomarkers that are useful in making a diagnosis" (Fischer & Buchanan, 2017, p. 5). Failure to diagnosis a psychiatric problem can lead to delays in treatment and result in a poorer prognosis.

Sikich (2013) recommends using developmentally and culturally appropriate language when assessing for psychotic symptoms. Direct screening questions include: "Have you seen visions or other things that other people did not see?" "Have you heard noises, sounds, or voices that other people did not hear?" "Do you ever feel as if people are following you or trying to hurt you in some way?" "Have you ever felt that you have special powers or found special messages from the radio or TV seemingly meant just for you?" (Hilt & Nussbaum, 2016, p. 94).

In order to meet the *DSM-5* (APA, 2013) criteria for schizophrenia, the following inclusion criteria must be met (Hilt & Nussbaum, 2016):

> 1. At least 6 months of continuous signs of disturbance, which may include prodromal or residual symptoms. 2. During at least 1 month of that period, at least *two* of the following symptoms are present, and at least *one* of the symptoms must be delusions, hallucinations, or disorganized speech. (p. 94)

Intercepting Problems for Children and Adolescents With Schizophrenia

Referring a child or adolescent with schizophrenia to a mental health specialist is vital. Otto (2017) recommends that early intervention to identify psychotic illness in children results in a better prognosis. Treatment for schizophrenia needs to be comprehensive and include medications, case management, CBT, and supportive interventions, along with education about the disorder for the family. Early intervention has been proven to decrease the risk of schizophrenia relapse. The author has one very strong recommendation that should be used to counsel adolescents and that is to avoid cannabis. Research has shown that "marijuana increases the risk of conversion to schizophrenia and the risk of relapse" (Otto, 2017, p. 1). The P-PCP and mental health specialist can co-manage the child and adolescent to treat symptoms and monitor medication side effects, while assisting with helping the child and family cope with the disabilities and stigma associated with schizophrenia (Fischer & Buchanan, 2017).

EBM and Treatment for Schizophrenia

Abidi (2013) explains schizophrenia to be a "chronic and persistent serious mental illness that requires ongoing treatment" (p. 297). Regardless of age, the treatment of schizophrenia is multifaceted, involving antipsychotic medications, family education and support, and behavioral and social skills training. Once treatment for psychosis begins with antipsychotic medications, therapy can occur, as children are better able to participate once starting the medications. The primary mechanism of action for psychotic medication is to decrease dopamine levels in the brain. Typical or first-generation antipsychotics (FGAs) can lead to extrapyramidal adverse effects in children because children are more susceptible to these effects. These symptoms include increased muscle tone in extremities, tremors, akathisia, and dystonic movement. In some cases, irreversibility of the adverse side effects can occur, so children are not typically prescribed any FGA medications.

Atypical or second-generation antipsychotics (SGAs) were developed to effectively treat children and adolescents by indirectly targeting dopamine and having less extrapyramidal adverse effects. However, due to SGAs also targeting histaminergic and cholinergic receptors, metabolic abnormalities like "weight gain, hypercholesterolemia, dyslipidemia, glucose intolerance, and cardiac abnormalities" are common (Abidi, 2013, p. 303). Due to the side effects of SGAs, akathisia and weight gain are the most common reported reasons for noncompliance of these drugs. The FDA has approved the following SGAs for the first-line treatment of EOS: risperidone (Risperdal), olanzapine (Zyprexa), quetiapine (Seroquel), aripiprazole (Abilify), and paliperidone (Invega).

■ TRAUMA AND STRESSOR-RELATED DISORDER

Posttraumatic stress disorder (PTSD) is defined as a "debilitating and often chronic mental disorder that develops in some children and adolescents following exposure to a traumatic event" (McLaughlin, 2017, p. 1). The majority of children will experience a traumatic event prior to adulthood. Surprisingly, only 16% of children will actually develop PTSD after exposure to a traumatic event. A study conducted in the United States with over 6,000 adolescents revealed that 62% of youths experienced at least one traumatic event in their lifetime, including interpersonal violence, serious accidents or injuries, natural disaster, and death of a loved one; 19% have experienced three or more such events (Finkelhor, Ormond, Turner, & Hamby, 2005).

Certain disruptive behavior disorders have been shown to place children at higher risk for experiencing traumatic events. These disorders include ADHD, ODD, and CD. Children with the above disorders are more likely to encounter interpersonal violence, accidents, and injuries as compared to children without any disruptive behavior disorders. In addition, children who only reside with one biological parent are at increased risk for experiencing all forms of trauma.

Also, girls when compared to boys are two to three times more likely to develop PTSD. Childhood comorbidities with PTSD include anxiety disorders, depression, externalizing behavior problems, and substance use during adolescence.

The four symptom clusters of PTSD include intrusion, avoidance, negative alterations in cognition and mood, and hyperarousal. Intrusion symptoms consist of "uncontrollable thoughts, dreams, and emotional reactions about a traumatic event" (McLaughlin, 2017, p. 4). Examples of internal trauma reminders include thoughts and memories. External trauma reminders may include sounds, smells, people, and places related to the traumatic event. The intrusive thoughts are involuntary and uncontrollable to the child. Repetitive play in young children is commonly how intrusive thoughts are demonstrated. Furthermore, avoiding situations related to the traumatic event becomes a child's way of avoiding distress.

Changes in thoughts and emotions can occur in children and can increase "negative emotions like fear, anger, guilt, and shame, as well as reductions in positive emotions like happiness, interest, and love" (McLaughlin, 2017, p. 5). Melnyk and Jensen (2013) explain negative alterations in cognition and mood associated with the traumatic event to include the inability to remember important aspects of the event; persistent negative beliefs about oneself; distorted cognitions about the cause of the traumatic event that lead the child to blame themselves or others; persistent negative emotional state of fear, horror, anger, guilt, or shame; diminished interest in significant activities; feelings of detachment from others; and persistent inability to experience positive emotions.

Marked alterations in arousal and reactivity associated with the traumatic event include irritable behavior and anger outbursts expressed as verbal or physical aggression toward people or objects; reckless or self-destructive behavior; hypervigilance; exaggerated startle response; problems with concentration; and sleep disturbances. Duration of the disturbance is more than 1 month. Disturbance causes clinically significant distress or impairment in social, occupational, or other important areas of functioning. The disturbance is not attributable to the physiological effects of a substance or other medical condition.

Assessment and Screening for PTSD

DSM-5 (APA, 2013) diagnostic criteria for PTSD contain two similar sections with diagnostic criteria listed for children older than 6 years and children 6 years and younger. PTSD symptoms appear differently in younger children as evidence demonstrates a "lower threshold of symptoms is more valid for diagnosing PTSD in this population" (McLaughlin, 2017, p. 6). Criteria for 6 years and older include exposure to actual or threatened death, serious injury, or sexual violence in one or more of the following ways: directly experiencing the traumatic event; witnessing the event that occurred to others; learning about traumatic events that occurred to a close family member or friend; and repeated exposure to details of the traumatic event. Presence of one or more of the previously listed intrusion symptoms that are associated with the traumatic event may include involuntary and recurring distressing memories of the traumatic event; recurrent dreams; dissociative reactions when the child feels as if the traumatic event were recurring; intense psychological distress at exposure to internal or external cues that resemble the traumatic event; and marked physiological reactions to internal and external cues that resemble an aspect of traumatic event. Persistent avoidance of stimuli associated with a traumatic event, beginning after the traumatic event occurred, by one or both of the following: avoidance of distressing memories or thoughts associated with the traumatic event and avoidance of external reminders that cause distressing memories associated with the traumatic event.

Intercepting Problems for Children and Adolescents With PTSD

When assessing a child for possible PTSD symptoms, the P-PCP needs to determine if the symptoms are related to a traumatic event or another type of mental disorder. P-PCPs should primarily "focus on intrusion symptoms, including intrusive thoughts, strong reactivity to trauma cues, nightmares, repetitive play; avoidance of trauma reminders; and hypervigilance" (McLaughlin, 2017, p. 9). Suicide risk assessment is also recommended to be performed in addition to evaluation of anxiety disorders, disruptive behavior problems, and substance use.

EBM for PTSD

The typical course of PTSD is extremely variable, with two-thirds recovering and one-third having chronic PTSD. Strawn and Keeshin (2017) explain the first-line treatment of PTSD in children is evidence-based trauma-focused psychotherapy. A referral is needed for the child to receive the appropriate care by a mental health specialist. There are currently no FDA-approved medications to treat PTSD in children or adolescents. Studies have proven most SSRIs are not effective in reducing PTSD symptoms in children. Furthermore, SSRIs may only be considered if the child or adolescent is also diagnosed with MDD or anxiety. Strawn and Keeshin note one uncontrolled trial that has shown evidence that "guanfacine may reduce intrusive and hyperarousal symptoms in children with PTSD symptoms" (Strawn & Keeshin, 2017, p. 4). Guanfacine and clonidine are not FDA approved to treat PTSD in children but their side effects profile in treating other mental health disorders has shown these medications to be well tolerated in children and adolescents. Prazosin is an alpha-1 adrenergic antagonist, prescribed at night, and has been proven beneficial in the treatment of sleep difficulties and nightmares in children. However, prazosin is not FDA approved for the treatment of sleep issues in children but does have FDA approval for the treatment of hypertension in children and adolescents. Last, evidence has not been proven for use of other medications like SGA, anticonvulsants, or SSRIs for treating PTSD symptoms in children, so they are not recommended due to their side effects (Strawn & Keeshin, 2017).

■ SUMMARY

In summary, improved access to mental behavioral health services for children and adolescents is greatly needed due to the high rate of mental and behavioral disorders that go untreated. Unfortunately, there are limited mental health resources in certain areas of the country and a shortage of mental health specialists to meet the demand. The P-PCP serving in the primary care role can assist children and adolescents in the early identification, diagnosis, treatment when appropriate, monitoring, and referral to appropriate mental health specialists when presented with behavioral, emotional, developmental, psychosocial, or educational concerns. The P-PCP needs to be competent and knowledgeable of the common mental health disorders. In addition to signs of common mental health disorders, the P-PCP must be aware of these indications for psychiatric specialty referral: suicidal ideation, psychotic features, impulsive or aggressive behaviors, functional impairments, comorbid conditions like ADHD, multiple failed medication trials, anxiety disorder or substance abuse, and recurrence of mood episodes. Collaboration with the mental health specialist and in some cases the school system is a vital part of helping these children with behavioral and mental health disorders to reach their fullest potential.

■ REFERENCES

Abidi, S. (2013). Psychosis in children and youth: Focus on early-onset schizophrenia. *Pediatrics in Review*, *34*(7), 296–306. doi:10.1542/pir.34-7-296

American Psychiatric Association. (2013). *The diagnostic and statistical manual of mental disorders* (5th ed.). Author.

Axelson, D. (2016). *Pediatric bipolar disorder: Overview of choosing treatment*. Retrieved from https://www.uptodate.com/contents/pediatric-bipolar-disorder-overview-of-choosing-treatment

Birmaher, B. (2016). *Pediatric bipolar disorder: Epidemiology, pathogenesis, clinical manifestations, and course*. Retrieved from https://www.uptodate.com/contents/pediatric-bipolar-disorder-epidemiology-pathogenesis-clinical-manifestations-and-course

Birmaher, B. (2017). *Bipolar disorder in children and adolescents: Assessment and diagnosis*. Retrieved from https://www.uptodate.com/contents/bipolar-disorder-in-children-and-adolescents-assessment-and-diagnosis

Black, D. (2016). *Antisocial personality disorder: Epidemiology, clinical manifestations, course and diagnosis*. Retrieved from https://www.uptodate.com/contents/antisocial-personality-disorder-epidemiology-clinical-manifestations-course-and-diagnosis

Black, D. (2017). *Treatment of antisocial personality disorder*. Retrieved from https://www.uptodate.com/contents/treatment-of-antisocial-personality-disorder

Bonin, L. (2016). *Pediatric unipolar depression: Epidemiology, clinical features, assessment, and diagnosis*. Retrieved from https://www.uptodate.com/contents/pediatric-unipolar-depression-epidemiology-clinical-features-assessment-and-diagnosis

Centers for Disease Control and Prevention. (2017). *Youth violence: Prevention strategies*. Retrieved from https://www.cdc.gov/violenceprevention/youthviolence/prevention.html

Finkelhor, D., Ormond, R., Turner, H., & Hamby, S. (2005). The victimization of children and youth: A comprehensive, national survey. *Child Maltreat*, *10*(5). doi:10.1177/1077559504271287

Fischer, B., & Buchanan, R. (2017). *Schizophrenia: Clinical manifestations, course, assessment, and diagnosis*. Retrieved from https://www.uptodate.com/contents/schizophrenia-clinical-manifestations-course-assessment-and-diagnosis

Hill, R. (2016). *Moody or aggressive kids. Partnership Access Line*. Retrieved from http://www.seattle-childrens.org/pal

Hilt, R. J., & Nussbaum, A. M. (2016). *DSM-5 pocket guide to child and adolescent mental health*. Arlington, VA: American Psychological Association Publishing.

LaRosa, A. (2017). *Developmental–behavioral surveillance and screening in primary care*. Retrieved from https://www.uptodate.com/contents/developmental-behavioral-surveillance-and-screening-in-primary-care

McLaughlin, K. (2017). *Posttraumatic stress disorder in children: Epidemiology, pathogenesis, clinical manifestations, course, assessment, and diagnosis*. Retrieved from https://www.uptodate.com/contents/posttraumatic-stress-disorder-in-children-epidemiology-pathogenesis-clinical-manifestations-course-assessment-and-diagnosis

Melnyk, B. M., & Jensen, P. (2013). *A practical guide to child and adolescent mental health screening, early intervention, and health promotion*. New York, NY: National Association of Pediatric Nurse Practitioners (NP-PCPAP).

Mitchell, A. M., Davies, M. A., Cassesse, C., & Curran, R. (2014). Antidepressant use in children, adolescents, and young adults: 10 years after the Food and Drug Administration black box warning. *The Journal for Nurse Practitioners*, 10(3), 149–156. doi:10.1016/j.nurpra.2013.08.012

Moses, S. (2017). Depression screening with Sig E Caps. *Family practice notebook*. Retrieved from http://www.fpnotebook.com/Psych/Exam/DprsnScrngWthSgECps.htm

Nierengarten, M. (2015). *Bipolar disorder in children: Assessment and diagnosis*. Retrieved from http://contemporarypediatrics.modernmedicine.com/contemporary-pediatrics/news/bipolar-disorder-children-assessment-and-diagnosis

Otto, M. A. (2017). Children with psychotic illness aren't treated soon enough. *Pediatric News*. Retrieved from http://www.mdedge.com/pediatricnews/article/130860/pediatrics/children-psychotic-illness-arent-treated-soon-enough?channel=248

PHQ-9. Retrieved from http://www.phqscreeners.com/sites/g/files/g10016261/f/201412/PHQ-9_English.pdf

Rosenberg, D. (2015). *Obsessive-compulsive disorder in children and adolescents: Epidemiology, pathogenesis, clinical manifestations, course, assessment, and diagnosis*. Retrieved from https://www.uptodate.com/contents/obessive-compulsive-disorder-in-children-and-adolescents-epidemiology-pathogenesis-clinical-manifestations-course-assessment-and-diagnosis

Rosenberg, D. (2016). *Treatment of obsessive-compulsive disorder in children and adolescents*. Retrieved from https://www.uptodate.com/contents/treatment-of-obsessive-compulsive-disorder-in-children-and-adolescents

Sarvet, B. (2013). Childhood obsessive-compulsive disorder. *Pediatrics in Review*, 34(19), 19–28. doi:10.1542/pir.34-1-19

Sikich, L. (2013). Diagnosis and evaluation of hallucinations and other psychotic symptoms in children and adolescents. *Child and Adolescent Psychiatric Clinics of North America*, 22(4), 655–673. doi:10.1016/j.chc.2013.06.005

Smiga, S. M., & Elliott, G. R. (2011). Psychopharmacology of depression in children and adolescents. *Pediatric Clinics of North America*, 58(1), 155–171. doi:10.1016/j.pcl.2010.11.007

Strawn, J., & Keeshin, B. (2017). *Pharmacotherapy for posttraumatic stress disorder in children and adolescents*. Retrieved from https://www.uptodate.com/contents/pharmacotherapy-for-posttraumatic-stress-disorder-in-children-and-adolescents

Tang, M. H., & Pinsky, E. G. (2015). Mood and affect disorders. *Pediatrics in Review*, 36(2), 52–61. doi:10.1542/pir.36-2-52

Windel, L., Anderko. L., & Konetzka, T. (2011). Transforming primary care: Improving on the medical home model. *Journal of Interprofessional Care*, 25, 305–307. doi:10.3109/13561820.2011/571316

Youngstrom, E., Meyers, O., Demeter, C., Youngstrom, J., Morello, L., Piiparinen, R., . . . Findling, R. L. (2005). Comparing diagnostic checklists for pediatric bipolar disorder in academic and community mental health settings. *Bipolar Disorder*, 7, 507. doi:10.1111/j.1399-5618.2005.00269.x

CHAPTER 26

Neurological Disorders: Neurofibromatosis Type 1 and Tourette Syndrome

BETH HEUER

Children with neurofibromatosis type 1 (NF-1) and Tourette syndrome (TS) may present with undiagnosed symptoms to the pediatric primary care office. Early identification of the symptoms, with diagnosis as early as possible with appropriate treatment interventions, is critical to meet the child's physical and behavioral healthcare needs. This chapter provides an in-depth discussion of the childhood presentations for NF-1 and TS with a focus on the cognitive, emotional, social, psychological, and developmental and behavioral health. Treatment strategies, including medical and behavioral therapy, are presented for children with these disorders to *intercept* behavioral health problems as early as possible with the goal of achieving behavioral health that enables the child to grow and interact within the family, school, and other community activities with a positive self-esteem and self-image.

■ NEUROFIBROMATOSIS TYPE 1

NF-1 is a genetic disorder that affects one in 3,000 to 4,000 persons worldwide (National Institute of Neurological Disorders and Stroke, 2011). The NF-1 gene (located on chromosome 17q11.2) encodes neurofibromin, a tumor suppressor gene that downregulates cell differentiation and proliferation along the "Ras signaling pathway." With an NF-1 gene mutation, a nonworking form of neurofibromin is made, leading the Ras cell signaling pathway into overdrive (Ratner & Miller, 2015). This enhanced cell proliferation is a central cause of tumor growth and other clinical features of NF-1. Fifty percent of cases of NF-1 are de novo mutations, and the other 50% are inherited in an autosomal dominant pattern. NF-1 is noted to have extremely variable gene expression, even within the same family. One family member can have significant physical or neurocognitive symptoms, while another family member may have only very mild symptoms (Pasmant, Vidaud, Vidaud, & Wolkenstein, 2012). Please see Box 26.1 for a case presentation on NF-1.

BOX 26.1

CASE STUDY: NF-1

Six-year-old Anna presents for well-child check as a new patient to your practice and is accompanied by her mother. Previous primary care has been sporadic, as her mother has moved five times in the past 4 years. Anna is in kindergarten, and her teachers report that Anna is inattentive and performing at well below grade level compared to her peers. She fidgets constantly and requires continuous redirection to stay in her seat and not disrupt her classmates as they work. Her mother is concerned that Anna is somewhat socially "awkward" and seems to have difficulty communicating easily with children her age.

On physical exam, Anna's height is <10th percentile on the WHO growth chart. She appears to be macrocephalic; a head circumference is obtained and is on the 95th percentile on the WHO growth chart. A Woods lamp evaluation reveals 19 café au lait macules >5 mm in size on trunk and extremities. Bilateral scattered inguinal freckling is noted. Her neurologic and musculoskeletal exams are within normal limits. As you discuss these skin findings with Anna's mother, she comments that Anna's biological father also had a number of these "birthmarks." You suspect that this child has neurofibromatosis type 1 (NF-1).

Questions:
1. How is the diagnosis of NF-1 confirmed?
2. What physical sequelae are associated with NF-1?
3. Are inattention and poor academic performance related to the physical diagnosis of NF-1?
4. What guidance can be provided to enhance a child's social, emotional, and cognitive development?

Note: Each of these questions is answered in the NF-1 information presented in this chapter.

Confirming a Diagnosis of NF-1

To establish a diagnosis of NF-1, children and adolescents must meet two (or more) of the criteria seen in Table 26.1. Genetic testing is available to confirm a clinical diagnosis (90%–95% detection rate) or to make a diagnosis when only one of the diagnostic criteria is met. Testing can resolve diagnostic ambiguity and set the stage for genetic counseling for reproductive decision making (Hirbe & Gutmann, 2014).

What Physical Sequelae Are Associated With NF-1?

The physical sequelae of NF-1 can cause a variety of significant impairments in a percentage of those affected (Hirbe & Gutmann, 2014). Children with NF-1 have a less than 20% risk of developing an optic pathway glioma, which is the most common type of central nervous system tumor in NF-1. While typically benign, optic pathway gliomas may cause visual loss. Multiple cutaneous and subcutaneous neurofibromas may cause disfigurement, pain, and dysfunction. Plexiform neurofibromas are neurofibromas that affect multiple branches of large nerves. They may be located deep under the skin and not become visible until they have grown significantly. They can also grow along the spinal column, causing vertebral erosion and spinal cord compression. Plexiform tumors can also transform into difficult-to-treat malignant peripheral nerve sheath tumors (MPNSTs). The cumulative lifetime risk of developing an MPNST in NF-1 is estimated at 8% to

TABLE 26.1

DIAGNOSTIC CRITERIA FOR NF-1

Individuals meet criteria for diagnosis when two or more of the following are present:

- ≥ Six café au lait macules (>5 mm in greatest diameter in prepubertal children; >15 mm in greatest diameter in post-pubertal individuals)
- Axillary and/or inguinal freckling
- Two or more neurofibromas of any type or one plexiform neurofibroma
- A distinctive bone abnormality (sphenoid dysplasia or thinning of long bone cortex, with or without pseudarthrosis)
- Optic nerve or optic pathway glioma
- Two or more Lisch nodules on slit lamp exam
- A first-degree relative (parent, sibling, or offspring) with NF-1 per these criteria

NF-1, neurofibromatosis type 1.

Source: From National Institute of Health. (1987). Neurofibromatosis. *NIH Consensus Statement Online 1987 July 13-15, 6*(12), 1–19.

13%. Approximately one third of patients with NF-1 will develop some type of bone abnormality, including sphenoid wing or long-bone dysplasia, dysplastic scoliosis, shorter stature, and macrocephaly (Hirbe & Gutmann, 2014).

Brain MRI findings often include T2 hyperintensities suggestive of dysmyelination. It remains unclear whether this dysmyelination contributes to cognitive difficulty in children with NF-1, and whether it may improve over time (Payne et al., 2014). Brain tumors such as astrocytomas as well as increased incidence of other malignancies (including myeloid leukemias and breast cancer) are also noted. Vascular malformations may include renal artery or pulmonary artery stenosis, coarctation of the aorta, and a type of cerebrovascular arterial blockage known as moya moya. Patients with NF-1 also have increased incidence of hypertension, migraines, and seizures (Hirbe & Gutmann, 2014). Approximately two thirds of patients with NF will never experience significant health problems. Life expectancy for patients with NF-1 is slightly reduced, often due to malignant tumors and vascular manifestations.

Cognitive Development in Children With NF-1

NF-1 is associated with impairments in cognitive, behavioral, and social domains. Many studies have shown a correlation between NF-1 and cognitive vulnerabilities (Marrus & Constantino, 2017; Walsh, et al., 2016). Some patients show strengths in verbal reasoning and weaknesses in working memory and processing speed. The majority of patients show average to low-average IQ scores. It is estimated that up to two thirds of patients with NF-1 will develop some form of learning disability. Learning disabilities represent the most significant cause of lifetime morbidity associated with this disease. Most commonly seen are deficits in attention, visual–spatial memory, and executive function. Executive function difficulty involves trouble with problem solving, abstract concept formation, planning/organization, shifting attention, and tasks that require mental flexibility (Plasschaert, Van Eylen,

Descheemaeker, Noens, Legius, & Steyaert, 2016). Deficits in visual–spatial–per-ceptual skills can result in reading, spelling, and written expressive learning dis-abilities. Poor fine-motor coordination is associated with poor handwriting skills (Marrus & Constantino, 2017; van der Vaart, et al., 2016).

Children with NF-1 may exhibit a higher degree of academic underachievement, often warranting a complete neuropsychological evaluation (Coutinho et al., 2016). Examples of appropriate testing may include the Weschler Intelligence Scales, the NEPSY, the Behavioral Rating Inventory of Executive Function (BRIEF), and the Kaufman Assessment Battery for Children (K-ABC). Age-appropriate testing can be done as early as preschool, and retesting is typically recommended during big transition periods for the child and adolescent (such as moving up academically into elementary, middle, or high school). Repeat testing is also helpful for older adolescents and young adults as they choose a career path and begin working.

Emotional Development in Children With NF-1

Increased emotional uncertainty can be seen in children, adolescents, and adults with NF-1. All individuals with NF-1 are at risk for increased concerns for body image, leading to lower self-esteem and isolation. Some children are reluctant to participate in gym or other physical activities in clothing that may expose signifi-cant numbers of café au lait macules or multiple cutaneous neurofibromas. When these concerns are noted, this is an opportunity for pediatric primary care pro-viders (P-PCPs) and specialists to *intercept* potential emotional health problems related to body image and self-esteem by providing guidance before issues arise, for example, about clothing to wear while participating in gym class, and advocat-ing for parents to speak with teachers in advance of the academic year to "solve problems" before they emerge (see Chapter 1).

Concerns for the future may include ongoing alterations in physical appear-ance leading to disfigurement, family planning concerns due to autosomal domi-nant nature of the disease, and long-term sequelae including malignancies and potential decreased life span.

Social Development and NF-1

Children with NF-1 often have impairments in functional communication and social skills (Allen, Willard, Anderson, Hardy, & Bonner, 2016; Klein-Tasman, Janke, Luo, & Casnar, 2013). Children with NF-1 are at an elevated risk for dif-ficulty with social competence skills and can have difficulty developing and main-taining friendships. Language impairments may include phonologic speech errors and expressive/receptive language delay. Articulation skills can be impaired by the presence of oral neurofibromas or facial plexiform tumors. Early evaluation and treatment with speech therapy services also can intercept these problems by enhancing language and communication skills.

Pediatric speech therapy centers and pediatric hospital settings may offer therapeutic groups for children who need assistance in building social communi-cation skills to interact and communicate more effectively with others. These skills may include learning to problem solve, active listening, taking turns and maintain-ing a topic during conversation, and understanding and expressing feelings.

Physical differences, including short stature, bony abnormalities, or disfiguring plexiform neurofibromas, may further cause social difficulty. Children may be rejected by peers or bullied. School-based counseling can be an excellent adjunct for addressing social concerns. Local and national NF support organizations, including the NF Clinics Association, can offer activities, summer camps, retreats, and support groups for children and their families.

Psychological Development and NF-1

Children with NF-1 have a high prevalence of other psychological comorbidities (Lewis, Porter, Williams, North, & Payne, 2016). On parent and teacher behavioral rating forms, many children with NF show a higher incidence of internalizing, externalizing, and thought problems (Lehtonen, Howie, Trump, & Huson, 2013).

Researchers postulate that there is a three- to 12-fold increased risk of ADHD in children with NF-1 when compared to the 5% prevalence in children in the general population (Potvin, Hardy, & Walsh, 2015). Studies using the clinical diagnostic criteria for attention deficit hyperactivity disorder (ADHD) suggest that the incidence of this disorder among children with NF-1 is as high as 40% to 50% (Lehtonen et al., 2013). Inhibitory control is often more problematic. Treatment principles are the same as with the general population with ADHD, including behavioral modification therapy, medication management, and accommodations in school and home settings. Management strategies for attention deficit hyperactivity disorder (ADHD) are discussed in Chapters 15 and 18.

Children with NF-1 may also have an increased incidence of autism spectrum disorder (ASD) in comparison to children without NF-1 (Garg et al., 2013). See Chapters 15 and 27 for further information on ASD. The delays in social, executive, and language skills that are inherent in NF-1 may confuse the diagnosis of autism, and a thorough assessment is required. Use of the Autism Diagnostic Observation Schedule-2 (ADOS-2) can help better delineate an appropriate diagnosis in this population (Garg et al., 2015).

■ TIC DISORDERS AND TS

Tics are characterized as brief, rapid, nonrhythmic, involuntary, and purposeless movements (motor tics) or vocalizations (vocal) tics. Early symptoms appear in childhood, with average onset between ages 3 and 9 years. Tics will typically peak in severity in early adolescence (between ages 10 and 12) and can vary in frequency and severity across the life span. More than 18% of all children have one or more tics at some point in their development (National Institute of Neurological Disorders and Stroke, 2012). Tics are three times more common in males than females. They can be influenced by internal and external factors such as fatigue, excitement, stress, or the reactions of others to one's tics. Tics can be simple (involving one movement or sound) or complex. A complex tic involves a coordinated movement produced by several muscle groups (motor tic) or linguistically meaningful vocalizations (vocal tic). Contrary to widespread belief, copropraxia (obscene movements or gestures) and copralalia (utterance of profanity or slurs) are less common. Please see Box 26.2 for a case presentation on TS.

BOX 26.2

CASE STUDY: TOURETTE SYNDROME

Anthony is a 9-year-old boy who presents for a well-child check. He has previously been in good health. He is currently in fourth grade. He was previously described as a straight-A student and a bit of a "perfectionist." When last seen in the office at 7 years of age, his father had reported that Anthony had several motor tics, including eye rolling and shoulder shrugging. His parents note today that these tics have increased in frequency and severity. For the past 14 months, Anthony has been making vocalizations that include throat clearing and humming noises. He is becoming increasing anxious and self-conscious about these movements and vocalizations. He has been exhibiting school-avoidance behaviors over the past 3 months, leading to a decline in his grades.

Questions:
1. Does this child meet criteria for diagnosis of Tourette syndrome based on clinical history and presentation?
2. What common comorbidities are associated with tics and Tourette syndrome?
3. When do pharmacologic and behavioral interventions become necessary to treat tics and Tourette syndrome?

Note: Each of these questions are answered in the TS information presented in this chapter.

Diagnostic Criteria for TS

TS is characterized by the presence of multiple motoric and vocal tics, developing during childhood and persisting for greater than a year (see Table 26.2). Evidence from twin and family studies suggests that TS is an inherited disorder. Scharf et al. (2015) published a meta-analysis that suggests a population prevalence of TS in children of 0.3% to 0.9%. The mean age at onset of TS is 7 years old.

Tics are thought to originate in the basal ganglia, a part of the brain that matures around 10 years of age. Recent MRI studies measuring gray matter and white matter volume differences between children with and without TS have suggested morphological differences in children with tic disorders. Some children demonstrate lower white matter volume bilaterally in the prefrontal cortex. The prefrontal cortex is the region of the brain where voluntary control over our actions occurs. Research MRIs also suggest increased gray matter volume in the hypothalamus, posterior thalamus, and midbrain (Greene, Williams, Koller, Schlaggar, & Black, 2016).

Comorbid Conditions in Children and Adolescents With TS

The most common neurologic and psychiatric comorbid conditions associated with tics and TS are ADHD (Chapter 29), anxiety and obsessive-compulsive disorder (OCD; Chapter 48), depression (Chapter 29), seizures disorders, and sleep disorders (Bellini et al., 2013). Approximately 7% of children with ADHD have TS, yet about 60% of children with TS have ADHD. Studies have shown a four-fold increase in migraines in children and adolescents diagnosed with TS (Bellini et al., 2013).

TABLE 26.2

TOURETTE SYNDROME DIAGNOSTIC CRITERIA

- Presence of two or more motor tics (for example, blinking or shrugging the shoulders) *and* at least one vocal tic (for example, humming, clearing the throat, or yelling out a word or phrase), although they might not always happen simultaneously
Symptoms must develop before the age of 18 years
- Tics must occur multiple times per day nearly every day or intermittently for at least 1 year
- Tics must not be due to the direct physiological effects of a substance or general medical condition

Source: Adapted from American Psychiatric Association. (2013). *Diagnostic and statistical manual of mental disorders* (5th ed.). Washington, DC: Author.

Cognitive Development in Children With TS

It is unclear whether children with TS alone have increased risk for a learning disability. Most studies have not isolated children with tics alone from children presenting with tics and comorbid ADHD or other impairments. Children with TS may be more likely to have math, written expressive, and other learning disabilities compared to non-TS peers (Sulkowski, McGuire, & Tesoro, 2016). Difficulty with visual–motor integration may impact handwriting and ease in copying from the blackboard or Smartboard. Classroom performance can be affected by the presence of tics. Reading activities and handwriting can be disrupted by motor tics of the eyes, head, and neck. Children with vocal tics may have more difficulty reading aloud in class. Using the diagnosis of "other health impairment," they may qualify for an individualized education plan (IEP) under the Individuals with Disabilities Education Act (IDEA) or for a Section 504 accommodation plan.

Classroom accommodations may include:

- Excusing child, as his/her request, to nurse's office or other private area to "release" the tics
- Untimed testing to reduce stress/anxiety
- Oral exams and reduced written assignments when the child's tics interfere with his/her handwriting ability

Social and Emotional Development for Individuals With TS

Frustration, anxiety, depressed mood, and hopelessness are commonly reported by children, adolescents, and adults with TS and other chronic tic disorders (Evans, Seri, & Cavanna et al., 2016). These symptoms are often multifactorial in nature and may be managed with behavioral therapy and medication, as indicated.

Tic behaviors can be disruptive in the classroom and social settings, leading to stigmatization. The nature of TS symptoms and the confusion between "voluntary" and "involuntary" behaviors adds to the vulnerability of children with this condition. Up to 26% of children and adolescents with TS report being victimized or bullied (Zinner, Conelea, Glew, Woods, & Budman, 2012; see Chapter 21 in this book for details on bullying). Children who are victimized can exhibit increased tic severity, anxiety, depression, explosive behaviors, and poorer psychosocial function. Victim status has been associated with greater tic frequency, complexity, and severity; explosive outbursts; internalizing symptoms; and lower quality of life. Behavioral or conduct issues can be seen in more than 25% of children with TS. Anticipatory guidance, specific bullying screening and prevention, and social skills training may be necessary to intercept potential problem behaviors in children with a diagnosis of TS (Zinner et al., 2012).

Psychological Development in TS

Young people with TS have reported poorer perception of their quality of life (Evans, Seri, & Cavanna, 2016). Anxiety, frustration, hopelessness, and low mood are commonly reported by patients with TS or other chronic tic disorders and appear to be multifactorial in origin. Although most individuals with TS experience a significant decline in their tics in later adolescence/early adulthood, the associated neurobehavioral sequelae (including ADHD, depression, generalized anxiety, mood swings, OCD, and panic attacks) may persist into adulthood. Dealing with these comorbid conditions can create a state of tension or anxiety that further exacerbates tics (Capriotti, Himle, & Woods, 2014). Due to the waxing/waning characteristics of tics, however, it is not always necessary to look for a specific psychological trigger for a tic exacerbation.

Treatment Strategies for TS

Considerations for treatment of tics include impairment of daily function, psychological distress, pain or injury related to movements, negative impact on school performance, and interference with social function. The main treatment strategies for tics involve medication and behavioral interventions. A recent systematic review of treatment strategies indicates that antipsychotics and alpha-adrenergic agonist medications, along with therapy (notably habit reversal therapy [HRT] and comprehensive behavioral intervention for tics [CBIT]), can effectively reduce tic frequency and severity (Hollis et al., 2016).

Medication Therapy for TS

There are no drugs of choice for treatment of TS. Medication strategies are highly individualized. The basis of medication therapy for tics is to use drugs that modulate the dopaminergic system, blocking post-synaptic D2-receptors (Gilbert & Jankovic, 2014). Other neurotransmitters (such as serotonin) are also important in the pathophysiology of both the tics and other comorbid conditions. Although combined pharmacotherapy is a more complicated approach, the advantages can include (a) reduced doses of each medication, thus minimizing the likelihood of side effects associated with higher doses of single agents, and (b) synergistic effects related to combined medications.

Alpha-adrenergic agonists (guanfacine and clonidine) have shown modest efficacy in tics on placebo-controlled trials. Guanfacine is less sedating for daytime use, but clonidine can reduce comorbid sleep disturbances. Side effects may include fatigue, sedation, dizziness, depression, headache, irritability, hypotension, constipation, and dry mouth.

Typical antipsychotics (haloperidol [Haldol] and pimozide [Orap]) cause strong blockade of D2 dopamine receptors, but are associated with higher incidence of extrapyramidal symptoms. Other associated side effects are fatigue, weight gain, muscle rigidity, tardive dyskinesia, depression, and cognitive "dulling."

A class of medications used more frequently for tics are the atypical antipsychotic medications, including risperidone (Risperdal) and aripiprazole (Abilify). Risperidone has a high affinity for D2 and 5HT2 receptors but may be a less desirable option due to side effects of hyperglycemia, dyslipidemia, fatigue, hypotension, hyperprolactinemia, and weight gain. Aripiprazole has D2 receptor binding and partial agonist effects. Side effects can include weight gain, nausea, akathisia (feeling of restlessness or agitation), and sedation (Takemoto, Hodding, & Kraus, 2016).

Several antiepileptic drugs (AEDs) are also used in the treatment of tic disorders. Gamma-aminobutyric acid (GABA) is the primary inhibitory neurotransmitter released by the globus pallidus internus within the brain. AEDs act at the GABA receptors, reducing involuntary movements. Topiramate (Topamax) was effective in reducing tic frequency/severity in a double-blind, placebo-controlled trial (Jankovic, Jimejez-Shahed, & Brown et al., 2010). Zonisamide (Zonegran), levetiracetam (Keppra), valproic acid, and other AEDs have also been utilized. Side effects of AEDs can be dose-related and may include vision changes, fatigue, unsteadiness, cognitive dulling, and sedation. Zonisamide has notably been associated with behavioral changes. Benzodiazepines have been sparingly used short-term for acute tic exacerbations (Kurlan, 2014).

Targeted botulinum toxin injections have been utilized to relax specific muscle groups in well-localized motor tics, but have been less effective in vocal tics. Botulinum toxin blocks acetylcholine release and temporarily weakens the associated muscle group, making it impossible to perform the tic. Some providers suggest supplementation with magnesium and vitamin B_6 (pyridoxine) to reduce tic frequency/severity. Magnesium reduces neuromuscular hyperexcitability, and vitamin B_6 is associated with decarboxylation of glutamic acid to GABA, DOPA to dopamine, and 5-hydroxytryptophan to serotonin. One open-label study (Garcia-Lopez et al., 2009) indicated possible effectiveness for this supplement combination, and the low side effect profile of these supplements can make this combination desirable in children.

Due to the high comorbid incidence of ADHD and TS, the question arises as to whether stimulant medications (which may exacerbate tics) can be utilized effectively. Many patients with TS tolerate stimulants well. Basic tenets of stimulant therapy for children with TS and ADHD are as follows: (a) if the child is already diagnosed with TS, a cautious trial of stimulant medication may be helpful and (b) if the child has already been diagnosed with ADHD and treated with stimulants and significant tics develop, the family can choose from several options. One option is that the clinician/family may elect to stop treatment with stimulants until the tics are treated and under control. Once controlled, the stimulants may then be added back in to treat the ADHD symptoms. Another option is to add in a second medication to manage the tics. Atomoxetine is a frequently prescribed stimulant for children who have ADHD and comorbid tic disorder diagnoses. A

2017 literature review (Yang, Li, Gao, & Zhao, 2017) suggested that atomoxetine may, however, induce or exacerbate tic symptoms in a small number of patients.

Behavioral Therapy for TS

A number of generalized behavioral/psychological interventions (including anger management training, family therapy, individual and group counseling, psychotherapy, and relaxation training) can help reduce tic triggers and decrease the impact of comorbid diagnoses.

Interventions that educate and provide social support can help with development of effective coping strategies, build resilience, and enhance self-esteem. Two therapies that have garnered empirical support are HRT and CBIT (McGuire et al., 2014).

HRT is one component of the more extensive CBIT protocol. Both HRT and CBIT are based on the following characteristics of tic disorders: (a) tics can get better and worse on their own; (b) tics are often done in response to a premonitory urge (a sensation that a tic is about to occur); and (c) tics can often be suppressed, at least for a brief time. Releasing the tic will briefly relieve the often-unpleasant sensation associated with the premonitory urge. CBIT breaks the premonitory urge > tic > relief feedback cycle. The use of CBIT and HRT has been supported across numerous randomized controlled trials. A pediatric study published in the *Journal of the American Medical Association* (Piacentini et al., 2010) indicated that 52.5% of the child participants who received CBIT showed significant symptom improvement compared to 18.5% receiving the control treatment. Improvement was sustained for at least 6 months after the end of the study.

CBIT requires a self-aware individual who can recognize his/her awareness of the tic premonitory urge. In children, self-awareness typically matures at about the age of 10 (+/-2 years). Until then children are generally aware that they tic, but do not realize when they are about to perform a tic. The therapeutic components of CBIT are described in Table 26.3.

Additional Treatment Considerations for TS

Treatment strategies that have been discussed to help reduce or eliminate tics in children are available in the literature. Transcranial magnetic stimulation is a non-invasive approach using a magnetic current delivered by a transducer wand. The magnet reportedly causes intra-cortical motor inhibition, causing a downstream improvement on basal ganglia activity and reducing tic symptoms. Preliminary studies have indicated that it is safe and may reduce tics. *There are no current published studies related to use of transcranial magnetic stimulant in pediatric TS.*

Deep brain stimulation (DBS) involves electrical stimulation of specific regions of the brain using surgically implanted electrodes. There are strict criteria for consideration for this experimental surgical approach, and *it has not been approved for trial in pediatric populations.*

Biofeedback is another noninvasive approach to tic management. Patients learn to manipulate a physiological measure to improve emotion/cognition and lessen triggers for tics. Acupuncture has also been utilized to alleviate muscle tension and create a generalized sense of well-being. Finally, there has been discussion as

TABLE 26.3

COMPONENTS OF CBIT

1. **Psychoeducation:** Assessment of what situations tend to exacerbate and alleviate tics. The child or adolescent can then learn to avoid tic triggers or find ways to lessen their impact. The child can also purposefully seek out situations that lessen tic activity.
2. **Self-awareness training:** Education to help the child recognize tic premonitory urges or early tic movements.
3. **Relaxation techniques:** Development of strategies to minimize stress and manage tics. Examples may include progressive muscle relaxation, guided imagery, and deep breathing techniques.
4. **Tic analysis:** Identification of the tic/movement causing the child the most distress or discomfort. The therapist works with the child to recognize the premonitory urge preceding that particular tic, then helps the child to "break down" the tic into individual components. The child identifies the precise muscle movements involved in the tic from start to finish.
5. **Competing response:** Identification of a new competing action that the child does in place of the tic. The muscles used to do the new action would make it impossible to perform the old habit. For example, instead of performing an eye blink tic, a child can very gently close his eyelids and hold them closed for 10 seconds. If the child has an urge to clear his throat loudly and repeatedly, doing a soft swallow or a deep breath instead will prevent the tic from happening.
6. **Social support:** Rallying of support for the child, family, friends, and educators is essential in achieving and maintaining success with tic management strategies. Effective positive reinforcement strategies are developed to enhance use of competing responses.

CBIT, comprehensive behavioral intervention for tics.
Source: Adapted from Pally, S. (2015). Basic concepts of CBIT: Comprehensive behavior intervention for tics. Retrieved from http://www.CBITinfo.ca

to whether tetrahydrocannabinol (THC) is effective in tic reduction, *but no published controlled studies to date have involved pediatric patients.*

■ SUMMARY

Neurodevelopmental disorders such as NF-1 and TS are associated with numerous emotional, cognitive, behavioral, and psychological impairments. The key to intercepting behavioral health problems in children with NF-1 or TS is early identification and treatment of the conditions, recognition of potential problems, and implementation of evidence-based interventions. These actions can reduce symptoms and distress for the children and adolescents with NF-1 or TS and may help to improve their quality of life during childhood and as they enter and live in the adult world.

■ REFERENCES

Allen, T., Willard, V. W., Anderson, L. M., Hardy, K. K., & Bonner, M. J. (2016). Social functioning and facial expression recognition in children with neurofibromatosis type 1. *Journal of Intellectual Disability Research*, 60(3), 282–293. doi:10.1111/jir.12248

American Psychiatric Association. (2013). *Diagnostic and statistical manual of mental disorders* (5th ed.). Washington, DC: Author.

Bellini, B., Arruda, M., Cescut, A., Saulle, C., Persico, A., Carotenuto, M., . . . & Tozzi, E. (2013). Headache and comorbidity in children and adolescents. *The Journal of Headache and Pain, 14*(1), 79. doi:10.1186/1129-2377-14-79

Capriotti, M., Himle, M., & Woods, D. (2014). Behavioral treatments for Tourette syndrome. *Journal of Obsessive-Compulsive and Related Disorders, 3,* 415–420. doi:10.1016.j.ocrd.2014.03.007

Coutinho, V., Kemlin, I., Dorison, N., deVillemeur, T., Rodriguez, D., & Delatollas, G. (2016). Neuropsychological evaluation and parental assessment of behavioral and motor difficulties in children with neurofibromatosis type 1. *Research in Developmental Disabilities, 48,* 220–230. doi:10.1016/j.ridd.2015.11.010

Evans, J., Seri, S., & Cavanna, A. E. (2016). The effects of Gilles de la Tourette syndrome and other chronic tic disorders on quality of life across the lifespan: Asystematic review. *European Child & Adolescent Psychiatry, 25*(9), 939–948. doi:10.1007/s00787-016-0823-8.

Garcia-Lopez, R., Perea-Milla, E., Garcia, C., Rivas-Ruiz, F., Romero-Gonzalez, J., Moreno, J. L., . . . & Diaz, J. (2009). New therapeutic approach to Tourette syndrome in children based on a randomized placebo-controlled double-blind phase IV study of the effectiveness and safety of magnesium and vitamin B6. *Trials, 10*(1), 16. doi:10.1186/1745-6215-10-16.

Garg, S., Green, J., Leadbitter, K., Emsley, R., Lehtonen, A., Evans, G., & Huson, S. (2013). Neurofibromatosis type 1 and autism spectrum disorder. *Pediatrics, 132* (6), e1642–e1648. doi:10.1542/peds.2013-1868

Garg, S., Plasschaert, E., Descheemaker, M., Huson, S., Borghgraef, M., Vogels, A., . . . & Green, J. (2015). Autism spectrum profile in neurofibromatosis type 1. *Journal of Autism and Developmental Disorders, 45*(6), 1549–1657. doi:10.1007/s10803-014-2321-5

Gilbert, D., & Jankovic, J. (2014). Pharmacological treatment of Tourette syndrome. *Journal of Obsessive-Compulsive and Related Disorders, 3,* 407–414. doi:10.1016/j.jocrd.2014.03.006

Greene, D., Williams, A., Koller, J., Schlaggar, B., & Black, K. (2016). Brain structure in pediatric Tourette syndrome. *Molecular Psychiatry, 22*(7), 972–980. doi:10.1038/mp.2016.194

Hirbe, A., & Gutmann, D. (2014). Neurofibromatosis type 1: A multidisciplinary approach to care. *The Lancet Neurology, 13*(8), 834–843. doi:10.1016/S1474-4422(14)70063-8

Hollis, C., Pennant, M., Cuenca, J., Glazebrook, C., Kendall, T., Whittington, C., . . . & Stern, J. (2016). Clinical effectiveness and patient perspectives of different treatment strategies for tics in children and adolescents with Tourette syndrome: A systematic review and qualitative analysis. *Health Technology Assessment, 20*(4). doi:10.3310/hta20040

Jankovic, J., Jimejez-Shahed, J., & Brown, L. (2010). A randomized, double-blind, placebo-controlled study of topiramate in the treatment of Tourette syndrome. *Journal of Neurology, Neurosurgery and Psychiatry, 81,* 70–73. doi:10.1136/jnnp.2009.185348

Klein-Tasman, B., Janke, K., Luo, W., & Casnar, C. (2013). Cognitive and psychosocial phenotype of young children with neurofibromatosis-1. *Journal of the International Neuropsychological Society, 20*(1), 88–98. doi:10.1017/S1355617713001227

Kurlan, R. (2014). Treatment of Tourette syndrome. *Neurotherapeutics, 11,* 161–165. doi:10.1007/s13311-013-0215-4

Lehtonen, A., Howie, E., Trump, D., & Huson, S. M. (2013). Behaviour in children with neurofibromatosis type 1: Cognition, executive function, attention, emotion, and social competence. *Developmental Medicine & Child Neurology, 55*(2), 111–125. doi:10.1111/j.1469-8749.2012.04399.x

Lewis, A. K., Porter, M. A., Williams, T. A., North, K. N., & Payne, J. M. (2016). Social competence in children with neurofibromatosis type 1: Relationships with psychopathology and cognitive ability. *Journal of Childhood & Developmental Disorders, 2*(2). doi:10.4172/2472-1786.100020

Marrus, N., & Constantino, J. (2017). Autism spectrum disorder. In J. Luby (Ed.), *Handbook of preschool mental health: Development, disorders, and treatment* (pp. 207–208). New York, NY: Guilford Press. ISBN-10: 146252785X

McGuire, J., Piacentini, J., Brennan, E., Lewin, A., Murphy, T., Small, B., & Storch, A. (2014). A meta-analysis of behavior therapy for Tourette syndrome. *Journal of Psychiatric Research, 50,* 106–112. doi:10.1016/j.jpscyhires.2013.12.009

National Institute of Health. (1987). Neurofibromatosis. *NIH Consensus Statement Online 1987 Jul 13–15, 6*(12), 1–19.

National Institute of Neurological Disorders and Stroke. (2011). *Neurofibromatosis Fact Sheet.* (NIH Publication No. 11-2126). Bethesda, MD: National Institutes of Health. Retrieved from https://www.ninds.nih.gov/Disorders/Patient-Caregiver-Education/Fact-Sheets/Tourette-Syndrome-Fact-Sheet

National Institute of Neurological Disorders and Stroke (2012). *Tourette syndrome fact sheet.* (NIH Publication No. 12-2163). Retrieved from https://www.ninds.nih.gov/Disorders/Patient-Caregiver-Education/Fact-Sheets/Tourette-Syndrome-Fact-Sheet

Pally, S. (2015). *Basic concepts of CBIT: Comprehensive behavior intervention for tics.* Retrieved from http://www.CBITinfo.ca

Pasmant, E., Vidaud, M., Vidaud, D., & Wolkenstein, P. (2012). Neurofibromatosis type 1: From genotype to phenotype. *Journal of Medical Genetics, 49*(8), 483–789. doi:10.1136/jmedgenet-2012-100978

Payne, J. M., Pickering, T., Porter, M., Oates, E. C., Walia, N., Prelog, K., & North, K. N. (2014). Longitudinal assessment of cognition and T2-hyperintensities in NF-1: An 18-year study. *American Journal of Medical Genetics Part A, 164*(3), 661–665.

Piacentini, J., Woods, D., Scahill, L., Wilhelm, S., Peterson, A., Chang, S., . . . & Walkup, J. (2010). Behavior therapy for children with Tourette disorder: A randomized controlled trial. *JAMA, 303*(19), 1929–1937. doi:10.1001/jama.2010.607

Plasschaert, E., Van Eylen, L., Descheemaeker, M. J., Noens, I., Legius, E., & Steyaert, J. (2016). Executive functioning deficits in children with neurofibromatosis type 1: The influence of intellectual and social functioning. *American Journal of Medical Genetics Part B: Neuropsychiatric Genetics.* doi:10.1002/ajmg.b.32414

Potvin, D., Hardy, K. K., & Walsh, K. S. (2015). The relation between ADHD and cognitive profiles of children with NF1. *Journal of Pediatric Neuropsychology, 1*(1–4), 42–49. doi:10.1007/s40817-015-0007-3

Ratner, N., & Miller, S. (2015). A RASopathy gene commonly mutated in cancer: The neurofibromatosis type 1 tumour suppressor. *Nature Reviews Cancer, 15,* 290–301. doi:10.1038/nrc3911

Scharf, J., Miller, L., Gauvin, C., Alabiso, J., Mathews, C., & Ben Shlomo, Y. (2015). Population prevalence of Tourette syndrome: A systematic review and metaanalysis. *Movement Disorders, 30*(2), 221–228. doi:10.1002/mds.26089

Sulkowski, M., McGuire, J., & Tesoro, A. (2016). Treating tics and Tourette's disorder in school settings. *Canadian Journal of School Psychology, 31*(1), 47–62. doi:10.1177/0829573515601820

Takemoto, C., Hodding, J., & Kraus, D (Eds.). (2016). *Pediatric & Neonatal Dosage Handbook* (23rd ed.). Hudson, OH: Lexi-Comp.

van der Vaart, T., Rietman, A. B., Plasschaert, E., Legius, E., Elgersma, Y., Moll, H. A., . . . Descheemaeker, M. J. (2016). Behavioral and cognitive outcomes for clinical trials in children with neurofibromatosis type 1. *Neurology, 86*(2), 154–160. doi:10.1212/WNL.0000000000002118

Walsh, K., Janusz, J., Wolters, P., Martin, S., Klein-Tasman, B., Toledo-Tamula, M., . . . Semerjian, C. (2016). Neurocognitive outcomes in neurofibromatosis clinical trials: Recommendations for the domain of attention. *Neurology, 87*(7 Suppl 1), S21–S30. doi:10.1212/WNL.0000000000002928

Yang, R., Li, R., Gao, W., & Zhao, Z. (2017). Tic symptoms induced by atomoxetine in treatment of ADHD: A case report and literature review. *Journal of Developmental Behavioral Pediatrics, 38*(2), 151–154. doi:10.1097/DBP.0000000000000371

Zinner, S. H., Conelea, C. A., Glew, G. M., Woods, D. W., & Budman, C. L. (2012). Peer victimization in youth with Tourette syndrome and other chronic tic disorders. *Child Psychiatry & Human Development, 43*(1), 124–136. doi:10.1007/s10578-011-0249-y

CHAPTER 27

Care Management of Adolescents With Autistic Spectrum Disorder in Residential Treatment Centers

THERESE W. HARRISON

Over the past quarter of a century since autism was first described, the indicative symptoms within the domains of social relatedness, communication/play, and restricted and repetitive activities/interests have changed as the diagnostic parameters of the *Diagnostic and Statistical Manual of Mental Disorders* (*DSM*) evolved. The *DSM-5* (American Psychiatric Association [APA], 2013) categories of Pervasive Developmental Disorders of Autistic Disorder, Asperger's Disorder, Rhett's Disorder, Childhood Disintegrative Disorder, and Pervasive Developmental Disorder Not Otherwise Specified are now revised into *DSM-5's* (APA, 2013) inclusive diagnosis Autism Spectrum Disorder (ASD). The three prominent features of this neurodevelopmental disorder remain as impaired language and communication, impaired or abnormal social interaction, and stereotypical and repetitive/restrictive behavior patterns (APA, 2013).

Often literal and concrete thinkers, ASD adolescents frequently have difficulty with abstract conceptual skills such as language and literacy, time, and number concepts. If they have learning disabilities as well, they may feel awkward and disrespected if others misunderstand what they need. Feelings of disrespect can quickly escalate to aggressive behavior. Their social interaction struggles may also include difficulty with interpersonal skills, social responsibility, self-esteem, naïveté with others (which can lead to victimization), social problem solving (which can lead to bullying; Sterzing, Shattuck, Narendorf, Wagner, & Cooper, 2012), gullibility/naïveté with false advertising (which leads to inappropriate purchases or demands for expensive and useless products), general safety issues (stranger safety, drownings, etc.), and the ability to follow socially conventional laws and rules (which can lead to inappropriate behaviors and arrests). ASD adolescents typically need help with activities of daily (ADL) living skills (personal care, showering/bathing, nail care), occupational/vocational skills, learning and assuming their personal healthcare responsibilities, travel/transportation training, and with self-direction such as making personal schedules/routines (and coping with transitioning changes in rote schedules), use of money (they often spend all their money with little insight for future needs), and appropriate and safe use of the phone/Internet (sexting, meeting with strangers, threatening others; Volkmere et al, 2014).

ASD adolescents tend to utilize higher rates of healthcare resources and are more often admitted to psychiatric hospitals for severe externalizing behaviors. They display a wide range of symptom expression along the continuum of the aforementioned ASD impairments. For those whose intelligence is within normal limits, these impairments may be quite subtle; early and correct identification of comorbidities may be missed. In adolescence, however, impairment expression and symptoms may become more severe and more likely to be attributed to comorbidities. Discerning symptomatology and comorbidities and how to manage and treat symptoms present challenging dilemmas. For example, if aggressive behavior is displayed, the question arises if it is an example of the strong resistance to change in those with ASD, or is it a symptom of oppositional defiant disorder, intermittent explosive disorder, posttraumatic stress disorder (PTSD), or anxiety disorder? If complex clinical symptoms include psychotic features, is it hallucinations, delusions, or is it magical thinking and fantasy world preoccupations common in ASD adolescents? An additional consideration is that the development of schizophrenia in later adolescence is not uncommon. Depending on the most apt diagnoses, psychiatric symptoms may be medically treated very differently. Accurately diagnosing comorbidity is especially of great consequence when prescribing psychotropic medications that may aggravate some comorbid symptoms in the ASD adolescent (Sadock, Sadock, & Ruiz, 2015).

This chapter presents the assessment, evaluation, and care management of children with a diagnosis of ASD who are residing in a residential treatment center (RTC).

■ EPIDEMIOLOGY

According to the Centers for Disease Control and Prevention (CDC) Surveillance Study of 2012 of 11 Network Sites, the combined estimated prevalence of ASD was one in 68 children aged 8 years old. Assuming there were no additionally identified adolescents since that time, in 2017 there are approximately one in 68 ASD adolescents aged 13 years old, with a significantly higher rate among boys than girls (4:1) and a higher rate among non-Hispanic white children (Centers for Disease Control and Prevention [CDC], 2017; Christensen et al, 2016).

■ ETIOLOGY

ASD is a central nervous system disorder influenced by a multitude of factors. There have been neurobiological studies using EEGs, MRI, and measurements of brain size to ascertain possible brain aberrations (Volkmere et al, 2014). Considering that positive responses and behavioral successes are evident with the use of neuroleptics, it is reasonable to suggest that problems with neurotransmitters may also be involved. In addition, environmental and genetic factors may be influential in the expression of ASD in the adolescent population.

■ ASD ADOLESCENTS IN RTCs

Adolescent RTCs provide a multifaceted, intensively structured residential therapeutic program for those with complex behavioral and psychiatric issues. The residential treatment team (RTT) can play a strategic role in delineating issues. Trained staff (a) provide trauma-informed care; (b) deliver crisis management; (c) identify and ameliorate triggers; (d) teach appropriate coping and self-regulation management skills; and (e) improve social skills. The staff understand the residents' behaviors within the contexts of both past and recent events, and work with the residents in building self-care and ADL skills. The RTT consists of residential direct care staff, healthcare professionals, clinicians, other multidisciplinary staff, residents, and their parents/guardians.

Residents have a treatment plan that addresses their individualized needs and triggers and capitalizes on their strengths. Although RTCs provide 24-hour staff supervision, they also allow for invaluable family input, home visits, and observing the adolescent within the school and residential settings. The primary care nurse practitioner (NP) plays a crucial role in participating in and monitoring RTT interventions, managing and coordinating healthcare, and advocating for the ASD adolescent and their family.

■ ASSESSMENT AND EVALUATION

History and Review of Systems

For a variety of reasons, it is increasingly apparent that many children, adolescents, and their families have encountered barriers in accessing mental health services (Van Cleve, Hawking-Walsh, & Shaffer, 2013). ASD adolescents who arrive at the RTC may have had their comorbidities misdiagnosed. Of additional importance, their diagnosis may have been based on *DSM-5* criteria (APA, 2013). For example, a resident may present at the RTC carrying a diagnosis of Asperger's, or pervasive developmental disorder not otherwise specified, and so forth. With the intention of ruling out medical causes as well as genetic components, it is paramount to obtain a comprehensive past medical and relevant psychiatric/psychosocial history for both the ASD adolescent and appropriate family members.

Physical, Medical, Genetic, or Environmental Factors

Physical causes of behavior are considered first. Are there any known physical/medical, genetic, or environmental factors? The NP must review all genetic testing results, corresponding referrals from specialist medical reports, and the history of all psychotropic medications and treatments with attention to treatment failures and effectiveness/successes. If not previously studied, all ASD adolescents should receive genetic testing referrals for Fragile X and chromosomal micro array (Blair, 2010; State 2010; Volkmere et al., 2014). Results are not only helpful for questions regarding recurrence rates in siblings, but parents often seek clarity for determining genetic causes.

Behavioral Disorders

The NP should also obtain relevant information regarding past hospitalizations, aggressive behaviors, triggers, hallucinations, medications, and past diagnoses with the *DSM-5* (APA, 2013). Imaging such as CT or MRI scans will usually be provided only if an organic/brain abnormality was previously suspected. Parents/guardians should routinely be questioned regarding any privately arranged consults with ongoing outside specialists and if they are pursuing alternative and complimentary therapies. If they are requesting dietary supplements or herbal remedies, the pharmacist should be consulted regarding drug interactions with prescribed psychotropic medications as well as other prescribed medications (Perrin et al., 2012).

Impaired Language and Communication

Regarding the core ASD symptoms of impaired language and communication, time and again, parents do not report periods of normal development. During history taking obtain information regarding symptomatology and whether there have been developmental gains or deteriorations. If there were deteriorations, enquire at what age they were first noticed and a timeline of decline. Ask how the resident makes his or her needs known, does he or she have appropriate facial expressions and can he or she correctly recognize other people's facial expressions and body language, does he or she engage in appropriate conversation, and does he or she initiate dialogue? Does the resident make appropriate eye contact? Does he or she have receptive and expressive language impairments/processing? Enquire if he or she needs longer processing time with questions and information, does he/she need explanations in simple terms and directions, and is he or she echolalic with questions. When the resident engages in conversation, does it appear to be scripted? Does he or she respond oversensitively to loud voices or specifically to male or female voices? Does the resident have past and current educational and behavioral assessments and interventions? Analyze IQ testing. It is not uncommon to have a wide variation of scores regarding cognitive abilities and intellectual functioning. Has he or she been referred to a neuropsychologist for evaluation of memory function, aphasia verses psychotic features, and cognitive strengths/weaknesses? Enquire about any increased anxiety with new examiner's questions and any episodes of catatonia or slowing of movement (Johnson, 2008).

Impaired or Abnormal Social Interactions

Regarding the core ASD symptoms of impaired or abnormal social interaction, enquire about friendships; are they superficial or awkward, or interactive and appropriate? Is there a persistent and sustained impairment in social/peer interaction and relationships? Does the ASD adolescent engage in bullying or experience victimization? Ask families how the ASD adolescent exercises self-regulatory controls and if he/she recognizes privileges pursuant to expected rules. Does the adolescent make reasonable attempts to comply with directives or is he or she usually oppositional? Ask if he or she is typically resistant or cooperative, and what behavioral interventions improve compliance or ameliorate triggers. Does the resident have appropriate insight into his or her obsessions, fantasies, preoccupations, or conflicts? Does the resident's specific interests or fixations interfere with learning and interacting with others? Is he or she ever allowed unsupervised Internet access, and if parents review visited websites, are the sites sexually inappropriate? During interviews with only the resident present, safety issues and bullying behaviors can be assessed by starting with general questions such as "Do you feel safe on campus?" "Do you feel safe at school?" "Do you feel safe at home?" "Is anyone hitting you, hurting you, making you feel badly about yourself, or touching you in an uncomfortable way?"

Stereotypical and Repetitive/Restrictive Behavior Patterns

Last, investigate the core ASD symptoms of stereotypical and repetitive/restrictive behavior patterns. Specifically enquire about self-injury and aggressive behaviors. These can include head banging; hand or arm biting; hair, gums, or fingernail picking; eye gouging or poking; face or head slapping or punching; skin picking, scratching, or pinching; forceful head shaking; dislocation of joints; rubbing body parts; and/or pica (persistent eating of non-nutritive substances). Can these behaviors be attributed to reactions to common physical concerns such as seizures, migraines or headaches, ear or throat or skin infections, dental pain, fractures, and/or gastrointestinal upsets such as cramping with constipation or diarrhea, or gastric reflux pain? Ask about depression, suicidal ideation, sleep disturbances, and frequency of injury or accidents (particularly those requiring emergency department visits and/or hospitalizations). Does the resident have motor deficits such as clumsiness, poor coordination, or tiptoe walking? Is he or she easily overwhelmed by sensory stimulation and then begins to display degrees of stereotypical behaviors? Inquire if the resident ever exhibits odd play or has limited spontaneous activity; does he or she typically prefer solitary interests (gaming or listening to music with earbuds)? When at home, is the resident preoccupied with specific videos, games, electronics, or movies, and if so, are they violent ones? Does the resident ever act them out? Does he or she restrict food regarding taste, smell, texture, or appearance (e.g., refusing fruits/vegetables, limiting all intake to peanut butter and jelly sandwiches or chicken nuggets, etc.)? Does he or she display a strong resistance to change in routine that is accompanied by heightened anxiety and/or aggression to maintain sameness? Does he or she display a preference for inanimate objects (e.g., stuffed animals, carrying odd "toys") or pictures or activities that can include repetitious fixation on fantasy and cartooning? Many ASD adolescents exhibit risky behavior, fall, are "clumsy," and have periodic strains/sprains. Since they may need periodic x-rays and CT scans, monitor cumulative imaging radiation exposure.

Supporting Autonomy

To support the development of greater responsibility and autonomy for the resident's choices and healthcare decisions, provide for teachable moments. This movement toward autonomy should be a dynamic and ongoing process even in those who are autistic and have comorbidities. Give repetitive information in simple terms and document participation in shared decision making in their plan of care.

■ PHYSICAL ASSESSMENT AND CONTINUED SURVEILLANCE

Perform a current complete review of systems, mental status exam, and physical exam.

Depending upon prescribed psychotropic medications that have side effects of weight gain, height/weight, body mass index (BMI), and waist circumference are monitored between 1 to every 6 months. Physical reasons for impaired speech and language may indicate more frequent hearing screenings and ear exams as well as necessitate a referral to an ear, nose, and throat (ENT) practitioner/audiologist for further evaluation. Hearing assessment is especially important for those ASD adolescents who frequently listen to earbuds/headphones with loud volume with the aim to self-soothe. Take notice during the history and physical if the resident demonstrates appropriate eye contact, has any facial expression, maintains reciprocal conversation, is echolalic or grunting answers to questions, or repeating idiosyncratic phrases/language. Do conversations appear to be scripted and one-sided and does the ASD resident use pronoun reversals? Notice if the resident is a very literal and concrete thinker, thus not understanding jokes, sarcasm, or abstract thoughts. As with any adolescent, enquire if he or she has friends or has any interest in peers. Note any stereotyped/repetitive and somewhat purposeless behaviors such as hand-flapping, body rocking, thigh rubbing, and fingernail biting. If present, does this behavior stop after he or she becomes comfortable with the NP, or continues throughout the history and physical? Are there persistent and repetitive, ritualistic, or perseverative interests or use of objects or a preoccupation with parts of objects (e.g., flipping through book pages but never reading a book, consistently asking for ears to be examined/cleaned)? Regarding sensoristimulation, during the physical exam is the ASD resident hypersensitive/tactily defensive (e.g., cannot cooperate with ear or oral examination) or indifferent to sensory input; can he or she correctly follow simple instructions regarding specific body parts (e.g., "point to what hurts you")? Improving cooperation and ameliorating sensitivity can be enhanced by asking the resident to place his/her hand over the examiner's and "guiding" the examination. Some ASD adolescents may display slowed or freezing activity during the physical exam that can be interrupted with verbal and/or body cues to continue their movements (Volkmere et al., 2014).

For those residents who must return for follow-up exams, note if they perseverate in restricted routines and if they become dysregulated by coming to the office for an exam. Oftentimes offering the option to reschedule the exam can ensure cooperation and returning to baseline regulatory behavior.

■ DIAGNOSIS OF ASD

Most adolescents arrive at RTCs having already been diagnosed with autism. Hopefully the diagnosis has been made at a very young age and after years of multidisciplinary treatment. If not previously diagnosed, several screening tools are available and assessment is usually done by the RTT, which includes a trained psychiatrist and/or psychologist and NP. There are several screenings as well as diagnostic tools available and many are available for free online.

TABLE 27.1

FUNCTIONAL IMPAIRMENT SYMPTOMS

PART A

Deficits in social communication and interaction across multiple contexts (both current as well as historical)

- **Social/Emotional Reciprocity Examples**
  - Difficulty waiting turns (e.g., jumping ahead of others or becoming dysregulated when having to wait)
  - Difficulty with "fairness" or losing a game (e.g., becoming dysregulated and/or aggressive if they do not win)
  - Lack of empathy when someone else is injured (e.g., ignoring others who are injured as well as not showing concern or assistance)
  - Lack of initiation of appropriateness with ongoing and reciprocal conversation (e.g., blurting unrelated talk or only answering questions)
  - Deficits in social communications such as greetings or concluding interactions (e.g., not saying hello or good bye, please or thank you)
  - Difficulty with using appropriate language with adults/peers (e.g., cursing, slurs)
  - Non-understanding of ambiguous meanings of language (e.g., being very literal and missing the meaning of jokes, repeatedly asking for clarification)
- **Nonverbal Communication Examples**
  - Difficulty playing with others and confusing "horseplay" with play (e.g., quickly escalating horseplay to aggression)
  - Poor eye contact (e.g., both initiating and sustaining)
  - Limited facial expression (e.g., limited smiling or frowning and difficulty understanding other's facial expressions)
  - Poor understanding of personal space (e.g., standing too close to others, touching others without permission)
- **Understanding Relationship Examples**
  - Deficits in developing, maintaining, and understanding appropriate relationships. Attempts to make friends are awkward and odd, and they often fail
  - They may have "boyfriends" and "girlfriends" to be socially appropriate. However, they often lack the understanding of appropriately consenting to sex activities, and may be easily led to participating without full understanding
  - Difficulty understanding their own family relationships and importance of past behaviors during home visits (e.g., placing importance of unfairness that some residents have weekend home visits while they do not)
  - Bullying behavior (both as the victim, the perpetrator, and/or as the witness)
  - Little or no interest in peers
  - Preference for solitary activity (e.g., such as gaming or listening to earbud music rather than initiate group games or exercise activity)

Source: American Psychiatric Association. (2013). *Diagnostic and Statistical Manual of Mental Disorders* (5th ed.). Washington, DC: Author. doi:10.1176/appi.books.9780890425596

See Table 27.1 for symptoms that are persistent and result in functional impairment for the ASD adolescent. See Table 27.2 for a list of behaviors of which at least two restricted, stereotypical repetitive patterns of behavior, interests, and activities must be present in ASD adolescents.

TABLE 27.2

FUNCTIONAL IMPAIRMENT SYMPTOMS

PART B

The ASD adolescent must display at least two of the restricted, stereotypical repetitive patterns of behavior, interests, and reactivities

- **Stereotypic motor movement examples**
  - Hand flapping, finger flicking, echolalia, flipping pages of books (some of these movements may appear to be self-soothing)
- **Resistance to transitions, need for ritualized routines examples**
  - Scripting conversations
  - Aggressive outbursts when transitions are interrupted by change in routines (e.g., dysregulation when nothing by mouth for fasting a.m. labs, not getting the expected treat immediately on a home visit, not having immediate access to electronics when arriving back at campus and instead being brought to an after-school activity)
  - Difficulty learning transitioning skills related to preparation for adult living/housing (e.g., oppositional or defiant behavior when instructed in self-care skills)
- **Restricted/fixated interest examples**
  - Limited flexibility with expanding interests in academic studies, recreational activities, etc. (e.g., wanting to only watch the weather-related channels on TV, hoarding-like behavior, avid collecting without social interest, persistence in carrying stuffed animals)
- **Hyper/hypo reactivity to sensory stimulation examples**
  - Great difficulty/aversion to touch (e.g., during physical exams; poor hygiene due to intolerance with the feel of the shower water or tooth brushing; difficulty with eating foods of specific odor, temperature, and texture; apparent indifference to pain; aversion to loud voices)

ASD, autism spectrum disorder.

Source: DSM-5 Diagnostic Criteria. American Psychiatric Association. (2013). *Diagnostic and Statistical Manual of Mental Disorders* (5th ed.; DSM-5). Washington, DC: Author. doi:10.1176/appi. books.9780890425596

■ PSYCHIATRIC COMORBIDITIES

Depending on their mood during the interview, ASD adolescents often present challenges in emotional lability and may withhold information. Accurately identifying psychiatric comorbidities versus autism symptoms can be quite perplexing and complex, particularly in the resident with a wide range of intellectual disability and communication difficulties. Comorbidities tend to be common and multiple in ASD residents (Coury et al, 2012; Simonoff et al., 2008).

See Table 27.3 for ASD common comorbidities in adolescents with ASD in an RTC.

■ GENERAL MANAGEMENT AND TREATMENT CONSIDERATIONS OF PSYCHIATRIC COMORBIDITIES

Not every treatment, even if evidence-based, works well with every resident. Selected treatment(s) must be individualized in their treatment plan. This plan

TABLE 27.3

ASD ADOLESCENT COMMON COMORBIDITIES

- Attentional disorders, including hyperactivity
  - This may be part of the ASD symptomatology or a separate diagnosis
- Obsessive-compulsive disorder
  - These behaviors arise from anxiety issues
- Ritualistic behaviors
  - These behaviors arise from self-soothing needs
- Aggression
  - Aggression internally directed
    - Self-injury/stimulation
      - e.g., cutting, picking, burning, rubbing skin, trichotillomania
  - Aggression externally directed
    - Bullying/victimization/witnessing
    - Violence directed at others
      - e.g., playful roughhousing with classmates and other residents can escalate quickly to violence/explosive behaviors
- Affective symptoms
  - Anxiety
    - Pacing; picking at skin, nails, and/or hair; nail biting; repetitive questions; perseverating on topics of conversation; aggressive behavior caused by difficulty with transitioning between routines or activities
    - ASD adolescents often have difficulty breaking perseverative thoughts and will continue to fixate on repeating thoughts. Those with high anxiety may exaggerate somatic symptoms (e.g., stomachaches, constipation) rather than perseverative thoughts and may have difficulty with remembering cues and frequency of their symptoms. It is helpful to point out any negative testing that they may have had.
    - Relaxation techniques and positive coping skills, such as those to be discussed in the "Behavior Management and Treatment" section, can be quite helpful: listening to quiet music, removing themselves from the anxiety-causing situation, telling an adult about their anxious feelings, holding a comforting object such as a stuffed toy, taking a walk, sitting in a quiet room, using guided imagery, and slow deep breathing
  - Depression
  - Bipolar disorder
  - Impaired emotional regulation
    - Under-reactive as well as over-reactive
      - Intermittent explosive disorder
- Oppositional/conduct disorder
- Enuresis
  - Note if enuresis is daytime and/or nocturnal
  - Note if enuresis is related to psychotropic(s) dose
  - Note if enuresis is related to constipation
- Encopresis
  - Note if encopresis is habitual or if there is leakage around a constipation impaction
- Tourette's syndrome
- Tic disorder
- Rhett's syndrome
- Sleep disturbance
- Inappropriate sexual behavior

ASD, autism spectrum disorder.

must be regarded as a living document that changes as the resident's needs change. Treatment options will include behavior therapy, speech/language therapy, occupational therapy, physical therapy, social skills therapy, special education interventions/services, vocational training, animal therapy, treatment of medical comorbidities, and psychotropics. Psychotropic interventions are aimed at ameliorating concerns with anxiety, mood disorders, aggressive behaviors, motor hyperactivity and attention deficit disorder (ADD)/attention deficit hyperactivity disorder (ADHD) symptoms, ritualistic repetitive behaviors that interfere with daily activity, sleep disturbances, inappropriate sexual behavior, and psychiatric comorbidities. For example, ASD residents may have difficulty regarding comprehending empathy; however, those with comorbid conduct disorder may have additional reasons for lack of empathy. Although aggressive outbursts may lessen with psychotropic medications, they will not increase the ASD resident's grasp of empathy. These residents still require behavior therapy in understanding the feelings of others (Sadock, Sadock, Ruiz, 2015).

▪ BEHAVIORAL MANAGEMENT AND TREATMENT

Individualized Treatment Plans

Depending on the diagnosis, severity of symptoms, and comorbidities, psychosocial behavioral management and treatment of symptoms are always used first and foremost before augmenting with psychotropic management. Success with co-management with psychotropic medications are often based on parent and caregiver reports as the ASD adolescent will often have difficulty articulating his/her needs.

Treatments are often multiple and may be influenced by the resident's medical insurance program as well as the expertise of the treatment team. There are volumes of published findings regarding multiple treatment modalities for treating adolescents with autism; however, more research is needed to be able to generalize findings and support robust conclusions. The RTT will provide a multifaceted, intensively structured residential therapeutic program that addresses each resident's complex behavioral and psychiatric issues. The resident's treatment plan will identify and address their individualized needs and triggers, provide crisis management when indicated, ameliorate triggers, teach appropriate coping and self-regulation management skills, and capitalize on their strengths while improving their social skills. Residents are often triggered by witnessing other residents in crisis. Removing them from the immediate situation as well as prompting them to use positive coping skills are usually quite helpful. They will need assistance in processing their emotions afterwards. Positive coping skills include time-outs; distracting themselves with music, video, reading, or journaling; deep breathing; positive self-talk; talking to responsive trusted adults who withhold judgement; practicing problem solving when the resident returns to self-regulated baseline; meditation/mindfulness; and physical activity (e.g., brisk walking, using the gym; Volkmere et al., 2014).

Behavior management also assists the resident in improving ADL skills and self-care abilities. The individualized treatment plan is a living document and should be formally reviewed at least every 6 months and updated on an ongoing basis. This plan differs from the specialized plan review (SPR) that is conducted with the parent/guardian, the resident, and the RTT. The SPR additionally focuses on the resident's progress at the RTC as well as with transition plans.

Recognizing that they have difficulty articulating their concerns, over time, the adolescents typically form trusting relationships with the primary care NP and will give consent/assent for the NP to discuss their concerns with their clinicians/therapists and/or psychiatrist. Clinicians/therapists will address anxiety, anger/aggression management, and auditory as well as sensory integration with a variety of methods that can include cognitive behavior therapy (CBT), dialectical behavior therapy (DBT), and so forth, and will share applicable interventions with the rest of the team on a need-to-know basis (Volkmere et al., 2014).

It is of paramount importance to remember that behaviors are meaningful and reflect the resident's needs. Challenging behaviors may be attempts for attention, power, or revenge, as well as failure avoidance. To best respond, adults should be aware of their own feelings, be aware of what the resident needs, neutralize the environment to control triggers and engage the resident to defuse his or her behavior, consistently and confidently exercise limit setting, give well-chosen directives, and give proportionate and enforceable consequences that are related to the misbehavior. When the resident is at baseline, calmly discuss the problematic behavior and help him or her to develop acceptable choices and consequences. Give firm eye contact and confident body posture.

■ PSYCHOTROPIC MANAGEMENT AND TREATMENT

Psychotropic co-management may be indicated in the treatment of autistic behaviors and comorbidities. It must be remembered that psychotropic treatment does not address the core symptoms of ASD, but rather manages the medical and psychiatric comorbidity symptoms. The generally targeted symptoms include anxiety, depression, aggression, explosive/anger and severe tantrums behavior, self-injury, hyperactivity and inattention (ADHD) symptoms, compulsive behaviors, repetitive/stereotypical behaviors, sleep disturbance, and inappropriate sexual behaviors (McDougle, 2017; Stahl, 2015).

Best practice guidelines include a complete high quality medical and psychiatric evaluation, behavioral treatment and management of the resident prior to starting psychotropic medications, developing an appropriate psychotropic treatment plan that includes monitoring, psychoeducation of the parent/guardian and resident regarding each proposed psychotropic, realistic expectations of outcomes, obtaining informed consents/assents, establishing an initiation of a psychotropic(s) with appropriate titration up and/or discontinuation, and management of the resident who does not respond as expected (Riddle, 2016).

Selection of the appropriate psychotropic is based on neuroscientific research that suggests associations of abnormalities in neuro-circuitry and/or abnormalities of the function of neurotransmitters, and/or abnormalities of the function of specific brain areas. At the decision-making stage of treatment, refer to the actions of each psychotropic. "Off-label" use may also need consideration for those who do not respond as expected to typically used psychotropic medications; however, prescribers should be mindful of requests for off-label use based on consumer advertising such as in magazine, television, and Internet searches. At this time, medical marijuana is avoided as it is not appropriate for ASD adolescents whose brains are still developing.

Special Considerations

Medication allergies, cardiac abnormalities, seizure/neurological abnormalities, personal medical histories, and family history of sudden unexplained death/malignant arrhythmias should be assessed. Required baseline laboratory testing and any imaging studies or ECGs should be obtained prior to initiating psychotropic interventions. The NP will be instrumental in coordinating collateral specialty input in managing ongoing surveillance of the psychotropic treatment plan. These plans should outline an initiation of medication starting with a low dose, proceeding with subsequent titrations of doses to achieve maximum response with minimized side effects, maintaining this balance, and eventually discontinuing the psychotropic(s) when clinically indicated by tapering the dose or eventually discontinuing the dose with minimizing the risk for relapse/reoccurrence of symptoms. The medication plan is done under the guidance of the psychiatrist (Riddle, 2016).

ASD residents will typically be initiated and tapered off psychotropic(s) at the RTC where they can be monitored frequently by the RTT for at least a week before going on home visits.

Typically, the psychiatrist is the prescriber of psychotropic medications. However, based on the NP's state scope of nursing practice, the psychiatric NP may be the prescriber as well as the monitor for risk verses benefit. Depending on comorbidities, whether they are mild or significant, combinations of psychotropic medications may be necessary. To limit polypharmacy, the general rule is to "start low and go slow." Paradoxical side effects can also be managed this way. Monotherapy is the most desirable goal, especially when one medication can appropriately treat a variety of symptoms; begin with the lowest effective dose and then titrate slowly to the maximum dose. Should the maximum dose of one psychotropic medication be ineffective in ameliorating symptoms, then switching to another medication within its classification should be tried before switching to another classification of psychotropic medication. Consultation with the pharmacist regarding safety of medication combinations is important for management of these complex behaviors in adolescents.

■ MONITORING COMPLIANCE: CHECKING BEHAVIOR CONCERNS

Staff must be consistent in checking the resident's open mouth to assure that medication was swallowed correctly and having the resident rinse his/her mouth with sufficient water. Some agency protocols require the resident to show an open mouth to the nurse and a caretaker. Do not give medication in opaque fluid such as milk, as the resident may spit the medication into the milk, thus making it appear to have been taken. This behavior is considered a medication refusal or noncompliance. Additionally, be aware of those who regurgitate medications when unobserved. Those residents may have to be in the presence of caretakers until enough time has elapsed to prevent regurgitation, or until this behavior stops. Some agencies will allow medications to be taken immediately with applesauce if they can be opened or crushed and sprinkled on food. Consult pharmacists and online resources when considering this option.

■ INFORMED CONSENTS AND SHARED DECISION MAKING

Foremost, shared decision making is key to best outcomes in the care of ASD adolescents with comorbidities. The RTT, adolescent, and the family are collaborative stakeholders in this ongoing process. The NP will be responsible in protecting these ASD adolescents' rights and to providing education and information, assessing their comprehension of said information, and assisting in obtaining ethical and legal informed consent. The process of obtaining consent is required particularly with regards to psychotropic interventions. When consenting or assenting, the ASD adolescent residents who are 18 years and older who can consent for themselves, along with surrogate legal guardians, should participate in making decisions regarding choices in care.

Informed consent includes information regarding diagnosis, purpose of each psychotropic medication, each option's risks and benefits, monitoring expected outcome, and includes the option of no treatment and its anticipated outcome, alternatives of treatment, decision discussion, and verification of choice. A legally valid informed consent is dated and signed by the competent 18-year-old resident, or his or her legal guardian, and the prescriber.

Information (e.g., specific psychotropic information sheets) is given to the parent/guardian. This information is also given to the resident in developmentally appropriate language that they can process and understand, therefore helping them share in making the appropriate healthcare decision. It is important to note that not all 18 years and older ASD adolescents can comprehend this information and make decisions.

When including the parent and ASD adolescents in the discussion and decision making, follow these guidelines (Elwyn et al., 2012; Farmer & Lundy, 2017; Volkmere et al., 2014):

- Signed informed consents are required prior to initiating any psychotropic, immunization, and sexually transmitted infection (STI)/HIV testing.
- This population is high risk for STIs and HIV for a variety of reasons, including withholding information for fear of punishment, misunderstanding, inability to give consent during sexual encounters, repression of memories due to PTSD, and victimization. Therefore, testing every 6 months is good standard practice.
- Ask them to repeat back to you in their own words what they understand you to have discussed with them. Although they may appear to be attentive and to follow your conversation, many ASD adolescents are quite literal, and it is their re-explanations that may indicate that they are incapable of giving informed consent.

■ Initial confusion can be readdressed and information rephrased. Often it is helpful to have another professional (e.g., their clinician or a nurse) present during education and/or information sessions and to witness signed informed consent.

■ Document your attention to their details in comprehending issues, assent/consent, or refusals of treatment with psychotropic medications.

■ Proposed psychotropic medications in general will have informed consent obtained by the prescribing psychiatrist and/or licensed independent provider (NP) within their state's Nurse's Scope of Practice Acts. Prior to beginning treatment, the consents should be kept in the medical record and a copy given to the parent/legal guardian. All informed consents should be accompanied by the written specific psychotropic information sheet.

■ Requests for informed consent should never be approached when the adolescent is in acute crisis.

■ At no time should an ASD adolescent be coerced or feel punished for not assenting or consenting to treatment that the RTT deems to be the best choice.

■ Always include information that drinking alcohol, using products that contain alcohol, and using substances may increase the side effects of prescribed psychotropic medications. If parents/guardians suspect that their child is using alcohol or drugs, they should contact the treatment team immediately. Safety plans should be in place at home, such as no guns/weapons or access to any medications, if their child is experiencing thoughts of suicide or self-harm.

Legal definitions and directives will vary state to state, and agency to agency; it is wise to consult with your state laws, authorizing agencies, and specific institutions regarding regulations and who can consent to treat, and the documentation. Again, informed consent for each prescribed psychotropic is mandatory. When providing psychotropic information, it is advisable to consult updated medication management guidelines that are available online, as well as to consult with pharmacists and/or online drug interaction websites. To improve medication compliance, assent for psychotropic medications should be considered for those residents younger than 18 years. Refer to Figure 27.1.

■ PSYCHOTROPIC MANAGEMENT OF ATTENTION DISORDERS

Very often, stimulants are ineffective as they may make ASD adolescents more aggressive and irritable. Additionally, they must be used with caution in those with sleep disturbance issues, in very slender youths with poor appetite, and those with tics or seizures.

First-line treatment is to consider alpha-2 agonists that may be more effective in ASD residents with ADD/ADHD. These psychotropic medications include guanfacine or clonidine. Complete a resident and family history for heart disease prior to initiating psychotropic treatment. If there is an underlying cardiac issue, then an ECG and/or referral for cardiac clearance is warranted. Ongoing cardiac

Informed consent for psychotropic medication

Resident's Name: _____

Date of Birth: _____

Your child's agency psychiatrist _____ has discussed the
possibility of placing your child on _____ in a dose range and
route of _____ for the symptoms of _____.

The Agency's Psychiatrist described the reasons (s)he thought the medication was worth a trial, the
potential benefits and side effects, and alternative options including no treatment. The anticipated
dosage range is individualized, and may be above or below the recommended range, but no
medication will be administered without your informed consent. Typically, standard references will
be used regarding dosages. You have also been given a medication Information Sheet regarding
this medication and have had opportunities to ask questions.

Your child will be under close observation to monitor any and all side effects. If any side effects are
observed, they will be dealt with appropriately. Sometimes the addition of another medication or
group of medications to help control the side effects may be required, and/or the discontinuation of
the medication may be done under the supervision of the Psychiatrist.

With some psychotropic medications, there can be irreversible side effects such as movement
disorders, breast growth, and diabetes and other metabolic issues. These have been discussed
with you by the agency's psychiatrist.

If you have any further questions pertaining to your child's treatment, we encourage you to contact
the Health Services Department and the staff will arrange for you to speak to the prescribing
psychiatrist.

I have read the above information and give permission for the use of _____.
I have received a medication Information Sheet in addition to discussion with
_____.
I also understand that I can withdraw my permission for the medication at any time.

_____

Resident's Name (Print) (18 and over)   Resident's Signature
    Date

_____

Parent/Guardian Name (Print)   Relationship to Resident   Parent/Guardian Signature
    Date

_____

Prescriber/Witness #1 Name (Print)   Prescriber/Witness # 1 Signature
    Date

_____

Witness #2 Name (Print) (for Verbal Consent)   Witness # 2 Signature
Date

FIGURE 27.1 Informed consent for psychotropic medication.

monitoring such as blood pressure and pulse will be necessary. This monitoring
can be daily for a week when initiated. If there are no adverse blood pressure or
pulse concerns, then monitor blood pressure and pulse weekly for a month or
two, followed by monthly monitoring afterwards. Usual side effects are sedation
and constipation. If alpha-2 agonists prove ineffective, the second line of treatment is to use a nonstimulant such as atomoxetine or bupropion. Atomoxetine also
helps with anxiety and mood comorbidities. It may take longer to see therapeutic
effects, and generally does not stimulate tics. Usual side effects include stomach
upset, sedation, and headache. Bupropion is not used in those with seizures, and

it can worsen tics. Usual side effects include constipation, dry mouth, and headache. A tricyclic can also be used, such as imipramine, as a third line of treatment. It is not used in those with seizures. Usual side effects include dry mouth, blurry vision, constipation, and cardiac arrhythmias. After these psychotropic trials prove ineffective, then stimulants can be considered as the last line of treatment. Stimulants are controlled substances that require monthly renewals, and they may act paradoxically by causing worsening of symptoms in the ASD population. Usual side effects include reduced appetite, insomnia, headache, and tics (French, 2015; McDougle, 2017; Riddle, 2016; Stahl, 2015).

▪ PSYCHOTROPIC MANAGEMENT OF OBSESSIVE-COMPULSIVE DISORDER (OCD) AND/OR RITUALISTIC BEHAVIORS

There are no psychotropic medications that improve the core symptoms of ASD, such as ritualistic behaviors. Although some selective serotonin reuptake inhibitors (SSRIs) are used to treat adolescents who have OCD, they do tend to make symptoms worse in those who also have ASD. They should by and large be avoided in treating OCD and/or ritualistic behaviors in ASD residents. These should not be given concomitantly with a monoamine oxidase inhibitor (MAOI), and residents should be monitored carefully for a possible increase of suicidal ideation/behavior. The SSRIs include fluoxetine, fluvoxamine, sertraline, paroxetine, citalopram, and escitalopram. Usual side effects include insomnia, sedation/somnolence, nausea, gastrointestinal discomfort/indigestion, sexual dysfunction, weight gain, dizziness, and constipation (Grados, Torrico, Frederick, & Riley, 2016; McDougle, 2017; Riddle, 2016; Stahl, 2015).

▪ PSYCHOTROPIC MANAGEMENT OF AGGRESSION

Internally Directed Aggression

Self-injury preoccupation and its accompanying irritability can be treated with one of the two FDA-approved atypical or second-generation antipsychotics for ASD adolescents: risperidone and/or aripiprazole. Both atypical psychotropic medications have a side effect of significant weight gain; however, aripiprazole has much less effect on prolactin levels than does risperidone. Aripiprazole must be started slowly and titrated slowly (Riddle, 2016; Stahl, 2015).

Externally Directed Aggression

The comorbidity of aggression and violence directed at others can be a significant concern in ASD adolescents. There can be severe tantrums or hurting others. Aggression can be managed with typical or first-generation antipsychotics such as haloperidol, thioridazine, or chlorpromazine. These drugs are also called neuroleptics and can have the severe side effects of tardive dyskinesia, neuroleptic malignant syndrome, or dystonia, and can also cause severe weight gain (Stahl, 2015).

Atypical or second-generation antipsychotics such as aripiprazole, risperidone, olanzapine, quetiapine, ziprasidone, and clozapine can also be used. Risperidone and aripiprazole work well with irritability, whereas clozapine works well with aggression but not with irritability and it must be used with caution in those with seizures. As it can cause significant drops in white blood cells (WBCs) and absolute neutrophil counts (ANC), clozapine requires clozaril registry (REMS) for each resident, and very careful and frequent WBC/ANC monitoring and recording on the REMS website. Olanzapine will have a significant impact on weight gain and residents must be monitored closely for metabolic syndrome. Although ziprasidone may cause less weight gain, it can have cardiac effects and should be avoided in those with known personal and/or family cardiac issues. Baseline and annual ECGs as well as referrals for cardiac clearance are warranted. Quetiapine also has a significant impact on weight gain and can cause significant daytime sleepiness and overall sedation (McDougle, 2017; Stahl, 2015).

Mood stabilizers such as lithium, carbamezepine, topiramate, and lamotrigine can also help with aggression. Although studies have shown that valproic acid has had no drug versus placebo difference with aggression, it is generally reserved for some ASD adolescents who have seizures as well as aggression. The use of mood stabilizers will require careful liver function tests (LFT)/monitoring. Weight gain and sedation are also common. Lithium is less commonly used for aggression and will require thyroid and kidney function monitoring; common side effects are weight gain and tremor. Carbamazepine will require psychotropic blood level testing, blood counts (WBC and ANC), and sodium level monitoring. Topiramate has less sedation and weight gain side effects but needs psychotropic blood level monitoring. Lamotrigine studies have also found no drug versus placebo difference, but it carries a risk for Stevens–Johnson skin rash, particularly when used with valproic acid. Alpha-2 agonists such as clonidine can be effective in treating aggression but may cause significant daytime sleepiness and overall sedation (McDougle, 2017; Riddle, 2016; Stahl, 2015).

■ PSYCHOTROPIC MANAGEMENT OF AFFECTIVE SYMPTOMS

Anxiety in the context of ASD will be observed in three broader domains: agitation/mood dysregulation (e.g., aggression, self-injury, irritability), hyperactivity/ADHD symptoms (e.g., impulsivity, inattention, distractibility), and general anxiety (e.g., perseverative thinking, repetitive/stereotypical behaviors, behavioral rigidity such as difficulty with transitioning from home visits to return to residential treatment and/or from residential life to school). Observed symptoms include pacing, picking at skin/nails/hair, nail biting, repetitive questions/perseverating on topics of conversation, and aggressive behavior caused by difficulty with transitioning. At times, the resident may think he or she is experiencing an asthma attack with chest tightness; however, he or she will have normal pulse oxometer findings. Those who experience anxiety symptoms but whose "jitteriness" is not improved with eating and drinking fluids may be experiencing an anxiety/panic attack. Psychotropics can include buspirone or mirtazapine. Usual side effects of mirtazapine include weight gain and sedation. As previously stated, although SSRIs are typically used as the first line of treatment for anxiety disorders, they often do not help and may worsen symptoms in ASD adolescents. Therefore, using an anxiolytic strategy may be more effective (Bandelow, Seidler-Brandler, Becker, Wedekind, & Ruther, 2007; Hacker, Picard, & Strawn, 2014; Riddle, 2016).

■ PSYCHOTROPIC MANAGEMENT OF DEPRESSION

Symptoms in the ASD adolescent can be those seen typically in the general population. Psychotropic management can include antidepressants such as bupropion, venlafaxine, or duloxetine, or tricyclic antidepressants such as imipramine. The second line of treatment can be an SSRI such as fluoxetine, fluvoxamine, sertraline, paroxetine, citalopram, or escitalopram. Again, SSRIs in general often worsen symptoms in ASD adolescents (Riddle, 2016; Stahl, 2015).

■ PSYCHOTROPIC MANAGEMENT OF BIPOLAR DISORDER

Psychotropic management can include mood stabilizers such as valproic acid, lithium, carbamazepine, gabapentin, topiramate, and lamotrigine. Valproic acid is usually not recommended as studies have demonstrated no difference with no drug versus placebo difference. It can however be useful in those with seizures and aggression. Should it be used, there is a need for LFT monitoring and psychotropic blood levels. Usual side effects include sedation and weight gain. Lithium will need monitoring for thyroid, cardiac (baseline ECG and annual thereafter), and kidney function. Lithium psychotropic blood levels also require monitoring. Usual side effects include weight gain, tremor, polydipsia, and polyuria. Carbamazepine will need blood count (WBC and ANC) monitoring, sodium level monitoring, and psychotropic blood levels. Usual side effects include dizziness and tics. Gabapentin is not very effective clinically, and usual side effects include weight gain and sedation. Topiramate usual side effects include sedation and cognitive dulling; however, it is usually not associated with weight gain. As it carries a risk for Stevens-Johnson rash, lamotrigine must be titrated up very slowly, especially if it is combined with valproic acid. It usually is not recommended as studies have demonstrated no difference with no drug versus placebo effect; however, it can be very useful when there is a comorbidity with seizure disorder (Riddle, 2016; Stahl, 2015; Ward, 2017).

■ PSYCHOTROPIC MANAGEMENT OF IMPAIRED EMOTIONAL REGULATION

ASD adolescents often display a wide variety of impaired emotional regulation behaviors, which can include intermittent explosive disorder (IED), severe tantrums, and self-injury behaviors. They may also include intentional and nonintentional violence directed at the self and/or at others, when there is an authority conflict and defiance toward parents and caretakers and/or teachers, fire-setting behavior, inappropriate sexual behavior, and homicidal/suicidal ideation and behavior. Typical antipsychotics can be used and include haloperidol, thioridazine, and chlorpromazine. Usual side effects can include sedation, weight gain, drooling, tardive dyskinesia, and acute extrapyramidal symptoms. Atypical antipsychotics can also be used and include clozapine, risperidone, olanzapine, quetiapine, ziprasidone, aripiprazole, and paliperidone (the primary metabolite of risperidone). Most of the atypicals have side effects of significant weight gain and risk abnormal glucose regulation, but less so for ziprasidone and paliperidone. They also have side effects of sedation. Aripiprazole and paliperidone have less elevation of prolactin levels. Mood stabilizers as mentioned in the "Psychotropic Management of Bipolar Disorder" section can also be useful, as can alpha-2 agonists as mentioned in the "Psychotropic Management of Attentional Disorders, Including Hyperactivity" section (Riddle, 2016; Stahl, 2015).

■ PSYCHOTROPIC MANAGEMENT OF TOURETTE'S SYNDROME, TIC DISORDER, AND RHETT'S SYNDROME

Referrals to neurologists to rule out organic causes are recommended. In general, the neurologist will recommend psychotropic management.

■ PSYCHOTROPIC MANAGEMENT OF SLEEP DISTURBANCES

ASD adolescents very often have sleep disturbance regarding falling asleep as well as waking often to pace. Routine behavioral approaches to improve sleep hygiene are warranted. These interventions include consistent bedtime hours, no electronics/TV 1 hour before sleep, and so forth. If these interventions are ineffective, melatonin, trazadone, or clonidine can be given at bedtime. Trazadone may adversely affect prolonged erections and males should be directed to go to the ER for erections lasting longer than 1 hour. An atypical antidepressant such as mirtazapine or a tricyclic antidepressant such as imipramine can also be tried. As benzodiazepines and diphenhydramine often cause paradoxical effects, they are not recommended to help with sleep disturbance. SSRIs can be useful but in general they exacerbate symptoms in those who also have ASD (Riddle, 2016; Sikora, Johnson, Clemons, & Katz, 2012; Stahl, 2015).

■ PSYCHOTROPIC MANAGEMENT OF INAPPROPRIATE SEXUAL BEHAVIORS

These behaviors can include sexually acting out, as well as preoccupation with sex and pornography. Refer to the previous section on "Psychotropic Management of Impaired Emotional Regulation." Behavioral strategies are strongly recommended.

GENERAL LABORATORY SURVEILLANCE AND CARDIAC CONSIDERATION FOR PSYCHOTROPIC MEDICATIONS

Depending on specific psychotropic management, obtain a baseline ECG and fasting laboratory work. Those with abnormal ECGs should have referrals to a cardiologist, and this specialist will advise on clearance for all psychotropic medications and activity participation, including physical education, sports, and so forth (see Table 27.4 for laboratory work recommendations).

The ASD adolescents can be quite aggressive and bite and cause bleeding injuries to others. Should this occur, they as well as the injured party should be monitored with a blood borne pathogens protocol: hepatitis B surface antibody quantitative, hepatitis C, and HIV testing within a week of the occurrence. The laboratory protocol is repeated at 1, 3, and 6 months after the biting incident.

MEDICAL COMORBIDITIES

Accurately identifying medical comorbidities can be quite perplexing and complex, particularly in the resident with a wide range of intellectual disabilities and communication difficulties. Comorbidities tend to be common and multiple in ASD residents due to poor self-care/hygiene concerns, self-limiting behaviors

TABLE 27.4

LABORATORY TESTING OFTEN COMPLETED FOR ADOLESCENTS WITH ASD IN RESIDENTIAL TREATMENT CENTERS

- Complete metabolic panel
- Complete blood count with differential (with attention to WBC/ANC for clozapine and carbamazepine)
- Lipid profile
- Thyroid profile + TSH
- Urinalysis
- HgbA$_1$C
- Psychotropic levels
  - Carbamazepine
  - Chlorpromazine
  - Clozapine
  - Lamotrigine
  - Lithium
  - Oxcarbazepine
  - Risperidone (when prescribed, there will inevitably be increased weight and higher prolactin levels. Those on risperidone should also have prolactin levels monitored, especially when there is evidence of gynecomastia). Prolactin will generally return to normal within a year of discontinuance. Healthy eating habits and improved exercise should be encouraged; however, there may be little impact on weight while on risperidone.
  - Valproic acid

ANC, absolute neutrophil counts; TSH, thyroid stimulating hormone; WBC, white blood cell.

TABLE 27.5

MEDICAL COMORBIDITIES IN ASD ADOLESCENTS

- Seizure disorders and other neurological concerns
- Metabolic syndrome and other endocrine concerns
  - Metabolic syndrome
    - Note if weight gain is related to psychotropic(s), emotional eating, and/or food preferences for carbohydrates/processed foods
  - Cushing syndrome
  - Delayed growth/bone health
  - Hypothyroidism
  - Gynecomastia
    - Note if gynecomastia is secondary to increased weight, or elevated prolactin levels
  - Sex hormone/PCOS monitoring
- General hygiene and tactile defensiveness
- Reproductive health: STI/HIV concerns
- Substance abuse
- Communication, speech, language, hearing
- Enuresis and constipation
- Sleep disorders and obstructive sleep apnea
- Cardiology concerns

ASD, autism spectrum disorder; HIV, human immunodeficiency virus; PCOS, polycystic ovary syndrome; STI, sexually transmitted infection.

regarding diet and exercise, as well as side effects of psychotropic management. Additionally, depending upon their mood and communication skills, these adolescents often present challenges in withholding information as well as the ability to accurately describe symptoms (McDougle, 2017; see Table 27.5 in this chapter for medical comorbidities).

■ GENERAL MANAGEMENT AND TREATMENT CONSIDERATIONS OF MEDICAL COMORBIDITIES

Immunization Considerations

As with all adolescents, a thorough and up-to-date immunization record is required for ASD adolescents in RTCs. Consult with the most recent CDC and specific state guidelines regarding immunization requirements. Additionally, at RTCs, titers hepatitis C should be drawn; and immunization records should be reviewed for prior status of hepatitis B, measles, mumps, rubella (MMR), and varicella. With parental consent, reimmunize with boosters or repeated series according to *Red Book Guidelines* when indicated. Tuberculosis testing with purified protein derivative (PPD) is recommended annually.

All residents should receive baseline labs on admission. If the resident is receiving psychotropics, and the baseline labs are within normal limits, then the following labs should be repeated every 6 months. Those who have abnormal results should have those labs repeated in 1 to 4 weeks, depending on the degree of abnormality. Those with grossly abnormal results, which are not due to lab error, should be immediately referred to the appropriate specialist for further evaluation and treatment. Additional specific recommended labs and tests can be found per the pharmaceutical company medication inserts.

- Complete metabolic panel
- Complete blood count with differential
- Lipid profile
- Urinalysis
- $HgbA_1C$

MEDICAL MANAGEMENT OF SEIZURE DISORDERS AND OTHER NEUROLOGICAL CONCERNS

ASD adolescents with seizure disorders and/or history of significant head injuries should be referred to neurologists for further evaluation and treatment. Include with the consult any information regarding staring episodes and descriptions of any seizure activity, as well as any imaging studies such as EEG, video EEG, and brain CT or MRI. In general, unless there is a question of seizure activity or neurologic deterioration, neuroimaging studies are not indicated for ASD adolescents and they should only be obtained if relevant (Klykylo, Bowers, Weston, & Jackson, 2014).

MEDICAL MANAGEMENT OF RELATED ENDOCRINE CONCERNS

Many psychotropic medications place the ASD resident at risk for metabolic syndrome. Additionally, preferences for more sedentary activity as well as diets high in processed foods and simple sugars put these residents at risk for significant weight gain. Perform baseline labs and then continued surveillance with $HgbA_1C$, CBC, CMP with differential, fasting insulin, fasting lipid profile, and 3-hour glucose tolerance test when indicated. Referrals to nutritionists are advisable if the resident can process nutritional information and guidance. Those with delayed growth, hypothyroidism, signs of polycystic ovary syndrome (PCOS), abnormal blood sugar/ $HgbA_1C$, and elevated prolactin with gynecomastia indications should be referred to endocrinologists for further evaluation and treatment.

Additional blood work and imaging may be indicated for these conditions prior to the endocrinologist evaluation:

Metabolic Syndrome
- Fasting insulin
- Gamma-glutamyl transferase (GGT)
- $HgbA_1C$
- Fasting glucose

Cushing Syndrome
- AM cortisol

Delayed Growth/Bone Health
- Vitamin D 25-hydroxy
- Wrist bone age

Hypothyroidism
- Thyroid panels: thyroid stimulating hormone (TSH), T4, free T4, T3, thyroid-peroxidase antibodies, antithyroglobulin antibodies

Gynecomastia
- DHEAs, testosterone, prolactin

Sex Hormone/PCOS Monitoring
- FSH, LH, testosterone, prolactin

The endocrinologist will indicate if additional tests and/or treatments such as these are indicated:

- Glucose tolerance testing
- Growth hormone injections
- Oral birth control
- Vitamin D-3 supplements
- Blood sugar medication such as Metformin and/or insulin injections

■ MEDICAL MANAGEMENT OF GENERAL HYGIENE AND TACTILE DEFENSIVENESS

Routine hygiene can be especially challenging for ASD residents. Dental work, tooth brushing, nail clipping/cleaning, facial cleaning, thorough showering/shampooing, wearing clean clothing, use of deodorant, and shaving must be supervised, and ADL skills addressed both developmentally and with attention to sensoristimulation tolerance. Very often, ASD adolescents are tactilely defensive; it is of the utmost importance to explain where you will touch them and receive their permission to examine body parts as you proceed with examinations. As with normally developing adolescents, continue to appraise them of normal findings and that the exam will conclude quickly. Reassure them that they are doing a good job with cooperating. For those who are severely tactilely defensive, it is helpful for them to place their hands over the NP's hands and "guide" the physical exam.

ASD adolescents who are tactilely defensive may need a desensitization program where the face or specific body parts are touched often over time. This desensitization program may assist with building tolerance for using a continuous positive airway pressure (CPAP) device for increasing lengths of time until it can be used throughout the night, in building tolerance to wear eyeglasses, and to improve cooperation with dental, orthodontic, and optic exams. Quite often, these adolescents have difficulty with the sensation of water during showering, drying themselves with towels, applying skin lotions, drying their feet, and so forth, and therefore present with a variety of other hygiene and secondary dermatology issues (see Table 27.6).

■ MEDICAL MANAGEMENT OF REPRODUCTIVE HEALTH STI AND HIV CONCERNS

ASD adolescents are at greater risk for STIs and HIV, as they are often less capable of giving appropriate sexual consents and may limit conveying information

TABLE 27.6

HYGIENE CONCERNS

Body Part	Concerns	Interventions
Head	Dandruff, seborrhea	ASD adolescents often are hypersensitive to the feeling of shower water on their body and may interrupt full showering too quickly. Flaking and dandruff may be residual shampoo. A health aide may be needed to supervise showering. Selenium sulfide shampoo two times a week; rinse off well after 10 minutes in the shower. Refer severe or resistant cases to a dermatologist.
Face	Acne, seborrhea	ASD adolescents often are hypersensitive to the feeling of soap and water on their face and may interrupt full washing too quickly. A health aide may be needed to supervise cleansing. Dry thoroughly, wipe with medicated pads as needed. Benzoyl peroxide or other acne/seborrhea medications as indicated. Males who need facial shaving should be closely supervised, or shaving completed while on home visits. Refer severe or resistant cases to a dermatologist.
Teeth	Gingivitis, dental caries, impacted teeth, plaque	ASD adolescents are often hypersensitive to complete dental cleaning as well as semiannual dental prophylaxis exams and treatment. Double-head toothbrush and supervised tooth brushing may be helpful. For those with orthodontics, frequently rinsing the mouth with water may be helpful. Attention should also be given to those who have orthodontics applied, as these residents at times break off brackets and wires that can be used for self-harm purposes. Those who complain of ear or jaw pain should be assessed for eruption/impaction of wisdom teeth. Medications in gummi form should be avoided as sticky residue is often left behind and may lead to dental caries. Refer for deeper cleaning under sedation as needed.
Eyes	Need for eye glasses	ASD adolescents are often hypersensitive to the feeling of eyeglasses on their faces. They can be helped by brief activities that desensitize the face and building up longer periods of tolerating eyeglasses. Those who self-harm or have unpredictable aggression will need eyeglasses without metal rods in the earpieces, and they should have high impact lenses.

(continued)

TABLE 27.6 *(CONTINUED)*

HYGIENE CONCERNS

Body Part	Concerns	Interventions
Ears	Cerumen impaction, hearing loss and pain	Often ASD adolescents will use earbuds to listen to music to self-soothe. This practice may result in hearing loss if the volume is loud and prolonged. Retesting hearing with an audioscope every 6 months is recommended. Those who wear hearing aids should remove them when listening to music with earbuds. Use of cotton-tipped swabs should be strongly discouraged. Many have a strong aversion to having their ear canals examined, while those with OCD may request very frequent exams. Always prepare them for the exam and ask permission to proceed. Having them hold the otoscope under the examiner's hand may be helpful. Only use ceruminolytics if hearing is impaired or if there is ear pain and the eardrum cannot be visualized. Refer to ENT as needed for complete impaction removal and to an audiologist for hearing evaluation if testing is failed. Those who experience self-aggression such as increased ear-slapping or head pounding should first be assessed for ear infection. If negative, assess for constipation and/or other body parts with infection or causes of pain, as these adolescents can demonstrate confusion with pain and other body parts (e.g., examine buttocks area for furuncles from poor toileting hygiene, as well as abdominal assessments for constipation pain).
Feet	Tinea pedis & unguum, ingrown toenails, pes planus, bunions	Epsom salt foot soaks daily. Vibrating foot baths may help to desensitize feet to being cleaned. Dry feet well and apply medicated ointments as needed. Wear clean, dry white socks and change twice daily. Keep socks and footwear on as much as possible to discourage picking at toenails. Apply foot powder to footwear daily. Check size of footwear for appropriate size. Air-dry footwear daily. Put on socks prior to underwear to prevent autoinoculation of the groin area. Wash/dry socks/underwear in hot water/dryer. May need an aide or nurse to assist in nail clipping. Refer those with deep callous, large warts, pes planus, bunions, and/or resistant nail infections to a podiatrist.
Skin	Hidradenitis suppurativa	Obese adolescents, particularly females who wear ill-fitted bras, may be prone to chronic lesions: check both axilla, under and between breasts, and in groin areas. Encourage looser clothing as needed. Refer those with chronic lesions to a dermatologist.

(continued)

TABLE 27.6 (CONTINUED)

HYGIENE CONCERNS

Body Part	Concerns	Interventions
Skin	Tinea corporis and cruris	Obese adolescents often are hypersensitive to the feeling of shower water on their body and may interrupt full showering and thorough drying too quickly. A health aide may be needed to supervise showering. Dry well and apply groin powder to skin fold areas as needed. Antifungal creams as needed; continue at least 1 week after tinea appears to be resolved. Males should be checked carefully for tinea as well as thorough cleaning under foreskins. Females should be reminded to not put soap inside the vagina, and to use plenty of plain water in the shower to clean themselves.
Weight gain	Emotional eating, boredom eating, psychotropic-related weight gain	ASD adolescents need to be reminded with simple explanations that there are no magic pills for weight loss. They often respond well to repetitive visual cues regarding portion-controlled meals. Helpful tips: Drink a full glass of plain water before each meal, and chew food slowly. Take a walk for 10 minutes before asking for second portions. No added simple sugars in food or beverages. Limit simple carbohydrates and processed food. Eat protein and vegetables before carbs and fruits. Have healthy snacks available. Encourage 30 minutes of activity daily.
General female reproductive health	Irregular menses, poor hygiene	ASD adolescents are quite vulnerable to false advertising and often request products aimed at their vulnerability. They will often ask for prescriptions for these unhelpful (and expensive) products. Simple explanations of normal menses cycles should be given, and LMP should always be asked in matter-of-fact interviews. Residential staff should monitor monthly cycles Use of tampons and vaginal douching are generally discouraged. U/A dips positive for WBC but negative for leukotrienes, and nitrates generally indicate poor hygiene and not a UTI. Encourage washing frequently with copious amounts of water, and re-dip only those who are symptomatic of UTI.

ASD, autism spectrum disorder; ENT, ear nose and throat; LMP, last menstrual period; OCD, obsessive-compulsive disorder; U/A, urinary analysis; UTI, urinary tract infection; WBC, white blood cell.

regarding sexual activity. Regardless of whether they admit to sexual activity, it is important to screen all ASD adolescents for STIs (RPR, U/G/CH) and HIV at baseline and every 6 months after receiving informed consent by the adolescent and/or parent/legal guardian.

■ MEDICAL MANAGEMENT OF SUBSTANCE ABUSE

Experimentation with drugs/alcohol peaks during adolescence, and this holds true for ASD adolescents as well. Comorbidity of drug/alcohol use is associated with ADHD, mood disorders, conduct disorders, anxiety disorders, and PTSD. Despite the ASD adolescents' difficulty with making and maintaining friendships, when on home visits or AWOL, they may try to "fit in," which may result in inappropriate risky behaviors such as sexual activity that coincides with alcohol and drug use and may also include the use of opiates. They may have great difficulty in declining to ingest drugs and alcohol. If the adolescent returns from AWOL and/or admits to using drugs/alcohol and/or appears under the influence, and/or is observed to use drugs/alcohol, a breathalyzer screen for initial alcohol level is advised. Be aware that this result is a "snapshot in time" and does not predict when or how high this level may rise. It is advisable to send the adolescent to the local emergency department for further evaluation and treatment. For those who continue to AWOL, the RTT may decide on the use of future random urine drug screening. This screening may be performed by the agency's substance abuse counselor or by the nurse. Typically, those who use synthetic cannabinoids will not protest urine drug screenings; at this time, synthetic cannabinoids are not traceable in the urine or blood toxicology screens. Adolescents who admit to their recent use should be referred to the local emergency department for ongoing evaluation and/or treatment as synthetics are often implicated in higher rates of seizures and medical complications and toxicity. Those needing naloxone should be treated immediately and 911 should be called. Symptoms to be particularly aware of include temperature regulation problems (especially high temperatures), diaphoresis, high or low blood pressure, tachycardia, nausea/vomiting, scleral injection, pupillary dilation, sensory perception concerns, agitation and aggression, and psychotic symptoms such as auditory and/or visual hallucinations, suicidal ideation, and self-harming. Acute intoxication usually resolves within 24 hours; however, recurrent symptoms may develop in those with PTSD and comorbidities of other psychotic disorders. There are a variety of validated screening tools available in assessing the adolescent on a routine basis (at least during regularly scheduled physicals). These residents often require complex systems of treatment such as referral to their clinicians and/or substance abuse counselors for behavioral interventions. The family remains an important stakeholder in these interventions (Bukstein, 2015; Hammond & Upadhyaya, 2015; Solages, 2015).

■ MEDICAL MANAGEMENT OF COMMUNICATION, SPEECH, LANGUAGE, AND HEARING CONCERNS

The teachers and school staff will address communication through the individualized education plan (IEP), with assistance as needed from a speech/language therapist. Those with severe speech problems should be assessed for hypertrophic tonsils and adenoids, and referrals made to an ENT and an audiologist as needed. These specialists will assess for neurological hearing deficits. Results should be shared with the school after receiving authorized consents and release of information from the parents/guardians or residents 18 years and older (Bukstein, 2015; Hammond & Upadhyaya, 2015; Solages, 2015).

■ MEDICAL MANAGEMENT OF ENURESIS AND CONSTIPATION

Many psychotropic medications result in constipation, and for some, this may be severe. The severity may influence enuresis episodes and require frequent evaluation. Constipation is often managed well by including high fiber diets, increased fluids, increased exercise, fiber supplements, stool softeners, and stool stimulating medications. Fecal impactions should be monitored. Periodic Miralax cleanouts are indicated: 12 scoops in 32 ounces of fluids, and drink over 4 hours. Those who have poor response should be referred to a gastroenterologist for further evaluation and treatment (Furuta et al., 2012).

Behavioral interventions for enuresis are tried before intervening with medication. Enuresis logs and limiting fluids after 6 p.m. should be used. The resident should be reminded to use the toilet every few hours and before bedtime. Trials with bell/alarm bed pads can be used to alert the resident to bed-wetting during the night. Adolescents with a history of ongoing nocturnal enuresis should be referred to a urologist and have urodynamic studies completed. Should these studies be within normal limits, desmopressin acetate (DDAVP) is typically ordered. Those who have no enuresis for at least 1 year can have a trial of lowering and then discontinuing the DDAVP. Those who have no episodes of enuresis may be kept off DDAVP; should enuresis episodes continue, then the DDAVP should be reinstated. Those who continue to have enuresis despite the reinstated previous dose should be referred to the urologist. For those residents receiving lithium and/or risperidone, very often the enuresis is related to the dosage. Lowering the dose may assist with urinary continence. The benefits of continuing the psychotropic medications are weighted against the need for DDAVP (Traisman, 2015).

■ MEDICAL MANAGEMENT OF SLEEP DISORDERS AND OBSTRUCTIVE SLEEP APNEA

Sleep problems persist in adolescents with ASD, and they often have problems with delayed sleep-onset as well as frequent nighttime awakenings and insomnia. Poor sleep hygiene can affect daytime behavior such as daytime sleepiness, irritability, aggression, self-injury behavior, and attention during school hours. In addition to inquiring about hours of sleep both during the weekday and on weekends, inquire about napping frequency, frequent awakenings to either use the toilet or to pace, and daytime sleepiness. Ask the resident about feeling fatigued during the day or feeling rested. This fatigue may be related to sleep disorders, depression, and/or psychotropic medications. For those who cannot clearly articulate their habits and needs, information can be gathered from parents, caretakers, and teachers (Goldman, Richdale, Clemons, & Malow, 2012).

If the ASD adolescent presents with daytime sleepiness, poor school functioning, and reports of snoring or frequent nighttime awakenings, they should be referred to an ENT and/or pulmonologist for sleep studies, assessment for obstructive sleep apnea, and the need for CPAP during sleep.

■ MEDICAL MANAGEMENT OF CARDIOLOGY CONCERNS

Those with identified cardiac risk factors, identified either through personal history, family history, or through baseline ECG testing. should be referred to a cardiologist for further evaluation, treatment, and follow-up with ECG, echocardiogram, and/or stress test. The cardiologist will clear for all activity such as routine physical education and/or sports clearance, limited activity, and the use of psychotropic medications. Future follow-up will be determined in conjunction with the cardiologist's recommendations. Those on known cardio-toxic medications such as lithium and ziprasidone will typically have an annual ECG (Stahl, 2015).

■ TRANSITION PLANNING

Transition planning involves the uninterrupted and purposeful planning to assist the ASD adolescent with developmentally appropriate transitions from adolescent services to assuming more adult roles and functions to the best of the adolescent's abilities. To help them process more as an adult, the goal is to recognize the ASD adolescents' maladaptive cognitive behaviors and concerns, and to maximize their positive abilities. Beginning at least by the age of 16 years, the residents should receive preparation for and assistance with transitioning to adult living. Depending on the adolescent's cognitive skills, developmental stage, age, and competency, the RTT will work with him or her and families on transition planning for adult housing, or return to family living arrangements. The RTT will continue to build on improving the ASD adolescent's self-esteem and positive strengths. Job coaches can properly train the adolescent in an appropriate field of his or her choice. The NP should continue to help connect the adolescent with community resources and mental health services. The NP should focus on the adolescent's concrete thinking and any other limitations in language skills in order to help him or her understand directions and adult responsibilities. The adolescent's comorbid physical conditions usually continue into adulthood and will need adult provider follow-up to provide continuity of care. The NP should guide the adolescent and his or her family to understand that this is not abandonment but rather a transitional process. They will need guidance in transitioning and obtaining adult community providers and accessing resources. Skill sets needed by the adolescent in this transition process can be found online, and the NP can work with the adolescent, the family, and the RTT in helping the adolescent to become more responsible for his or her healthcare. Assistance with developing a transition plan can be found at both state-specific as well as federal websites and the plans can be tailored to chronological and developmental ages. The NP should continue to encourage

ASD adolescents and provide them with guidance to the next phases of responsibility during noncrisis times. Parents and legal guardians in particular will need assistance with legal guardianship concerns that extend into adulthood (Volkmere et al., 2014).

■ SUMMARY

Accurately identifying psychiatric and medical comorbidities can be quite perplexing and complex, particularly in the ASD adolescent who presents with a wide range of intellectual disability and communication difficulties. Comorbidities tend to be common and multiple.

The NP who works with the ASD adolescent population in residential treatment will undoubtedly be presented with a challenging but very rewarding experience and have the opportunity to play a crucial role in participating in and monitoring RTT intervention, managing and coordinating healthcare, and advocating for ASD adolescents and their families.

■ REFERENCES

American Psychiatric Association. (2013). *Diagnostic and Statistical Manual of Mental Disorders* (5th ed.).Washington, DC: Author. doi:10.1176/appi.books.9780890425596

Bandelow, B., Seidler-Brandler, U., Becker, A., Wedekind, D., & Ruther, E. (2007). Meta-analysis of randomized controlled comparisons of psychopharmacological and psychological treatments for anxiety disorders. *The World Journal of Biological Psychiatry, 8*, 175–187. doi:10.1080/15622970601110273

Blair, R. J. (2010). Psychopathy, frustration, and reactive aggression: The role of ventromedial prefrontal cortex. *British Journal of Psychology, 101*(Pt3), 383–399. doi:10.1348/000712609X418480

Bukstein, O. (2015). Medication-assisted treatment (MAT) for adolescents with opiate use disorder. *Child and Adolescent Psychopharmacology News, 20*, 1–4, 8. doi:10.1521/capn.2015.20.2.1

Centers for Disease Control and Prevention. (2017). *Autism spectrum disorder (ASD)*. Retrieved from www.cdc.gov/ncbddd/autism/index.html

Christensen, D. L., Baio, J., Braub, K. V., Bilder, D., Charles, J., Constantino, J. N., . . . Yeargin-Allsopp, M. (2016). Prevalence and characteristics of autism spectrum disorder among children aged 8 years – Autism and developmental disabilities monitoring network, 11 sites, United States, 2012. *MMWR Surveillance Summaries. 65*(3), 1–23. doi:10.15585/mmwr.ss6503a1

Coury, D., Anagnostou, E., Manning-Courtney, P., Reynolds, A., Cole, L., McCoy, R., . . . Perrin, J. M. (2012). Use of psychotropic medication in children and adolescents with autism spectrum disorder. *Pediatrics, 130*, S69–S76. doi:10.1542/peds.2012-0900D

Elwyn, G., Frosch, D., Thompson, R., Joseph-Williams, N., Lloyd, A., Kinnersley, P., . . . Barry, M. (2012). Shared decision making: A model for clinical practice. *Journal of General Internal Medicine, 27*, 1361–1367. doi:10.1007/s11606-012-2007-6

Farmer, L., & Lundy, A. (2017). Informed consent: Ethical and legal considerations for advanced practice nurses. *The Journal for Nurse Practitioners, 13*, 124–130. doi:10.1016/j.nurpra.2016.08.011

French, W. P. (2015). Assessment and treatment of attention-deficit/hyperactivity disorder. *Pediatric Annals, 44*, 160–168. doi:10.3928/00904481-20150410-11

Furuta, G., Williams, K., Kooros, K., Kaul, A., Panzer, R., Coury, D., & Fuchs, G. (2012). Management of constipation in children and adolescents with autism spectrum disorders. *Pediatrics, 130*, S98–S105. doi:10.1542/peds.2012-0900H

Goldman, S., Richdale, A., Clemons, T., & Malow, B. (2012). Parental sleep concerns in autism spectrum disorders: Variations from childhood to adolescence. *Journal of Autism and Development Disorders, 42*, 531–538. doi:10.1007/s10803-011-1270-5

Grados, M., Torrico, H., Frederick, J., & Riley, T. (2016). Pediatric obsessive-compulsive disorder: A psychopharmacology update, *Child and Adolescent Psychopharmacology News, 21*, 1–5, 8. doi:10.1521/capn.2016.21.1.1

Hacker, J., Picard, L., & Strawn J. (2014). Treatment of anxiety disorders in children and adolescents. *Child and Adolescent Psychopharmacology News, 19,* 1–7. doi:10.1521/capn.2014.19.5.1

Hammond, C., & Upadhyaya, H. (2015). Adolescent substance use disorders: Principles for assessment and management. *Child and Adolescent Psychopharmacology News, 20,* 1–7. doi:10.1521/capn.2015.20.1.1

Johnson, C. (2008). Recognition of autism before age 2 years. *Pediatrics in Review, 29,* 86–95. doi:10.1542/pir.29-3-86

Klykylo, W., Bowers, R., Weston, C., & Jackson, J. (2014). *Green's Child & Adolescent Clinical Psychopharmacology* (5th ed.). Philadelphia, PA: Wolters Kluwer.

McDougle, C. (2017). Psychopharmacology of autism spectrum disorder. *CTAAP Webinar/Teleconference Series, 2017,* March 8.

Perrin, J., Coury, D., Hyman, S., Cole, L., Reynolds, A., & Clemons, T. (2012). Complementary and alternative medicine use in a large pediatric autism sample. *Pediatrics, 130,* 77–82. doi:10.1542/peds.2012-0900E

Riddle, M. (2016). *Pediatric psychopharmacology for primary care.* Elk Grove, IL: American Academy of Pediatrics.

Sadock, B., Sadock, V., & Ruiz, P. (2015). *Synopsis of psychiatry, behavioral sciences/clinical psychiatry* (11th ed.). New York, NY: Wolters Kluwer.

Sikora, D., Johnson, K., Clemons, T., & Katz, T. (2012). The relationship between sleep problems and daytime behavior in children of different ages with autism spectrum disorders. *Pediatrics, 130*(Suppl 2). http://pediatrics.aappublications.org/content/130/Supplement_2/S83.long

Simonoff, E., Pickles, A., Charman, T., Chandler, S., Loucas, T., & Baird, G. (2008). Psychiatric disorders in children with autism spectrum disorders: Prevalence, comorbidity, and associated factors in a population-derived sample. *Journal of the American Academy of Child and Adolescent Psychiatry, 47,* 921–929. doi:10.1097/CHI.0b013e318179964f

Solages, M. (2015). Synthetic cannabinoids. *Child and Adolescent Psychopharmacology News, 20,* 1–4, 8. doi:10.1521/capn.2015.20.5.1

Stahl, S. (2015). *Prescriber's guide: Stahl's essential psychopharmacology* (5th ed.). New York, NY: Cambridge University Press.

State, M. W. (2010). The genetics of child psychiatric disorders: Focus on autism and Tourette syndrome. *Neuron, 68,* 254–269. doi:10.1016/j.neuron.2010.10.004

Sterzing, P., Shattuck, P., Narendorf, S., Wagner, M., & Cooper, B. (2012). Prevalence and correlates of bullying involvement among adolescents with an autism spectrum disorder. *Archives of Pediatrics & Adolescent Medicine, 11,* 1058–1064. doi:10.1001/archpediatrics.2012.790

Traisman, E. (2015). Enuresis evaluation and treatment. *Pediatrics Annals, 44,* 133–137. doi:10.3928/00904481-20150410-03

Volkmere, F., Siegel, M., Woodbury-Smith, M., King, B., McCracken J., & State, M. (2014). Practice parameters for the assessment and treatment of children and adolescents with autism spectrum disorder. *Journal of the American Academy of Child and Adolescent Psychiatry, 53,* 237–257. doi:10.1016/j.jaac.2013.10.013

Ward, I. (2017). Managing bipolar disorder: pharmacologic options for treatment. *Clinical Advisor.* February: 17–24.

CHAPTER 28

Case Study: Adolescent With a Substance Use Disorder

KATELYN DALINA, MARY ELIZABETH KATINAS,
SAMAR MOHSEN ASHMAWI, AND DONNA HALLAS

CASE PRESENTATION

A 16-year-old male presents to the pediatric primary care office for a routine physical examination prior to returning to school for the start of the new academic year. While completing a routine adolescent screen (the SSHADESS Screen assessment tool: discussed under screening tools in this chapter; American Academy of Pediatrics [AAP], 2014), a red flag was raised for the initial question in the "Drugs and Substance Use" section of the tool. When asked: "Do any of your friends talk about smoking cigarettes, taking drugs, or drinking alcohol?" he responded "Yes." When asked, "Do you smoke cigarettes? Drink alcohol? Have you tried sniffing glue, smoking weed, or using pills or other drugs?" he hesitantly admitted to both: occasional drinking alcohol and experimenting with drugs with his friends, mostly on weekends.

■ CONFIDENTIALITY IS CRITICAL IN ADOLESCENT HEALTHCARE

Sigman, Silber, English, and Gans (1997) define confidentiality as "an agreement between patient and provider that information discussed during or after the encounter will not be shared with other parties without explicit permission of the patient" (p. 409). A confidentiality statement must be provided to adolescents at every healthcare visit. The confidentiality statement assures adolescents that information provided to the pediatric primary care provider (P-PCP) during the office visit is a standard of care that supports full disclosure and trust between the adolescent and the P-PCP, without punitive consequences for the adolescent. Additionally, establishing confidentiality affords adolescents an opportunity to gain independence in relation to their personal health, behavior, and treatment plan. The P-PCP *must* include one exception in the statement to all adolescents: "I will keep in confidence anything you tell me or we discuss about the use of alcohol, drugs, or sexual practices. The only time I can break a confidence is if you tell me that you are planning to hurt yourself or another individual."

P-PCPs must be knowledgeable about the laws in the state in which they practice to provide accurate information to the adolescents with admitted substance use problems. In New York State, the law states that a minor can receive nonmedical alcohol or substance abuse services without parental consent or notification (Feierman, Lieberman, Schissel, Diller, Kim, & Chu, n.d). This includes inpatient or outpatient medical treatment for alcohol or substance abuse. The services or treatment provided are mandated as confidential (Feierman et al., n.d.). In New York, P-PCPs who treat adolescents should also inform them of this law along with the confidentiality statement.

▪ HISTORY OF PRESENT ILLNESS

After assurance of confidentiality, the adolescent admitted to occasional use of alcohol with his high school and a few college friends, but did not "feel much while drinking." He also admitted to experimenting with some street drugs which gave him a "high, almost powerful feeling" every time. He likes this feeling and often thinks "I need to feel high this weekend."

Both of his parents have chronic back pain and two of his grandparents have arthritis. He borrowed some of their pain medications, including oxycontin, percocet, and a few other pills without his parents' or grandparents' awareness, shared them with his "weekend friends," and was able to try a few of their street drugs. He denies using injectable drugs but has used street-made cocaine.

▪ SCREENING TOOLS TO DETECT SUBSTANCE ABUSE

Overall, many of the screening tools for alcohol and drug use commonly used in clinical practice have not been rigorously studied in the adolescent population (Pilowsky & Wu, 2013). Thus, the validity and reliability of many of the screening instruments for drug and alcohol use have not been established for use with adolescents. Therefore, P-PCPs may be using screening instruments without strong scientific evidence that the screening instrument or tool has the same sensitivity and specificity in the adolescent population as it has in the adult population. Rigorously designed research studies should be conducted to establish the sensitivity and specificity for behavioral health screening tools currently used in clinical practice to minimize false positive and false negative screening results (Pilowsky & Wu, 2013). Additionally, adolescents who participate in risky behaviors are at increased risk for involvement in activities that may lead to severe behavioral problems. Risky adolescent behaviors include, but are not limited to, use of alcohol and illicit drugs, smoking marijuana, binge drinking, alcohol or drug use before sexual intercourse, and drinking and driving (Centers for Disease Control and Prevention [CDC], 2015), unprotected sexual intercourse, participation in gang activities including participation in violent activities, and possession of weapons, for example, knives and guns. It is particularly important to screen adolescents for substance use at all healthcare encounters to identify risk-taking behaviors in adolescents who are using alcohol and/or drugs. Identifying these adolescents early and *intercepting* their behaviors with evidence-based interventions may have beneficial outcomes such as reducing health risks, accidents, injuries (Bernstein & D'Onofrio, 2017), and risky behaviors, identified earlier, which are often a sequela to drug use.

SSHADESS Assessment

The American Academy of Pediatrics (AAP) recommends using the SSHADESS Screen as a tool to collect information on adolescent behaviors to assess risky behaviors and formulate an effective care plan to reduce risks (Levy & Williams, 2016). SSHADESS is a mnemonic that is an acronym for important topics to cover when interviewing an adolescent to obtain a comprehensive understanding of the adolescent's beliefs about him or herself. The SSHADESS Screen acronym stands for the following topics: Strengths, School, Home, Activities, Drugs/Substance Use, Emotions/Eating/Depression, Sexuality, and Safety (AAP, 2014). Each topic covers a variety of details as well. For example, to determine the adolescents' perception of their strengths, it is important to ask what they like doing, how the adolescents describe themselves, what are they proud of, and how would their friends describe them (AAP, 2014).

HEEADSSS Versus SSHADESS

For many years, the HEEADSSS screening instrument (Klein, Goldenring, & Adelman, 2014) has been used to obtain the psychosocial history for adolescents. The HEEADSSS interview focuses on assessment of the Home environment, Education and employment, Eating, peer-related Activities, Drugs, Sexuality, Suicide/depression, and Safety from injury and violence (Klein et al., 2014). Recently the HEEADSSS has been updated to include the media influence on adolescent behavioral health. However, the HEEADSSS and SSHADESS Screen differ as the SSHADESS is viewed as a "strength and resiliency based tool" while the HEEADSSS assessment is not (Levy & Williams, 2016). The "D" in SSHADESS provides opportunity for the provider to inquire about the patient's substance use along with information about use by his/her friends or household members (Levy & Williams, 2016). In conclusion, the SSHADESS instrument is a reliable guide to allow the provider to gain insight about the adolescents' holistic approach and triggers adolescents to provide pertinent information that may require immediate interventions by a provider and/or referral for behavioral health treatment interventions.

In this case study, the adolescent screened positive on the SSHADESS tool for use of drugs; therefore, immediate office-based interventions are needed. Details concerning the adolescent's responses are included in the history of present illness (HPI).

CRAFFT Screening Instrument

The CRAFFT instrument is used to collect additional history and information on the substance abuse, both alcohol and drug use, to determine if further conversation or interventions are warranted (Center for Adolescent Substance Abuse Research, [CeASAR], 2016; Stewart & Connors, 2004–2005). The CRAFFT instrument is the preferred instrument to use for adolescents, rather than the Audit-C, which is used for adults and adolescents. The Audit-C only asks questions about alcohol use.

Thus, drug use may be missed if only the Audit-C is used in the primary, urgent, and acute care settings that treat adolescents. In addition, the CRAFFT instrument is the most studied screening instrument for adolescents and has a sensitivity and specificity of 0.80/0.86 (Knight, Sherritt, Shier, & Chang, 2002).

The following questions are on the CRAFFT:
(www.integration.samhsa.gov/clinical-practice/sbirt/screening)

C– Have you ever ridden in a CAR driven by someone (including yourself) who was "high" or had been using alcohol or drugs?

R– Do you ever use alcohol or drugs to RELAX, feel better about yourself, or fit in?

A– Do you ever use alcohol/drugs while you are by yourself, ALONE?

F– Do you ever FORGET things you did while using alcohol or drugs?

F– Do your family or FRIENDS ever tell you that you should cut down on your drinking or drug use?

T– Have you gotten into TROUBLE while you were using alcohol or drugs?

SCORING THE CRAFFT SCREENING INSTRUMENT

The CRAFFT instrument is easy to administer and score. A "yes" answer to any question is scored as equal to 1. A total score of 2 or higher is a positive screen and warrants interventions (Knight et al., 2002). In this case study, the adolescent provided detailed information with questions asked in "**R**–relax"—that are included in the HPI on his drug use, the satisfaction of feeling high on drugs, and drinking with friends—thus scoring a 3, which is a positive screen warranting interventions and referral to treatment to prevent risk behaviors that can lead to harm, injuries, and even death.

■ PERSONAL HEALTH QUESTIONNAIRE (PHQ-2 AND PHQ-9)

The PHQ-2 contains two questions that, if positive, require the PHQ-9 to be completed to further assess the adolescent for depression. Completing depression and suicide screening is crucial during every adolescent visit. The PHQ-9 is a reliable and valid multipurpose instrument used to screen, diagnose, monitor, and measure the severity of depression (Kroenke, Spitzer, & Williams, 2001). If the adolescent answers "yes" to two or more of the questions, the screen is considered positive and additional assessments, referrals, and interventions are indicated (CeASAR, 2016). The PHQ-9 is also available on the SAMHSA website (www.integration.samhsa.gov/clinical-practice/sbirt/screening).

In this case study, the adolescent's responses to the PHQ-2 did not reveal any evidence of depression; however, based on presenting history of drug use, the PHQ-9 was also administered. No evidence of depression was revealed on the PHQ-9.

■ REVIEW OF SYSTEMS

Pertinent Positives

General: Reports generally healthy with a recent decrease in overall energy level and difficulty sleeping.

Head: Reports headaches for a few months intermittently. Denies dizziness, syncope, or blurred vision. Denies trauma, infestation, or hair loss.

Gastrointestinal: Reports a recent change in appetite with weight loss. A few reported episodes of nausea; denies emesis. Denies constipation or diarrhea.

Musculoskeletal: Reports feeling achy all over and decreased activity tolerance. Denies deformity or pain to joints. Denies changes in range of motion.

Neurological: Denies seizures, loss of consciousness, issues with balance and coordination, numbness or tingling.

Psychiatric: Reports increased difficulty in school and focusing on homework. Denies confusion, memory or mood changes, or thoughts of hurting oneself or others. Admits to drug use on weekends as described in the HPI. Admits to occasional alcohol use: prefers the "drug high" feeling.

Physical Examination

General: Cachexic, weak appearing adolescent, inattentive and fatigued during exam.

Eyes: Conjunctiva pale, injected sclera

Mouth: Evidence of caries bilaterally to left second and right third molars.

Cardiovascular: Apical pulse 101; sinus tachycardia without diaphoresis; regular rate and rhythm; normal S1/S2; no thrills, heaves, or taps; no bruits, murmurs, or irregular heart sounds noted; warm, and well perfused, cap refill <2 seconds, no clubbing noted

Gastrointestinal: Hypoactive bowel sounds; abdomen flat, soft, distended, nontender; no masses; no hepatosplenomegaly

Neurological: Mental Status: Alert, oriented; speech clear

Central Nerves: CN II-XII intact.

Motor: Moves extremities equally, fair bulk/tone.

Reflexes: DTRs intact +3 bilaterally and symmetric.

Sensory: Pinprick, and vibratory sense intact. Unable to identify light touch to upper or lower extremities.

Coordination: Refused to demonstrate rapid alternating hand or finger movements; dysmetria during finger to nose test and heel-knee to shin; Romberg absent

Gait/Stance: Posture normal. Gait with inconsistent ataxia during heel to toe and tandem gait.

Psychiatric: Apathy in the discussion of school, family, and friends; flat affect

Diagnosis

Drug use: Marijuana, and opioids, both prescribed for relatives, and street opioids

Manifestations of alcohol and/or drug use in physical findings may include reports by the adolescent of fatigue. Inattentive behaviors may be observed during the history activities or may be reported by a parent. The adolescent may look cachexic which is supported by a history of poor eating behaviors and weight loss when compared to previous health records. Hypoactive bowel sounds. Overall, the adolescent may be apathetic or flat during the history and physical examination. Eyes may be bloodshot, which may be consistent with recent marijuana use. Drug use also affects the teeth, with evidence of poor oral hygiene and increased incidence of cavities. Tachycardia may be present on physical examination. Subtle signs may be present in the neurological examination.

In this case, the adolescent's physical examination is consistent with a diagnosis of drug use in the areas of general appearance and presenting affect, eye and oral cavity findings, cardia tachycardia, and the neurological examination. In this case, all other diagnoses, such as depression, were excluded based on the presenting history and analysis of results from the screening tools.

■ OPIOID USE AMONG ADOLESCENTS AND YOUNG ADULTS

Substance use disorder (SUD) is the new term that is used by the *Diagnostic and Statistical Manual of Mental Disorders* (fifth edition; *DSM-5*) rather than substance abuse or substance dependence. In order to determine the level of severity of the diagnosis, SUD is categorized to mild, moderate, and severe. There are a number of criteria set by *DSM-5* to diagnose an individual with SUD (American Psychiatric Association [APA], 2013). The cause of substance use disorder among adolescents is unknown but there are many contributing factors that increase the incidence of developing such diagnosis, including experiencing negative events, having genetic predisposition or family history, having a poor/weak relationship with their families, and existence of other psychiatric disorders, for example, depression, conduct disorder, or attention deficit hyperactivity disorder (ADHD). Moreover, a study conducted by group of researchers used a self-reported survey evaluating two risk factors: having impulsivity trait and history of behavioral addiction (food, sex, Internet), and in the past 6 months using of marijuana, alcohol, or tobacco. There were 1,612 high school students who filled out the survey: 48% of them reported high impulsivity rate; 38% endorsed three behavioral addictions (Chuang et al., 2017). The study shows that there is an association between having impulsivity trait or any addiction behaviors (food addiction, Internet addiction) and increasing the incidence of future or current drug use among adolescents. In general, the study concludes that existence of behavioral addiction or impulsivity trait alone significantly increases the likelihood of drug use among adolescents.

It is essential for the P-PCP to recognize the signs and symptoms of SUD and to carefully listen in a nonjudgmental manner during taking history and assessment. SUD signs and symptoms might be behavioral changes such as getting into trouble or illegal activities, not going to school or lacking in academic performance, being unreasonably angry, and changes in mood, sleep, appetite, and sexual desire. They also might be physical changes such as sudden change in weight either by loss or gain, unusual breath odor, dilated or constricted pupils, slurred speech, and fine tremors.

The number of adolescents and young adults using opioids has increased significantly in the past few years resulting in increases in adolescents and young adults experiencing overdoses and dying from both prescription opioids and illicit drug use. Ten states are participating in the State Unintentional Drug Overdose Reporting System (SUDORS), which was designed to track fatal opioid overdoses (O'Donnel, Halpin, Mattson, Goldberger, & Gladden, 2016). Data from this reporting system revealed that between July and December 2016, the number of opioid deaths was almost 3,000 individuals who tested positive for fentanyl and over 700 opioid overdose deaths tested positive for fentanyl analogs, including an extremely potent fentanyl analog, carfentanil, which is used to sedate large animals (O'Donnel et al., 2016).

McCabe, West, and Boyd, (2013) reported the results of a recent survey of U.S. high school seniors. Thirteen percent reported nonmedical use of prescription opioids (NMUPO) and 8.7% reported using NMUPO in the past 12 months. Emergency room visits for NMUPO more than doubled between 2004 and 2008 for patients younger than 21 years old (McCabe et al., 2013). Data further revealed that dentists, primary care providers, and emergency medicine physicians were the leading prescribers of opioids among adolescents and young adults in the United States (McCabe et al., 2013). Opioid prescriptions written for adolescents, ages 15 to 19, have doubled since 1994. Furthermore, in one study of illicit drug use among adolescents, the researchers reported that 100% of adolescent-related drug deaths were from the use of opioids (Schechter & Walco, 2016).

Opioids include legal prescription pain relief medications such as oxycodone, hydrocodone, codeine, morphine, hydromorphone, and fentanyl, in addition to illicit street drugs, such as heroin, and combination street-made drugs, of which today many are laced with fentanyl. The mechanism of action for opioids involves the opioid receptors in the nervous system that relieve pain and produce euphoria. Continued use of one or more opioids leads to tolerance and dependence that results in an increased need for higher and/or more frequent dosages to obtain the same reward and feelings of euphoria (Lobmaier, Gossop, Waal, & Bramness, 2010). Discontinuing the drugs results in withdrawal symptoms (e.g., nausea, vomiting, headache, and tremors), which anyone addicted to opioids tries desperately to avoid. Individuals experiencing initial withdrawal symptoms will "do anything" to obtain relief: take prescription drugs from relatives, seek prescription drugs from healthcare providers, and often become the victims of drug dealers.

■ INITIATIVES TO FIGHT DRUG ABUSE

In 1992, Congress established the Substance Abuse and Mental Health Administration (SAMHSA; www.samhsa.gov) as a major national initiative to make readily available to the public and healthcare providers information about substance use, information on mental health disorders and services, as well as research. Today, SAMHSA operates as part of the Department of Health and Human Services and provides national leadership with the goal of advancing behavioral health in the United States. "SAMHSA's mission is to reduce the impact of substance abuse and mental illness on America's communities" (www.samhsa.gov/about-us).

All healthcare providers must be astutely aware of the opioid crisis in adolescents and ways to assess each adolescent for drug use at every healthcare visit, inclusive of primary care practices, emergency departments, urgent care centers, dental offices, school health center offices, and hospitals. It is the concerted efforts by all healthcare providers in collaboration with the communities in which the adolescents live, work, and play that may make a difference in reducing the current incidence and prevalence of drug use among the adolescent population.

■ PARENTAL ROLE

Early warning signs of adolescent drug and alcohol use include behavior changes, decline in grades, erratic or irrational behavior, and/or changes in friends and group participation (Shahid et al., 2011). As adolescents continue to use drugs, more obvious signs emerge, including a lack of motivation, depression, apathy, and mood instability (Shahid et al., 2011).

Parent education on signs of drug and alcohol use by adolescents is important, as a parent may not recognize the early, more subtle warning signs of a potential drug use problem. Parents can be directed to the SAMHSA website (www.samhsa .gov/) as part of routine anticipatory guidance prior to the time a child becomes an adolescent to become actively involved in prevention of drug use in their own homes. Parents may not realize the importance of preventing extended access to opioids in their own home from prescriptions they or the adolescent may have received to manage a short-term problem, such as extraction of wisdom teeth, a sports injury, or a parent's personal injury. Parents should question the provider when pain management is needed for their adolescent and ask for a non-opioid prescription for short-term pain management.

In this case study, the adolescent admitted to beginning with the use of pain medication found in his home. He had easy access and no one paid attention to his use of the prescription drugs. Indeed, the adolescent may even initially think it is acceptable to take a drug prescribed by a trusted healthcare provider. Then, within a short time frame, the adolescent develops a physiological need for the drug, as previously described, which was the presentation in this case study.

■ THE ROLE OF P-PCPs

There are numerous warning signs that P-PCPs can identify during the intake history and physical examination. The home and environment are critical factors in adolescent development. Poor parental supervision, family tensions and conflicts, inconsistent household rules or policies, lower socioeconomic status, adolescent day to day exposure to neighborhoods where crime and violence are the norm are all warning signs that may lead to adolescent drug use (Shahid et al., 2011). Adolescents are also influenced by their parents' behaviors. If parents use drugs or alcohol, then the adolescent may view his/her personal use as acceptable.

P-PCPs who are knowledgeable about drug use among adolescents can *intercept* potential drug problems from escalating by working with adolescents who admit to using one drug by providing immediate counseling and referral to treatment, as it is well known that adolescents who use one substance are more likely to use another substance and become polysubstance users (Russell, Trudeau, & Leland, 2015). Russell et al. (2015) surveyed 31 high school students enrolled in a recovery program. Study results revealed that children who began substance use as early as 8 years old came from drug abusing families and were pressured by their peer culture to engage in substance use. In addition, these study participants reported that their engagement in polysubstance use, including opioids, was the outcome of peer pressure over several years (Russell et al., 2015). Hallas

(2017) discussed the value of the interprofessional collaborative care model in all settings to proactively address the healthcare needs of the individual patient, family, and community to reverse the current upward trends in opioid use.

■ TREATMENT

Screenings, Brief Office-Based Interventions, and Referral to Treatment

Healthcare providers can be educated and trained to perform screenings, brief office-based interventions, and referral to treatment (SBIRT) in primary care offices, emergency departments, urgent care centers, college health centers, and in any healthcare environment that treats adolescents, young adults, and all adults who are potentially or actively using drugs and/or alcohol. Providers who use SBIRT can immediately influence the individual with a brief office discussion about the identified problem and immediately refer the individual for individualized treatment. A full description of SBIRT is available on the SAMHSA website (www.samhsa.gov/sbirt). It is highly recommended that all healthcare professionals become trained to use SBIRT as part of routine practice protocols.

Medication-Assisted Treatment

Another recognized office-based treatment strategy is medication-assisted treatment (MAT), which is the addition of medications to behavioral therapy for the treatment of opioid use disorder, also available on the SAMHSA website (www.samhsa.gov/medication-assisted-treatment). On July 22, 2016, President Obama signed the Comprehensive Addiction and Recovery Act (CARA) into law as Public Law 114-198 (www.samhsa.gov/medication-assisted-treatment/qualify-nps-pas-waivers). Under this law, nurse practitioners and physician assistants may apply to complete the CARA 24-hour course to prescribe buprenorphine in office-based practices.

To combat the crisis in New York State, all prescribers who hold a Drug Enforcement Agency (DEA) registration number to prescribe controlled substances must complete a required 3-hour course in pain management, palliative care, and addiction (Bureau of Narcotic Enforcement [BNE], 2017). Prescriber awareness from this New York State law may alter current practices. For example, Hadland, Wood, and Levy (2016) reported that many addiction treatment centers do not use medications as treatment for opioid use disorder. In addition, Hadland et al. (2016) reported that the majority of pediatric patients with opioid use disorder do not receive treatment of any kind, and when treatment is initiated, it most often does not include evidence-based medication management. To successfully treat opioid addiction, combination therapy is required, which consists of pharmacotherapy and behavioral or psychosocial counseling (Lobmaier et al., 2010). Providing MAT services in primary care centers by qualified behavioral and mental health specialists, or specially trained primary care providers, has the benefit of providing access to drug treatment without the stigma that is often associated with a drug treatment center (Hadland et al., 2016).

Medications

Methadone is a full opioid agonist with a long half-life. Buprenorphine is a partial opioid agonist with strong affinity for the opioid receptor. Both methadone and buprenorphine can alter the intense highs and lows associated with opioids that have short half-lives. Naltrexone is an opioid antagonist that also has a strong affinity for the opioid receptor. A benefit of naltrexone is that as an opioid antagonist, it has a very limited potential for addiction, misuse, or diversion (AAP Committee on Substance Use and Prevention, 2016).

Recommendations from the AAP policy statement on MAT include the following: (a) resources should be increased to provide access to MAT in both primary care and outpatient treatment centers; (b) pediatricians (and P-PCPs) should offer MAT to adolescents with severe opioid use disorder or discuss referrals; and (c) further research is needed to be done on treatment of SUDs in the pediatric population (AAP Committee on Substance Use and Prevention, 2016).

Narcan

Narcan availability is also an important initiative to decrease drug overdose deaths in the United States. On November 18, 2015, the U.S. Food and Drug Administration (FDA) approved Narcan nasal spray, the first FDA-approved nasal spray version of naloxone hydrochloride (National Institute on Drug Abuse, 2015). A nasal spray formulation of Narcan is easier to deliver and eliminates the risk of a contaminated needle stick. Narcan can stop or reverse the effects of an opioid overdose. Narcan use saves lives. Narcan will not stop the opioid crisis, but it will save lives.

▪ SUMMARY

The incidence and prevalence of adolescents and adults using opioids and dying from opioid overdoses is astounding. To combat this crisis, initiatives at the national, state, and local levels have been implemented, and yet, our youth continue to die on the streets in every state in the United States. P-PCPs play a key role in identifying with appropriate screening instruments adolescents at risk for drug use and those who are using both prescription drugs and illicit drugs to "feel high," and then initiating SBIRT as an intervention in the practice as soon as a drug problem is identified. The key to intercepting these behaviors is effective office-based screenings and an immediate intervention with prompt referral to treatment *and* interprofessional collaborative initiatives at the national, state, and local community levels. Steadfast follow-up care is essential; since adolescents are protected by confidentiality laws, they may not have parental support to continue treatment plans unless the adolescent consents to informing his/her parents or guardians of his/her personal drug use.

▪ REFERENCES

American Academy of Pediatrics. (2014). *Reaching teens: Strength-based communication strategies to build resilience and support healthy adolescent development.* Retrieved from https://www.aap.org/en-us/professional-resources/Reaching-Teens/Documents/Private/SSHADESS_handout.pdf

American Academy of Pediatrics, Committee on Substance Use and Prevention. (2016). Medication-assisted treatment of adolescents with opioid use disorder. *Peidatrics, 138,* 1–4. doi:10.1542/peds.2016-1893

American Psychiatric Association. (2013). *Diagnostic and statistical manual of mental disorders* (5th ed.). Arlington, VA: American Psychiatric Association.

Bernstein, S., & D'Onofrio, G. (2017). Screening, treatment initiation, and referral for substance use disorders. *Addiction Science and Clinical Practice, 12,* 18. doi:10.1186/s13722-017-0083-z

Bureau of Narcotic Enforcement. (2017). *Mandate prescriber education.* Retrieved from https://www.health.ny.gov/professionals/narcotic/mandatory_prescriber_education/

Center for Adolescent Substance Abuse Research. (2016). The *CRAFFT screening tool.* Retrieved from http://www.ceasar-boston.org/CRAFFT/index.php

Centers for Disease Control and Prevention. (2015). *Youth risk behavior surveillance United States 2015.* Retrieved from https://www.cdc.gov/healthyyouth/data/yrbs/pdf/2015/ss6506_updated.pdf

Chuang, C. I., Sussman, S., Stone, M. D., Pang, R. D., Chou, C., Leventhal, A. M., & Kirkpatrick, M. G. (2017). Impulsivity and history of behavioral addictions are associated with drug use in adolescents. *Addictive Behaviors, 74,* 41–47. doi:10.1016/j.addbeh.2017.05.021

Feierman, J., Lieberman, D., Schissel, A., Diller, R., Kim, J., & Chu, Y. (ND). *Teenagers, health care & the law: A guide to the law on minors' rights in New York State* (2nd ed., pp. 7–99). New York, NY: New York Civil Liberties Union.

Hadland, S. E., Wood, E., & Levy, S. (2016). How the pediatric workforce can address the opioid crisis. *Lancet, 388,* 1260–1261. Retrieved from https://www.ncbi.nlm.nih.gov/pmc/articles/PMC5046819

Hallas, D. (2017). Opioids: The menace in our midst. *Contemporary Pediatrics.* Retrieved from http://contemporarypediatrics.modernmedicine.com/contemporary-pediatrics/news/opioids-menace-our-midst

Klein, D. A., Goldenring, J. M., & Adelman, W. P. (2014). HEEADSSS 3.0: The psychosocial interview for adolescents updated for a new century fueled by media. *Contemporary Pediatrics.* Retrieved from http://contemporarypediatrics.modernmedicine.com/contemporary-pediatrics/content/tags/adolescent-medicine/heeadsss-30-psychosocial-interview-adolesce?page=full

Knight, K., Sherritt, L., Shier, L. A., & Chang, G. (2002). Validity of the CRAFFT substance screening test among adolescent clinic patients. *Archives of Pediatrics & Adolescent Medicine, 156,* 607–614. Retrieved from https://www.ncbi.nlm.nih.gov/pmc/articles/PMC3623552/ doi:10.1001/archpedi.156.6.607

Kroenke, K., Spitzer, R., & Williams, W. (2001). Validity of a brief depression severity measure. *Journal of General Internal Medicine, 16,* 606–616. Retrieved from http://www.cqaimh.org/pdf/tool_phq9.pdf doi:10.1046/j.1525-1497.2001.016009606.x

Levy, S., & Williams, J. (2016). Substance use screening, brief intervention, and referral to treatment. *American Academy of Pediatrics, 138,* e1–e15. doi:10.1542/peds.2016-1211

Lobmaier, P., Gossop, M., Waal, H., & Bramness, J. (2010). The pharmacological treatment of opioid addiction—a clinical perspective. *European Journal of Clinical Pharmacology, 66,* 537–545. doi:10.1007/s00228-010-0793-6

McCabe, S. E., West, B. T., & Boyd, C. J. (2013). Leftover prescription opioids and nonmedical use among high school seniors: A multi-cohort national study. *Journal of Adolescent Health, 52,* 480-485. doi:10.1016/j.jadolhealth.2012.08.007

National Institute on Drug Abuse. (2015). FDA approves naloxone nasal spray to reverse opioid overdose. Retrieved from https://www.drugabuse.gov/news-events/news-releases/2015/11/fda-approves-naloxone-nasal-spray-to-reverse-opioid-overdosess

O'Donnel, J. K., Halpin, J., Mattson, C. L., Goldberger, B. A., & Gladden, R. M. (2016). Deaths involving fentanyl, fentanyl analogs, and U-47700—10 states. *Morbidity and Mortality Weekly Report, 66,* 1197–1202. doi:10.15585/mmwr.mm6643e1

Pilowsky, D., & Wu, Li-Tzy. (2013). Screening instruments for substance use and brief interventions targeting adolescents in primary care: A literature review. *Addictive Behaviour, 38,* 2146–2153. doi:10.1016/j.addbeh.2013.01.015

Russell, B.S., Trudeau, J. J., & Leland, A.J. (2015). Social influence on adolescent polysubstance use: The escalation to opioid use. *Substance Use and Misuse, 50,* 1335–1331. doi:10.3109/10826084.2015.1013128

Schechter, N., & Walco, G. (2016). The potential impact on children of the CDC guideline for prescribing opioids for chronic pain. *JAMA Pediatric, 170,* 425–426. doi:10.1001/jamapediatrics.2016.0504

Shahid, A., Mouton, C., Jabeen, S., Ofoemezie, E., Bailey, R, Shahid, M., & Zeng, Q. (2011). Early detection of illicit drug use in teenagers. *Innovations in Clinical Neuroscience*, *8*, 24–28. Retrieved from https://www.ncbi.nlm.nih.gov/pmc/articles/PMC3257983

Sigman, G., Silber, T., English, A., & Gans, J. (1997). Confidential health care for adolescents: Position paper of the Society for Adolescent Medicine. *Journal of Adolescent Health*, *21*, 408–415. doi:10.1016/S1054-139X(97)00171-7

Stewart, S. H., & Connors, G. J. (2004–2005). Screening for alcohol problems: What makes a test effective? *Alcohol Res Health*, *28*, 5–16. Retrieved from https://www.ncbi.nlm.nih.gov/pmc/articles/PMC3623552

Child Population

CHAPTER 29

Child Behaviors Within Military Families*

JENNIFER HENSLEY

U.S. Armed Forces service members are heroes and selflessly serve with personal sacrifice and extended time away from loved ones. Military spouses are the silent heroes and work tirelessly to keep the family and household stable on the home front. Military children and adolescents are the unsung heroes, learning at a very young age that life is full of change and transition. Healthcare providers caring for military families should be educated on the military culture and be prepared to provide world-class medical care to our nation's heroes. This chapter provides insight and evidence for pediatric and adult primary care providers, as well as behavioral health and mental health providers, about the unique social–emotional and behavioral healthcare needs of military children.

■ HISTORY OF FAMILIES ON THE HOME FRONT

In 1971, the 37th president of the United States of America, Richard Nixon, signed a law transforming the U.S. military forces from a draft, obligatory enlistment, to an all-volunteer force (AVF) with standby selective service. The following 46 years resulted in the most powerful and resilient military force in the world. Immediately following President Nixon's signature of the AVF law, senior military leaders were charged to develop recruitment tools to attract high-quality youths to volunteer to serve. The results of this new law included pay increases, diverse career opportunities, incentive bonuses, educational opportunities, and, for the first time ever, the military became "family friendly." As a "family-friendly" entity, the Department of Defense improved the quality of military housing, increased the availability of childcare, expanded healthcare benefits for military families, established military installation stores, and developed family advocacy programs. As quality-of-life measures improved for service members, more service members opted to marry and ultimately raise children in the military (Rostker, 2006).

---

*The views expressed in this chapter are those of the author and do not reflect the official policy or position of the Department of the Army, Department of the Navy, Department of Defense, or the U.S. government.

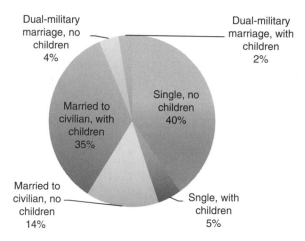

FIGURE 29.1 Active duty family member status: $N = 1{,}326{,}273$.

Note: Single includes annulled, divorced, and widowed. Children include minor dependents 20 years or younger or dependents 22 years and younger enrolled as full-time students. Percentages may not total to 100 due to rounding.

Source: Caliber and ICF Consulting Company. DMDC Active Duty Military Family File (September 2014); DMDC Active Duty Military Personnel Master File (September 2014).

According to the Office of the Deputy Assistant Secretary of Defense 2014 demographic profile of the military community, there are over 3.5 million military personnel stationed all over the world. Approximately 42% (Figure 29.1) of all service members have family responsibilities to about 1.8 million military children. Approximately 35% of service members are married to a civilian with children, 5% are single with children, and 2% are dual military with children. The military child population is comprised of 38% of children 0 to 5 years; 31% of children 6 to 11 years; 24% of children 12 to 18 years; and 7% of children 19 to 22 years (Figure 29.2).

Since 2001, approximately 2.3 million service members have been deployed to Iraq and Afghanistan, some for up to 18 months at a time. Some service members have done multiple deployments with little time home in between deployments. As a result, approximately 2 million military children have experienced the deployment of a loved one since the War on Terror began (Siegel & Davis, 2013).

■ MILITARY CHILDREN: ALWAYS ON THE MOVE

Regional conflicts have put our service members through multiple deployments and extended periods of time away from their families. Service members and their families live a life not many understand, with transition and stress that is a part of their everyday lives. Military families move more often than civilian families and most military families will have at least one overseas move. Military children are expected to move often, transition to new schools, make new friends at each duty station, send parents off to war, and be resilient. Providing healthcare for military children should be approached differently than the general pediatric population.

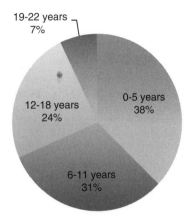

FIGURE 29.2 Age of military children: $N = 1,819,659$.

Note: Children of ages 21 to 22 must be enrolled as full-time students in order to qualify as dependents. Percentages may not total to 100 due to rounding.

Source: Caliber and ICF Consulting Company. DMDC Active Duty Military Family File (September 2014); DMDC Reserve Components Family File (September 2014).

More than half of all military children receive primary care from civilian pediatricians (Siegel & Davis, 2013). Therefore, it is critical that pediatric primary care providers (P-PCPs) are prepared to provide primary healthcare including behavioral health services to children and adolescents of military families.

■ HEALTHCARE FOR MILITARY CHILDREN

A primary care provider can be a safe, nonjudgmental source of communication and compassion. A study by Eide, Gorman, and Hisle-Gorman (2010) concluded that children with married military parents were seen more frequently by their P-PCPs for acute and well visits during deployment. P-PCPs should afford service members and families time for open dialogue to listen and respond to the needs and concerns of children and parents. Comprehensive records documenting a child's emotional, developmental, behavioral, and physical health help ease the transition as military families face recurrent moves (Howard, 2008). P-PCPs provide an essential role and should encourage open communication with both the caregiver on the home front and the deployed parent, recommend for the family to keep routines, and encourage healthy behaviors and exercise (Siegel & Davis, 2013). Identifying children on the home front who are at risk for social, emotional, and behavioral health problems is an essential skill of P-PCPs. Currently, the trend in pediatric healthcare is to transition to the patient-centered, family-centered, medical healthcare in both the civilian sector and military treatment facilities. This primary healthcare model is utilized to identify behavioral and mental health concerns with a team-based approach to care.

Currently, there are no evidenced-based screening tools to specifically screen military children for their unique social, emotional, and behavioral healthcare needs. Planned use of available behavioral and mental health screening tools, utilizing military resources as identified in Table 29.1, astute clinical skills, and

TABLE 29.1

RESOURCES FOR MILITARY CHILDREN

Web Link	Website
https://bluestarfam.org/resources/family-life/blue-star-museums	Blue Star Families
http://www.militarychild.org	Military Child
http://militaryonesource.com	Military One Source
http://www.militaryfamily.org	Military Family
http://realwarriors.net	Real Warriors
http://www.dcoe.healthmmil	Defense Center of Excellence
http://Zerotothree.org	Zero to Three
http://operationpurple.org	Operation Purple
http://militaryfamily.org	Military Family
http://militaryhomefront.dod.mil	Military Homefront
http://aap.org/sections/uniformedservices/deployment/videos.html	American Academy of Pediatrics
https://www.aap.org/en-us/about-the-aap/Committees-Councils-Sections/Section-on-Uniformed-Services/Pages/Information-for-Families.aspx	American Academy of Pediatrics
http://focusproject.org	Focus Project
http://sesameworkshop.org/tlc	Sesame Workshop
http://www.deploymentkids.com	Deployment Kids
http://www.cfs.purdue.edu/mfri/pages/military/deployment_support.html	Military Family Institute at Purdue
http://www.homebase.org	Homebase
http://militarykidsconnect.dcoe.mil/educators/coping/coping-video	Military Kids Connect

awareness of status of emotional cycle of deployment will enable the P-PCP to provide comprehensive military child healthcare. A 14-year review of studies related to military child behaviors related to deployment included increase in stress, mental health problems, academic struggles, and child maltreatment (Alfano et al., 2015). When Chan et al. (2013) reviewed studies, emerging concerns for child substance abuse and child maltreatment were identified. A general screening tool with a parent report and self-report to identify at-risk military children with psychosocial

Emotional Cycle of Deployment

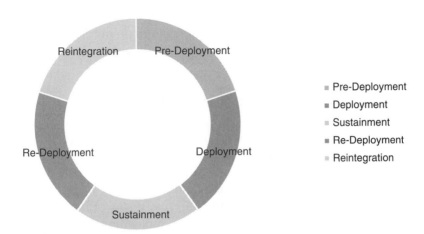

FIGURE 29.3 The emotional cycle of deployment.

symptoms during a deployment is recommended (Aranda, Middleton, Flake, & Davis, 2011). Identifying the stage of the emotional cycle of deployment (Figure 29.3) that the family is in will assist to identify if the child has additional healthcare needs. Healthcare providers should remember that even after the service member returns home, effects of the deployment can have a cumulative effect on military children and continued evaluations are necessary (Lester et al., 2010).

P-PCPs should consider submitting a referral to an outpatient behavioral or mental health provider if a child has any of the following: significant changes in behavior, drop in grades, child has increased negativity, teenager is continually not home, home-front parent is struggling to cope, death or injury of parent, child's behaviors have become more extreme, and it has been more than 3 months since deployed parent has returned (Siegel & Davis, 2013). In addition, a referral should be made by the P-PCP if the P-PCP is unsure of his or her skills to treat child, the parent, or the family (Siegel & Davis, 2013).

■ TRICARE HEALTH BENEFIT

Uniformed service members and dependent families, National Guard/Reserve members and immediate families, survivors, former spouses, and Medal of Honor recipients and immediate families are guaranteed healthcare coverage with TRICARE, a medical and mental healthcare insurance benefit. The service member must enroll in the Defense Enrollment Eligibility Reporting System (DEERS) and subsequently can choose from TRICARE Prime, an all-inclusive healthcare benefit utilizing TRICARE selected network providers without any out-of-pocket expense to the service member, or TRICARE Standard, optional utilization of non-network providers, which includes a yearly deductible (TRICARE, 2017). A comprehensive ophthalmologic exam is included annually for active duty military families and every 2 years for retiree families. Dental insurance requires an additional nominal fee for biannual dental cleanings and a co-pay for additional dental work for both active duty and retirees. Service members and their families have direct access to mental healthcare by self-referral and do not need a primary care provider referral or prior authorization for up to eight visits.

■ THE EMOTIONAL CYCLE OF DEPLOYMENT

Since 2001, military families have been living life with a degree of uncertainty due to the Global War on Terror. Military families are at high risk for psychosocial effects. Pincus, House, Christenson, and Alder (2001) developed the emotional cycle of deployment to assist with understanding military families who experience a separation of more than 6 months. The five stages of the emotional cycle of deployment cycle include pre-deployment, deployment, sustainment, redeployment, and reintegration (post-deployment). Each phase of this cycle has an assigned time line and emotional challenges (Figure 29.3).

Stage 1: Pre-deployment is the phase when the service member is going through additional training and preparation for the mission. Families experience anticipation of loss versus denial, and the length of this stage can be variable. The service member may have long work hours, and marital stress and arguments may increase with concurrent increase in mental and physical distance (Pincus et al. 2001). Families may experience shock, stress, confusion, disbelief, and anxiety surrounding the anticipated departure (Esposito-Smythers et al., 2011).

Stage 2: Deployment is the phase when the service member has physically moved away from their home installation and to their assigned mission. This time can be very difficult for military families as there is now a physical separation that can be months or years. The family often feels a void during this stage and a sense of abandonment. This phase can feel like a roller coaster with a mix of emotions (Pincus et al., 2001).

Stage 3: Sustainment is when the shock and anticipation has now ended and new routines are established. This phase lasts from 1 month until the end of the separation. Families depend on their military support network called the Family Readiness Group (FRG), family, churches, or community. Spouses become more confident during this stage. When a parent is deployed for long periods of time, children may display negative behaviors. Infants may refuse to eat, toddlers may cry or have tantrums, preschoolers may have secondary enuresis, school-age children may be clingy or whiney, and teenagers may isolate themselves or participate in risky adolescent behaviors (Pincus et al., 2001).

Stage 4: Redeployment is when there is excitement in anticipation of homecoming. The spouse may start "nesting" in preparation to have the service member home. The time frame is the month prior to return of the service member. There can also be a surge of emotions during this phase with difficultly in decision making for parents and apprehension for all family members (Pincus et al., 2001).

Stage 5: Reintegration (post-deployment) phase includes return of the service member to their families, community, and regular military unit. This stage can last 3 to 6 months and begins with reunion of service member and family

(Pincus et al., 2001). Additional support services may be needed for the service member or family members because this can be a time of additional stress (Military Deployment Guide, Department of Defense). Military families will experience intense feelings of elation initially but then may transition into reintegration struggles and have difficulties redefining new roles, routines, and responsibilities (Esposito-Smythers et al., 2011). The relational turbulence model was utilized to evaluate the relationship climate between parents and military children. Parents reported difficulty with depressive symptoms, relationship uncertainty, and partner interference with their children struggling with reintegration (Knobloch, Knoblock-Fedders, Yorgason, Ebata, & McGlaughlin, 2017).

■ PARENTING MILITARY CHILDREN

In addition to typical parenting strife, military parents experience deployment-related transitions and uncertainties. Devoe and Ross (2012) developed the Parenting Cycle of Deployment, which is a step-by-step process to assist parents with deployments during each phase of the deployment cycle. The steps include thinking ahead, saying goodbye, parenting from the home front, parenting from the war zone, facing reality, and moving forward. During pre-deployment, parents must think ahead to the future to maintain family stability and prepare to say goodbye. During deployment, parents focus on parenting from the home front and parenting from the war zone while developing new routines with ambiguous times and limited communication. Finally, with reintegration, parents face reality and move forward with negotiations and restructuring with new roles and duties as the family reunites (DeVoe & Ross, 2012).

For an active duty service member, there are many factors that influence the level of stress experienced. Some of these factors may include the deployment schedule, rank, unit cohesiveness, mission, and roles in theater and at home (DeVoe & Ross, 2012). Service members are often unaware of the struggles that the family is experiencing back home. Psychological well-being of parents diminishes during long deployments, especially among military fathers (DeVoe & Ross, 2012). An increase in the length of the deployment of the service member results in an increase in difficulty to manage home life for the child (Chandra et al., 2010).

Stresses that may influence the spouse on the home front include media coverage of the war, community support against the war mission, lack of support of military unit, and the ability of the community to respond to the needs of the military family (DeVoe & Ross, 2012). Chandra et al. (2010) found that caregivers with mental health challenges and extended deployments directly correlated with behavioral health challenges in their children. Army wives with deployed spouses reported a 19% increase in mental health services during 1 to 11 months deployments and 27% increase in mental health services during a deployment lasting longer than 11 months (Mansfield et al., 2010). A study by Flake, Davis, Johnson, and Middleton (2009) determined that approximately 50% of home-front spouses experience "clinically significant" stress during a deployment. This research study also concluded that stress of military parents and military children is more than double the national average. Jensen et al. (1990) studied 134 children in a military psychiatric clinic and reported that parental psychopathology, specifically, maternal psychopathology, was the biggest risk factor for child psychopathology.

■ INFANTS ON THE HOME FRONT

Infancy is a time of tremendous physical and mental growth. During the first year of life, children learn how to walk, talk, and self-advocate. Attachment and preference for a specific caregiver occurs during the first year of life. There have been limited studies conducted on military infants on the home front. According to Chartrand, Frank, White, and Shope (2008), when the family structure changes during a military deployment, infants seem to handle deployments the best of all age groups. Consistent caretaking is essential for infant development at a fragile time of life when a person is dependent on caregivers for all basic needs (Osofsky & Chartrand, 2013). During a deployment, an infant is not only separated from a primary caregiver, he or she is also left with a caregiver that is experiencing distress as he or she copes with the separation of a spouse. Signs of deployment distress in an infant may be listlessness and refusal to eat (Esposito-Smythers et al., 2011). Separating young children from parents can result in a break in attachment and may result in extreme behaviors and anxieties (Osofsky & Chartrand, 2013). It is important during deployment for parents and caregivers of infants to keep routines consistent and to stay connected to the deployed service member through innovative ways. Examples may include viewing visual images of parents, allowing the infant to listen to prerecorded voice tapings of the deployed parent, and allowing the infant to view prerecorded videos of the infant and deployed parent playing together and cuddling (Osofsky & Chartrand, 2013). These opportunities allow the infant to be connected to their own emotions and their deployed parent.

■ TODDLERS AND PRESCHOOLERS ON THE HOME FRONT

Toddlers explore their environment but like to stay close to their primary caregiver. Negotiation and cooperation are learned during this stage of life. Toddlers and preschoolers can retain visual images of parents, even if separated for a deployment. A child between 2 to 4 years of age has the ability to verbally communicate and establish secure attachment relationships (Hallas, Koslap-Petraco, & Fletcher, 2017; Osofsky & Chartrand, 2013). Children between the ages 3 and 5 years exhibit the most frequent behavioral health concerns during a parent's deployment (Chartrand et al., 2008). If a child does not have a secure attachment relationship with a caregiver during this time, ongoing struggles with attachment could persist throughout life. If the home-front parent struggles with mental instability during the deployment or the service member returns from deployment with mental instability, this instability can also affect the child's ability to develop bonds and healthy attachments (Osofsky & Chartrand, 2013). Signs of deployment distress in a toddler/preschooler may be crying, tantrums, and secondary enuresis (Esposito-Smothers, et al., 2011). A cross-sectional study at a large Marine base showed an increase in behavioral symptoms and clinically significant depression scores in children 3 years and older when a parent is deployed as compared to other children without a deployed parent (Chartrand et al., 2008). Parents of toddlers/preschoolers should listen to the child's concerns, talk to the child about what is happening in simple language, acknowledge the child's personal feelings, allow the child to stay connected to the deployed family member through daily routines, identify and match feelings, and create an environment to share emotions with the child (Osofsky & Chartrand, 2013).

■ SCHOOL-AGE CHILD ON THE HOME FRONT

School-age children are concrete thinkers. A parent going to war, for this age group, means extended periods of time away from the child. Confusion about war and stories from other children may increase stress and worries in the school-age child with a deployed parent. Most studies conducted on military children are on the school-age population. One third of military children between ages 5 and 12 experiencing a deployment are "high risk" for psychosocial morbidity with internalizing symptoms more common than attention on externalizing symptoms (Flake et al., 2009). Mansfield, Kaufman, Engel, and Gaynes (2011) concluded during a nonrandomized cohort study of 6,579 military children of deployed parents, between ages 5 and 17, that there was an increase in mental health diagnoses during the study period associated with deployment during Operation Iraqi Freedom and Operation Enduring Freedom. Males and females were equally affected, and the most frequent diagnoses included stress, depression, anxiety, sleep disorders, and other behavioral health problems. A study in a military treatment facility by Jensen, Bloedau, Degroot, Ussery, and Davis (1990) analyzed military children's symptomology. This study concluded that parent psychopathology and life stress increased military child symptoms (Jensen et al., 1990). Children are most vulnerable when the mental health of the parents is compromised and the parent cannot fulfill parental obligations (DeVoe & Ross, 2012). The child may feel responsible for the deployed parent and the home-front parent may try to shield the child from the details of the deployment (Siegel & Davis, 2013). Specifically, boys and younger children show an increase in vulnerability during deployment and should be monitored closely for secondary effects (Jensen, Martin, & Watanabe, 1996).

■ ADOLESCENTS ON THE HOME FRONT

Adolescence is an emotionally charged stage of life with the potential for tremendous growth and development. Abstract thinking abilities develop during the adolescent years. As teenagers mature toward adulthood, they naturally take on more responsibility. In addition to previously established adolescent roles and responsibilities, parents often increase family responsibilities for adolescents on the home front during deployments.

Additional duties at home may include grocery shopping, yard work, cleaning, cooking, pet care, home protection, and transportation requirements. Adolescents often assume a caregiver role and are responsible for the safety, well-being, tutoring, and mentoring of younger siblings for extended times. In 2009, a research team at Johns Hopkins School of Public Health compared 11 different focus groups from five military installations and concluded that adolescents had an increase in stress and anxiety related to changes of roles and responsibilities at home during a parental deployment (Mmari, Roche, Sudhinaraset, & Blum, 2009). An increase in stress and anxiety can negatively impact multiple domains of development. An adolescent may demonstrate social–behavioral and academic maladjustments during long deployments, which is especially true for male adolescents (Nicosia, Wong, Shier, Massacre, & Datar, 2016). It is common during deployments for teenagers to feel angry and sad (Siegel & Davis, 2013). With extreme emotional reactions, risky adolescent behaviors may increase during deployments to include social isolation and drug abuse (Esposito-Smythers et al., 2011). Parents of adolescents on the home front reported that their adolescent children became targets and experienced an increase in bullying from antiwar peers. This same research study identified that school personnel did not feel adequately prepared to assist adolescents on the home front with deployment-related concerns, potentially leaving the adolescent without proper school-based support services (Mmari et al., 2009).

Suggestions that may help *intercept* some of the problems and concerns for adolescents during the deployment cycle include (a) coping mechanisms should be in place for all stages of the emotional cycle of deployment; (b) teachers should have additional training on military children and the deployment cycle; and (c) support groups for adolescents should be readily available (Mmari et al., 2009). It is common for adolescents to seek support from peers versus family members during deployments (Siegel & Davis, 2013). Establishment of a healthy network of peers is essential for children of all ages, especially teens as they turn to one another for support.

■ EXCEPTIONAL MILITARY CHILDREN ON THE HOME FRONT

There are additional subgroups of military children that have not been addressed in this chapter, and although they are the silent minority, it is essential to mention them as they face challenges beyond the typical military child. Exceptional military families include children of dual military parents, National Guard and Reserve, single parents, active duty mothers, combat wounded veterans, divorced parents, deceased parent due to military conflict, and children with special healthcare needs. A study by Eide et al. (2010) concluded that children of young, single military parents were seen in primary care for acute and well-child care less frequently during a deployment. If the child is seen less often due to family constraints, then it is critical to assess how the child is coping with the deployment at every visit. All subsets of military children require additional support and there is limited research to address their specific healthcare needs. Healthcare providers should provide additional time and attention to these military families as deployment and transition may cause an increase in turbulence for these families.

When caring for a military dependent with a chronic health condition, the active duty member is required to enroll their dependent into the Exceptional

Family Member Program (EFMP). The DD Form 2792 should be completed by a qualified civilian or military medical professional healthcare provider and can be found here: www.dtic.mil/whs/directives/forms/eforms/dd2792.pdf. Once a qualified medical provider completes this form, the service member or spouse will submit this form to the military EFMP office for review. By enrolling dependents into the EFMP program, the service member will be stationed only in locations with adequate healthcare for the exceptional healthcare needs of the family.

▪ SERVICES FOR CHILDREN ON THE HOME FRONT

Over the recent years, there have been a growing number of resources to assist military children to cope with deployment during each phase of the deployment cycle. Generally, military families are resilient; however, healthcare providers should be able to assess and identify when additional support is necessary and know how to access the resources available for these families. Parents should be encouraged to elicit teacher- and school-based support for a child when needed (Siegel & Davis, 2013). Only 4.7% of military children attend a Department of Defense Educational Activity school. The other 95.3% of military children attend public school, private school, or are homeschooled. About 80% of military children attend school in a public military-connected school district and receive Federal Impact Aid dollars to support military children by educating staff members and providing support groups (De Pedro et al., 2011).

Resources to Intercept Behavioral Problems

There are a multitude of resources for family members, such as online workshops, videos, blogs, support groups, and educational materials/resources and handouts. Zero to Three, a nonprofit organization that educates and supports parents and professionals to improve the lives of children birth to 3 years old, also provides additional resources and support for military families (Osofsky & Chartrand, 2013). Sesame Street has developed Talk, Listen, and Connect for preschool-age children of military families. The goal of the developers was to provide practical tools for deployment with a focus on love and laughter (www.sesameworkshop.org/what-we-do/our-initiatives/military-families). Operation Military Kids has created community partnerships with local Boys and Girls Clubs, 4-H, and youth clubs throughout the country. Prevention programs such as Operation Purple and family retreats include evidence-based resiliency activities (Esposito-Smythers et al., 2011). FOCUS-Resilience Training for Military Families is a web-based telehealth resource for military families that assists with emotional regulation, communication, problem solving, goal setting, and managing deployment reminders (Mogil et al., 2015). Homebase is a Red Sox Foundation and Massachusetts General Hospital program dedicated to healing invisible wounds of post-9/11 veterans, service members, and families, and it offers educational information and support for clinicians (www.homebase.org). These programs are just a few of the many resources available for military families.

Evidence-based treatment approaches with skill-building techniques and skills training for military youth to assist with coping with deployment should be considered.

Education for nondeployed parents to manage stress, watch for warning signs for military child distress; reintegration with service member, group-based support groups; interventions sensitive for military culture; evidence-based techniques to address emotional and behavioral repercussions associated with deployment; and sustainable and accessible care endorsed by the military is essential (Esposito-Smythers et al., 2011). Children and adolescents who screen positive on any of the standard anxiety or depression screening tools should be referred for counseling and therapeutic interventions. The earlier the children and adolescents are identified and referred for therapeutic interventions, the more likely potential emotional and behavioral problems can be *intercepted* with the goal of improving the well-being of the military children, adolescents, and their family unit.

■ SUMMARY

Military families are in a constant state of uncertainty with increased demands on service members and recurrent deployments. The life of the military family can be turbulent. P-PCPs are often the first line of contact for military children in distress. It is essential for both civilian and military healthcare providers to be sensitive to the military culture, to be knowledgeable about the emotional cycle of deployment, to screen children and adolescents appropriately to identify a child in crisis, and to intercept potential problems using evidence-based practice for treatment. During the emotional cycle of deployment, there can be struggles for military members, spouses, and military children; however, deployment of a parent can also provide positive outcomes for children and adolescents by encouraging maturity, emotional growth, independence, and flexibility, strengthening family bonds, and bringing awareness to the importance of civic duty (Pincus et al., 2001). Although certainly there are resources available to assist military children, many are still being evaluated and have not been proven effective, warranting the need for rigorous research studies to better inform P-PCPs about care management for military families and their children.

CASE PRESENTATION

Reason for the Visit: Jonah Noble just turned 10 years old when he arrived at the primary care clinic accompanied by his mother for his yearly well-child visit.

Family history revealed that Jonah's father is a combat engineer, deployed 1 month ago for his third tour to an active war zone. Jonah, his mother, and his 16-year-old brother, Harold, live in a single-family home on a base in Georgia.

(continued)

Social History: Jonah's mother works up to 12 hours a day and weekends at a local hair salon. Harold preferred to be out with friends rather than at home. Often, Jonah was home alone, without supervision or interactions with peers.

Jonah's Affect: During the clinic visit, Jonah was solemn. He spoke when he was spoken to but otherwise remained rather quiet, and when asked a question, refused to make eye contact with the examiner, holding his head down.

Mother's Affect: His mother was also rather quiet and offered little information, and both initially stated when asked that they were doing well while Jonah's father was deployed.

Jonah's Personal History: Jonah was asked by the P-PCP how he was sleeping at nighttime. Jonah continued to look down and did not answer. The P-PCP asked Jonah again how he was sleeping at nighttime and Jonah looked toward the P-PCP, but then quickly looked away. The P-PCP asked Jonah and his mother if it would be okay to talk in private with Jonah while the mother was out of the room. Both mother and Jonah agreed.

Jonah's Story: As soon as Jonah's mother left the room, Jonah started to cry. He stated his older brother babysat him after school and as soon as he would get home his brother would start to torture him. He would yank his legs so hard when he was sitting on the couch that he would fall onto the floor and bang his head. He further revealed that it was routine for Harold to curse at him. Harold also demanded that Jonah do all of Harold's chores, leaving little time for him to do his homework or play with friends. Jonah admitted that he was too scared of Harold to tell his mother what happened while she was at work. As soon as his mother got home from work at 7 p.m., Harold would behave but Jonah knew that it would start all over again the next day after school. Jonah didn't want to be home anymore. After further questions, Jonah admitted to suicidal ideations. As a matter of fact, he didn't want to even live anymore. He tried several times to wrap his video game cord around his neck and put one end attached to the door handle and then slam it shut to try to kill himself.

Questions that you should consider:

1. *What clinical concerns should the P-PCP consider?*
   The P-PCP should consider an immediate risk assessment for suicidal/homicidal ideations.
2. *Describe the stage of the emotional cycle of deployment for Jonah and his family? Provide a rationale for your answer.*

Deployment is the phase when service members have physically moved away from their home installation and to their assigned mission. This time can be very difficult for military families as there is now a physical separation which can be months or years. The family often feels a void during this stage and a sense of abandonment. This phase can feel like a roller coaster with a mix of emotions.

3. *What type of an assessment should be performed to best evaluate Jonah's current behavioral health and mental health status?*
   A general mental health questionnaire with both the option for a parent report and a self-report is the appropriate assessment to perform for this child.
4. *What resources are available for Jonah and his family?*

The following resources are available: (a) Military One Source; (b) Behavioral Health Referral; (c) American Academy of Pediatrics; (d) Operation Purple

■ REFERENCES

Alfano, C. A., Lau, S., Balderas, J., Bunnell, B. E., & Beidel, D. C. (2014). The impact of military deployment on children: Placing developmental risk in context. *Clinical Psychology Review, 43,* 17–29. doi:10.1016/j.cpr.2015.11.003

Aranda, M.C., Middleton, L.S., Flake, E., & Davis, B.E. (2011). Psychosocial screening in children with wartime-deployed parents. *Military Medicine, 176,* 402–407. doi:10.7205/MILMED-D-10-00202

Caliber and ICF Consulting Company. (2014). *2014 Demographic profile of the Military Community Office of the Deputy Under Secretary of Defense (Military community and family policy)*. Retrieved from http://download.militaryonesource.mil/12038/MOS/Reports/2014-Demographics-Report.pdf

Chandra, A., Lara-Cinisomo, S., Jaycox, L. H., Tanielian, T., Burns, R. M., Ruder, T., & Han, B. (2010). Children on the homefront: The experience of children from military families. *Pediatrics, 125*(1), e2002-e2015. doi:10.1542/peds.2009-1180

Chartrand, M. M., Frank, D. A., White, L. F., & Shope, T. R. (2008). Effect of parents' wartime deployment on the behavior of children in military families. *Archives of Pediatric Adolescent Medicine, 162*(11), 1009–1014. doi:10.1001/archpedi.162.11.1009

De Pedro, K. M. T., Astor, R. A., Benbenishty, R., Estrada, J., Dejoie Smith, G. R., & Esqueda, M. C. (2011). The children of military service members: Challenge, supports, and future. *Educational Research, 81*, 566–618. doi:10.3102/0034654311423537

DeVoe, E. R., & Ross, A. (2012). The parenting cycle of deployment. *Military Medicine, 177*, 184–190. doi:10.7205/MILMED-D-11-00292

Eide, M., Gorman, G., & Hisle-Gorman, E. (2010). Effects of parental military deployment on pediatric outpatient and well-child visit rates. *Pediatrics, 126*(1), 1–6. doi:10.1542/peds.2009-2704

Esposito-Smythers, C., Wolff, J., Lemmon, K. M., Bodzy, M., Swenson, R. R., & Spirito, A. (2011). Military youth and the deployment cycle: Emotional health consequences and recommendations for interventions. *Journal Family Psychology, 25*, 497–507. doi:10.1037/a0024534

Exceptional Family Member Program. (2017) Retrieved from http://www.dtic.mil/whs/directives/forms/eforms/dd2792.pdf

Family Resilience Training for Military Families. (2017). Retrieved from www.focusproject.org

Flake, E. M., Davis, B. E., Johnson, P. L., & Middleton, L. S. (2009). The psychosocial effects of deployment on military children. *Journal Developmental Behavioral Pediatrics, 30*, 271–278. doi:10.1097/DBP.0b013e3181aac6e4

Homebase. (2017). Retrieved from http://www.homebase.com

Howard, B. J. (2008). Tune in to special needs of military families. (Behavioral Consult). *Pediatric News, 34*. doi:10.1016/S0031-398X(08)70072-9

Jensen, P. S., Bloedau, L., Degroot, J., Ussery, T., & Davis, H. (1990). Children at risk: Risk factors and child symptomatology. *Journal of the American Academy of Child and Adolescent Psychiatry, 29*(1), 51–59. doi:10.1097/00004583-199001000-00010

Jensen, P. S., Martin, D., & Watanabe, H. (1996). Children's response to parental separation during Operation Desert Storm. *Journal of the American Academy of Child and Adolescent Psychiatry, 35*, 433–441. doi:10.1097/00004583-199604000-00009

Knobloch, L. K., Knoblock-Fedders, L. M., Yorgason, J. B., Ebata, A. T., & McGlaughlin, P. C. (2017). Military children's difficulty with reintegration after deployment: A relational turbulence model perspective. *Journal of Family Psychology, 31*(5), 542–552. doi:10.1037/fam0000299

Lester, P., Peterson, K., Reeves, J., Knauss, L., Glover, D., Mogil, C., . . . Beardslee, W. (2010). The long war and parental combat deployment: Effects on military children and at-home spouses. *Journal of the American Academy of Child and Adolescent Psychiatry, 49*(4), 838–845. doi:10.1097/00004583-201004000-00006

Mansfield, A. J., Kaufman, J. S., Engel, C. C., & Gaynes, B. N. (2011). Deployment and mental health diagnoses among children of U.S. Army personnel. *Archives of Pediatric and Adolescent Medicine, 165*, 999–1005. doi:10.1001/archpediatrics.2011.123

Mansfield, A. J., Kaufman, J. S., Marshal, S. W., Marshall, S. W., Gaynes, B. N., Morrissey, J. P., & Engel, C. C. (2010). Deployment and the use of mental health services among U.S. army wives. *The New England Journal of Medicine, 363*(2), 101–109. doi:10.1056/NEJMoa0900177

Mmari, K., Roche, K. M., Sudhinaraset, M., & Blum, R. (2009). When a parent goes off to war: Exploring the issues faced by adolescents and their families. *Johns Hopkins Bloomberg School of Public Health, Youth and Society, 40*(4), 455–475. doi:10.1177/0044118X08327873

Mogil, C., Hajal, N., Garcia, E., Kiff, C., Paley, B., Milburn, N., & Lester, P. (2015). FOCUS for early childhood: A virtual home visiting program for military families with young children. *Contemporary Family Therapy, 37*(3), 199–208. doi:10.1007/s10591-015-9327-9

Nicosia, N., Wong, E., Shier, V., Massacre, S., & Datar, A. (2016). Parental deployment, adolescent academic and social–behavioral maladjustment, and parental psychological well-being in military families. *Public Health Reports 2017, 132*(1), 93–105. doi:10.1177/0033354916679995

Osofsky, J. D., & Chartrand, M. M. (2013). Military children from birth to five years. *The Future of Children, 23*, 61–73. doi:10.1353/foc.2013.0011

Pincus, S. H., House, R., Christenson, J., & Alder, L. E. (2001). *The emotional cycle of deployment: A military family perspective.* Retrieved from http://www.hooah4health.com/deployment/family matters/emotionalcycle.htm

Rostker, B. (2006). *The evolution of the all-volunteer force, Research Brief* (Document number: RB-9195-RC). Retrieved from http://www.rand.org/pubs/research_briefs/RB9195.html

Siegel, B. S., & Davis, B. E. (2013). Health and mental health needs of children in U.S. military families. *Pediatrics, 131,* e2002–e2015. doi:10.1542/peds.2013-0940

TRICARE. (2017). Retrieved from www.tricare.mil/Plans/Eligibility.

CHAPTER 30

Child Abuse: Intercepting Behavioral Health Issues

MARY WEGLARZ, EILEEN CORCORAN, DEBORAH
GUTTER, PAULA BARBEL, STEPHANIE BROWN,
JAMES T. MULHOLLAND, AND NINA B. COLABELLI

Childhood maltreatment is a global, national, state, and local problem (Annie E. Casey Foundation, 2017; U.S. Department of Health & Human Services, Administration for Children and Families, Administration on Children, Youth and Families, & Children's Bureau, 2017; World Health Organization and International Society for Prevention of Child Abuse and Neglect, 2006). In the United States alone, child welfare agencies respond to more than 4 million calls for suspected abuse and neglect of children annually (Annie E. Casey Foundation, 2017; U.S. Department of Health & Human Services, Administration for Children and Families, Administration on Children, Youth and Families, & Children's Bureau, 2017). The federal government began overseeing state child welfare agencies in 1974 when Congress passed the Child Abuse Prevention and Treatment Act (CAPTA, U.S. Congress, 1974), key federal legislation addressing child abuse and neglect. The most recent revision of CAPTA (U.S. Department of Health & Human Services, Administration for Children and Families, Administration on Children, Youth and Families, & Children's Bureau, 2016) provides federal funding to states in support of prevention, assessment, investigation, prosecution, and treatment activities, and provides grants to public agencies and nonprofit organizations, including Indian tribes and tribal organizations, for demonstration programs and projects, and monitors the incidence of abuse and neglect through the creation the National Center on Child Abuse and Neglect (NCCAN).

Child maltreatment is physical, sexual, or psychological abuse or neglect of any child younger than 18 years of age by his or her parent, caregiver, guardian or any adult that can cause death, injury, or impact to the child's physical and mental health (Fortson, Klevens, Merrick, Gilbert, & Alexander, 2016; Leeb, Paulozzi, Melanson, Simon, & Arias, 2008). Physical abuse is any intentional physical act such as punching, beating, throwing, or pushing that may potentially cause harm. Sexual abuse consists of sexual penetration, sexual touch, and noncontact sexual abuse including exposure of the child to sexual activity, pornography, or prostitution. Psychological or emotional abuse is intermittent or ongoing behavior that communicates to the child a wide range of harmful feelings that can damage the child's psychological and emotional development. Child neglect fails to meet the child's physical, emotional, or educational needs (Fortson et al., 2016; Leeb et al., 2008). The Centers for Disease Control and Prevention (CDC; Fortson et al., 2016) defines abuse and neglect so that the federal government, states, child welfare agencies, and their community partners, including pediatric primary care providers (P-PCPs), can uniformly monitor and plan their response to reports of maltreatment.

P-PCPs are obligated to report evidence of child abuse and neglect. They do not need to be experts, but they do need knowledge and skills to identify the signs of potential abuse and neglect. Their attention to children and families, and partnerships with child welfare, social services, and community providers, can protect children and aid in the prevention of abuse and neglect's adverse effects (Christian & Committee on Child Abuse and Neglect, 2015). Maltreatment is a significant problem and failure to prevent, address, and treat threatens the future of our children and their adult life. Intentional acts of maltreatment impact the surviving child's emotional, behavioral, and mental health throughout their life span (Fortson et al., 2016; Leeb et al., 2008). This chapter presents the evidence that places children at risk for maltreatment, its consequences, and methods for screening, assessment, and care with a goal of *intercepting* the adverse effects of child maltreatment.

■ FACTORS THAT RENDER CHILDREN VULNERABLE TO MALTREATMENT

Social determinants of health and disparities linked to social disadvantage can place a child at greater risk for abuse and neglect (Zimmerman & Mercy, 2010). Low-income children and minorities are at greatest risk for abuse and neglect and involvement with child protective services (Lanier, Jonson-Reid, Stahlschmidt, Drake, & Constantino, 2010). However, even though this health disparity exists, child abusers do not discriminate, and maltreatment is found in every socioeconomic, racial, and ethnic group. The vast majority (91.6%) of abusers are one or both parents; 13.3% of victims are abused by nonparents; and 2.8% are unknown (U.S. Department of Health & Human Services, Administration for Children and Families, Administration on Children, Youth and Families, & Children's Bureau, 2017). Parental, child, and environmental factors are known to place a child at risk for abuse and neglect. Not every indicator is a red flag, but identification of a risk factor warrants attentionand additional services might help prevent disruption of the family unit (Table 30.1).

Parental substance use and domestic violence expose the child to high-risk behavior and place them at risk for abuse and neglect. Also, parents who are challenged by their own chronic physical or mental illness have difficulty meeting the needs of their children. Other risk factors for maltreatment include parents with their own history of maltreatment as a child, parental age, cognitive ability, education level, and lack of knowledge about child development. Sadly, some parents verbalize a negative attitude toward the child, or the fact that the child was from an unwanted pregnancy (Gelles, 2009; McCoy & Keen, 2009). Consideration needs to be given to the parent and child within a family and household structure. Single parent households, large family size, marital conflict, domestic violence, stress, housing insecurity, and low socioeconomic status place a strain on family dynamics

TABLE 30.1

RISK FACTORS FOR CHILD ABUSE AND NEGLECT

Parental Factors	Child Factors	Environmental Factors
Substance use	Premature infants	Poverty
Minor parents	Multiple births	Resides in a high-crime area
Mental illness	Infants with congenital malformations/genetic disorders/chronic disease	Chaotic homes
Developmental disability	Challenging behavior	Domestic violence
Parent with a chronic illness that could impact their ability to meet the day-to-day needs of their children	Child of an unwanted pregnancy	Lack of family or community support
History of abuse as child	Home schooling	Life changes: death, separation, divorce, military deployment

and contribute to the risk for maltreatment (Gelles, 2009; McCoy & Keen, 2009; Taylor, Washington, Artinian, & Lichtenberg, 2007).

Known characteristics of children that place them at greater risk include infants and toddlers, especially the infant with a difficult temperament. Also, children with disabilities, such as those who suffer from a cognitive impairment, emotional disturbance, visual or hearing impairment, learning disability, physical disability, behavioral problems, poor communication skills, a difficult temperament, or chronic illness are known to have greater vulnerability (U.S. Department of Health & Human Services, Administration for Children and Families, Administration on Children, Youth and Families, & Children's Bureau, 2017).

The community where the child lives can place him or her at risk for abuse and neglect. Impoverished communities with a high density of vacant housing, above average unemployment rates, and community violence have been known to be associated with maltreatment. These communities generally lack social resources and cohesion (Connell, Bergeron, Katz, Saunders, & Tebes, 2007; Egan, Tannahill, Petticrew, & Thomas, 2008). Awareness of these red flags and careful assessment skills are necessary for P-PCPs to guard the safety and health of children.

■ CONSEQUENCES OF ABUSE AND NEGLECT

The physical and mental health of a child can be harmed by maltreatment. Some periods of child growth and development are more critical than others, such as younger than 4 years of age. During early development, children are particularly vulnerable. Brain development and myelination of the spinal cord and nerves are necessary for development of language, fine and gross motor skills, social and emotional development, and cognition and learning. Positive and negative experiences during early years of life help shape the brain and the connections that the brain makes. This rapid growth and development makes infants and young children vulnerable to developmental delays, illness or injury, and requires careful surveillance by parents, caregivers, healthcare providers, and the community to guard the health of infants and young children (Zimmerman & Mercy, 2010). Later in childhood, the trauma of maltreatment can lead to poor academic achievement, mental illness, antisocial behavior, and high-risk behaviors, which for an adolescent increases their exposure to communicable disease (Szilagyi, 2012). Children need emotional stability, social competency, and cognitive growth for brain development and ongoing development (National Scientific Council on the Developing Child, 2007).

The long-term consequences of child maltreatment on health include poorer control of chronic health conditions among adults, such as cardiovascular disease, high blood pressure, diabetes, respiratory illness, liver disease, poor nutritional status including obesity, and vision problems (Felitti & Anda, 2009; Felitti et al., 1998; Widom, Czaja, Bentley, & Johnson, 2012). Furthermore, maltreated children have been noted to transition into adulthood with mental illness including suicide attempts and substance abuse (Felitti & Anda, 2009). Child maltreatment impacts future abilities, choices, and life course trajectories (National Scientific Council on the Developing Child, 2007). Positioned within the community, the P-PCP is looked upon for guidance and to aid in the protection of children. At every encounter with a child, P-PCPs must screen and assess for suspected abuse and neglect.

■ ASSESSMENT

Children are brought to their primary provider for routine well-child care, which provides the opportunity for preventive dental, physical, and emotional care. Each encounter with a family and child has its own rhythm. The family has needs they want fulfilled during the visit and the provider has expectations to meet during the same visit. This develops into the shared agenda for the appointment (Hagan, Shaw, & Duncan, 2017). However, if the P-PCP's initial assessment indicates acute life-threatening injury, the P-PCP should secure transport to an emergency department (ED) and ensure the health and safety of the child while waiting for emergency medical services. Furthermore, if the P-PCP does not have the expertise to examine the genitalia of a child with suspected sexual abuse, the P-PCP should refer the child to the ED or a specialist in the area (Jenny, Crawford-Jakubiak, & Committee on Child Abuse and Neglect, 2013). The P-PCP obtains information about the injury from the child or parent and explains to the parent the P-PCP's responsibility to the child. Even though the ED may report the injury to Child Protective Services (CPS), the P-PCP is also expected to call in a referral (Christian & Committee on Child Abuse and Neglect, 2015).

If there are no immediate health and safety concerns, during the assessment process, the P-PCP evaluates the family strengths and considers if risk factors are present. Parental resilience, social connections, knowledge of parenting and child development, concrete supports in time of need, and the social–emotional competence of children are protective factors the P-PCP can help families attain and grow (for more information on protective factors, see Chapter 6). Knowledge of family stressors and the protective factors that support families who may be at risk for child maltreatment can inform interventions to improve health and reduce the risk of future child welfare involvement (Campbell, Myrup, & Svedin, 2017).

■ HISTORY

History assists the P-PCP with screening for abuse and neglect, deciding whether an injury was accidental or not, and determining the necessity to report to CPS. If a referral is made to CPS, investigators will question the child and all involved in the child's care in detail. Prior to any thoughts of referring to CPS, the P-PCP conducts an initial interview and may choose to question the parents and children together or separately. All questions should be nonjudgmental, nonleading, and open ended (Christian & Committee on Child Abuse and Neglect, 2015).

Current history includes asking about the reason for the visit. If an injury is reported, the child's activity level before, during, and after is noted. In the absence of a witnessed injury, specifics about when the child last appeared normal can provide information about timing of the injury. When neglect is a concern, history of present illness and medications addresses length of time child has been ill, symptoms, and treatments offered to the child (Christian & Committee on Child Abuse and Neglect, 2015).

Routine medical history and a review of systems (see Chapter 31, Table 31.2 for additional questions to add to the reveiw of systems [ROS]) detail medical, birth and family history, development, education, and social history. When thinking about abuse and neglect, consider the following questions. Does the child have a primary medical home, or does it appear that the child has none or that the parents are jumping around between providers? When was the child last seen for care? Was the infant born prematurely, were there complications or substance use during the pregnancy? What developmental milestones are the parents reporting? What is the child's temperament? Who is the child's primary caregiver: a parent, daycare provider, or babysitter? What school does the child attend, and what is his or her grade level? How is the child doing in school? Are there reports of truancy or bullying? What does the family schedule look like? Does the family have support from family or community? Is there a history of substance use, mental or chronic illness, or domestic violence? Has the family been referred to CPS previously? Is there financial need for food, housing, or transportation?

■ SCREENING

Screening tools are used during well-child care visits and can also be used during episodic visits (see Chapter 6, Table 6.1 for specific screening tools to use during a visit). These tools will provide the P-PCP with insight into parental health and household stress. Screening is part of routine pediatric care even if parents have no concerns (Christian & Committee on Child Abuse and Neglect, 2015). Likewise, the main reason for the visit may be an injury or illness, or parents may be worried about changes in the child that may signal injury, or the child might report that they have been hurt. With every encounter, P-PCPs should listen, ask questions, observe, and be alert for signs of abuse and neglect (Table 30.2).

If the chief complaint is an injury, listen to the explanation. Can it be explained or was it not witnessed? Is the history vague, or inconsistent with the injury or developmental age of the child? As you ask more questions, does the story change? If the child is able to speak, does the parent allow the child to share his or her explanation? If you want to speak to the child separately, does the parent object? When did the injury happen? Did the parent delay seeking treatment? Is the family known to your practice, or is this their first encounter with you? If there is no overt sign of trauma but a change in activity level, ask when the child was last behaving normally.

Some encounters might indicate that the child is being neglected. The P-PCP should think about neglect if the family seeks care only when the child is sick. Does the child have frequent visits to the ED, or hospitalizations for a condition that can be controlled with medication and outpatient treatment? Does the child lack immunizations, well-child care, and dental care? How is the child's hygiene? Does the child appear well nourished? If observations and questions are suspicious for abuse or neglect, additional history should be obtained, and continue with your assessment.

TABLE 30.2

SIGNS OF ABUSE AND NEGLECT

Physical Abuse	Sexual Abuse	Neglect
Any injury in a nonmobile infant	Pain, discharge, or odor in genital area	Failure to thrive
Injuries to torso, ears, and neck in a toddler	Recurrent urinary tract infections	Malnutrition, feeding disorders
Injuries that are at different stages of healing	Sexually transmitted infection	Poor hygiene
Injuries without explanation	Pregnancy	Lack of healthcare
Human bite marks	Enuresis or encopresis	Truancy
Injury to the oral frena in infants		Enuresis
Patterned bruising (belt, electrical cords)		Sleep disorders
Submersion or cigarette burns		

■ PHYSICAL EXAMINATION

Physical examination links information obtained through history and screening, further evaluates the child's health, and completes the P-PCP's assessment of the child. If abuse or neglect is suspected, the child should be unclothed and placed in an examination gown (Christian & Committee on Child Abuse and Neglect, 2015). The child's vital signs and growth parameters are measured and plotted to assist the P-PCP with determining whether the child is healthy, following his/her growth curve, or failing to thrive. Observe the child's appearance, alertness, and interactions. Is he or she responsive, or lethargic and withdrawn? Also, while examining the child, note the parents' emotions. Are they angry, stressed, overwhelmed, or fatigued? Assess the child's development and determine the milestones that the child has attained. Is the child's development delayed, does his or her development align with what the parents are reporting, or would it be impossible for the child to sustain the injury based upon the developmental level?

Carefully examine the child from head to toe. Examine the fontanelles of infants, look for alopecia or wounds on the scalp; check eyes for red reflex, and response to light; and assess tympanic membranes, nasal and oral mucosa, and dentition for signs of illness, injury, or poor hygiene (Fisher-Owens, Lukefahr, Tate, American Academy of Pediatrics, Section on Oral Health, Committee on Child Abuse and Neglect, American Academy of Pediatric Dentistry, Council on Clinical Affairs, Council on Scientific Affairs, & Ad Hoc Work Group on Child Abuse and Neglect, 2017). Throughout this process, inspect the skin, looking at hidden areas, such as behind the ears, or in the scalp. Is the skin clear, clean, and intact, or are there bruises, burns, or bite marks? Document any marks, noting the location, size, shape, induration, and age. Listen to breath sounds, and palpate the chest, abdomen, and extremities for any evidence of fracture or injury. Complete the physical exam with a neurological assessment of reflexes and cranial nerves. If assessment reveals suspected abuse or neglect, discuss concerns with the parents and intervene on behalf of the child by reporting to CPS (Christian & Committee on Child Abuse and Neglect, 2015).

■ REPORTING

The primary goal of reporting is to ensure safety and prevent further injury or neglect to the child. Also, calling CPS might actually help the family receive additional supports (Christian & Committee on Child Abuse and Neglect, 2015; Fisher-Owens et al., 2017). P-PCPs should know the telephone number for reporting to CPS and be familiar with the child abuse experts in their area who are available for consultation. However, even though a child may be referred to a specialist or ED, the P-PCP is still responsible for reporting their suspected concerns to CPS (Christian & Committee on Child Abuse and Neglect, 2015).

Reporting can be made anonymously, and information reported to CPS is kept confidential. However, sharing your name, address, and telephone number is preferable since it will allow CPS to follow up with you as they investigate allegations should additional information be needed. A P-PCP should be prepared to provide CPS with as much information as possible. CPS will ask for the P-PCP's name, if they are willing to share; the child's and parents' names, ages, and address; if known the name of the person who is inflicting the abuse or neglect and what their relationship is to the child; the P-PCP's concerns; and the type of abuse or neglect the P-PCP is reporting. Furthermore, if the P-PCP is reporting an injury, CPS will ask if it is current and are there previous injuries, and when does the P-PCP think the abuse occurred and where it happened. Last, CPS will ask where is the child now, at home or the ED; what is the urgency of the call; and is the child in imminent danger?

Involvement with and investigations by CPS is stressful for families, and suspecting that a child has been abused or neglected is disturbing for P-PCPs. Reporting can disrupt the relationship between the P-PCP and the family. The P-PCP's discussion with parents about their concerns will be difficult, but being transparent and explaining the P-PCP's mandatory responsibility by law to report might ease that tension. Some families might leave the practice, but the P-PCP can help those who stay through cooperation with CPS during the investigation and advocating for support services for the family (Christian & Committee on Child Abuse and Neglect, 2015; Fisher-Owens et al., 2017; Jenny et al., 2013).

■ PREVENTION

Families look to their P-PCP for care and advice about the health of their children. The P-PCP can aid in prevention of child maltreatment during each encounter with a family through a comprehensive assessment of the family's strengths and needs (Christian & Committee on Child Abuse and Neglect, 2015). This assessment requires the P-PCP to ask families to complete screening tools and to review the findings. Are the parents struggling with finances, substance use, or their own physical and mental health? Is the youth encountering bullying? Does the P-PCP suspect human trafficking? If the P-PCP does not ask, they will not know. With knowledge of family needs, the P-PCP can promote health through anticipatory guidance and offer community supports for families.

■ SUMMARY

Children are vulnerable to maltreatment, which has long-term consequences for their health and well-being (Lanier et al., 2010). Through a comprehensive assessment of child and family strengths and needs, the P-PCP can play a role in intercepting the adverse effects of abuse and neglect. The P-PCP's routine screening for abuse and neglect, interventions, and advocacy will contribute to ensuring that children will grow up and thrive in a safe, nurturing environment.

■ REFERENCES

Annie E. Casey Foundation. (2017). *Kids count data book*. Baltimore, MD. Retrieved from http://www. aecf.org/resources/2017-kids-count-data-book/

Campbell, K. A., Myrup, T., & Svedin, L. (2017). Parsing language and measures around child maltreatment. *Pediatrics, 139*(1), e20163475. doi:10.1542/peds.2016-3475

Christian, C. W., & Committee on Child Abuse and Neglect. (2015). The evaluation of suspected child abuse. *Pediatrics*, *135*(5), e1337–e1354. doi:10.1542/peds.2015-0356

Connell, C. M., Bergeron, N., Katz, K. H., Saunders, L., & Tebes, J. K. (2007). Re-referral to child protective services: The influence of child, family, and case characteristics on risk status. *Child Abuse and Neglect*, *31*(5), 573–588. doi:10.1016/j.chiabu.2006.12.004

Egan, M., Tannahill, C., Petticrew, M., & Thomas, S. (2008). Psychosocial risk factors in home and community settings and their associations with population health and health inequalities: A systematic meta-review. *BMC Public Health*, *8*, 239. doi:10.1186/1471-2458-8-239

Felitti, V. J., & Anda, R. (2009). The relationship of adverse childhood experiences to adult medical disease, psychiatric disorders, and sexual behavior: Implications for healthcare. In R. Lanius, E. Vermetten, & C. Pain (Eds.), *The hidden epidemic: The impact of early life trauma on health and disease*. Retrieved from http://www.acestudy.org/yahoo_site_admin/assets/docs/LaniusVermetten_FINAL_8-26-09.12892303.pdf

Felitti, V. J., Anda, R. F., Nordenberg, D., Williamson, D. F., Spitz, A. M., Edwards, V., . . . Marks, J. S. (1998). Relationship of childhood abuse and household dysfunction to many of the leading causes of death in adults. The Adverse Childhood Experiences (ACE) Study. *American Journal of Preventive Medicine*, *14*(4), 245–258. doi:10.1016/S0749-3797(98)00017-8

Fisher-Owens, S. A., Lukefahr, J. L., Tate, A. R., American Academy of Pediatrics, Section on Oral Health, Committee on Child Abuse and Neglect, American Academy of Pediatric Dentistry, Council on Clinical Affairs, Council on Scientific Affairs, & Ad Hoc Work Group on Child Abuse and Neglect. (2017). Oral and dental aspects of child abuse and neglect. *Pediatrics*, e20171487. doi:10.1542/peds.2017-1487

Fortson, B. L., Klevens, J., Merrick, M. T., Gilbert, L. K., & Alexander, S. P. (2016). *Preventing child abuse and neglect: A technical package for policy, norm, and programmatic activities*. Retrieved from National Center for Injury Prevention and Control, Centers for Disease Control and Prevention; https://www.cdc.gov/violenceprevention/pdf/CAN-Prevention-Technical-Package.pdf doi:10.15620/cdc.38864

Gelles, R. J. (2009). Violence, abuse, and neglect in families and intimate relationships. In S. J. Price, C. A. Price & McKenry (Eds), *Families and change: Coping with stressful events and transitions* (pp. 119–139). Thousand Oaks, CA: Sage Publications.

Hagan, H. F., Shaw, J. S., & Duncan, P. M. (2017). *Bright futures: Guidelines for health supervision of infants, children and adolescents* (4th ed.). Elk Grove Village, IL: American Academy of Pediatrics.

Jenny, C., Crawford-Jakubiak, J., & Committee on Child Abuse and Neglect. (2013). The evaluation of children in the primary care setting when sexual abuse is suspected. *Pediatrics*, *132*(2), e558–e567. doi:10.1542/peds.2013-1741

Lanier, P., Jonson-Reid, M., Stahlschmidt, M. J., Drake, B., & Constantino, J. (2010). Child maltreatment and pediatric health outcomes: A longitudinal study of low-income children. *Journal of Pediatric Psychology*, *35*(5), 511–522. doi:10.1093/jpepsy/jsp086

Leeb, R. T., Paulozzi, L., Melanson, C., Simon, T., & Arias, I. (2008). *Child maltreatment surveillance: Uniform definitions for public health and recommended data elements, version 1.0*. Retrieved from Centers for Disease Control and Prevention, National Center for Injury Prevention and Control; http://www.cdc.gov/violenceprevention/pdf/CM_Surveillance-a.pdf

McCoy, M. L., & Keen, S. M. (2009). Risk factors for child maltreatment. In M. L. McCoy & S. M. Keen, *Abuse and neglect* (pp. 19–30). Philadelphia, PA: Taylor and Francis Group, LLC.

National Scientific Council on the Developing Child. (2007). *The science of early childhood development*. Retrieved from http://www.developingchild.net

Szilagyi, M. (2012). The pediatric role in the care of children in foster and kinship care. *Pediatrics in Review*, *33*(11), 496–508. doi:10.1542/pir.33-11-496

Taylor, J. Y., Washington, O. G., Artinian, N. T., & Lichtenberg, P. (2007). Parental stress among African American parents and grandparents. *Issues in Mental Health Nursing*, *28*(4), 373–387. doi:10.1080/01612840701244466

U.S. Congress. (1974). *Child abuse prevention and treatment Act: Public law 93-247: S. 1191*. Retrieved from http://www.gpo.gov/fdsys/pkg/STATUTE-88/pdf/STATUTE-88-Pg4.pdf

U.S. Department of Health & Human Services, Administration for Children and Families, Administration on Children, Youth and Families, & Children's Bureau. (2016). *Child abuse prevention and treatment Act: As amended by P.L. 114-22 and P.L. 114-198*. Retrieved from https://www.acf.hhs.gov/sites/default/files/cb/capta2016.pdf

U.S. Department of Health & Human Services, Administration for Children and Families, Administration on Children, Youth and Families, & Children's Bureau. (2017). *Child maltreatment 2015*. Retrieved from https://www.acf.hhs.gov/sites/default/files/cb/cm2015.pdf

Widom, C., Czaja, S., Bentley, T., & Johnson, M. (2012). A prospective investigation of physical health outcomes in abused and neglected children: New findings from a 30-year follow-up. *American Journal of Public Health*, *102*(6), 1135–1144. doi:10.2105/AJPH.2011.300636

World Health Organization and International Society for Prevention of Child Abuse and Neglect. (2006). *Preventing child maltreatment: A guide to taking action and generating evidence.* Retrieved from http://whqlibdoc.who.int/publications/2006/9241594365_eng.pdf

Zimmerman, F., & Mercy, J. A. (2010). A better start: Child maltreatment prevention as a public health priority. *Zero to Three.* Retrieved from http://www.zerotothree.org/maltreatment/child-abuse-neglect/30-5-zimmerman.pd

CHAPTER 31

Foster Care Children: Intercepting Behavioral Health Issues

MARY WEGLARZ, EILEEN CORCORAN, DEBORAH GUTTER, AND NINA B. COLABELLI

The health and well-being of children, particularly vulnerable children, is one of the major national health priorities identified in Healthy People 2020 (U.S. Department of Health & Human Services [DHHS], 2013). Children within the child welfare systems represent a significant population of concern. Pediatric primary care providers (P-PCPs) who are educated to screen, assess, diagnose, and treat children are also mandated to report evidence of child maltreatment, neglect, and abuse. Abuse and neglect of any child by a parent, caregiver, guardian, or any adult who interacts with the child (i.e., school personnel, religious affiliations, sport coaches), whose actions may result in an injury or death, is maltreatment. Intentional acts of maltreatment can impact the surviving child's emotional, behavioral, and mental health throughout their life span (Leeb, Paulozzi, Melanson, Simon, & Arias, 2008). Children who are placed within the foster care system most often have experienced one or more of the following: abuse, neglect, maltreatment, and exposure to dysfunctional family life, including drugs, alcohol, domestic violence, and/or a parent remanded to jail. This chapter describes the current best available evidence for care of children in foster care, including the initial comprehensive physical and behavioral health assessments, screenings, and treatment plans, with a goal of identifying and *intercepting* permanent emotional trauma from the adverse effects from prior life experiences.

■ FOSTER CARE: THE MOST VULNERABLE CHILDREN

The most recent child health statistical data revealed more than 3 million children are investigated for reports of abuse and neglect annually, with approximately 700,000 of these children substantiated for maltreatment (Department of Health & Human Services [DHHS], 2014, 2015). More than 75% of the cases substantiated for maltreatment are classified as neglect, with an additional 17% substantiated as physical abuse, and 8% as sexual abuse (DHHS, 2014). Furthermore, these data showed that maltreated children have higher rates of physical, mental, and developmental conditions that are undetected, undertreated, and chronic in nature, often due to the multiple negative social determinants of health factors impacting their daily lives (American Academy of Pediatrics [AAP], 2005).

Considerable numbers of children move through the child welfare system spending significant time during their childhood in foster care until it has been determined that they can safely return home or are ready for adoption. According to state child welfare annual agency reports submitted to the Adoption and Foster Care Analysis and Reporting Systems (AFCARS), over 400,000 of those 700,000 children whose caregivers were substantiated for abuse and neglect are living in foster care, with 269,000 entering and 243,000 exiting foster care (DHHS, 2014). Half of the children leaving care were reunited with their primary caregiver (DHHS, 2015).

■ TEAM-BASED CARE TO IMPROVE OUTCOMES

Children enter the foster care system with a plethora of physical, emotional, behavioral, and mental health diagnoses, comorbidities, and complications (Simms, Dubowitz, & Szilagyi, 2000; Stahmer et al., 2005; Steele & Buchi, 2008; Sullivan & van Zyl, 2008; Szilagyi, 2012). Placement in foster care occurs most often as an abrupt separation of children from their parents or relatives and their home that elicits significant stress and fear by the children, despite unsafe factors in their home environment, and may further impair their coping skills, attachment behaviors, ability to develop their identity, and as an adolescent/young adult, to achieve their independence (Kools & Kennedy, 2003).

The Child Welfare League of America (CWLA) and the American Academy of Pediatrics (AAP) recommend a coordinated system of healthcare management to monitor services children receive while in foster care to promote optimal health and well-being (AAP, 2005; Child Welfare League of America [CWLA], 2007). A comprehensive, trauma-informed, team-based approach to healthcare management is essential to meet the children's primary healthcare needs. The healthcare team includes caseworkers, psychologists, foster parents, and community service providers, child advocates and/or legal guardians, nursing case managers,and primary and specialty care providers. The biological parents should be included as part of the child's health team; however, the parents often require comprehensive services to be better prepared to understand the complexities of maltreatment, neglect, or other parental adverse behaviors, such as drug or alcohol use or criminal behaviors, to correct their behaviors and prepare to safely care for their children. Open communication and collaboration is essential for the success of the healthcare team to achieve the outcome goal of optimal physical, emotional, and behavioral health for the children.

■ HEALTHCARE VISITS

Foster children should receive preventative pediatric healthcare visits according to the AAP periodicity schedule (American Academy of Pediatrics [AAP], 2017), as well as additional visits are recommended to assess a child prior to placement and at a greater frequency (Table 31.1). Goals for initial, maintenance, and follow-up healthcare visits include: (a) identify medical, behavioral, emotional, developmental, and educational problems; (b) intercept identified problems through screening and implementation of evidence-based guidelines; (c) assess adjustment to foster home and monitor for abuse and neglect; (d) support child and foster parents; and (e) promote health and well-being of the children (AAP, 2005; Szilagyi, Rosen, Rubin, & Zlotnik, 2015).

■ PLACEMENT EXAMINATIONS

An assessment by a P-PCP is recommended prior to placing a child into foster care. The examination includes a detailed history (if family members are present), review of systems (ROS; Table 31.2), physical, behavioral, and mental health assessments and identification of issues that require immediate medical or emergent attention (AAP, 2005; Szilagyi et al., 2015). A team-based approach to care assures that the results of these assessments are shared with the caseworker to ensure the child's safety and well-being and the foster parent's ability to meet the child's specific needs.

■ THE COMPLEXITY OF THE COMPREHENSIVE EXAMINATION

A child's medical and mental health diagnoses upon entry into foster care are often unknown. Most often children enter the foster care system with little or no details

TABLE 31.1

AAP WELL-CHILD PERIODICITY VISITS COMPARED TO VISITS FOR CHILDREN IN FOSTER CARE

Age	Varies from AAP	Frequency	Periodicity Schedule
Birth to 6 months	Yes	1, 2, 4, 6 months	Monthly visits
9 months to 12 months	No	9 and 12 months	9 and 12 months
15 to 24 months	Yes	15, 18, 24 months	21 months
Over 24 months	Yes	Annual	Every 6 months
Behavioral health problems	Yes	Not on table	Every 1 to 2 months until stable, then every 6 months

AAP, American Academy of Pediatrics.

TABLE 31.2

CRITICAL QUESTIONS TO ADD TO THE STANDARD ROS FOR FOSTER CARE CHILDREN

System	Critical Questions
General	Inconsistent growth measurements, unusual dietary patterns, overall activity level, sleep disturbance, medications
Skin and lymph	Bruises, lesions, itching, uneven skin tone or texture, rashes in unusual locations or at unusual ages, bites, scars
Hair and nails	Abnormal hair growth or loss, absence or change in nail structure
Head	Abnormal shape and/or size
Eyes	Loss of vision, swelling of eyes, squinting, glasses
Ears	Loss of hearing, discharge from ear, swelling of ear, pain, hearing aids
Nose and sinuses	Difficulty with nasal breathing, nasal deformity, nosebleeds, nasal discharge, pain, snoring, misshapen nose, allergies
Mouth and throat	Dental issues—loss of teeth, caries, fluoride, sealants, braces Odor, difficulty swallowing, oral cavity injuries
Cardiac	Previous murmur, chest pain, abnormal anatomy, cyanosis, racing heart
Respiratory	Flu vaccine status, tuberculosis screening, choking, wheezing, cough, trouble breathing
Gastrointestinal	Dietary restrictions, appetite, weight change, abdominal pain, nausea, vomiting, diarrhea, constipation, encopresis, stool smearing
Urinary	Toilet habits, enuresis
Hematology	Lead exposure, iron deficiency anemia, sickle cell anemia, exposure to HIV, hepatitis B or C exposure, hemophilia, thalassemia
Reproductive	Age-appropriate knowledge level
Female	Menstrual difficulties, onset, discomfort, discharge, LMP, pregnancies, terminations
Male	Puberty onset, discharge, discomfort, undescended testicles, swelling of testicles, emissions, erections
Both	Tanner stages, sexual activity—with whom, protection, sexually transmitted infections
Musculoskeletal	Abnormal gait, weakness, clumsiness, swelling of joints, fractures
Neurologic	Head injury, seizures, learning problems, attention span, school grade level, school supports
Endocrine	Skin, hair, voice changes, cold/heat intolerance

LMP, last menstrual period; ROS, review of systems.

about their past medical history, behavioral health history, and/or current state of health including immunization records and screening test results. To understand the complexity of the health status of vulnerable children entering the foster care system, case workers, social workers, nurse case manager, P-PCPs, child and adolescent psychologists, and psychiatrists use team-based efforts to capture the presenting health status of the child by obtaining and analyzing the birth history, medical, behavioral health, laboratory test results, immunization, and educational records. The biological parents may provide important information to develop the diagnoses and treatment plans, but often the biological parents are either not available or resistant to participation. A comprehensive medical examination is completed for each child (Table 31.3). An analysis of the results from the comprehensive physical examination and diagnostic testing builds the foundation for both medical and behavioral diagnoses and treatment plans.

■ THE COMPLEXITY OF THE BEHAVIORAL HEALTH EXAMINATION

Children who enter foster care have been exposed to adverse conditions prior to removal (Szilagyi et al., 2015). The degree, length of exposure, and developmental age can have a significant impact on a child's health (see Chapter 32). The importance of identifying exposures to alcohol and illicit substances, domestic violence, homelessness, poverty, and caregivers with chronic physical and mental health disorders cannot be understated. Very young children can present with developmental delays in the areas of language development, social and adaptive skills, and fine motor development. As children age in the foster care system, the impact of adverse childhood experiences upon health begins to emerge (Deutsch et al., 2015).

Screening for Behavioral Health Problems

Foster parents and verbal children often report changes in sleep patterns, diet, toileting, and behavior related to separation from family. Screening with developmentally appropriate tools for impact on behavioral and mental health of the child at the time of admission is critical to generating differential diagnosis and determining strategies to correct presenting behavioral problems and intercept adverse behavioral outcomes. Screening tools and resources, which may assist in diagnosis and treatment planning, are in Table 31.4 (AAP, 2014a, 2014b, 2014c; American Academy of Pediatrics and American Academy of Pediatric Dentistry, 1999; Baker & Donahue, 2016; Centers for Disease Control and Prevention [CDC], 2017; Perrin, Sheldrick, Visco, & Mattern, 2016).

Complexities of Diagnosing Foster Care Children

Children involved in the foster care system have a greater incidence of chronic illnesses, developmental delays, mental illness, and comorbidities when compared with their peers. Common illnesses among foster care children include respiratory infections, asthma, developmental disorders, dental infections, fever of unknown origin, allergic reactions, viral infections, gastrointestinal

TABLE 31.3

COMPREHENSIVE PHYSICAL EXAMINATION

Schedule within 30 to 60 days of placement: preferably the first week
Conduct a diligent search for previous healthcare providers and/or birth records to obtain the following histories:
  Past medical history
  Medical and surgical
  Hospitalization
  Abuse, neglect, maltreatment
  Dental care
  Medications, past and present
  Immunization
  Social and developmental history
  Family history

  Additional history the child may provide (age dependent):
    Allergies to medications, foods, environment
    Nutrition
    Usual elimination patterns
    Behavioral patterns
    School history

Screen for physical, emotional, and behavioral health problems: hearing and vision; height; weight; growth velocity; vital signs

Perform an initial comprehensive physical examination

Diagnostic testing: routine blood work (age and history dependent): urinalysis; TB testing; additional blood work based on history and presentation and if the child is or will be placed on psychotropic medications: anemia panel; chemistry panel, including lipid screen; thyroid function studies and thyroid stimulating hormone; lead level (age dependent)

TB, tuberculosis.

Sources: American Academy of Pediatrics. (2005). *Fostering health: Health care for children and adolescents in foster care* (2nd ed.). New York, NY: Task Force on Health Care of Children in Foster Care; Szilagyi, M., Rosen, D., Rubin, D., & Zlotnik, S. (2015) Health care issues for children and adolescents in foster care and kinship care. *Pediatrics, 136*(4), e1142–e1166.

disorders, nutritional and endocrine disorders, eye disorders, and superficial injuries (Center for Mental Health Services and Center for Substance Abuse Treatment, Substance Abuse and Mental Health Services Administration [CMHS, SAMHSA], 2013).

Comorbid mental health diagnoses include attention deficit hyperactivity disorder (ADHD), conduct disorder (CD) and oppositional defiant disorder (ODD), adjustment disorder, anxiety and mood disorders, and substance related disorders (CMHS, SAMHSA, 2013). Children in foster care are diagnosed with anxiety, behavioral problems, and depression at a rate at least five times greater than children who reside with their families (Turney & Wildeman, 2016). However, many behavioral health issues are often misdiagnosed in foster care children since the examiner may not have considered the adverse events the children experienced prior to placement. Behaviors that are responsive to trauma and placement require appropriate interventions prior to making a diagnosis of a behavioral or

TABLE 31.4

SCREENING TOOLS FOR PHYSICAL AND BEHAVIORAL HEALTH ASSESSMENTS

Area of Focus	Tool	Website
General	Height, weight, head circumference, BMI, blood pressure, lead level, anemia, dyslipidemia, HIV	https://www.aap.org/en-us/Documents/periodicity_schedule.pdf
Development	AAP recommendation	https://www.cdc.gov/ncbddd/childdevelopment/documents/screening-chart.pdf
	Ages and Stages Questionnaires (ASQ)–3, ASQ Social and Emotional Questionnaires	http://www.brookespublishing.com/resource-center/screening-and-assessment/asq
	Learn the Signs. Act Early	https://www.cdc.gov/ncbddd/actearly/milestones/index.html
Mental Health	The Survey of Well-being of Young Children (SWYC) tools, age specific	https://sites.google.com/site/swyc2016/Age-Specific-Forms
	ADHD—Vanderbilt Assessment	http://www.chadd.org/Understanding-ADHD/For-Professionals/For-Healthcare-Professionals/Clinical-Practice-Tools/Evaluation-and-Assessment-Tools.aspx
	Pediatric Symptom Checklist	https://www.brightfutures.org/mentalhealth/pdf/professionals/ped_sympton_chklst.pdf
Immunizations	Recommended and Catch Up Immunization Schedule for Children and Adolescents	https://www.cdc.gov/vaccines/schedules/index.html
Hearing	Audiometer	https://www.cdc.gov/ncbddd/hearingloss/recommendations.html
Vision	Optotypes, Critical Line Screening, Snellen Chart	http://pediatrics.aappublications.org/content/pediatrics/early/2015/12/07/peds.2015-3597.full.pdf
Dental	Oral health risk assessment tool, pediatric oral and dental abuse and neglect screen	http://www2.aap.org/oralhealth/RiskAssessmentTool.html http://pediatrics.aappublications.org/content/pediatrics/104/2/348.full.pdf

ADHD, attention deficit hyperactivity disorder.

mental health disorder (Chasnoff, Wells, & King, 2015). Collaboration and communication among the entire healthcare team is critical for accurate diagnosis and development of an appropriate healthcare plan.

■ HEALTH PLAN

A foster child's health plan is child and family centered. Begin the plan by addressing immediate healthcare concerns such as delayed immunizations, current infections, and injuries. Continue to develop the plan to meet all of the child's health needs. Components of the behavioral health plan include referrals, education, advocacy, follow-up/reassessment, and transition planning.

Behavioral Health Plan

Each child entering the foster care system should have an assessment to determine his or her current behavioral health status and to establish a behavioral health plan. Interventions may be emergently required, with an immediate referral to a behavioral health specialist, or if nonemergent may be planned after the foster parent and child have had time for interactions to better describe the child's behavioral health needs. Behavioral health assessments and screenings have been described in each of the opening chapters for the specific development age of the child (see also Table 31.4).

Based on the screening results for each foster care child, specific behavioral health interventions should be planned. The goal is to provide careful and gentle guidance for the child within a family-centered home supported by interactions among the child, the foster family, and health professional team to enable the child to adjust and normalize his or her behavioral health status. For example, a child who steals may have lived in a home where stealing was the norm for survival. Recognition of the stealing behavior along with assurance that the child's needs will be met may then alter the course of stealing behaviors. If a child steals because he/she is hungry, then assuring that there is food in the foster home that the child likes to eat and the child has funds to purchase food at school may put an end to the behavior. Critical to intercepting the cycle of stealing is to help the child understand the behavior and become engaged in ways to change the stealing behaviors. If the stealing behaviors do not respond to such guidance, the child should be referred for individual counseling with a member of the healthcare team.

■ REFERRALS

Referrals to specialists for treatment and community support services are routine for children in foster care. The chronic illnesses and behavioral health problems that cannot be managed within primary care and the usual lack of care prior to foster placement require collaboration with specialists and timely appointments. A referral to a psychiatrist and/or an in-home therapist for a foster care child with ADHD and comorbid behavioral problems will secure treatment for symptoms before further decline. A child's escalating behaviors without professional interventions cause difficulties in the foster home and can lead to a failed placement.

■ P-PCPs: LEADING THE HEALTHCARE TEAM

The P-PCPs lead the healthcare team providing guidance and education to all team members including anticipatory guidance. The caseworker and foster parent share a responsibility for the child and must understand all of the child's needs and how to assist the child dealing with illness, separation from family and friends, and the unknown. Empowering the caregiver to advocate for the child's needs and best interests will contribute to better healthcare outcomes. Encourage engagement of the children for their own care to build resiliency skills and a knowledge base for their own personal physical, emotional, and behavioral health.

For example, an adolescent who is truant and ignores foster home curfew hours should be evaluated for the cause of the behavior. Often, lack of general house rules and lack of concern from the biological parents have contributed to these behaviors. Another consideration is whether the adolescent is using drugs or alcohol and/or has feelings of depression, or the demands of the educational system may be frustrating to the child. Screening for depression (PHQ-2, PHQ-4, and PHQ-9) and alcohol and drug use (CRAFFT Tool) and a school educational evaluation are the essential steps toward problem identification, followed by accurate diagnosis, and *interception* of the problem by implementation of evidence-based plans of care.

■ ADVOCACY

As a member of the child's team, the P-PCP advocates across systems for the child. Timely appointments with specialists and behavioral/mental health and developmental evaluations are needed for all foster care children. In-home support services help maintain placement; however, they require advocacy with insurance companies or child welfare if not covered through insurance. Encouraging consistency in team leadership is accomplished when the P-PCP and case worker maintain their roles, rather than transferring care to another provider. The case worker is responsible to working with the child and family to have the first foster placement be the only placement. Additionally, the child should be placed in their own community for day care or school, which promotes the child's feeling of security (Lockwood, Friedman, & Christian, 2015; Table 31.5).

■ FOLLOW-UP REASSESSMENT

Planning for the unexpected is one of the basic components of caring for children in foster care. Numerous factors can lead to poor follow-up of physical and behavioral healthcare. Unanticipated cancellations, changes in placement location, or caseworker assignment may lead to delay or missed care. Additionally, gaps in insurance, lack of specialized services, appointment availability,

TABLE 31.5

RESOURCES FOR MANAGEMENT OF CHILDREN IN FOSTER CARE

Administration for Children and Families: https://www.acf.hhs.gov
American Academy of Pediatrics: www.aap.org/fostercare
American Academy of Pediatrics: https://www.aap.org/en-us/advocacy-and-policy/aap-health-initiatives/healthy-foster-care-america/Pages/Primary-Care-Tools.aspx
American Academy of Pediatrics: https://www.aap.org/en-us/advocacy-and-policy/aap-health-initiatives/healthy-foster-care-america/Pages/default.aspx
Child Welfare Information Gateway: https://www.childwelfare.gov
Child Welfare League of America: www.cwla.org
National Association of Pediatric Nurse Practitioners: https://www.napnap.org
Substance Abuse and Mental Health Service Administration: https://www.samhsa.gov
The National Child Traumatic Stress Network: www.nctsn.org

caregiver schedules, problems with transportation, or lack of knowledge impact follow-up care. Early identification of any of these possible issues is beneficial in the reassessment process and maintains continuity of care. The healthcare team is responsible for the health outcomes of every foster care child, and the P-PCP team leader is accountable for implementing plans to help overcome all obstacles.

Reassessment for the foster child is needed to monitor the adjustment to the foster home, to assess his or her interactions with the foster parent, and to monitor responses to treatment. Any concerns about the care provided by the foster parent are communicated to the caseworker. Measurement of the child's growth parameters can alert the nurse practitioner to a poor adjustment to foster care, responses to treatment for chronic healthcare conditions, or a side effect of a psychotropic medication. Planned repeat screenings for depression and all behavioral health problems must be the standard of care for all foster care children to identify as early as possible the behavioral health problems and plan strategies to intercept the problems.

The P-PCP refers foster children to psychiatrists or psychiatric advanced practice nurses for evaluation and treatment of possible mental illnesses that are beyond the scope of the P-PCP (Pediatric Nursing Certification Board [PNCB], 2017). The P-PCP collaborates by sharing pertinent exam findings, including growth parameters, metabolic monitoring, and reported behavioral changes. A thorough follow-up and reassessment by the P-PCP will open avenues of advocacy for the child. Input from the entire team—caseworker, P-PCP, therapist, specialists, psychiatrist, psychiatric advanced practice nurse—will lead to an accurate diagnosis and treatment plan for the behavioral/mental health needs of the child in foster care.

■ TRANSITION PLANNING

Foster children encounter multiple transitions. These occur when a child enters care, moves foster placements, visits with biological parents, and approaches reunification with family, adoption, or aging out of foster care. The nurse practitioner can ease these transitions through education and collaboration. Foster parents must understand how to care for the children in their home; biological parents need preparation to care for their child upon reunification; and youth aging out of foster care must work with the case worker to establish community connections.

Evidence-based knowledge and P-PCP clinical skills guide the physical and behavioral health plan. Communication and collaboration among the child's healthcare team are key to a successful health plan. Becoming familiar with the available resources will assist the P-PCP with an understanding of the child welfare system and ways to partner to improve the healthcare outcomes for foster care children.

■ PREVENTING FOSTER CARE PLACEMENT

So how can we prevent foster care placement? At every healthcare visit for all children, PCPs must assess family dynamics and identify family issues that signal a child is at risk for foster care placement. Questions that may lead to intercepting the issues before they escalate are difficult to ask but essential for the health and well-being of the child. Questions about food and housing insecurity, family supports, substance use, domestic violence, and mental illness should be included in all healthcare assessments. Assessments using valid and reliable screening tools are the standard for practice. Screenings promote early identification of these concerns and connection for the families with community support services may identify behavioral health problems for the entire family and help prevent disruption of the family unit. P-PCPs play a critical role in preventing foster care placement.

■ SUMMARY

Foster children deserve comprehensive trauma-informed care from P-PCPs (refer to Chapter 33). Understanding the special needs of this vulnerable population, their behavioral health problems, strategies to intercept and intervene to treat behavioral health problems, the benefits of collaborative team-based care, and advocacy for the child and family will improve the children's experience in foster care and enable them to achieve their optimal state of physical and behavioral health. P-PCPs have a unique opportunity to lead team-based care efforts to provide high-quality primary, behavioral, and specialty care for foster care children.

■ REFERENCES

American Academy of Pediatrics. (2005). *Fostering health: Health care for children and adolescents in foster care* (2nd ed.). New York, NY: Task Force on Health Care of Children in Foster Care.

American Academy of Pediatrics. (2014a). Clinical report: Fluoride use in caries prevention in the primary care setting. *Pediatrics, 134,* 626–633. doi:10.1542/peds.2014-1699

American Academy of Pediatrics. (2014b). Clinical report: Management of dental trauma in a primary care setting. *Pediatrics, 133,* e466–e476. doi:10.1542/peds.2013-3792

American Academy of Pediatrics. (2014c). Policy statement: Maintaining and improving the oral health of young children. *Pediatrics, 134,* 1224–1229. doi:10.1542/peds.2014-2984

American Academy of Pediatrics. (2017). *Recommendations for preventive pediatric health care.* Retrieved from https://www.aap.org/en-us/Documents/periodicity_schedule.pdf

American Academy of Pediatrics and American Academy of Pediatric Dentistry. (1999). Joint statement: Oral and dental aspects of child abuse and neglect. *Pediatrics, 104*(2). Retrieved from http://pediatrics.aappublications.org/content/pediatrics/104/2/348.full.pdf

Baker, C. N., & Donahue, S. P. (2016). Procedures for the evaluation of the visual system by pediatricians. *Pediatrics, 137*(1). Retrieved from http://pediatrics.aappublications.org/content/pediatrics/early/2015/12/07/peds.2015-3597.full.pdf

Center for Mental Health Services and Center for Substance Abuse Treatment, Substance Abuse and Mental Health Services Administration. (2013). *Diagnoses and health care utilization of children who are in foster care and covered by Medicaid.* HHS Publication No. (SMA) 13-4804. Rockville, MD.

Centers for Disease Control and Prevention. (2017). *Immunization schedules.* Retrieved from https://www.cdc.gov/vaccines/schedules/hcp/imz/child-adolescent.html

Chasnoff, I. J., Wells, A.M., & King, L. (2015). Misdiagnosis and missed diagnoses in foster and adopted children with prenatal alcohol exposure. *Pediatrics, 135*(2), 264–270. doi:10.1542/peds.2014-2171

Child Welfare League of America. (2007). *Standards of excellence for health care services for children in out-of-home care.* Retrieved from http://www.cwla.org/programs/standards/cwsstandardshealthcare.htm

Deutsch, S. A., Lynch, A., Zlotnik, S., Matone, M., Kreider, A., & Noonan, K. (2015) Mental health, behavioral and developmental issues for youth in foster care. *Current Problems in Pediatric and Adolescent Health Care, 45*(10), 292–297. doi:10.1016/j.cppeds.2015.08.00

Kools, S., & Kennedy, C. (2003). Foster child health and development: Implications for primary care. *Pediatric nursing, 29*(1), 39–41, 44–36.

Leeb, R. T., Paulozzi, L., Melanson, C., Simon, T., & Arias, I. (2008). *Child maltreatment surveillance: Uniform definitions for public health and recommended data elements, version 1.0.* Retrieved from Centers for Disease Control and Prevention, National Center for Injury Prevention and Control; http://www.cdc.gov/violenceprevention/pdf/CM_Surveillance-a.pdf

Lockwood, K. K., Friedman, S., & Christian, C. W. (2015). Permanency and the foster care system. *Current Problems in Pediatric and Adolescent Health Care, 45,* (10), 306–315. doi:10.1016/j.cppeds.2015.08.005

Pediatric Nursing Certification Board. (2017). *The pediatric primary care mental health specialist: Role, settings and ethics.* Retrieved from https://pncb.org/pmhs-role?_ga=2.33672801.1309449709.1494530487-54572078.1494530053

Perrin, E.C., Sheldrick, C., Visco, Z., & Mattern, B. (2016). *User's manual: The survey of well-being of young children.* Retrieved from https://www.floatinghospital.org/-/media/Brochures/Floating%20Hospital/SWYC/SWYC%20Manual%20v101%20Web%20Format%2033016.ashx

Simms, M. D., Dubowitz, H., & Szilagyi, M. A. (2000). Health care needs of children in the foster care system. *Pediatrics, 106*(Supplement 3), 909–918.

Stahmer, A. C., Leslie, L. K., Hurlburt, M., Barth, R. P., Webb, M. B., Landsverk, J., & Zhang, J. (2005). Developmental and behavioral needs and service use for young children in child welfare. *Pediatrics, 116*(4), 891–900. doi:10.1542/peds.2004-2135

Steele, J. S., & Buchi, K. F. (2008). Medical and mental health of children entering the Utah foster care system. *Pediatrics, 122*(3), e703–e709. doi:10.1542/peds.2008-0360

Sullivan, D., & van Zyl, M. (2008). The well-being of children in foster care: Exploring physical and mental health needs. *Children and Youth Services Review, 30*(7), 774–786. doi:10.1016/j.childyouth.2007.12.005

Szilagyi, M. (2012). The pediatric role in the care of children in foster and kinship care. *Pediatrics in Review.* Retrieved from http://pedsinreview.aappulications.org/content/33/11/496 doi:10.1542/pir.33-11-496

Szilagyi, M., Rosen, D., Rubin, D., & Zlotnik, S. (2015) Health care issues for children and adolescents in foster care and kinship care. *Pediatrics, 136*(4), e1142–e1166. doi:10.1542/peds.2015-2656

Turney, K., & Wildeman, C. (2016). Mental and physical health of children in foster care. *Pediatrics, 138*(5). doi:10.1542/peds.2016-1118

U.S. Department of Health & Human Services. (2013). *Healthy people 2020*. Retrieved from https://www.healthypeople.gov/2020/About-Healthy-People

U.S. Department of Health & Human Services, Administration for Children and Families, Administration on Children, Youth and Families, & Children's Bureau, (2015). *Child maltreatment, 2015 report*. Retrieved from http://www.acf.hhs.gov/programs/cb/research-data-technology/statisticsresearch/child-maltreatment

U.S. Department of Health & Human Services, Administration for Children and Families, Administration on Children, Youth and Families, Children's Bureau, National Child Abuse and Neglect Data System, NCANDS Child File, FFY. (2014). *KIDS COUNT data center, Children who are confirmed by child protective services as victims of maltreatment by maltreatment type*. Retrieved from http://datacenter.kidscount.org/data/tables/6222-children-who-are-confirmed-by-child-protective-services-as-victims-of-maltreatment-by-maltreament-type

CHAPTER 32

Toxic Stress

HILLARY FAIRBANKS

A thorough understanding of toxic stress is a critical pathway for the diagnosis and treatment of behavioral and mental health conditions such as attention deficient hyperactivity disorder (ADHD), conduct disorder, and violent sociopathy as well as depression, anxiety, and substance use disorders. This chapter reviews research on toxic stress, available screening tools, and evidence-based approaches for intervention.

■ BACKGROUND: THE ADVERSE CHILDHOOD EXPERIENCE STUDY

In the 1980s, Dr. Vincent Felitti, then chief of Kaiser Permanente's Department of Preventive Medicine, conducted a program for adult obese patients (Stevens, 2012). The program attrition rate was approximately 50%, and many of the patients were losing weight at the time they left the program. This high attrition rate dramatically impacted Dr. Felitti's ability to positively intervene with this patient population, and the active weight loss at the time of last visit made the attrition more surprising. In his quest to understand this phenomenon, Dr. Felitti explored the medical records of the obese patients (weighing more than 300 pounds). The data showed that they had normal weight at birth and had appropriate weight gain patterns throughout childhood. Abnormal gains in weight occurred acutely at a later point in life and led to a persistent struggle with overweight and obesity. He then opted to interview patients who left the program. During the interview process, a disturbingly high prevalence of reported childhood sexual abuse was identified among the patients who had dropped out. This finding, a possible association between a traumatic event in childhood and the persistence of a problematic medical outcome, led to a more in-depth investigation that became the Adverse Childhood Experience (ACE) Study conducted from 1995 to 1997 in collaboration with Dr. Robert Anda, from the Centers for Disease Control and Prevention.

The original ACE study was conducted in two waves and surveyed over 17,000 Kaiser Permanente members via a health questionnaire that elicited information on history of abuse (i.e., physical, emotional, and sexual) and stressful household exposures (i.e., substance abuse, mental illness, mother treated violently, and household members with criminal behavior) as well as current quality of life markers (About the CDC–Kaiser ACE Study, n.d.; Felitti et al., 1998). The researchers then compared prevalence of ACEs (number of ACEs) with prevalence in morbidity rates for a wide range of physical and mental health outcomes. Overall, Felitti and Anda found a graded relationship between the number of ACEs and the prevalence of adverse health and social outcomes including substance use disorders, smoking, depression, suicidality, high-risk sexual activity, physical inactivity, obesity, cardiovascular disorders, cancer, chronic lung disease, skeletal fractures, and liver disease (Felitti et al., 1998). Subsequent research has both supported these findings and added to the body of knowledge on the ACE comorbid paradigm for physical, behavioral, and mental health problems.

■ TOXIC STRESS: A NEURODEVELOPMENTAL DISORDER

The term "toxic stress" is used to describe the phenomenon of prenatal and early childhood stressors causing permanent changes in the architecture of the developing brain (Garner et al., 2012; Shonkoff et al., 2012). Examples of toxic stressors include maternal depression, parental substance use, domestic/community violence, food scarcity, poverty, poor social connectedness, and a history of neglect or abuse. The impact of these stressors on the developing brain is a powerful, complex phenomenon.

The brain continues to grow and develop throughout the first 25 years of life. The period of most intense growth in both weight and complexity occur in the first 2 years of life, with total brain weight tripling by 5 years of life. During this time, there is significant myelination occurring as well as increases in the number of synapses created and the pruning of redundant neurons (Horner, 2015). Under optimal biological and environmental circumstances, these activities proceed in a healthy fashion supporting optimal neurological, cognitive, and emotional development. Under exposure to toxic stress, these processes are altered.

Exposure to toxic stress leads to an activation of the hypothalamic–pituitary–adrenocortical (HPA) axis as well as the sympathetic-adrenomedullary system (Shonkoff et al., 2012). Excitation of the HPA axis leads to increased release of corticotropin-releasing hormone (CRH) from the hypothalamus followed by the release of adrenocortropic hormone (ACTH) that stimulates the release of glucocorticoid (cortisol) from the adrenal gland. As the HPA axis incorporates a feedback loop, higher cortisol levels lead to periods of suppression and subsequent excessive secretion. In essence, cortisol levels become dysregulated. Periods of hypercortisolinemia excite the sympathetic system leading to the release of norepinephrine and epinephrine. Prolonged or repeated bathing of the brain and nervous system in these chemical mediators has been shown to cause permanent changes in brain architecture—a heightened response system similar to "fight or flight" that is engaged at even low levels of stress or uncertainty.

The structures of the brain that are most impacted include the amygdala, hippocampus, and prefrontal cortex as they have large amounts of glucocorticoid receptors (Shonkoff et al., 2012). The amygdala is a key player in the physiological stress response; it becomes hypertrophied as a result of glucocorticoid stimulation (Shonkoff et al., 2012). The hippocampus and prefrontal cortex are key players in executive function and emotional regulation; glucocorticoid stimulation leads to a loss of neurons and neuronal connections in these areas (Shonkoff et al., 2012). Another region of the brain affected is the ventral tegmental area of the nucleus accumbens. The dose-related exposure of this area of the brain to neurochemical mediators, as described, leads to changes in dopamine receptor activity and can permanently alter the reward system (Pechtel & Pizzagalli, 2011). This alteration predisposes the impacted individual toward high-risk behaviors and substance use. Overall, learning, memory, the reward system, and emotional regulation are all affected by toxic stress.

The charts (Figure 32.1) provide insights from the original ACE study into how dose-related exposures to toxic stress correlate with later behavioral and mental health conditions.

Cortisol also plays a major role in regulating the immune system and metabolic processes. When cortisol levels are erratic, there is a subsequent dysregulation in the inflammatory response as well as in glucose storage and metabolism (Slopen, McLaughlin, & Shonkoff, 2014). The higher prevalence of cardiovascular and metabolic disorders as well as autoimmune disorders, asthma, chronic obstructive pulmonary disease (COPD), diabetes, and cancer in individuals exposed to toxic stress may be partially explained by these pathophysiological mechanisms.

The alterations set in motion by toxic stress are epigenetic in nature—they imprint in the individual's DNA, changing how it is read and transcribed, and contributing to differential gene expression (Burke Harris, 2015). These epigenetic modifications begin as early as the prenatal period and continue through early childhood and throughout the life span (Burke Harris, 2015; Shonkoff et al., 2012). Further research is needed to determine the exact mechanism for these epigenetic modifications.

■ ECOBIODEVELOPMENTAL FRAMEWORK

Given scientific developments in the field of toxic stress, the American Academy of Pediatrics (AAP) identified the need for a new "pediatric paradigm to promote health and prevent disease" (Shonkoff et al., 2012, p. e238). The ecobiodevelopmental (EBD) framework was established to provide structure for this new paradigm. The EBD framework (see Shonkoff et al., 2012; http://pediatrics.aap-publications.org/content/129/1/e232) promotes an understanding of the constant interactions between the social and physical environment, physiological adaptation and disruption, and health and development (Shonkoff et al., 2012, p. e234). The EBD framework supports the hypothesis that these interactions begin prenatally and continue through infancy and childhood. Through this framework, it becomes more readily apparent how childhood adversity can contribute to lifelong

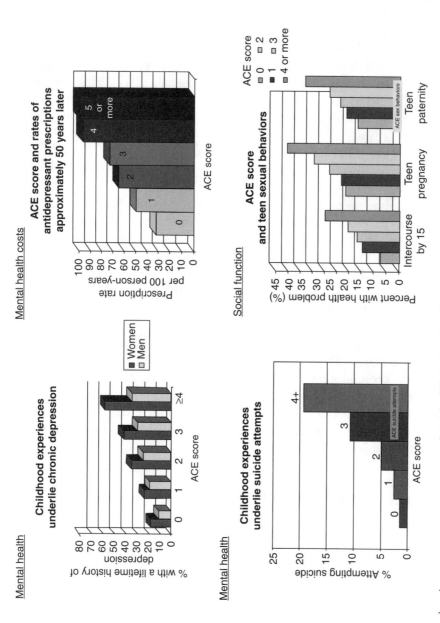

FIGURE 32.1 Toxic stress exposures as correlated with behavioral/mental health outcomes.

ACE, adverse childhood experience.

Source: Lanius, R. A., Vermetten, E., & Pain, C. (Eds.). (2010). *The Impact of early life trauma on health and disease: The hidden epidemic.* New York, NY: Cambridge University Press. © Cambridge University Press, 2010.

impairment. The EBD framework also states that it is the absence or insufficiency of protective relationships in the presence of significant adversity that leads to disruptive physiologic responses (Garner et al., 2012). Therefore, there is an imperative to screen for and identify toxic stressors as early as possible in order to support and enhance those protective relationships and intervene effectively to positively impact life course.

■ SCREENING FOR TOXIC STRESS

The AAP (American Academy of Pediatrics: The Resilience Project, n.d.) and Bright Futures (American Academy of Pediatrics [AAP], 2017) promote screening as a means to support providers in their efforts to effectively identify and care for children and adolescents exposed to toxic stress. The AAP provides a listing of suggested tools for reference and/or use; see Table 32.1. Two of the tools listed here will be explored in greater depth.

Many of the screening tools are designed for parents to complete in which questions are directed to elicit information about the parents' lives—history of ACEs, family patterns and behaviors, and parental resilience. One such tool is the SEEK PQ-R (Safe Environment for Every Kid Parent Questionnaire-R) developed by Dr. Howard Dubowitz with the University of Maryland School of Medicine. The SEEK PQ-R was designed to identify psychosocial challenges among parents that are associated with child maltreatment (child abuse and neglect). These challenges include parental depression, substance abuse, stress, intimate partner violence, utilization of harsh punishment, and food insecurity (Dubowitz, 2014). The tool was designed to be used in primary care with families with children aged birth to 5 years; suggested screening points include the 2-, 9-, and 15-month well-child visits and the 2-, 3-, 4-, and 5-year well-child visits (The SEEK Model, n.d.). The SEEK PQ-R is part of the SEEK model which includes training for primary care providers (PCPs) to support assessment and engagement as well as increase competency in addressing identified parental risk factors and problems (The SEEK Model, n.d.). Online provider training is available via the website www.seekwellbeing. com/the-seek-online-training-description.

There are fewer available tools designed to elicit information from the child or adolescent's point of view—to screen for child/adolescent adverse experiences and toxic exposures. One available set of tools is the Center for Youth Wellness Adverse Childhood Experiences Questionnaire (ACE-Q) developed by Dr. Nadine Burke Harris and the Center for Youth Wellness. These screening tools are accessible from the Center for Youth Wellness (CYW) website following a brief registration process (http://centerforyouthwellness.org/CYW-ACE-Q-and-User-Guide). The CYW is "part of a national effort to revolutionize pediatric medicine and transform the way society responds to kids exposed to significant ACEs and toxic stress." (About Us—Overview—Center for Youth Wellness, n.d.).

The difference in point of view can be seen when comparing questions eliciting similar risk factors, for example, "Has a partner threatened, shoved, hit or kicked you or hurt you physically in any way?" (SEEK PQ-R) versus asking if "your child

TABLE 32.1

AAP SUGGESTED SCREENING TOOLS FOR REFERENCE AND/OR USE

Screening Tool	Notes for Use in Practice	Link to Tool
ACEs Family Health History and Health Appraisal Questionnaire (original questionnaire used in the ACE study)	Parent completes the tool. Screens for parental ACEs and socio-behavioral factors.	https://www.cdc.gov/violenceprevention/acestudy/pdf/fhhflorna.pdf
The Parental ACEs Screening Tool	Parent completes the tool. Screens for parental ACEs; also includes a parental resilience questionnaire.	https://www.aap.org/en-us/Documents/resilience_ace_screening_parents.pdf
Resilience Questionnaire	Parent completes the tool. Screens for parental resilience.	https://www.aap.org/en-us/_layouts/15/WopiFrame.aspx?sourcedoc=/en-us/Documents/RESILIENCE_Questionnaire-1.docx&action=default
Parental Questionnaire: A Safe Environment for Every Kid (SEEK PQ-R)	Parent completes the tool. Screens for current parental risk factors that can impact parenting.	http://www.seekwellbeing.com/the-seek-parent-questionnaire-
The Pediatric Intake Form (also known as the Family Psychosocial Screening Form)	Parent completes the tool. Broader psychosocial screening tool. Screens for family history, functioning, and concerns. Screens parental risk factors that impact parenting, parental history of abuse, and social supports.	https://www.brightfutures.org/mentalhealth/pdf/professionals/ped_intake_form.pdf
The Child Stress Disorders Checklist	Parent completes the tool. Screens for exposure of the child/adolescent to frightening or traumatic events as well as related feelings and behaviors.	http://www.nctsnet.org/nctsn_assets/acp/hospital/CSDC.pdf
Center for Youth Wellness Adverse Childhood Experiences Questionnaire (ACE-Q)	Parent completes the tool. Adolescent completes his or her own tool. Screens for child/adolescent's exposures to toxic stressors.	http://centerforyouthwellness.org/CYW-ACE-Q-and-User-Guide

AAP, American Academy of Pediatrics; ACEs, adverse childhood experiences.

Source: https://www.aap.org/en-us/advocacy-and-policy/aap-health-initiatives/resilience/Pages/Clinical-Assessment-Tools.aspx; American Academy of Pediatrics: The Resilience Project. (n.d.). *Clinical assessment tools.* Retrieved from https://www.aap.org/en-us/advocacy-and-policy/aap-health-initiatives/resilience/Pages/Clinical-Assessment-Tools.aspx. Additional tools can be found on the National Child Traumatic Stress Network website (http://www.nctsnet.org/content/identifying-and-providing-services-young-children-who-have-been-exposed-trauma-professionals).

saw or heard household members hurt or threaten to hurt each other?" (CYW ACE-Q Child and Teen). In the first, the focus is placed on the parent's experience which results in the child or adolescent's exposure. In the second, the focus is placed on the child or adolescent's experience and is not specific to the parent.

Burke Harris, pediatrician and founder of CYW, recommends screenings be administered without having the children or parents identify which specific ACE they experienced, simply the total number of ACEs experienced (Burke Harris, 2015). This recommendation is consistent with the findings from the original ACE study which found a graded relationship between the number of ACEs and the prevalence of adverse health and social outcomes (Felitti et al., 1998). The goal is to screen for total dose of exposure, rather than identifying specific exposures. An added benefit is that the tool does not require a parent or adolescent to acknowledge and reveal specific potentially painful experiences, thereby eliminating a possible barrier in the screening process. A score of four or higher on the ACE indicates a positive screen requiring intervention. A score of one suggests the need for anticipatory guidance for the client and family around ACEs.

It is highly recommended that ACE screening tools are integrated as a part of each semiannual or annual child health maintenance visit to identify the children or adolescents who may be adversely affected by exposure to toxic stress and are in need of an evidence-based intervention (EBI). There is also strong evidence to support screening as part of a behavioral or mental health evaluation. There is a need for rigorous research psychometric studies to establish validity and reliability for many of the available tools. Until best practices are established, providers and practices are encouraged to review available resources to determine how they will integrate screening given the strong imperative to identify children and adolescents in their care impacted by toxic stress.

■ INTERCEPTING TOXIC STRESS TO IMPROVE OUTCOMES

Toxic stress in early childhood profoundly disrupts the physical and emotional development of exposed children. Without effective intervention, these disruptions lead to biological changes with lifelong impact at significant personal and societal costs. Toxic stress contributes to some of the costliest societal challenges, including limited educational achievement, diminished economic productivity, criminality, and disparities in health (Shonkoff et al., 2012). There is a strong imperative to intercept this trajectory. Interception strategies include the integration of anticipatory guidance, implementing routine screenings and early identification, enhancement of protective factors, and integration and referral of effective interventions.

■ ANTICIPATORY GUIDANCE ON TOXIC STRESS

Though well established, the science of toxic stress is not well known. Pediatric providers can take a lead role in educating their families by integrating the topic into well visits. In addition, providers can take leadership and advocacy roles to heighten awareness among the entities that make up the socioeconomic and political context for families, including childcare providers, school professionals, service providers, community leaders, and policy makers (Shonkoff et al., 2012). A widespread effort to support prevention, early recognition, and the appropriate intercept requires broad interprofessional support and advocacy.

■ IMPLEMENTING ROUTINE SCREENINGS AND EARLY IDENTIFICATION

Routine screening for toxic stress is critical for early identification. Early identification allows providers to intercept the potential for permanent changes in brain architecture, the immune system, and the other organ systems. Examples of tools were addressed earlier in the chapter. These tools can be implemented at all routine pediatric well visits. In addition, they can be integrated as concerns arise. This tool integration is particularly relevant for the providers addressing behavioral, mental health, and emotional concerns in the pediatric population. It is critical to assess for a history of toxic stress as this will impact the management plan. Without doing so, the management plan may prove ineffective and a lost opportunity results.

■ ENHANCEMENT OF PROTECTIVE FACTORS

Protective factors have been shown to support resiliency and positive life trajectories in children and adolescents exposed to toxic stressors. Positive community connections and school cohesion have been found to have a strong buffering effect (Bethell, Newacheck, Hawes, & Halfon, 2014; Cleveland, Feinberg, Bontempo, & Greenberg, 2008; Schofield, Lee, & Merrick, 2013). Providers are encouraged to identify community and school programming, build referral relationships, and connect children and adolescents with a positive ACE score to these programs. Supporting parental resilience can be instrumental as well. If issues are identified that are impacting parenting—parental history of ACEs, mental health or substance use challenges, limited support, or poor coping strategies—it is important to support parental resilience with a strength-based approach and connecting parents to additional resources. It is important to highlight that providers can advocate for and support efforts in the local community and school programming to maximize the benefit of protective factors for affected children and families.

Schofield et al. (2013) conducted a meta-analysis on intergenerational "maltreatment." Findings from their study revealed that safe, stable, nurturing relationships (SSNRs) for the child and the parent positively impacted family dynamics, coping, and life trajectory. Providers are encouraged to assist children and adolescents with positive ACE scores to identify actual or potential safe, stable, nurturing adults in their lives with whom they can experience a positive, supportive relationship. An established relationship with healthcare providers in a family-centered medical home can be considered one of the SSNRs and has been strongly correlated with a high level of resilience (Bethell et al., 2014). Through that relationship with the medical home providers can also support parental resilience and enhance parental capacity to be an SSNR for their children.

■ REFERRAL FOR EVIDENCE-BASED INTERVENTIONS

Research has shown that integrating supportive programming into the plan of care positively impacts outcome for children and families exposed to toxic stress. Slopen et al. (2014) note there is evidence to support a physiological basis for this impact—a potential lowering of the cortisol level to baseline following participation in supportive interventions. They acknowledge that further research is necessary. That being said, it is clear that interventions that complement the child's care plan can mitigate the impact of toxic stress with the potential to impact both short- and long-term health and social outcomes.

Excellent evidence-based community resources to support parents and families can be found on the Substance Abuse and Mental Health Services (SAMHSA) National Registry of Evidence-based Programs and Practices (NREPP) website: http://nrepp.samhsa.gov/01_landing.aspx. The interventions listed were designed to create protective forces that support resiliency in families and children across a wide range of need including mental health, substance use, and wellness promotion. Search features allow providers to filter by age of child, gender, special populations (i.e., youth transitioning out of foster care, lesbian, gay, bisexual, transgender and questioning [LGBTQ] youth), and by outcome rating. Interventions are not listed by zip code; therefore, providers need to identify the EBIs first, then search by EBI for availability in their community.

Targeted interventions for the treatment of trauma include trauma-focused cognitive behavioral therapy and eye movement desensitization and reprocessing for the affected child, parent–child interactive therapy, child–parent psychotherapy, and family therapy for the family unit (Horner, 2015). In addition, researchers are examining interventions that address good nutrition, regular exercise, healthy sleep, healthy relationships, relaxation techniques, mindfulness meditation techniques, and a range of cognitive behavioral therapies to determine their relationship to positive changes after a diagnosis of childhood exposure to toxic stress. All interventions should be directed to support both generations impacted by toxic stress: the child and caregiver.

■ SUMMARY

Toxic stress is considered a neurodevelopmental disorder that can lead to potentially permanent changes in learning, behavior, emotional regulation, and physiology (Shonkoff et al., 2012). Routine screening for toxic stress should be integrated into well-child maintenance visits. When children and adolescents present with physical, behavioral, or mental health concerns, providers should consider the possibility that toxic stress may be a contributing factor and screen appropriately. *Early identification is critical to intercept and improve both short- and long-term outcomes.*

PCPs are encouraged to offer a strength-based, trauma-informed approach to the care of the child and family affected by toxic stress that encourages safe, stable and nurturing relationships. PCPs need to identify supportive programs within community and school settings as well as identify EBIs available in their areas. PCPs should also develop interprofessional collaborative relationships to provide the highest quality of care to positively *intercept* the adverse effects of toxic stress on the child's and family well-being. See Table 32.2 for helpful websites regarding information and resources on toxic stress.

TABLE 32.2

HELPFUL WEBSITES: INFORMATION AND RESOURCES ADDRESSING TOXIC STRESS

Name of Website	Website Address
CDC: Adverse Childhood Experiences	https://www.cdc.gov/violenceprevention/acestudy
Harvard Center for the Developing Child	http://developingchild.harvard.edu
AAP: Center on Healthy, Resilient Children	https://www.aap.org/en-us/advocacy-and-policy/aap-health-initiatives/CHRC/Pages/Default.aspx
AAP: Healthy Foster Care America Pediatrics for the 21st Century Conference: The Trauma-Informed Pediatrician: Identifying Toxic Stress and Promoting Resilience	https://www.aap.org/en-us/advocacy-and-policy/aap-health-initiatives/healthy-foster-care-america/Pages/Peds21-Trauma.aspx
AAP: The Resilience Project: We Can Stop Toxic Stress	https://www.aap.org/en-us/advocacy-and-policy/aap-health-initiatives/resilience/Pages/default.aspx
ACEs Too High	https://acestoohigh.com/got-your-ace-score/
Substance Abuse and Mental Health Service Administration: National Repository for Evidence-based Programs and Practices	http://nrepp.samhsa.gov/01_landing.aspx
National Child Traumatic Stress Network	http://www.nctsn.org/resources/topics/trauma-informed-screening-assessment/trauma-screening
Center for Youth Wellness	http://centerforyouthwellness.org
University of Maryland, School of Social Work, The Institute for Innovation and Implementation, SEEK Overview	http://www.seekwellbeing.com/overview

ACEs, adverse childhood experiences; AAP, American Academy of Pediatrics; CDC, Centers for Disease Control and Prevention; SEEK, Safe Environment for Every Kid.

CASE PRESENTATION

A 4.5-year-old male presents to the primary care practice with his mother who reports that the child acts out at home and school. The preschool teacher reports that he is disruptive in school, gets up from his seat, and fails to complete activities. She and the teacher have established rules and consequences but they have not been effective. She further reports that the teacher and school psychologist have said that he may have attention deficit hyperactivity disorder (ADHD) and recommended an evaluation. The child's last healthcare visit was 3 months ago with another provider in the same practice. History and physical examination were unremarkable. The diagnosis was normal growing child. Complete blood count, serum lead level, and urinalysis were within normal limits (WNL). Hearing and vision were normal and the Denver Developmental Screening Tool was WNL.

How Should the PCP Manage This Case?
Consider the following:
1. What is the most likely diagnosis?
2. Are there additional screening tools that should be ordered?
3. What is the most appropriate treatment plan?

Case Resolution
This case is a typical presentation of ADHD in a preschool-age child. It is best practice to pursue the initial stages of evaluation. A PCP should provide the parent with an age-appropriate screening tool for ADHD. The provider would also engage the teacher and ask that he/she complete the school version of the tool. The results are likely to demonstrate that the child does meet the criteria for an ADHD diagnosis—impulsivity/hyperactive type.

Now consider these questions: What if the provider also included an ACE screening and found that the child had a positive score? Is it possible that the symptoms of impulsivity and distraction could be related to an easily activated stress response? How might this impact monitoring and management at this point in time? What about in the future? The ACE study clearly indicated that a positive ACE score correlates with higher risk of multiple medical disorders—cardiovascular, metabolic, and immune system mediated—as well as mental health disorders, particularly substance use. How might one monitor this child over time? How might this impact care of the child's siblings and caregivers?

With regard to ADHD, it is worth noting that from the preschool ADHD treatment study, the researchers found that the majority of children identified with ADHD in the preschool years continue to show signs and symptoms throughout school age and adolescence; they added that the majority of participants who had been prescribed medication still met the diagnostic criteria for ADHD 6 years after initiating therapy (Riddle et al., 2013). It is possible that ADHD is highly persistent. Is it also possible that there was an etiology that contributed to its persistence that was not being addressed?

The Imperative to Integrate Developmental Science of Toxic Stress Into Practice
Much of the toxic stress literature points to the need for full integration into primary care. There is also a critical need for full integration into the fields of behavioral and mental health. Symptoms of toxic stress are similar to those consistent with common behavioral and mental health disorders including sleep disturbances, developmental regression, school failure, aggression, and poor impulse control. Given the overlaps in symptomatology, it is highly apparent that an accurate diagnosis would require an ACE screening. Management and treatment planning would then be built on best practices available for addressing toxic stress as well as the specific mental/behavioral health diagnosis (see Chapters 24 and 31).

ACE, adverse childhood experience; PCP, primary care physician.

■ REFERENCES

About the CDC–Kaiser ACE Study. (n.d.). Retrieved from https://www.cdc.gov/violenceprevention/acestudy/about.html

About Us—Overview—Center for Youth Wellness. (n.d.). Retrieved from http://www.centerforyouthwellness.org/about/overview

American Academy of Pediatrics. (2017). *Bright futures: Guidelines for health supervision of infants, children, and adolescents*. (4th ed.). Elk Grove Village, IL: Author.

American Academy of Pediatrics: The Resilience Project. (n.d.). *Clinical assessment tools*. Retrieved from https://www.aap.org/en-us/advocacy-and-policy/aap-health-initiatives/resilience/Pages/Clinical-Assessment-Tools.aspx

Bethell, C. D., Newacheck, P., Hawes, E., & Halfon, N. (2014). Adverse childhood experiences: Assessing the impact on health and school engagement and the mitigating role of resilience. *Health Affairs*, *33*(12), 2106–2115. doi:10.1377/hlthaff.2014.0914

Burke Harris, N. (2015). *An unhealthy dose of stress* [YouTube video]. Retrieved from American Academy of Pediatrics, Pediatrics for the 21st Century Conference on the Trauma-informed Pediatrician: Identifying Toxic Stress and Promoting Resilience; https://www.aap.org/en-us/advocacy-and-policy/aap-health-initiatives/healthy-foster-care-america/Pages/Peds21-Trauma.aspx

Burke Harris, N., & Renschler, T. (2015). *Center for Youth Wellness ACE-Questionnaire (CYW ACE-Q Child, Teen, Teen SR) Version 7/2015*. San Francisco, CA: Center for Youth Wellness.

Cleveland, M. J., Feinberg, M. E., Bontempo, D. E., & Greenberg, M. T. (2008). The role of risk and protective factors in substance use across adolescence. *Journal of Adolescent Health*, *43*(2), 157–164. doi:10.1016/j.jadohealth.2008.01.015

Dubowitz, H. (2014). The safe environment for every kid model: Promotion of children's health, development, and safety, and prevention of child neglect. *Pediatric Annals*, *43*(11), e271–e277. doi:10.3928/00904481-20141022-11

Dubowitz, H., Feigelman, S., Lane, W., & Kim, J. (2009). Pediatric primary care to help prevent child maltreatment: The safe environment for every kid (SEEK) model. *Pediatrics*, *123*(3), 858–864. doi:10.1542/peds.2008-1376

Dubowitz, H., Lane, W., Semiatin, J., & Magder, L. (2012). The SEEK model of pediatric primary care: Can child maltreatment be prevented in a low-risk population? *Academic Pediatrics*, *12*(4), 259–268. doi:10.1016/j.acap.2012.03.005

Felitti, V. J., Anda, R. F., Nordenberg, D., Williamson, D. F., Spitz, A. M., Edwards, V., . . . Marks, J. S. (1998). Relationship of childhood abuse and household dysfunction to many of the leading causes of death in adults: The adverse childhood experiences (ACE) study. *American Journal of Preventive Medicine*, *14*(4), 245–258. doi:10.1016/S0749-3797(98)00017-8

Garner, A. S., Shonkoff, J. P., Siegel, B. S., Dobbins, M. I., Earls, M. F., Garner, A. S., . . . Wood, D. L. (2012). Early childhood adversity, toxic stress, and the role of the pediatrician: Translating developmental science into lifelong health. *Pediatrics*, *129*(1), e224–e231. doi:10.1542/peds.2011-2662

Horner, G. (2015). Childhood trauma exposure and toxic stress: What the PNP needs to know. *Journal of Pediatric Health Care*, *29*(2), 191–198. doi:10.1016/j.pedhc.2014.09.006

Pechtel, P., & Pizzagalli, D. A. (2011). Effects of early life stress on cognitive and affective function: An integrated review of human literature. *Psychopharmacology*, *214*(1), 55–70. doi:10.1007/s00213-010-2009-2

Riddle, M. A., Yershova, K., Lazzaretto, D., Paykina, N., Yenokyan, G., Greenhill, L., . . . Posner, K. (2013). The preschool attention-deficit/hyperactivity disorder treatment study (PATS) 6-year follow-up. *Journal of the American Academy of Child & Adolescent Psychiatry*, *52*(3), 264–278.e2. doi:10.1016/j.jaac.2012.12.007

Schofield, T. J., Lee, R. D., & Merrick, M. T. (2013). Safe, stable, nurturing relationships as a moderator of intergenerational continuity of child maltreatment: A meta-analysis. *Journal of Adolescent Health*, *53*, S32–S38. doi:10.1016/j.jadohealth.2013.05.004

SEEK Model. (n.d.). Retrieved from http://www.seekwellbeing.com/theseekmodel

SEEK Parent Questionnaire (PQ, formerly Parent Screening Questionnaire or PSQ). (n.d.). Retrieved from http://www.seekwellbeing.com/the-seek-parent-questionnaire-

Shonkoff, J. P., & Garner, A. S., Committee on Psychosocial Aspects of Child and Family Health, Committee on Early Childhood, Adoption, and Dependent Care, and Section on Developmental and

Behavioral Pediatrics, Siegel, B. S., Dobbins, M. I., Earls, M. F., . . . Wood, D. L. (2012). The life-long effects of early childhood adversity and toxic stress. *Pediatrics*, *129*(1), e232–e246. doi:10.1542/peds.2011-2663

Slopen, N., McLaughlin, K., & Shonkoff, J. (2014). Interventions to improve cortisol regulation in children: A systematic review. *Pediatrics*, *133*, 312–326. doi:10.1542/peds.2013-163

Stevens, J. E. (2012). *The adverse childhood experiences study—the largest, most important public health study you never heard of—began in an obesity clinic.* Retrieved from https://acestoohigh .com/2012/10/03/the-adverse-childhood-experiences-study-the-largest-most-important-public -health-study-you-never-heard-of-began-in-an-obesity-clinic

CHAPTER 33

Trauma-Informed Care: Responding to Childhood Trauma

MARY WEGLARZ, NINA B. COLABELLI, DEBORAH GUTTER, AND EILEEN CORCORAN

Exposure to traumatic experiences during childhood is pervasive in our society. Children are most vulnerable to trauma. Traumatic events may include but are not limited to physical and sexual abuse, neglect, bullying, family violence, natural disasters, terrorism, and war. In addition, exposure to community-based violence, poverty, and parenting by someone with a chronic physical or mental/behavioral illness can be traumatizing to the child and to other family members (Centers for Disease Control and Prevention [CDC], 2016). Everyone reacts to trauma differently. Pediatric primary care providers (P-PCPs), who are educated about trauma, screen and assess for trauma and are better prepared to respond in a manner that helps mitigate the adverse effect of trauma exposure on the child. Adverse childhood events impact the developing child's physical, emotional, behavioral, and mental health into adulthood. This chapter educates P-PCPs about trauma and offers evidence for a trauma-informed approach to care with the aim of responding to the child who has experienced trauma in a manner that *intercepts* further trauma and has the potential to improve outcomes for the child and their family members.

■ ADVERSE CHILDHOOD EXPERIENCES (ACEs): TRAUMA

The landmark ACEs study conducted by the Centers for Disease Control and Prevention (CDC, 2016) in conjunction with Kaiser Permanente's Health Appraisal Clinic in San Diego revealed that almost 60% of middle-aged, middle-class Americans of both genders were exposed to at least one traumatic event as children. (For further discussion on ACEs, see Chapter 32). The study provides evidence for the known strong relationship between ACEs and adult physical and/ or mental health issues. Many communities have incorporated the information from the ACE study into their own health planning. Philadelphia surveyed its residents using the ACE questionnaire, adding four additional questions particular to an urban population. The sample size was much smaller than the original, but almost 70% of the Philadelphia respondents had experienced at least one traumatic event as a child (Public Health Management Corporation, 2013).

The Substance Abuse and Mental Health Services Administration (SAMHSA) is the agency within the U.S. Department of Health & Human Services (DHHS) that is charged with reducing the impact of substance abuse and mental illness in America. In collaboration with mental and behavioral health experts, SAMSHA has developed a working definition of trauma:

> *Individual* trauma results from an event, series of events, or set of circumstances that is experienced by an *individual* as physically or emotionally harmful or threatening and that has lasting adverse effects on the *individual's* functioning and physical, social, emotional, or spiritual well-being. (SAMSHA, 2014a, p.7)

The second National Survey of Children's Exposure to Violence (NatSCEV) confirmed the findings from the first NatSCEV (Finkelhor, Turner, Ormrod, Hamby, & Krache, 2009) that approximately 60% of children have been victims or witnessed one or more of these traumas: assaults and bullying, sexual victimization, maltreatment by a caregiver, property crime, or witnessing trauma. Multiple exposures of six or more traumas were experienced by 11% of the youth, regardless of age or gender (Finkelhor, Turner, Shattuck, & Hamby, 2013). The more traumatic events experienced as children, the more likely those adults will be diagnosed with a chronic physical ailment or a behavioral/mental health diagnosis, including substance abuse (CDC, 2016).

■ A TRAUMA-INFORMED APPROACH TO CARE

SAMHSA aims to reduce the pervasive, harmful, and costly health impact of trauma by integrating trauma-informed approaches to primary care throughout behavioral health systems.

To incorporate a trauma-informed approach to care in their practice, P-PCPs will:

> *Realize* the widespread impact of trauma and understand potential paths for recovery; *recognize* the signs and symptoms of trauma in clients, families, staff, and others involved with the system; *respond* by fully integrating knowledge about trauma into policies, procedures, and practices; and seek to actively *resist* re-traumatization. (SAMHSA, 2014a, p.9)

SAMHSA recognizes six principles of a trauma-informed approach: "safety; transparency and trustworthiness; peer support; collaboration and mutuality; empowerment, voice, and choice; and cultural, historical, and gender issues" (SAMHSA, 2014a, p.10). A trauma-informed approach to care is different from trauma-specific treatment or therapy. A P-PCP can incorporate a trauma-informed approach to assessment, screening, and developing treatment plans for children when knowledgeable about the principles of trauma-informed care.

■ PRINCIPLES OF TRAUMA-INFORMED CARE

The six principles of trauma-informed care (Figure 33.1) are interrelated and codependent on each other. The principles guide practice in any P-PCP setting or specialty. For example, once the principle of safety is established for the child and family as well as the P-PCP, clients participate in their own care as P-PCPs listen and respect client issues. When peers provide support to children and families and the P-PCPs, collaboration across disciplines is welcomed. Understanding the historical context of traumatic events on healthcare is possible when the child or family feels safe to tell the story and the P-PCP is safe in the professional setting (SAMHSA, 2014a, 2014b, 2014c).

Safety

Safety is the first principle of trauma-informed approach to care. Safety aims to ensure the physical and psychological safety of the child and family (Fallot & Harris, 2009). Feelings of safety begin when the reception, waiting, interview, and exam rooms are welcoming and child friendly. Families should understand the goal and mission of pediatric care: prevention of illness and injury, and promotion of optimal health and well-being for their children (American Nurses Association, National Association of Pediatric Nurse Practitioners, and Society of Pediatric Nurses, 2015). A safe environment should comfort the parent and child and help

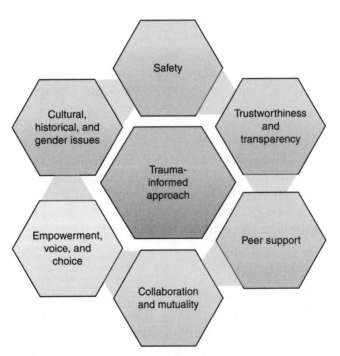

FIGURE 33.1 Trauma-informed approach to care.

Source: Designed by the chapter authors using the principles of trauma-informed care (SAMHSA, 2014a) and showing the interdependence of the basic tenets.

them openly communicate their concerns with the P-PCP. Safety for the P-PCP includes the physical as it relates to the availability of office-based security and the lighting of an office building. Also, safety is enhanced when the P-PCP has the ability to recognize triggers in themselves and families that might escalate conversations and the P-PCP responds appropriately.

Transparency and Trustworthiness

Transparency and trustworthiness lay the foundation for the P-PCP's practice (Fallot & Harris, 2009). This principle may present a challenge for individuals who have difficulty trusting others; however, a trauma-informed approach that includes transparency can help the child and family trust that their needs will be met by the P-PCP. Begin accomplishing trust by ensuring that the child and family assent to care from the P-PCP. The P-PCP must explain to the child and family the P-PCP's role as the healthcare provider, and their responsibilities as the parent or child. When providing treatment, inform the child and family of their options and the related risks and benefits. Active listening by the P-PCP and efforts to understand the family's life challenges helps the family form realistic expectations for follow-up care. Furthermore, the child and parent will develop trust in the P-PCP if communication is consistent, appointments are kept on time, and follow-up is delivered as planned.

Peer Support

A child's peer group impacts his or her growth, development, and well-being. However, peer support for the child requires him or her to seek assistance from members who they identify as his or her peer group. The child might include individuals who are dealing with the same chronic illness, behavioral/mental illness, or substance use disorder. Families may experience the same challenges as their children. The P-PCP must encourage families to seek support of other family members and the community in which they work, live, and recreate (SAMSHA, 2014a, 2014c).

Parents need to be aware of the influence the child's peer group has on the child's choices. The nurse practitioner (NP) should advise parents to have an awareness of the child's friends at school and in the community and welcome the child's friends into their home. The P-PCP's peer group are not only members of the child and family's healthcare team and their professional affiliations but may also include other trauma survivors.

Collaboration and Mutuality

Collaboration and mutuality create a shared responsibility for the health and well-being of the child (Fallot & Harris, 2009). It requires the P-PCP to partner with the child, family, and other healthcare providers. A trauma-informed P-PCP considers how each member of the team can participate in the child's care and advocates for the child's age-appropriate involvement in his or her care. Asking a child to describe his or her preferences for health and behavioral healthcare delivery is a more acceptable way for treating the child and often is less traumatizing. P-PCPs should listen to the child and family, respect their experiences, and incorporate them into the plan of care. This portion of trauma-informed care is consistent with the principles of shared decision making (Burns et al., 2017).

Empowerment, Voice, and Choice

Empowerment, voice, and choice recognize strengths, abilities, and needs of the child and family (Fallot & Harris, 2009). A comprehensive assessment of a child supports the child's plan of care and validates the child and family's experience. Identifying preferences assists with offering the choice of when treatment starts and ends, and where care is provided. Choices help the child and family feel safe and in control. Although sometimes time consuming, the benefits of encouraging choices when possible will help to minimize conflict and build self-confidence.

Depending on the child's developmental stage, the P-PCP can teach a child self-care, including the basics of nutrition, rest, personal hygiene, safety, and the importance of school. This guidance will help the child recognize personal attributes and improve his/her potential. Parents should be engaged and identify their strengths that can assist with the health plan for the child. Provide tools to help families follow the health plan and be successful and offer feedback on their progress.

Cultural, Historical, and Gender Issues

Cultural, historical, and gender issues should support, not hinder, trauma-informed care (SAMHSA, 2014b). The diversity of a child and family must be respected and assessed without judgment. P-PCPs can improve communication through the use of translators and translation lines for families in which English is not their native language. Culturally appropriate anticipatory guidance and education must be provided to the children and families. Respect is evident if the P-PCP has an understanding of the culture within the practice and reflects upon his or her own personal culture and history. P-PCPs should make every effort to understand the cultural beliefs of individuals in their practice. P-PCPs who lack specific knowledge about a culture may be providing inappropriate anticipatory guidance, which leads to nonadherence by the child and family. One strategy to improve cultural knowledge is for P-PCPs to invite community leaders to a meeting in their practice to discuss common medical beliefs, concerns, and practices.

Gender issues are now on the forefront of healthcare. Individuals of all ages are exploring their personal preferences for gender identity and their personal beliefs about the family unit. Chapter 34 provides an in-depth discussion on health-related issues related to gender identity for children and adolescents and also provides insights into providing quality healthcare for individuals who are either lesbian, gay, bisexual, or transgender (LGBT).

■ RESPONDING TO TRAUMA

The trauma-informed P-PCP realizes and recognizes trauma in families served and *responds* in a manner that avoids re-traumatization. The P-PCP needs to understand what trauma the child and/or family has experienced. Recognition of the child and family experience guides the treatment plan.

During each encounter with children and families, P-PCPs screen children and ask families about their concerns. The Survey of Well-Being of Young Children (SWYC) and the Pediatric Symptom Checklist (PSC/Y-PSC) are valid and reliable screening tools designed to recognize cognitive, emotional, and behavioral problems in children. Screening helps ensure that appropriate mental health intervention is initiated for a child as early as possible (CDC, 2017). Furthermore, the SWYC screens families for depression, substance use, family discord, and food insecurity (Survey of Well-Being of Young Children [SWYC], 2016).

P-PCPs must be aware of community resources (Table 33.1) that offer evidence-based trauma-specific interventions to assist them with appropriate referrals. Furthermore, P-PCPs may wish to educate themselves in one of these trauma-specific models as a means of providing further support to children and families (Table 33.2).

■ SUMMARY

P-PCPs develop relationships with children and families over time. All children deserve to receive primary care services that provide opportunities for an early assessment, diagnosis, and treatment for all real and potential healthcare problems. Using a trauma-informed approach to care for all children reduces the risk of failing to diagnose a child who has been exposed to a trauma and needs services to *intercept* the adverse effects of trauma experiences. SAMHSA (2014a) recognizes six principles of trauma-informed care. P-PCPs should be familiar with these principles and apply them to their practices on a daily basis. This application of the principles is the first step in P-PCPs' efforts to improve outcomes for all children

TABLE 33.1

TRAUMA-SPECIFIC INTERVENTION SERVICES		
Service	Web-Based Information	Brief Description
Addiction and Trauma Recovery Integration Model (ATRIUM)	https://alamedacountytraumainformedcare.org/atrium-addictions-and-trauma-recovery-integration-model/	12-week session recovery interprofessional model for groups or individuals
Essence of Being Real	https://alamedacountytraumainformedcare.org/essence-of-being-real-relational-peer-support-for-men-and-women/	Peer-to-peer approach to address the effects of trauma and learn to create a safe group
Service Model®	http://sanctuaryweb.com/TheSanctuaryModel.aspx	To teach individuals and organizations non-violent lives and non-violent systems

TABLE 33.2

ADDITIONAL TRAUMA-SPECIFIC INTERVENTION SERVICES

Service	Web-Based Information	Brief Description
Seeking Safety	http://www.treatment-innovations.org/ss-description.html	Evidence-based consulting model to keep people be safe from trauma and substance abuse
Trauma, Addiction, Mental Health, and Recovery (TAMAR)	https://www.nasmhpd.org/content/trauma-addictions-mental-health-and-recovery-tamar-treatment-manual-and-modules	15 learning modules to work with women who experienced trauma
Trauma Affect Regulation: Guide for Education and Therapy (TARGET)	https://www.crimesolutions.gov/ProgramDetails.aspx?ID=145	Trauma focused psychotherapy for adolescents and women with posttraumatic stress disorder (PTSD)
Trauma Recovery and Empowerment Model (TREM and M-TREM)	http://www.nrcpfc.org/ebp/downloads/AdditionalEBPs/Trauma_Recovery_and_Empowerment_Model_(TREM)_8.26.13.pdf	Group instruction for women who have been physically and sexually abused

who have experienced or are experiencing one or more of the identified childhood traumas: assaults and bullying, sexual victimization, maltreatment by a caregiver, property crime, or witnessing crime.

■ REFERENCES

American Nurses Association, National Association of Pediatric Nurse Practitioners, and Society of Pediatric Nurses. (2015). *Pediatric nursing: Scope and standards of practice* (2nd ed.). Silver Spring, MD: Nursesbooks.org.

Burns, C. E., Dunn, A. M, Brady, M. A., Starr, B. B., Blosser, C. G., & Garzon, D. W. (2017). *Pediatric primary care* (6th ed.). St. Louis, MO: Elsevier.

Centers for Disease Control and Prevention. (2016). *Adverse childhood experiences (ACE) study*. Retrieved from https://www.cdc.gov/violenceprevention/acestudy/index.html

Centers for Disease Control and Prevention. (2017). *Developmental monitoring and screening*. Retrieved from https://www.cdc.gov/ncbddd/childdevelopment/screening.html

Fallot, R., & Harris, M. (2009). *Proceedings from community connections: Creating cultures of trauma-informed care*. Retrieved from http://sfbhn.org/misc%20pdf/Fallot%20Tool%20Explanation%20TIC.pdf

Finkelhor, D., Turner, H. A., Ormrod, R., Hamby, S., & Krache, K. (2009). *OJJDP Bulletin* (pp. 1–11). Retrieved from Office of Juvenile Justice and Delinquency Prevention; https://www.ncjrs.gov/pdffiles1/ojjdp/227744.pdf

Finkelhor, D., Turner, H. A., Shattuck, A. M., & Hamby, S. L. (2013). Violence, crime, and abuse exposure in a national sample of children and youth: An update. *Pediatrics, 167*(7), 614–621. doi:10.1001/jamapediatrics.2013.42

Public Health Management Corporation. (2013). *Philadelphia urban ACE survey.* Retrieved from http://www.rwjf.org/content/dam/farm/reports/reports/2013/rwjf407836

Substance Abuse and Mental Health Services Administration. (2014a). *SAMHSA's concept of trauma and guidance for a trauma-informed approach.* Retrieved from http://store.samhsa.gov/shin/content//SMA14-4884/SMA14-4884.pdf

Substance Abuse and Mental Health Services Administration. (2014b). *TIP 59: Improving cultural competence.* Retrieved from http://store.samhsa.gov/product/Improving-Cultural-Competence/SMA16-4931

Substance Abuse and Mental Health Services Administration. (2014c). *Trauma-informed care in behavioral health services.* Treatment Improvement Protocol (TIP) Series 57. HHS Publication No. (SMA) 13-4801. Rockville, MD: Substance Abuse and Mental Health Services Administration.

Survey of Well-Being of Young Children. (2016). *User's manual.* Retrieve from https://www.floatinghospital.org/The-Survey-of-Wellbeing-of-Young-Children/Overview.aspx

CHAPTER 34

Supporting the Lesbian, Gay, Bisexual, or Transgender Child or Adolescent

CAROLINE DORSEN, MILES HARRIS, AND SHYVON PAUL

The vast majority of lesbian, gay, bisexual, transgender, and queer (LGBTQ+; note: a plus sign signifies to the LGBTQ+ community that the acronym is inclusive of those who do not identify with LGBT or Q) children face similar developmental hurdles as their heterosexual and cisgender (non-transgender) peers, and grow up to be happy, healthy, resilient adults (Levine, 2013). However, research suggests that LGBTQ+ children also face a number of special challenges that may impact self-esteem, social–emotional development, behavioral risk taking, and mental and physical health (Graham et al., 2011; Levine, 2013). Influential adults, including parents, healthcare providers (HCPs), nurses, social workers, psychologists, teachers, and others, are in a unique position to positively impact the lives and development of LGBTQ+ youth (Puckett, Woodward, Mereish, & Pantalone, 2015; Ryan, Russell, Huebner, Diaz, & Sanchez, 2010). This chapter synthesizes available evidence to help *identify* and *intercept* issues related to sexual orientation and gender identity among children and adolescents and offers suggestions for caring for this increasingly visible, vulnerable, and wonderful population.

■ DEMOGRAPHICS AND DEFINING TERMS

It is a common myth that the majority of LGBTQ+ persons are White from upper-middle-class backgrounds in urban areas. In fact, LGBTQ+ persons live in every state in the United States and come from every religious, ethnic, and socioeconomic background (Gates, 2014; Graham et al., 2011). Due to a lack of national data, and differences in how researchers have historically collected data related to sexual orientation and gender identity, the exact number of LGBTQ+ people in the United States is not known (Graham et al., 2011; Gates, 2014). However, studies suggest that approximately 4% of the population, or more than 10 million people, identify as LGBTQ+ (Gates, 2014). Perhaps due to a changing social landscape that is more accepting of LGBTQ+ persons, the number of people who identify as LGBTQ+ seems to be increasing, with higher numbers of young people identifying as LGBTQ+ during childhood and adolescence than previously recorded (Brown, 2017).

■ GENDER IDENTITY AND SEXUAL ORIENTATION

Gender identity formation and sexual orientation identification are ongoing processes that occur over a person's childhood and adolescence and may emerge or be fluid over a person's entire lifetime. However, it is generally thought that gender identity is formed by age 4 (Levine, 2013) and that self-identified same-sex sexual attraction is often noted by age 9 or 10, although individuals may not "come out" for many years after self-awareness is noted, if at all (see section on "coming out"; Coleman, 1982). Thus, identifying and intercepting potential physical and mental health issues among LGBTQ+ persons is an ongoing process that begins in early childhood and may continue throughout adulthood.

Although included in one acronym, the LGBTQ+ community is, in fact, comprised of multiple distinct communities based on sex, sexual orientation, gender identity, and/or gender expression. Although some of the physical and mental health issues within these disparate groups overlap, there may be special issues for each LGBTQ+ subgroup. For example, overweight and obesity are common issues for lesbian, bisexual, and queer identified women, but are not a pervasive issue among gay, bisexual, or queer identified men or transgender/gender nonconforming (T/GNC) folks (Boehmer, Bowen, & Bauer, 2007; Graham et al., 2011; McClain & Peebles, 2016). Conversely, altered body image, binge eating and purging, and anorexia may be more common among sexual minority men and transgender men and women, than among other LGBTQ+ groups (Graham et al., 2011; McClain & Peebles, 2016).

Likewise, it is important to recognize that LGBTQ+ persons' identity is not solely defined by their sexual orientation or gender identity (SOGI). Research is increasingly recognizing the ways that multiple identities intersect and combine to influence individual experience (Bowleg, 2012; Crenshaw, 1991). Thus, for example, an LGBTQ+ person of color or an LGBTQ+ person with disabilities may have a very different experience and have different physical and mental health needs than a White LGBTQ+ individual or an LGBTQ+ person without physical challenges (Kuper et al., 2014). Being an ally to the LGBTQ+ community means being open and inclusive to the multiple ways that individuals define themselves and experience the world.

Understanding the fast-changing, sometimes overlapping, terms used in this community is essential for working with LGBTQ+ youth in a thoughtful, culturally sensitive way. Below are some of the common definitions currently used in the LGBTQ+ community (Human Rights Campaign, n.d.). It is especially important to note that sexual orientation and gender identity are separate concepts, and that T/GNC persons may identify as gay, bisexual, straight, or other (see Table 34.1).

■ HEALTH DISPARITIES IN LGBTQ+ COMMUNITIES

Despite growing social acceptance and legal protections, LGBTQ+ persons have numerous health disparities as compared to the general population (Graham

TABLE 34.1

KEY TERMS (ADAPTED FROM HUMAN RIGHTS CAMPAIGN)

Ally: A person who is not LGBTQ but shows support for LGBTQ people and promotes equality in a variety of ways.

Asexual: The lack of a sexual attraction or desire for other people.

Biphobia: Prejudice, fear, or hatred directed toward bisexual people.

Bisexual: A person emotionally, romantically, or sexually attracted to more than one sex, gender, or gender identity though not necessarily simultaneously, in the same way or to the same degree.

Cisgender: A term used to describe a person whose gender identity aligns with those typically associated with the sex assigned to them at birth.

Closeted: Describes an LGBTQ person who has not disclosed their sexual orientation or gender identity.

Coming out: The process in which a person first acknowledges, accepts, and appreciates his or her sexual orientation or gender identity and begins to share that with others.

Gay: A person who is emotionally, romantically, or sexually attracted to members of the same gender.

Gender dysphoria: Clinically significant distress caused when a person's assigned birth gender is not the same as the one with which they identify. According to the American Psychiatric Association's *Diagnostic and Statistical Manual of Mental Disorders* (*DSM*), the term—which replaces Gender Identity Disorder—"is intended to better characterize the experiences of affected children, adolescents, and adults."

Gender-expansive: Conveys a wider, more flexible range of gender identity and/or expression than typically associated with the binary gender system.

Gender expression: External appearance of one's gender identity, usually expressed through behavior, clothing, haircut, or voice, and which may or may not conform to socially defined behaviors and characteristics typically associated with being either masculine or feminine.

Gender-fluid: According to the Oxford English Dictionary, a person who does not identify with a single fixed gender; of or relating to a person having or expressing a fluid or unfixed gender identity.

Gender identity: One's innermost concept of self as male, female, a blend of both or neither—how individuals perceive themselves and what they call themselves. One's gender identity can be the same or different from his or her sex assigned at birth.

Gender nonconforming: A broad term referring to people who do not behave in a way that conforms to the traditional expectations of their gender, or whose gender expression does not fit neatly into a category.

Genderqueer: Genderqueer people typically reject notions of static categories of gender and embrace a fluidity of gender identity and often, though not always, sexual orientation. People who identify as "genderqueer" may see themselves as being both male and female, neither male nor female, or as falling completely outside these categories.

Gender transition: The process by which some people strive to more closely align their internal knowledge of gender with its outward appearance. Some people socially transition, whereby they might begin dressing, using names and pronouns and/or be socially recognized as another gender. Others undergo physical transitions in which they modify their bodies through medical interventions.

(continued)

TABLE 34.1 (CONTINUED)

KEY TERMS (ADAPTED FROM HUMAN RIGHTS CAMPAIGN)

Homophobia: The fear and hatred of or discomfort with people who are attracted to members of the same sex.

Lesbian: A woman who is emotionally, romantically, or sexually attracted to other women.

Outing: Exposing someone's lesbian, gay, bisexual, or transgender identity to others without their permission. Outing someone can have serious repercussions on employment, economic stability, personal safety, or religious or family situations.

Queer: A term people often use to express fluid identities and orientations. Often used interchangeably with "LGBTQ."

Sexual orientation: An inherent or immutable enduring emotional, romantic, or sexual attraction to other people.

Transgender: An umbrella term for people whose gender identity and/or expression is different from cultural expectations based on the sex they were assigned at birth. Being transgender does not imply any specific sexual orientation. Therefore, transgender people may identify as straight, gay, lesbian, bisexual, etc.

Transphobia: The fear and hatred of, or discomfort with, transgender people.

et al., 2011). None of these inequalities are due to being LGBTQ+ per se; rather, research suggests that these inequities are mostly due to the stigma and marginalization experienced by members of this community and the impact that external and internalized stigma has on behavioral risk taking, access to healthcare, utilization of care, stress, and social disparities, such as poverty, housing instability, un- and underemployment, and insurance status (Fredriksen-Goldsen et al., 2014; Graham et al., 2011; WHO Commission on Social Determinants of Health & World Health Organization, 2008). Although there is much we don't know about the health and well-being of LGBTQ+ persons, existing research strongly suggests that LGBTQ+ adults have higher rates of mental health concerns than their heterosexual peers, including an increased incidence of depression, anxiety, and suicidality (Graham et al., 2011; Remafedi, French, Story, Resnick, & Blum, 1998; Roberts, Austin, Corliss, Vandermorris, & Koenen, 2010). Moreover, substance use remains a serious issue within the LGBTQ+ community with higher rates of use than heterosexuals of tobacco, alcohol, and illicit drugs, including MDMA (ecstasy or molly), cocaine, and methamphetamines (crystal meth), a drug that has been closely linked to HIV transmission and infection among men who have sex with men (MSM; Hughes, 2005; Lee, Griffin, & Melvin, 2009; McCabe, Hughes, Bostwick, West, & Boyd, 2009). Further evidence suggests that LGBTQ+ persons are less likely than their peers to utilize preventive health services and primary care than heterosexuals and cisgender persons, and that because of this, LGBTQ+ persons may not benefit from evidence-based disease prevention strategies or early detection and treatment of certain diseases, including cardiovascular disease, diabetes, and cancer (Caceres et al., 2017; Wender, Sharpe, Westmaas, & Patel, 2016). More research is needed on the incidence and impact of chronic disease and malignancies in the LGBTQ+ community. Lastly, it is well known that the global burden of HIV/AIDS has disproportionately impacted MSM, as has syphilis and other sexually transmitted infections (STIs; Beyrer et al., 2012). Worldwide, 70 million people have been infected with HIV over the course of the epidemic, resulting in approximately 35 million deaths (WHO, n.d.).

■ HEALTH DISPARITIES AMONG LGBTQ+ CHILDREN AND ADOLESCENTS

Many of the health disparities seen among LGBTQ+ adults are apparent among LGBTQ+ youth as well. In fact, research suggests that LGBTQ+ young people are particularly vulnerable to the impact of societal judgment and stigma related to SOGI, which may be experienced as familial and peer rejection, negative messages in the media and on social media, and through harassment and victimization (Almeida, Johnson, Corliss, Molnar, & Azrael, 2009; Nadal et al., 2011). Although overt homophobia is clearly harmful, it is important to note that less obvious forms of discrimination, such as heteronormativity and heterosexism (the belief that heterosexuality is "normal" and thus, being LGBTQ+ is "abnormal"), may cause significant harm as well. Microaggressions is a term commonly used to describe the potential cumulative effect of small, hurtful experiences such as name calling or subconscious exclusion (Nadal et al., 2011).

Research suggests that structural and individual stressors may result in increased substance use among LGBTQ+ youth (Hatzenbuehler & Pachankis, 2016; Hatzenbuehler, Wieringa, & Keyes, 2011; Newcomb, Ryan, Greene, Garofalo, & Mustanski, 2014). A recent study by Human Rights Campaign (HRC) found that LGBTQ+ youth are twice as likely than their heterosexual/cisgender peers to use alcohol and drugs (Corliss et al., 2010; HRC, 2011). Tobacco use is also higher among LGBTQ+ youth than the general population (Hatzenbuehler et al., 2011). LGBTQ+ youth are more likely to feel depressed, sad, and/or hopeless than non-LGBTQ+ youth (Levine, 2013; Russell & Fish, 2016) and twice as likely to have considered suicide in the past year (Bostwick et al., 2014). LGBTQ+ youth are more likely to be sexually active than their heterosexual/cisgender peers and less likely to practice safe sex (Everett, McCabe, & Hughes, 2017; Levine, 2013). Sexual, emotional, and physical victimization may also be higher among LGBTQ+ youth than the general population (Espelage, Aragon, Birkett, & Koenig, 2008; Russell, Ryan, Toomey, Diaz, & Sanchez, 2011). Lastly, homelessness is higher among LGBTQ+ adolescents than in the general population, as some LGBTQ+ teens may be forced to leave their homes due to issues related to SOGI and the subsequent, previously mentioned, struggles with substance use, risky sexual behaviors, and mental health (Keuroghlian, Shtasel, & Bassuk, 2014).

■ SUPPORTING THE LGBTQ+ CHILD OR ADOLESCENT

Creating a Safe and Inclusive Environment

Despite the real challenges that LGBTQ+ youth face, many of the concerns in this community can be prevented or lessened with the support of trusted adults and peers (Espelage, et al., 2008; Heck et al., 2014; Ryan et al., 2010). The singularly most important way that influential adults can intercept potential issues with LGBTQ+ youth is to create a nonjudgmental environment where children feel seen and supported and are able to ask questions and openly discuss issues that may be concerning them. Research has consistently shown the impact of familial acceptance or rejection on the mental health of LGBTQ+ young people, with studies suggesting that a higher rate of parental rejection toward sexual orientation or gender expression is significantly associated with higher rates of suicide ideations and attempts, drug use, HIV infection, unprotected sexual intercourse, depression, anxiety, and poor physical health (Puckett et al., 2015; Ryan, Huebner, Diaz, & Sanchez, 2009; Ryan et al., 2010).

In healthcare or school environments, simply having a visible symbol of LGBTQ+ acceptance, such as a rainbow triangle or poster depicting a same-sex couple or T/GNC person, lets youth know that you offer a safe place to discuss their physical, emotional, and social concerns (Poynter & Tubbs, 2008). Likewise, avoiding assumptions about sexual orientation or gender on intake and other forms and using nongendered language when asking questions allows children and teens the space to identify who they are and speak openly and honestly about their lives (for more information on asking about SOGI, please refer to Fenway Institute Training Modules at www.fenwayinstitute,org; Badgett, 2009).

Coming Out

Contrary to the pop culture idea of "coming out" as a singular event, an LGBTQ+ child will "come out" dozens, if not hundreds, of times throughout the course of their life. The first adult a child comes out to—or discloses their SOGI to—will likely be one they perceive to be an ally, and from who they hope to receive a supportive and loving response. This adult may have a wide variety of personal reactions to the disclosure of the LGBTQ+ child: shock, relief, fear, joy, or others. Regardless, the interaction should remain focused on feelings and needs of the child, not of the adult. The adult should validate that children are able to know their identity, convey support to them, and inquire if they have any specific requests or needs. When asking questions of the child, the adult must consider if these questions help provide support or are motivated by curiosity. It is vital to maintaining the agency of LGBTQ+ children by allowing them to determine to whom they disclose their SOGI, and when. Children may want to come out to some friends but not others, or to only certain family members. Clarify with the child, who, if anyone, the adult may comfortably share this information with. HCPs encounter situations in which children come out to them as LGBTQ+ but request that this not be part of their medical records or shared with other members of the healthcare team. In this situation, the HCP and/or pediatric primary care provider (P-PCP) can explore a particular fear of patients (e.g., their parents will accidentally find out), reassure them of the confidentiality of their medical information, and explain why this information is important to their healthcare (American Academy of Pediatrics [AAP], 2016).

An adult may be an important figure in the life of a child who they suspect may be LGBTQ+ but has not yet come out. The decision on whether or not to initiate a conversation regarding the child's SOGI should be based on the child's safety and well-being. If the child is engaging in risky or harmful behaviors (for example, an age-inappropriate same-sex relationship) then it is the trusted adult's responsibility to intervene. Additionally, adults can normalize behaviors that GNC children may try to conceal, without directly addressing the child's identity. For example, if a parent is aware the child is secretly trying on his or her mother's high heels, the parent can tell the child it doesn't need to be done in secret and he or she can ask to borrow them.

Ally-Ship

Being an ally for an LGBTQ+ child is not an all-or-nothing premise. The Riddle Scale (Table 34.2) provides an interpretation of stages of ally-ship, with "tolerance" and "acceptance" being stages on the way to "admiration" and "nurturance" (Riddle, 1996). An adult, especially one who is new to supporting LGBTQ children, should make an honest self-assessment of where he or she falls on this scale. While the support of allies is important to all LGBTQ+ individuals, it is vital for LGBTQ+ children, who have less control over their day-to-day lives and thus unable to choose to avoid homophobic and transphobic people and situations.

By far, the most common discrimination faced by LGBTQ+ children is peer bullying (see Chapter 21 on bullying; Russell et al., 2011). Bullying behaviors

TABLE 34.2

THE RIDDLE SCALE

Negative levels of attitudes

1. Repulsion: Homosexuality is a sin. LGBTQ+ persons are sick, crazy, etc.
2. Pity: Heterosexuality is preferable to being LGBTQ+.
3. Tolerance: LGBTQ+ is a phase that many people grow out of.
4. Acceptance: LGBTQ+ is something to accept; what you do is your business, etc.

Postive levels of attitudes

1. Support: Aware of homphobic climate and discrimination but still personally uncomfortable
2. Admiration: Acknowledges how hard it is to be LGBTQ+ in a nonaccepting society; willing to examine own beliefs, attitudes, and behaviors
3. Appreciation: Value diversity of people and see LGBTQ+ people as part of that; willing to work to combat homophobia
4. Nurturance: Sees LGBTQ+ people as indispensible part of society; allies and advocates

Source: Riddle Homophobia Scale adapted from Wall, V. (1995). *Beyond tolerance: Gays, lesbians and bisexuals on campus. A handbook of structured experiences and exercises for training and development.* American College Personnel Association.

range from social ostracization and name-calling to physical and sexual assault. An LGBTQ+ child may be reticent to bring these experiences to the attention of an adult, thinking that they are unavoidable, inevitable, or even deserved (Bouris, Everett, Heath, Elsaesser, & Neilands, 2016). The onus is on the part of the trusted adults of an LGBTQ+ child to regularly inquire if he or she feels physically and emotionally safe in all parts of his or her life. Depending on the adult's role, he or she may be in a place to intervene, or may need to contact an administrator, coach, or others to address the bullying concerns. Adults faced with leadership that is unresponsive to their bullying concerns may involve outside resources like the American Civil Liberties Union (www.ACLU.org) or the Gay, Lesbian and Straight Education Network (www.GLSEN.org) among others.

An integral component of developing skills to be a better LGBTQ+ ally is processing one's own attitudes, thoughts, and experiences (Dillon & Worthington, 2003). While mixed or negative reactions to a child's coming out are part of the process for many allies, it is vital to avoid processing these thoughts with the child. Connecting with adults in similar roles, such parents, social workers, or HCPs, provides space to ask for help and process shared experiences. Numerous local and national organizations have educational and support systems set up to assist adults as they support LGBTQ+ children. For more information, consult Parents and Friends of Lesbians and Gays (www.PFLAG.org).

■ T/GNC CHILDREN AND ADOLESCENTS

A transgender child may request to be addressed by a name and pronouns that better fit their gender identity. For example, a transgender girl may ask to be addressed as "Johanna" instead of "John" and "she" instead of "he." Some children, such as those who identify as gender non-binary (i.e., not male or female, or embodying both the masculine and feminine), may prefer the non-gendered pronouns "they" and "them." As with coming out, the child may not want to make this change with everyone in their life at the same time. Additionally, the name and pronoun preferences of the child may change over time; this fluidity is a normal part of the child's development. Those from whom the child has requested a change in name and/or pronouns should consistently use the child's desired name and pronouns, even when the child is not physically present, provided this does not "out" the child to someone.

Mistakes With Names and Pronouns: What to Do?

Making mistakes with names and pronouns is inevitable. If catching oneself using the incorrect (nonpreferred) name or pronoun, the best practice is to correct oneself and move on in the conversation. Effusive and lengthy apologies may result in the child feeling compelled to console the adult, shifting the burden of role as supporter onto the child. Another important part of being an ally to a trans or gender nonbinary child is correcting others who use the incorrect name or pronoun for the child. Correcting others is a constant struggle for many T/GNC children; when others step in to provide the correct name and pronoun, they demonstrate visible and direct support for the child (Zimman, 2017).

Clothing Choices

Throughout childhood, many children, regardless of SOGI, will try on gender non-conforming clothing, or play with toys associated with the "opposite" gender. A child's SOGI cannot be inferred from their gender expression (REF). Regardless, adults should support the LGBTQ+ child in wearing the clothing that makes him or her most comfortable and playing with toys he or she prefers. A parent or teacher may struggle to decide if an outfit is "appropriate" for a GNC child; often, the best strategy is to consider if this outfit was worn by a gender-*conforming* child would it be considered acceptable? However, attention to certain issues may merit special allowances: a transmasculine child might choose baggy shirts to de-emphasize his breasts, a transfeminine child might want to wear make-up to conceal beard stubble.

Gender-Binary Spaces and Activities

Gender-binary spaces and activities are pervasive, often more so in the lives of children. Bathrooms are the most frequently encountered example of gender-binary spaces, and one in which many T/GNC children feel especially vulnerable. Children may choose a different gendered bathrooms depending on the context and perceived safety. Providing access to gender-neutral, single-stall toilets allows T/GNC children to use the bathroom without entering single-gender spaces and may positively impact their short- and long-term mental health (Seelman, 2016).

■ SCREENING FOR COMMON HEALTH ISSUES IN THE LGBTQ+ ISSUES

All teens should have a comprehensive evidence-based psychosocial assessment at yearly visits, using a tool such as the HEEADSSS interview instrument (Klein, Goldenring, & Adelman, 2014). However, providers should have a high index of suspicion for mental health concerns, bullying and other forms of victimization, substance use, risky sexual behaviors, and other physical and mental health issues among LGBTQ+ youth. Screening for anxiety (SCARED screening too), depression, and suicidality (PHQ-9) should be performed regularly using a validated tool for adolescents (Levine, 2013). Likewise, screening for online and in-person bullying and other forms of victimization should be a regular part of mental health assessments with LGBTQ+ adolescents. Providers and other adults should ask LGBTQ+ youth about home and school atmosphere and existence of social supports, including individual peers and peer support groups, such as gay–straight alliances (Espelage et al., 2008; Heck et al., 2014). Honest discussions about use of drugs, alcohol, and tobacco, from a harm reduction perspective, must be integrated into every visit. Providers and other influential adults should also consider higher rates of disordered eating among LGBTQ+ persons and include interview questions about eating habits and body image, and evidence-based measures of weight, such as body mass index (BMI) measurements and physical activity regularly (Lock, J., La Via, M. C., & American Academy of Child and Adolescent Psychiatry [AACAP] Committee on Quality Issues [CQI], 2015). As with all adolescents, conversations about healthy sexual expression and relationships should be ongoing, with a reminder to focus less on how LGBTQ+ young people *identify* (i.e., the words they use to describe themselves), and more on their *behaviors* (i.e., what they are doing, and with whom) in an effort to prevent STIs and unwanted pregnancy. It is important to note that a significant percentage of gay/queer identified men have sex with women, and vice versa. In fact, studies suggest that incidence of unintended pregnancy may be higher among LGBTQ+ youth than heterosexuals (Brakman, Ellsworth, & Gold, 2015; Everett et al., 2017).

■ SUMMARY

There are significant gaps in the research on wellness, prevention, and care of LGBTQ+ young people, especially regarding subpopulations within the general LGBTQ+ umbrella, including T/GNC youth, LGBTQ+ young persons of color, LGBTQ+ youth living in rural areas, LGBTQ+ immigrants, and others (Graham et al., 2011). Many LGBT people continue to face oppression and discrimination despite the laws that were put in place to protect their basic human rights, making it difficult to access healthcare and other services (Bockting, 2013; Graham et al., 2011; Harper & Schneider, 2003). Even when LGBTQ+ people have access

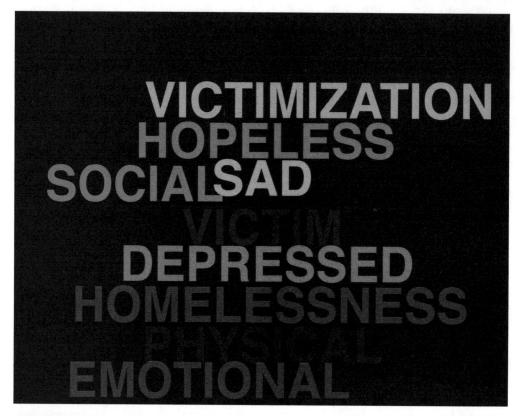

FIGURE 34.1 External and internal experiences of stigma and marginalization.

to medical care it is often not adequate due to provider bias or lack of aware-ness regarding LGBTQ+ issues (Dorsen, 2012; Dorsen & Van Devanter, 2016; Sanchez, Sanchez, & Danoff, 2009).

LGBTQ+ youth face dual challenges—the expected developmental and social hurdles of childhood and adolescence combined with the struggles inherent in recognizing and accepting one's sexual orientation and/or gender identity, includ-ing external and internal experiences of stigma and marginalization (Figure 34.1). To effectively *intercept* some of the common medical and mental health concerns faced by this community, adults are encouraged to reflect on their own attitudes and biases toward LGBTQ+ persons, to increase their knowledge about LGBTQ+ culture, experiences, and unique health needs, and to familiarize themselves with local, national, and online resources to support this resilient community. Indeed, research suggests that even one supportive and trusted adult can make all the dif-ference in the life of a child.

■ REFERENCES

Almeida, J., Johnson, R. M., Corliss, H. L., Molnar, B. E., & Azrael, D. (2009). Emotional distress among LGBT youth: The influence of perceived discrimination based on sexual orientation. *Journal of Youth and Adolescence*, 38(7), 1001–1014. doi:10.1007/s10964-009-9397-9

American Academy of Pediatrics. (2016). Confidentiality protections for adolescents and young adults in the health care billing and insurance claims process. *Journal of Adolescent Health*, 58(3), 374–377. doi:10.1016/j.jadohealth.2015.12.009

Beyrer, C., Baral, S. D., Van Griensven, F., Goodreau, S. M., Chariyalertsak, S., Wirtz, A. L., & Brookmeyer, R. (2012). Global epidemiology of HIV infection in men who have sex with men. *The Lancet*, 380(9839), 367–377. doi:10.1016/S0140-6736(12)60821-6

Bockting, W. O. (2013). Stigma, mental health, and resilience in an online sample of the U.S. transgender population. *American Journal of Public Health*, 103(5), 943–951. doi:10.2105/AJPH.2013.301241

Boehmer, U., Bowen, D. J., & Bauer, G. R. (2007). Overweight and obesity in sexual-minority women: Evidence from population-based data. *American Journal of Public Health*, 97(6), 1134–1140. doi:10.2105/AJPH.2006.088419

Bostwick, W. B., Meyer, I., Aranda, F., Russell, S., Hughes, T., Birkett, M., & Mustanski, B. (2014). Mental health and suicidality among racially/ethnically diverse sexual minority youths. *American Journal of Public Health, 104*(6), 1129–1136.

Bouris, A., Everett, B. G., Heath, R. D., Elsaesser, C. E., & Neilands, T. B. (2016). Effects of victimiza-tion and violence on suicidal ideation and behaviors among sexual minority and heterosexual adoles-cents. *LGBT Health*, 3(2), 153–161. doi:10.1089/lgbt.2015.0037

Bowleg, L. (2012). The problem with the phrase women and minorities: Intersectionality—an impor-tant theoretical framework for public health. *American Journal of Public Health*, 102(7), 1267–1273. doi:10.2105/AJPH.2012.300750

Brakman, A., Ellsworth, T. R., & Gold, M. (2015). Gay, lesbian, and bisexual youth grouped, show increased risk for unintended pregnancy. *Contraceptive Technology Update*, 36(9), 106–107.

Brown, A. (2017). *5 key findings about LGBT Americans*. Fact tank. Retrieved from http://www.pewre-search.org/fact-tank/2017/06/13/5-key-findings-about-lgbt-americans/

Caceres, B. A., Brody, A., Luscombe, R. E., Primiano, J. E., Marusca, P., Sitts, E. M., & Chyun, D. (2017). A systematic review of cardiovascular disease in sexual minorities. *American Journal of Public Health*, 107(4), e13–e21. doi:10.2105/AJPH.2016.303630a

Coleman, E. (1982). Developmental stages of the coming out process. *Journal of Homosexuality*, 7(2–3), 31–43. doi:10.1300/J082v07n02_06

Corliss, H. L., Rosario, M., Wypij, D., Wylie, S. A., Frazier, A. L., & Austin, S. B. (2010). Sexual orien-tation and drug use in a longitudinal cohort study of U.S. adolescents. *Addictive Behaviors*, 35(5), 517–521. doi:10.1016/j.addbeh.2009.12.019

Crenshaw, K. (1991). Mapping the margins: Intersectionality, identity politics, and violence against women of color. *Stanford Law Review*, 43(6), 1241–1299. doi:10.2307/1229039

Dillon, F., & Worthington, R. L. (2003). The lesbian, gay and bisexual affirmative counseling self-efficacy inventory (LGB-CSI): Development, validation, and training implications. *Journal of Counseling Psychology, 50*(2), 235. doi:10.1037/0022-0167.50.2.235

Dorsen, C. (2012). An integrative review of nurse attitudes towards lesbian, gay, bisexual, and transgender patients. *CJNR (Canadian Journal of Nursing Research), 44*(3), 18–43.

Dorsen, C., & Van Devanter, N. (2016). Open arms, conflicted hearts: Nurse-practitioner's attitudes towards working with lesbian, gay and bisexual patients. *Journal of Clinical Nursing, 25*(23–24), 3716–3727. doi:10.1111/jocn.13464

Espelage, D. L., Aragon, S. R., Birkett, M., & Koenig, B. W. (2008). Homophobic teasing, psychological outcomes, and sexual orientation among high school students: What influence do parents and schools have? *School Psychology Review, 37*(2), 202.

Everett, B. G., McCabe, K. F., & Hughes, T. L. (2017). Sexual orientation disparities in mistimed and unwanted pregnancy among adult women. *Perspectives on Sexual and Reproductive Health.* doi:10.1363/psrh.12032

Fredriksen-Goldsen, K. I., Simoni, J. M., Kim, H. J., Lehavot, K., Walters, K. L., Yang, J., . . . Muraco, A. (2014). The health equity promotion model: Reconceptualization of lesbian, gay, bisexual, and transgender (LGBT) health disparities. *American Journal of Orthopsychiatry, 84*(6), 653. doi:10.1037/ort0000030

Gates, G. (2014). *LGBT Demographics: Comparisons among population-based surveys.* Retrieved from https://williamsinstitute.law.ucla.edu/research/census-lgbt-demographics-studies/lgbt-demogs-sep-2014/

Graham, R., Berkowitz, B., Blum, R., Bockting, W., Bradford, J., de Vries, B., . . . Makadon, H. (2011). *The health of lesbian, gay, bisexual, and transgender people: Building a foundation for better understanding.* Washington, DC: Institute of Medicine.

Harper, G. W., & Schneider, M. (2003). Oppression and discrimination among lesbian, gay, bisexual, and transgendered people and communities: A challenge for community psychology. *American Journal of Community Psychology, 31*(3–4), 243–252.

Hatzenbuehler, M. L., & Pachankis, J. E. (2016). Stigma and minority stress as social determinants of health among lesbian, gay, bisexual, and transgender youth. *Pediatric Clinics, 63*(6), 985–997. doi:10.1016/j.pcl.2016.07.003

Hatzenbuehler, M. L., Wieringa, N. F., & Keyes, K. M. (2011). Community-level determinants of tobacco use disparities in lesbian, gay, and bisexual youth: Results from a population-based study. *Archives of Pediatrics & Adolescent Medicine, 165*(6), 527–532. doi:10.1001/archpediatrics.2011.64

Heck, N. C., Livingston, N. A., Flentje, A., Oost, K., Stewart, B. T., & Cochran, B. N. (2014). Reducing risk for illicit drug use and prescription drug misuse: High school gay–straight alliances and lesbian, gay, bisexual, and transgender youth. *Addictive Behaviors, 39*(4), 824–828. doi:10.1016/j.addbeh.2014.01.007

Hughes, T. L. (2005). Alcohol use and alcohol-related problems among lesbians and gay men. *Annual Review of Nursing Research, 23*, 283–325.

Human Rights Campaign. (n.d.). *Glossary of terms.* Retrieved from https://www.hrc.org/resources/glossary-of-terms

Human Rights Campaign. (2011). Growing up LGBT in America. Retrieved from https://www.hrc.org/youth-report

Keuroghlian, A. S., Shtasel, D., & Bassuk, E. L. (2014). Out on the street: A public health and policy agenda for lesbian, gay, bisexual, and transgender youth who are homeless. *American Journal of Orthopsychiatry, 84*(1), 66. doi:10.1037/h0098852

Klein, D. A., Goldenring, J. M., & Adelman, W. P. (2014). HEEADSSS 3.0: The psychosocial interview for adolescents updated for a new century fueled by media.

Kuper, L. E., Coleman, B. R., & Mustanski, B. S. (2014). Coping with LGBT and racial–ethnic-related stressors: A mixed-methods study of LGBT youth of color. *Journal of Research on Adolescence, 24*(4), 703–719. doi:10.1111/jora.12079

Lee, G. L., Griffin, G. K., & Melvin, C. L. (2009). Tobacco use among sexual minorities in the USA: 1987 to May 2007: A systematic review. *Tobacco Control, 18*, 275–282. doi:10.1136/tc.2008.028241

Levine, D. A. (2013). Office-based care for lesbian, gay, bisexual, transgender, and questioning youth. *Pediatrics, 132*(1), e297–e313. doi:10.1542/peds.2013-1283

Lock, J., La Via, M. C., & American Academy of Child and Adolescent Psychiatry Committee on Quality Issues. (2015). Practice parameter for the assessment and treatment of children and adolescents with eating disorders. *Focus, 14*(1), 75–89. doi:10.1176/appi.focus.140107

McCabe, S. E., Hughes, T. L., Bostwick, W. B., West, B. T., & Boyd, C. J. (2009). Sexual orientation, substance use behaviors and substance dependence in the United States. *Addiction, 104*(8), 1333–1345. doi:10.1111/j.1360-0443.2009.02596.x

McClain, Z., & Peebles, R. (2016). Body image and eating disorders among lesbian, gay, bisexual, and transgender youth. *Pediatric Clinics, 63*(6), 1079–1090. doi:10.1016/j.pcl.2016.07.008

Nadal, K. L., Issa, M. A., Leon, J., Meterko, V., Wideman, M., & Wong, Y. (2011). Sexual orientation microaggressions: "Death by a thousand cuts" for lesbian, gay, and bisexual youth. *Journal of LGBT Youth, 8*(3), 234–259. doi:10.1080/19361653.2011.584204

Newcomb, M. E., Ryan, D. T., Greene, G. J., Garofalo, R., & Mustanski, B. (2014). Prevalence and patterns of smoking, alcohol use, and illicit drug use in young men who have sex with men. *Drug and Alcohol Dependence, 141*, 65–71. doi:10.1016/j.drugalcdep.2014.05.005

Poynter, K. J., & Tubbs, N. J. (2008). Safe zones: Creating LGBT safe space ally programs. *Journal of LGBT Youth, 5*(1), 121–132.

Puckett, J. A., Woodward, E. N., Mereish, E. H., & Pantalone, D. W. (2015). Parental rejection following sexual orientation disclosure: Impact on internalized homophobia, social support, and mental health. *LGBT Health, 2*(3), 265–269. doi:10.1089/lgbt.2013.0024

Remafedi, G., French, S., Story, M., Resnick, M. D., & Blum, R. (1998). The relationship between suicide risk and sexual orientation: Results of a population-based study. *American Journal of Public Health, 88*(1), 57–60. doi:10.2105/AJPH.88.1.57

Riddle, D. (1996). Riddle homophobia scale. In *Social diversity and social justice: Gay, lesbian and bisexual oppression* (p. 31).

Roberts, A. L., Austin, S. B., Corliss, H. L., Vandermorris, A. K., & Koenen, K. C. (2010). Pervasive trauma exposure among U.S. sexual orientation minority adults and risk of posttraumatic stress disorder. *American Journal of Public Health, 100*(12), 2433–2441. doi:10.2105/AJPH.2009.168971

Russell, S. T., & Fish, J. N. (2016). Mental health in lesbian, gay, bisexual, and transgender (LGBT) youth. *Annual Review of Clinical Psychology, 12*, 465–487. doi:10.1146/annurev-clinpsy-021815-093153

Russell, S. T., Ryan, C., Toomey, R. B., Diaz, R. M., & Sanchez, J. (2011). Lesbian, gay, bisexual, and transgender adolescent school victimization: Implications for young adult health and adjustment. *Journal of School Health, 81*(5), 223–230. doi:10.1111/j.1746-1561.2011.00583.x

Ryan, C., Huebner, D., Diaz, R. M., & Sanchez, J. (2009). Family rejection as a predictor of negative health outcomes in white and Latino lesbian, gay, and bisexual young adults. *Pediatrics, 123*(1), 346–352. doi:10.1542/peds.2007-3524

Ryan, C., Russell, S. T., Huebner, D., Diaz, R., & Sanchez, J. (2010). Family acceptance in adolescence and the health of LGBT young adults. *Journal of Child and Adolescent Psychiatric Nursing, 23*(4), 205–213. doi:10.1111/j.1744-6171.2010.00246.x

Sanchez, N. F., Sanchez, J. P., & Danoff, A. (2009). Health care utilization, barriers to care, and hormone usage among male-to-female transgender persons in New York City. *American Journal of Public Health, 99*(4), 713–719. doi:10.2105/AJPH.2007.132035

Seelman, K. L. (2016). Transgender adults' access to college bathrooms and housing and the relationship to suicidality. *Journal of Homosexuality, 63*(10), 1378–1399. doi:10.1080/00918369.2016.1157998

Wender, R., Sharpe, K. B., Westmaas, J. L., & Patel, A. V. (2016). The American Cancer Society's approach to addressing the cancer burden in the LGBT community. *LGBT Health, 3*(1), 15–18.

Williams Institute. (2009). Best practices for asking questions about sexual orientation on surveys. Retrieved from https://williamsinstitute.law.ucla.edu/wp-content/uploads/SMART-FINAL-Nov-2009.pdf

World Health Organization. (n.d.). Global health observatory (GHO) data: HIV/AIDS. Retrieved from http://www.who.int/gho/hiv/en

WHO Commission on Social Determinants of Health, & World Health Organization. (2008). *Closing the gap in a generation: Health equity through action on the social determinants of health: Commission on Social Determinants of Health final report.* Geneva: Author.

Zimman, L. (2017). Transgender language reform: Some challenges and strategies for promoting trans-affirming, gender-inclusive language. *Journal of Language and Discrimination, 1*(1), 84–105. doi:10.1558/jld.33139

CHAPTER 35

Holistic Care, Integrative Medicine, and Behavioral Health

EMILY SCHADT

The human body is an incredibly complex system with a wide variety of healing capabilities. Over the course of time, human beings have been able to tolerate and heal physical, behavioral, and mental illnesses through a vast array of mechanisms. Although Western medicine plays a tremendous role in how practitioners provide patient care, improvements and recent advances in the field of epigenetics and integrative medicine are also impacting healthcare. Patients are much more aware of their bodies and the alternative treatments and therapies available for certain disease and illness states. This chapter provides insights into the general concepts of holistic and patient-centered care with a focus on improving behavioral health in the pediatric, adolescent, and young adult populations. Pediatric primary care providers (P-PCPs) must understand the concepts of complementary, alternative, and integrative medical practices and the impact these modalities may have on *intercepting* adverse behaviors in these populations. The principles of epigenetics are also discussed in this chapter.

■ COMPLEMENTARY, ALTERNATIVE, AND INTEGRATIVE MEDICINE

Complementary, alternative, and integrative medicine are terms that are generally used interchangeably. However, each one uses a different model and approach for improving healthcare. The foundation for complementary medicine practices is based on both Western medicine and unconventional practices to provide a combination of care dependent on disease states. For example, a patient practicing complementary medicine may utilize natural products for headaches or generalized body aches and pains, but seek Western medical management for treatment of a severe infection, such as a urinary tract infection or ruptured appendix. The term alternative medicine refers to patients who use organic and nontraditional practices for all disease states; however, most people select a combination therapy of complementary medicine. Integrative medicine refers to the conjunction of complementary and alternative medical models used in a synchronized approach to reach the best possible patient outcomes. Integrative medicine aims to provide individualized holistic care that not only nurtures the physical aspects of health but also the psychological characteristics that center on healing (National Center for Complementary and Integrative Health [NCCIH], 2016a).

Although major advances in the field of Western medicine have allowed for life-saving procedures and cures for some disease states, a major problem with the medical model is the chronic disease state and symptomatic treatment. P-PCPs often overprescribe medications and merely bandage symptoms rather than cure diseases. Most providers do not have formal training in the field of integrative medicine. Thus, providers lack knowledge of how remarkable the human body is, and that the body innately recognizes how to restore itself. More patients are interested in the body's natural healing potentials and unconventional medical practices for treatment. Thus, the use of an integrative medical model of health-care has increased. Therefore, it is imperative providers of this new generation embrace and understand medical management that falls outside of the commonly practiced Westernized medicine (Kanherkar et al., 2017).

■ EPIGENETICS

To understand the perspective of patients who seek integrative medicine, P-PCPs must *first be knowledgeable about* the topic of epigenetics. Recently, advances in the field of epigenetics have demonstrated the way environmental factors may influence and change genetic makeup. Epigenetics, by definition, is an additional change to the genetic sequencing due to modification of gene expression that does not cause a change in underlying genetic material (Labonte & Turecki, 2012). In essence, epigenetics is the study of determining what turns gene expression "on" and "off." Since the emergence of epigenetics as a field of study, researchers have been investigating relationships between physical and psychological illness, as well as methods to explain how the environment affects genomic structures (Labonte & Turecki, 2012).

Multiple mechanisms involved in causing genomic alterations occur naturally. If the genomic alterations occur out of balance through over- or underproduction, large effects and major alterations may be seen in the genome. Two of the best-known processes are DNA methylation and chromatin modification, which have been linked to increased disease states and cancer. Mechanisms involved in epigenetics act as on/off switches and are actively altered by environmental factors. For example, when DNA has a methyl group added or removed, genetic reprogramming can be seen; this reprogramming has been linked to increases in rates of disease. Environmental factors affect each individual differently. Since there are numerous factors linked to alterations, it is difficult to generalize ways to avoid "switches" being distorted. The field of epigenetics needs well-designed, rigorous research studies to determine the impact of epigenetics on disease states and the ability to cure diseases. If researchers identify exact links, there is the potential for paradigm shifts in the care for individuals with physical, emotional, behavioral, or mental health illnesses (Weinhold, 2006).

Families and individuals who seek alternative medical practices versus Western medicine believe that their genetic makeup was altered by environmental factors leading to physical, emotional, behavioral, or mental health illnesses. Therefore, P-PCPs who understand the individuals' or families' viewpoints and the best available research evidence for their beliefs are better able to provide holistic and empathetic care. Environmental factors linked to altering the genome and causing cancer, autism, allergies, and other disease states include (a) consuming genetically modified organisms; (b) consuming inorganic foods that have been treated with pesticides or animal products treated with antibiotics; (c) being exposed to chemicals like glyphosate; and (d) injecting metals directly into the blood stream. When an individual or family presents with any of these fears or worries, the P-PCP should research their statements, consult with specialists, and provide them with the most up-to-date research-based information.

▨ PHARMACOGENOMICS

Advances in technology have improved healthcare delivery systems, with changes rapidly occurring in the field of pharmacogenomics. Individuality, genetic changes, and epigenetic factors affect how each individual metabolizes medications. Pharmacogenomics has provided the methods for practitioners to identify how each individual's genome affects his or her response to medications, therefore removing the generalities (adult dosing based on 150-pound male) and the guesswork (i.e., administer 20–40 mg/kg) that can occur in prescribing medications. Although drug research studies provide clinically recommended dosages for medications, there is no one-size-fits-all approach to Western medicine; many patients have adverse reactions to small doses of medications, whereas others may be on the largest recommended dosage and have no beneficial effect. Although the science and research of pharmacogenomics is in the early stages of development, there is a promising outlook that genetic testing may be advantageous to patients suffering from physical, psychological, emotional, and behavioral and mental health disorders.

▨ INTEGRATIVE MEDICAL PRACTICES

Numerous methods and approaches to healthcare are utilized through integrative medical practices that begin at the cellular level and progress through physiological and psychological issues. Integrative medical practices must be customized for each patient based on epigenetic factors and patient individuality. Integrative providers review a patient's unique set of circumstances and attempt to restore health and rid the body of illnesses, disorders, and diseases. Integrative practices are considered whole-system care, with the overarching goal of reducing symptoms and identifying underlying causes, while treating the body in a holistic, mind–body fashion. The following practices are examples of integrative medical routes of care management providers. They are categorized into three practices: natural products, mind and body practices, and other complementary health approaches (Kanherkar et al., 2017).

Natural Products

The use of natural products such as vitamins and herbs is not a new trend in health-care. These products are readily available in malls, supermarkets, pharmacies, and for online purchase without a prescription. Natural products do not have Food and Drug Administration (FDA) approval and may have unknown adverse side effects (Patridge, Gareiss, Kinch, & Hoyer, 2016). PCPs must question patients about their use and consider possible interactions with prescribed medications which may include reducing the effectiveness of the drug or increasing the risks of an adverse reaction. PCPs must also know that some patients may choose to self-medicate and incorrectly utilize these products. PCPs must know the recommendations for use of natural products and understand the consequences of possible adverse effects or medication interactions with other pharmaceutical grade medications they may be prescribing.

VITAMINS, MINERALS, AND PROBIOTICS

The majority of vitamins, minerals, and probiotics can be bought over the counter and have various usages. For patients incurring physical and psychological disorders or disease, some of the natural medications can have large benefits for improving outcomes. Research studies provide evidence that improving overall physical health entails proper nutrition. Vitamins, minerals, and probiotics may help improve physical health. For example, research has shown that adding natural supplements to the diet can improve brain health. The most common supplements recommended for brain health include omega-3s, vitamins D and B-12, l-methylfolate, and s-adenosyl methionine. Research studies have shown improvements in some aspects of physical and psychological health through the use of vitamins, minerals, and/or probiotics; however, data is limited and there is no specific evidence that these products will cure a disease. Thus, vitamins, minerals, and probiotics are currently only recommended as supplements (Group, 2014).

HERBALISM

Herbs have been used in medicine for thousands of years. Herbalism refers to plant-derived medications that are available in a variety of different forms. Herbs can be applied topically, ingested, or inhaled aromatically. In recent years, there has been an increase in the use of essential oils. There are mixed feelings but many states now support the use of cannabis and have enacted policies and laws for medicinal use. In addition, there is support for cannabis to be rescheduled by the FDA to permit research studies to evaluate the benefits and adverse effects of prescribing cannabis. Other well-known herbs for use in mental health include St. John's wort, valerian, and ginkgo.

Mind and Body Practices

Mind and body practices comprise the next group of integrative medicine practices and are typically taught or performed by trained professionals. Popularity of these practices has increased in recent years in the United States. Many of these practices are derived from ancient rituals. Mind and body practices affect patients individually and allow for diverse possibilities and options for care.

AROMATHERAPY

The science of aromatherapy is a long-standing process that, although not well studied, has been linked to improvements of overall mental and physical health. Aromatherapy utilizes oils in different ways to help improve health by activating neurotransmitters in the brain; oils may be directly massaged into the skin or placed in baths for soaking, inhaled via steam, or directly ingested. Unfortunately, no formal training is required to practice aromatherapy, which makes it difficult for patients to find providers, and usually ends with patients' self-treating. Although the majority of oils used for aromatherapy are safe, if used incorrectly, adverse effects can occur. Therefore, providers must ensure patients understand the consequences of misusing aromatherapy. Although therapy may be beneficial for helping to aid in mind–body health, there has been no clear benefit for using the therapy alone as treatment for illness (Sanchez-Vidana et al., 2017).

ACUPUNCTURE

Acupuncture involves the insertion of multiple needles into certain points of the body to help relieve physical and/or mental symptoms and disease. Acupuncturists restore appropriate body flows ("qi" and "chi") to patients. By restoring equilibrium, acupuncture is thought to repair mind and body disturbances, which leads to an improved state of health. A few research studies have shown that anxiety and depression can be treated appropriately with acupuncture and is relatively safe (Kanherkar et al., 2017). However, further rigorous research studies need to be conducted to identify better correlations between acupuncture and improvement in mental health status.

TAI CHI

Tai chi is an old Chinese practice that incorporates breathing, relaxation, and meditation techniques into an exercise to help with mind–body adaptation. The practice is generally safe and has been indicated in treating and preventing psychosomatic disorders. Research has indicated that tai chi promotes relaxation and decreases sympathetic output, which would benefit patients suffering from depression and anxiety, as well as other various physical diseases. Due to the relative safety and promising effects of the practice, tai chi is increasing in popularity for integrative medicine (Abbott & Lavretsky, 2013).

BIOFIELD THERAPIES

Biofield therapies are types of integrative medicine that include healing touch, therapeutic touch, spiritual touch, qigong (similar to yoga and tai chi), and reiki. Therapies utilize nonphysical energy to activate and heal the mind–body complex; therapists or individuals channel energy through the means of physical touch and laying of hands. Like most of the previously reviewed practices, biofield therapy has been practiced for thousands of years. Recently, Western medicine has begun to examine the techniques practiced during biofield therapy. Some research studies have shown that biofield therapies may have some beneficial effects in the treatment of physical ailments associated with chronic pain and cancer treatments (Jain & Mills, 2010). However, studies showing a relationship between biofield therapy and improvements in mental health are limited (Jain

& Mills, 2010) and need to be conducted to determine links and/or beneficial relationships.

YOGA

Yoga is a form of exercise that activates the mind–body response to help restore and maintain health. While yoga is typically practiced during instructor-led sessions, participants who practice yoga are often able to transfer lessons learned in practice sessions to real-life personal and workplace relationships. As a result, most individuals who practice yoga are able to self-regulate their emotions more quickly than those who do not, and have a better grasp on coping mechanisms they can apply toward daily stressors. Researchers investigating the possible healing benefits of yoga have reported clear links to improving overall health by lowering stress and improving autonomic responses (Kanherkar et al., 2017). The practice is highly recommended and has numerous benefits for overall mind–body health (Kanherkar et al., 2017).

BODY MASSAGE

The goal of massage therapy is to alleviate pain and improve overall mind–body health. Numerous benefits have been suggested in relation to therapeutic massage. These benefits include reduction in chronic pain for various diseases, improving muscle tone (Wang, 2017), reducing stress, and improving overall health of preterm infants (Alvarez et al., 2017). During massage therapy, soft body tissue is manipulated. Some research studies have demonstrated a positive relationship between mental health effects of massage and a reduction in symptoms of depression and anxiety, as well as lowering overall stress hormones in the body.

CHIROPRACTIC CARE

Chiropractic care focuses on holistic health through the noninvasive manipulation of the musculoskeletal and nervous systems. Chiropractors study the body as a whole and perform procedures through the manipulation of subluxations. Chiropractic care aims to restore balance in the body, which in turn is thought to help maintain physical and psychological health. Chiropractic care has been linked to improvements in almost every major system in the human body, from reductions in abnormal gastrointestinal issues to improved mental health. However, care is individualized, and not every patient reports the same or even similar benefits. Chiropractic care may benefit patients seeking integrative medical practices.

HYPNOTHERAPY

Hypnotherapy is one of the oldest forms of psychotherapy practiced in Western medicine. Correlations between hypnotherapy and improved health have not been established in research studies; however, hypnotherapy may be beneficial to some individuals. Through the induction of a sleep-like trance, hypnotherapy stimulates subconscious mind–body changes that are thought to eventually activate behavioral changes to improve overall health. Although the body goes through a dream-like state, hypnosis actually heightens concentration to promote the healing of unresolved issues that may subconsciously be leading to physical or mental ailments. Hypnotherapy is typically the most efficient at reducing chronic pain, abuse or misuse of medications or substances, headaches, and anxiety.

GUIDED IMAGERY

Guided imagery is a therapeutic treatment that stimulates psychological capabilities to overcome illness and disease. Therapists use relaxation techniques to tap into the subconscious of a patient, enabling them to visualize their healing process and the steps needed to promote overall well-being. Therapists utilize the mind–body complex to actively engage a patient at the psychological level to create a desired physical response. Guided imagery has been found to improve numerous mental illnesses, as well as issues with chronic pain.

MEDITATION

Meditation is a common integrative medical approach used to stimulate the patient's subconscious through a tranquil state. Meditation may be accomplished in many different forms. Through the use of a practitioner or with self-induction, patients can become more aware of their surroundings and help dictate how their body will react to stressors and physical conditions. Meditation is thought to activate limbic and parietal centers in the brain that help reduce stress and promote health and healing. Although meditation may combat illness, many patients will seek to utilize the therapy to maintain homeostasis and avoid illness altogether. Recent studies have shown that patients who utilize meditation are more apt to have positive epigenetic changes in their genome that may help combat physical and mental disease (Kanherkar et al., 2017).

Other Complementary Health Approaches

The last classification of integrative medical approaches to healthcare includes homeopathy, naturopathy, and Ayurveda. Although these approaches may be similar to those previously discussed, they do not fit into the same category and are thus separated. The final category is based on the foundation that the body can be healed through the use of herbal products, appropriate nutrition, and the right spiritual mind frame. The natural homeostasis and balance of the body is incorporated into overall health according to the final category.

HOMEOPATHY

Homeopathy is an integrative medical approach that believes in feeding disease. The underpinnings for homeopathy are predicated on the following beliefs: (a) if a substance can cause a disease, the substance can also cure it; (b) a minute dose of medication offers the greatest benefit. Homeopathic medications are found organically in nature and may include substances from animals, plants, or minerals, which can be ingested, inhaled, or applied topically. The field of homeopathy has been inadequately researched as a complementary therapy, and is thus only weakly supported in medical literature (National Center for Complementary and Integrative Health [NCCIH], 2016b).

NATUROPATHY

Naturopathy is a form of integrative medicine that utilizes a combination of previously described treatments, as well as naturopathic practitioners, to provide primary and acute care to patients. Naturopaths aim to treat the entire person, strive for holistic care, and attempt to be proactive in treating disease versus reactive in treating symptoms. Although similar to Western practitioners, naturopathic practitioners attempt to rely on organic forms of medical management like herbal products, massage, dietary management, detoxification, yoga, and chiropractic care. Naturopathy and the lifestyle modification the practice involves have proven to be beneficial with some medical and psychological disease states, including anxiety, depression, and physical ailments rooted in poor nutrition (Breed & Bereznay, 2017).

AYURVEDA

Ayurvedic medicine is one of the oldest forms of healthcare, and even today is the most practiced mode of medical management in Eastern countries. The practice of Ayurveda focuses on the mind–body complex and is deeply rooted in the universal ideology of connecting people with the universe. Ayurveda is extremely individualized and utilizes a variety of principles including tridoshas (ideologies of body, structure, and movement), gunas (psychological qualities), and prakriti (components of energy). Treatment modalities for disease focus on diet and lifestyle management. Medication management may include prescribing herbs, metals, and minerals. The use of some metals and minerals, such as lead, make treatments dangerous and possibly toxic if used incorrectly by Western medical providers. Patients who want to use Ayurvedic medicine should only seek care from trained Ayurvedic medical professionals. Despite the possible issues with toxic effects, if used incorrectly, Ayurvedic medicine has been shown to have positive benefits for physical and psychological diseases, including arthritis, gastrointestinal disorders, depression, and anxiety (Kanherkar et al., 2017).

■ SUMMARY

The human body is a tremendously complex system that has the ability to self-regulate and is impacted through the mind–body complex. Although Western medicine is the traditional form of treatment for most patients in the United States, current trends toward more holistic care have led to a surge in the practice of integrative medicine. To provide the most appropriate care for their patients, PCPs must have a basic understanding of the different types of integrative medical management available for patients. They should inform patients about all available therapies for treatment of physical and mental health illnesses, including alternative and complementary modes of therapy that may benefit their particular condition. PCPs should be comfortable in assisting or referring patients, if requested, to help avoid patient-led self-treatment, which can be dangerous. PCPs must also understand the field of epigenetics and utilize the latest research in the field to enable patients to make informed decisions about their care. Although providers may not always agree on alternative or complementary forms of treatment, they do need to be knowledgeable about alternative options and provide as much supporting evidence to patients to help complement the integrative medical surge.

■ REFERENCES

Abbott, R., & Lavretsky, H. (2013). Tai chi and qigong for the treatment and prevention of mental disorders. *The Psychiatric Clinics of North America*, 36(1), 109–119. doi:10.1016/j.psc.2013.01.011

Alvarez, M. J., Fernández, D., Gómez-Salgado, J., Rodríguez-González, D., Rosón, M., & Lapeña, S. (2017). The effects of massage therapy in hospitalized preterm neonates: A systematic review. *International Journal of Nursing Studies*, 69, 119–136. doi:10.1016/j.ijnurstu.2017.02.009

Breed, B., & Bereznay, C. (2017). Treatment of depression and anxiety by naturopathic physicians: An observational study of naturopathic medicine within an integrated multidisciplinary community health center. *The Journal of Alternative and Complementary Medicine*, 21(7), 395–400. doi:10.1089/acm.2016.0232

Group, E. (2014). *Nutritional approaches to mental health.* Retrieved from http://www.globalhealing-center.com/natural-health/nutritional-approaches-to-mental-health/

Jain, S., & Mills, P. J. (2010). Biofield therapies: Helpful or full of hype? A best evidence synthesis. *International Journal of Behavioral Medicine*, 17(1), 1–16. doi:10.1007/s12529-009-9062-4

Kanherkar, R. R., Stair, S. E., Bhatia-Dey, N., Mills, P. J., Chopra, D., & Csoka, A. B. (2017). Epigenetic mechanisms of integrative medicine. *Evidence-Based Complementary and Alternative Medicine*, 2017, 19. doi:10.1155/2017/4365429

Labonte, B., & Turecki, G. (2012). Epigenetic: A link between environment and genome. *Sante Mentale Au Quebec*, 37(2), 31–44.

National Center for Complementary and Integrative Health. (2016a). *Complementary, alternative, or integrative health: What's in a name?* Retrieved from https://nccih.nih.gov/health/integrative-health

National Center for Complementary and Integrative Health. (2016b). *Homeopathy.* Retrieved from https://nccih.nih.gov/health/homeopathy

Patridge, E., Gareiss, P., Kinch, M. S., & Hoyer, D. (2016). An analysis of FDA-approved drugs: Natural products and their derivatives. *Drug Discovery Today*, 21, 204–207. doi:10.1016/j.drudis.2015.009. (Epun 2015 Jan 21)

Sanchez-Vidana, D. I., Ngai, S. P., He, W., Chow, J. K., Lau, B. W., & Tsang, H. W. (2017). The effectiveness of aromatherapy for depressive symptoms: A systematic review. *Evidence-Based Complementary and Alternative Medicine*, 2017, 1–21. doi:10.1155/2017/5869315

Wang, J. (2017). Therapeutic effects of massage and electrotherapy on muscle tone, stiffness and muscle contraction following gastrocnemius muscle fatigue. *Journal of Physical Therapy Science*, 29(1), 144–147. doi:10.1589/jpts.29.144

Weinhold, B. (2006). Epigenetics: The science of change. *Environmental Health Perspectives*, 114(3), 160–167. doi:10.1289/ehp.114-a160

Index

strength, school, home, activities, drugs/
substance abuse, emotions/eating/
depression, sexuality, and safety
(SSHADESS) assessment, 293,
295–297, 377
"strengthening families" approach
child's social and emotional competence,
58
concrete assistance, 57
parent knowledge of child development,
57–58
parental resilience, 57
social connections, 57
stress
and adverse childhood experiences,
20–21
military children, 395
Stressful Life Events Questionnaire, 204
substance abuse
autism spectrum disorder adolescents,
369
CRAFFT instrument, 377–378
diagnosis, 379–380
HEEADSSS screening instrument,
377
history, 376
medication-assisted treatment, 383
medications, 384
Narcan availability, 384
opioid use, 380–381
parental role, 382
pediatric primary care providers' role,
382–383
Personal Health Questionnaire, 378
pertinent positives, 378–379
physical examination, 379
SAMHSA initiative, 381
SBIRT, 383
SSHADESS assessment, 377
Substance Abuse and Mental Health
Service Administration (SAMHSA),
62, 279, 444
substance use disorder (SUD), 380–381
substance abuse, 50–51
SUD. See substance use disorder
SUDORS. See State Unintentional Drug
Overdose Reporting System
Survey of Well-Being of Young Children
(SWYC), 448
SWYC. See Survey of Well-Being of Young
Children

tai chi, 469
TAMAR. See Trauma, Addiction, Mental
Health, and Recovery
TARGET. See Trauma Affect Regulation:
Guide for Education and Therapy
TCQ. See Toddler Care Questionnaire
temper tantrums, 186, 194–195
temperament, 145–147
Test of Infant Motor Performance (TIMP),
71
time-out for toddlers, 150
TIMP. See Test of Infant Motor
Performance
Toddler Care Questionnaire (TCQ), 145,
190
toddlers
anticipatory guidance, 149–151
assessment for behavioral problems,
147–149
autism spectrum disorder (see autism
spectrum disorder)
cognitive development, 144
impulsive behavior, 190–195
military deployment, 396–397
receptive and expressive language
development, 143–144
social and emotional development,
144–145
temper tantrums, 151–152
temperament, 145–147
toilet training, 155–160
toilet training
accidents, 159
Azrin and Foxx's method, 158
behavioral and developmental
differences, 157
Brazelton's approach, 157–158
challenges, 159
chronic illness, 157
cultural considerations, 156–157
environmental factors, 157
gender, 156
physiological milestones, 155
resistance, 160
timing of, 155–156
tolerable stress, 20
topiramate
aggression, 359
bipolar disorder, 360
Tourette syndrome
acupuncture, 338